STOELTI'

HANDBOOK Ol

Pharmacology and Physiology in Anesthetic Practice

THIRD EDITION

STOELTING'S

HANDBOOK OF
Pharmacology and Physiology in Anesthetic Practice

THIRD EDITION

Robert K. Stoelting, MD

Emeritus Professor
Department of Anesthesia
Indiana University School of Medicine
Indianapolis, Indiana

James P. Rathmell, MD

Executive Vice Chair and Chief, Division of
*   Pain Medicine*
Department of Anesthesia, Critical Care
*   and Pain Medicine*
Massachusetts General Hospital
Henry Knowles Beecher Professor of
*   Anaesthesia, Harvard Medical School*
Boston, Massachusetts

Pamela Flood, MD, MA

Professor of Anesthesiology, Perioperative
*   and Pain Medicine*
Stanford University
Palo Alto, California

Steven Shafer, MD

Professor of Anesthesiology, Perioperative
*   and Pain Medicine*
Stanford University
Palo Alto, California

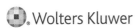

Philadelphia • Baltimore • New York • London
Buenos Aires • Hong Kong • Sydney • Tokyo

Acquisitions Editor: Brian Brown
Product Development Editor: Nicole Dernoski
Editorial Assistant: Lindsay Burgess
Senior Production Project Manager: Alicia Jackson
Design Coordinator: Stephen Druding
Illustration Coordinator: Jennifer Clements
Manufacturing Coordinator: Beth Welsh
Marketing Manager: Daniel Dressler
Prepress Vendor: Absolute Service, Inc.

Third Edition

Library of Congress Cataloging-in-Publication Data

Stoelting, Robert K., author.
 [Handbook of pharmacology & physiology in anesthetic practice]
 Stoelting's handbook of pharmacology and physiology in anesthetic practice / Robert K. Stoelting, Steven Shafer, James P. Rathmell, Pamela Flood. — Third edition.
   p. ; cm.
 Handbook of pharmacology and physiology in anesthetic practice
 Accompanies Stoelting's pharmacology and physiology in anesthetic practice / [edited by] Steven Shafer, James P. Rathmell, Pamela Flood. Fifth edition. 2015.
 Preceded by Handbook of pharmacology & physiology in anesthetic practice / by Robert K. Stoelting, Simon C. Hillier. 2nd ed. c2006.
 Includes bibliographical references and indexes.
 ISBN 978-1-60547-549-3 (alk. paper)
 I. Shafer, Steven L., author. II. Rathmell, James P., author. III. Flood, Pamela, 1963- , author. IV. Stoelting's pharmacology and physiology in anesthetic practice. Fifth edition. Guide to (work): V. Title. VI. Title: Handbook of pharmacology and physiology in anesthetic practice.
 [DNLM: 1. Anesthetics—pharmacology—Handbooks. 2. Anesthetics—pharmacology—Outlines. 3. Anesthesia—methods—Handbooks. 4. Anesthesia—methods—Outlines. 5. Physiological Phenomena—Handbooks. 6. Physiological Phenomena—Outlines. QV 39]
 RD82.2
 615.7'81—dc23

                                                                    2014039931

PREFACE

Stoelting's Handbook of Pharmacology and Physiology in Anesthetic Practice is intended to provide a rapid and accurate source of information relevant to the pharmacology of drugs encountered during anesthesia and the physiologic responses that impact the anesthetic experience. The handbook uses a format that follows the identical chapters and headings in the fifth edition of *Stoelting's Pharmacology and Physiology in Anesthetic Practice*, thus permitting the reader to refer to corresponding areas of the more detailed information in the textbook. As such, the intent of the handbook is to serve as a companion and to provide a practical cross-reference to *Stoelting's Pharmacology and Physiology in Anesthetic Practice* and its more in-depth discussion of drugs and physiology. This design provides rapid visibility of pertinent aspects of pharmacology and physiology that can be readily assessed at sites other than the individual's personal library.

Robert K. Stoelting, MD

ACKNOWLEDGMENT

The authors would like to gratefully acknowledge the efforts of the contributors to the fifth edition of the textbook ***Stoelting's Pharmacology and Physiology in Anesthetic Practice***.

Nicholas Anast, MD

Bihua Bie, MD, PhD

Mark Burbridge, MD

Kenneth Cummings III, MD, MS

Hesham Elsharkawy, MD, MSc

Pamela Flood, MD, MA

Sumeet Goswami, MD, MPH

David A. Grossblatt, MD

Jonathan Hastie, MD

Maya Jalbout Hastie, MD

Bessie Kachulis, MD

Mihir M. Kamdar, MD

Joseph Kwok, MD

Barrett Larson, MD

Jerrold H. Levy, MD

Sansan S. Lo, MD

Kamal Maheshwari, MD

Jillian A. Maloney, MD

Steven Miller, MD

Vivek K. Moitra, MD

Teresa A. Mulaikal, MD

Michael J. Murray, MD, PhD

Mohamed A. Naguib, MD, MSc, FFARCSI

Carter Peatross, MD

James Ramsay, MD

James P. Rathmell, MD

Carl E. Rosow, MD, PhD

Steven Shafer, MD

Jack S. Shanewise, MD, FASE
Peter Slinger, MD, FRCPC
Sarah C. Smith, MD
Jessica Spellman, MD
Hui Yang, MD, PhD

CONTENTS

PART VII:
Endocrine System

PART VIII:
Miscellaneous

PART IX:
Special Populations

CHAPTER 1

Basic Principles of Physiology

This chapter reviews the basic principles of the composition of the body and the structure of cells.

I. **Body Composition**
   A. Water accounts for about 60% of the weight in an adult man, about 50% of the body weight in an adult woman (reflects increased body fat in women), and up to 70% of body weight in a neonate (Table 1-1).
   B. Body fluids can be divided into intracellular and extracellular fluid, depending on their location relative to the cell membrane (Fig. 1-1).
      1. Interstitial fluid is present in the spaces between cells.
      2. Plasma is in dynamic equilibrium with the interstitial fluid through pores in the capillaries; the interstitial fluid serves as a reservoir from which water and electrolytes can be mobilized into the circulation.
      3. The normal daily intake of water (drinks and internal product of food metabolism) by an adult averages 2.5 L of which about 1.5 L is excreted as urine, 100 mL is lost in sweat, and 100 mL is present in feces.

II. **Blood Volume**
   A. The average blood volume of an adult is 5 L, comprising about 3 L of plasma and 2 L of erythrocytes (varies with age, weight, and gender).
      1. In nonobese individuals, the blood volume varies in direct proportion to the body weight, averaging 70 mL/kg for lean men and women.
      2. The greater the ratio of fat to body weight, the less is the blood volume in milliliters per kilogram because adipose tissue has a decreased vascular supply.

| Table 1-1 | | |

Total Body Water by Age and Gender

| | Total Body Water | |
Age (yrs)	Men (%)	Women (%)
18–40	61	51
40–60	55	47
>60	52	46

  B. The normal hematocrit is about 45% for men and post-menopausal women and about 38% for menstruating women, with a range of approximately ±5%.

III. Constituents of Body Fluid Compartments (Fig. 1-2)
  A. An unequal distribution of ions results in establishment of a potential (voltage) difference across cell membranes.
  B. The constituents of extracellular fluid are carefully regulated by the kidneys so that cells are bathed in a fluid containing the proper concentrations of electrolytes and nutrients.
  C. Trauma is associated with progressive loss of potassium through the kidneys due, in large part, to the increased secretion of vasopressin and, in variable part (depending on the type of surgery), to the role of nasogastric suctioning and direct potassium loss.

IV. Osmosis is the movement of water (solvent molecules) across a semipermeable membrane from a compartment in which the nondiffusible solute (ion) concentration is lower to a compartment in which the solute concentration is higher (Fig. 1-3).

V. Tonicity of Fluids
  A. A solution of 5% glucose in water is initially isotonic when infused, but glucose is metabolized so the net effect is that of infusing a hypotonic solution.
  B. Lactated Ringer's solution plus 5% glucose is initially hypertonic (about 560 mOsm/L), but as glucose is metabolized, the solution becomes less hypertonic.

VI. Fluid Management
  A. The goal of fluid management is to maintain normovolemia and hemodynamic stability.

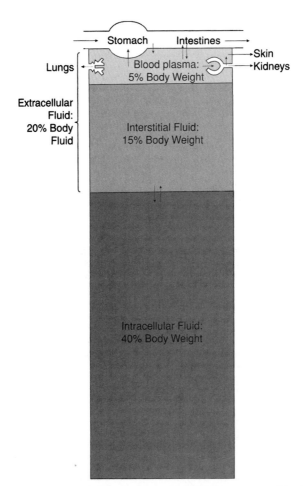

FIGURE 1-1 Body fluid compartments and the percentage of body weight represented by each compartment. The location relative to the capillary membrane divides extracellular fluid into plasma or interstitial fluid. *Arrows* represent fluid movement between compartments. (From Gamble JL. *Chemical Anatomy, Physiology, and Pathology of Extracellular Fluid.* 6th ed. Boston, MA: Harvard University Press; 1954, with permission.)

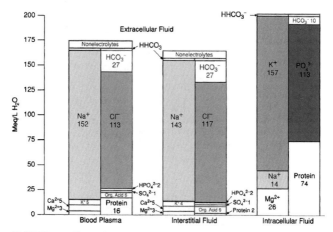

FIGURE 1-2 Electrolyte composition of body fluid compartments. (From Leaf A, Newburgh LH. *Significance of the Body Fluids in Clinical Medicine.* 2nd ed. Springfield, IL: Thomas; 1955, with permission.)

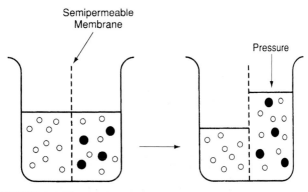

FIGURE 1-3 Diagrammatic representation of osmosis depicting water molecules *(open circles)* and solute molecules *(solid circles)* separated by a semipermeable membrane. Water molecules move across the semipermeable membrane to the area of higher concentration of solute molecules. Osmotic pressure is the pressure that would have to be applied to prevent continued movement of water molecules. (From Ganong WF. *Review of Medical Physiology.* 21st ed. New York, NY: Lange Medical Books/McGraw-Hill; 2003.)

B. After 20 to 30 minutes, an estimated 75% to 80% of an isotonic saline or a lactate-containing solution will have distributed outside the confines of the circulation, thus limiting the efficacy of these solutions in treating hypovolemia (ability of crystalloids to restore perfusion in the microcirculation is doubtful).

VII. Dehydration

A. Loss of water by gastrointestinal or renal routes or by diaphoresis (excessive sweating) is associated with an initial deficit in extracellular fluid volume.

B. The ratio of extracellular fluid to intracellular fluid is greater in infants than adults (dehydration develops more rapidly and is often more severe in the very young).

C. Clinical signs of dehydration are likely when about 5% to 10% (severe dehydration) of total body fluids have been lost in a brief period of time.

1. Physiologic mechanisms can usually compensate for acute loss of 15% to 25% of the intravascular fluid volume.

2. A greater loss places the patient at risk for hemodynamic decompensation.

VIII. **Cell Structure and Function. The basic living unit of the body is the cell. (It is estimated that the entire body consists of 100 trillion or more cells of which about 25 trillion are red blood cells.)**

A. **Cell Anatomy** (Fig. 1-4)

B. **Cell Membrane**

1. Each cell is surrounded by a lipid bilayer that acts as a permeability barrier, allowing the cell to maintain a cytoplasmic composition different from the extracellular fluid (Table 1-2).

2. Lipid bilayers are nearly impermeable to water-soluble substances, such as ions and glucose. Conversely, fat-soluble substances (steroids) and gases readily cross cell membranes.

C. **Transfer of Molecules through Cell Membranes**

1. **Diffusion**. Oxygen, carbon dioxide, and nitrogen move through cell membranes by simple diffusion through the lipid bilayer (Table 1-3).

2. **Endocytosis and exocytosis** transfer molecules such as nutrients across cell membranes without the molecule actually passing through the cell membrane (Fig. 1-5). Neurotransmitters are ejected from cells by exocytosis, a

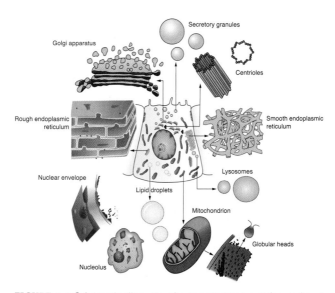

FIGURE 1-4 Schematic diagram of a hypothetical cell *(center)* and its organelles.

Table 1-2

Cell Membrane Composition

Phospholipids
   Lecithins (phosphatidylcholines)
   Sphingomyelins
   Amino phospholipids (phosphatidylethanolamine)
Proteins
   Structural proteins (microtubules)
   Transport proteins (sodium–potassium ATPase)
   Ion channels
   Receptors
   Enzymes (adenylate cyclase)

ATPase, adenosine triphosphatase.

Table 1-3

Predicted Relationship between Diffusion Distance and Time

Diffusion Distance (mm)	Time Required for Diffusion
0.001	0.5 min
0.01	50 min
0.1	5 s
1	498 s
10	14 h

process that requires calcium ions and resembles endocytosis in reverse.

3. **Sodium–potassium ATPase** (sodium–potassium pump) is an ATP-dependent sodium and potassium transporter on the cell membrane that ejects three sodium ions from the cell in exchange for the import of two potassium ions (Fig. 1-6).

4. **Ion channels** are transmembrane proteins that generate electrical signals in the brain, nerves, heart, and skeletal muscles (Fig. 1-7).

5. Some channels are highly specific with respect to ions allowed to pass (sodium, potassium), whereas other channels allow all ions below a certain size to pass (Table 1-4).

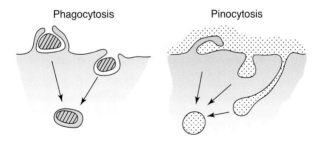

Phagocytosis   Pinocytosis

FIGURE 1-5 Schematic depiction of phagocytosis (ingestion of solid particles) and pinocytosis (ingestion of dissolved particles).

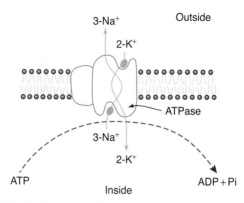

FIGURE 1-6 Sodium–potassium adenosine triphosphatase is an enzyme present in all cells that catalyzes the conversion of adenosine triphosphate (ATP) to adenosine diphosphate (ADP). The resulting energy is used by the active transport carrier system (sodium–potassium pump) that is responsible for the outward movement of three sodium ions across the cell membrane for every two potassium ions that pass inward.

     6. Genes encoding the protein ion channels may be defective, leading to diseases such as cystic fibrosis (chloride channel defects) and long Q-T interval syndrome (mutant potassium or, less commonly, sodium channels).
- D. **Nucleus** is primarily made up of the 46 chromosomes, except the nucleus of the egg cell, which contains 23.
  1. **Structure and Function of DNA and RNA** (Fig. 1-8)
     a. The genetic message is determined by the sequence of nucleotides.
     b. The human genome is composed of 20,000 to 25,000 genes (the protein encoding genes account for only 1% to 2% of our DNA).
  2. **Cytoplasm** consists of water; electrolytes; and proteins, including enzymes, lipids, and carbohydrates; and also contains numerous organelles.
     a. **Mitochondria** are the power-generating units of cells containing both the enzymes and substrates of the tricarboxylic acid cycle (Krebs cycle) and the electron transport chain.
     b. **Endoplasmic reticulum** is a complex lipid bilayer that folds and creates vesicles in the cytoplasm. The

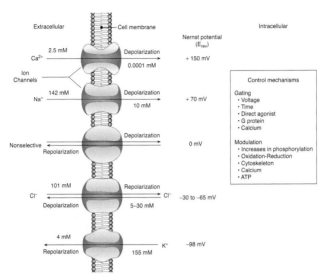

FIGURE 1-7 The five major types of protein ion channels are calcium, sodium, nonselective, chloride, and potassium. Flow of ions through these channels (calcium and sodium into cells and potassium outward) determines the transmembrane potential of cells.

Table 1-4

Diameters of Ions, Molecules, and Channels

	Diameter (nm)[a]
Channel (average)	0.80
Water	0.30
Sodium (hydrated)	0.51
Potassium (hydrated)	0.40
Chloride (hydrated)	0.39
Glucose	0.86

[a]1 nm = 10 Å.

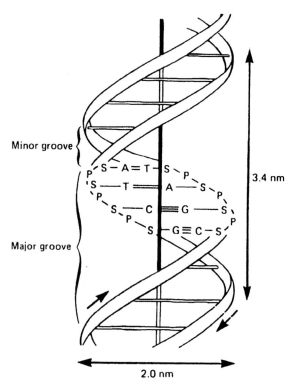

FIGURE 1-8 Double helical structure of DNA with adenine (A) bonding to thymine (T) and cytosine (C) to guanine (G). (From Murray RK, Granner DK, Mayes PA, et al. *Harper's Biochemistry.* 21st ed. Norwalk, CT: Appleton & Lange; 1988, with permission.)

portion of the membrane containing these ribosomes is known as the *rough endoplasmic reticulum.* The part of the membrane that lacks ribosomes is the *smooth endoplasmic reticulum.* This smooth portion of the endoplasmic reticulum membrane functions in the synthesis of lipids, metabolism of carbohydrates, and other enzymatic processes. The sarcoplasmic reticulum is found in muscle cells, where it serves as a reservoir for calcium.

CHAPTER 2

Basic Principles of Pharmacology

This chapter presents a foundation for pharmacology and fundamental principles of drug behavior and drug interaction that govern our daily practice of anesthesia.

I. **Receptor Theory**
   A. A drug that activates a receptor by binding to the receptor (a protein) is called an *agonist* (combination usually reversible).
   B. When the receptor is bound to the agonist ligand, the effect of the drug is produced (Fig. 2-1).
   C. An *antagonist* is a drug that binds to the receptor without activating the receptor (Fig. 2-2).
      1. Antagonists block the action of agonists simply by getting in the way of the agonist, preventing the agonist from binding to the receptor and producing the drug effect.
      2. *Competitive antagonism* is present when increasing concentrations of the antagonist progressively inhibit the response to the agonist.
      3. *Noncompetitive antagonism* is present when, after administration of an antagonist, even high concentrations of agonist cannot completely overcome the antagonism.
   D. Although this simple view of activated and inactivated receptors explains agonists and antagonists, it has a more difficult time with *partial agonists* and *inverse agonists*. It turns out that receptors have many natural conformations, and they naturally fluctuate between these different conformations (Figs. 2-3 and 2-4).

II. **Receptor Action**
   A. The number of receptors in cell membranes is dynamic and increases (upregulates) or decreases (downregulates) in response to specific stimuli.

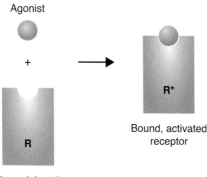

Agonist

+

R

Unbound, inactive
receptor

R*

Bound, activated
receptor

FIGURE 2-1 The interaction of a receptor with an agonist may be portrayed as a binary bound versus unbound receptor. The unbound receptor is portrayed as inactive. When the receptor is bound to the agonist ligand, it becomes the activated, R^*, and mediates the drug effect. This view is too simplistic, but it permits understanding of basic agonist behavior.

    B. Changing receptor numbers is one of many mechanisms that contribute to variability in response to drugs.

III. **Receptor Types**
    A. Many of the receptors thought to be the most critical for anesthetic interaction are located in the lipid bilayer of cell membranes (opioids, intravenous sedative hypnotics, benzodiazepines, beta blockers, catecholamines, muscle relaxants) and interact with membrane bound receptors.
    B. Other receptors are intracellular proteins and interact with insulin and steroids.
    C. Proteins function in the body as small machines, catalyzing enzymatic reactions and acting as ion channels.
       1. When a drug binds to a receptor, it changes the activity of the machine, typically by enhancing its activity (propofol increases the sensitivity of the γ-aminobutyric acid receptor [GABA$_A$] to GABA, the endogenous ligand), decreasing its activity (ketamine decreases the activity of the N-methyl-D-aspartate [NMDA] receptor), or triggering a chain reaction (opioid binding to the

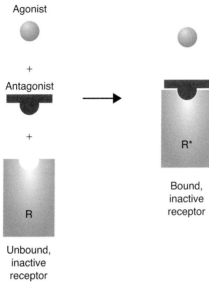

FIGURE 2-2 The simple view of receptor activation also explains the action of antagonist. In this case, the antagonist *(red)* binds to the receptor, but the binding does not cause activation. However, the binding of the antagonist blocks the agonist from binding, and thus blocks agonist drug effect. If the binding is reversible, this is competitive antagonism. If it is not reversible, then it is noncompetitive antagonism.

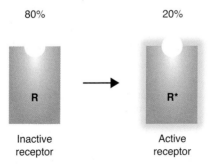

FIGURE 2-3 Receptors have multiple states, and they switch spontaneously between them. In this case, the receptor has just two states. It spends 80% of the time in the inactive state and 20% of the time in the active state in the absence of any ligand.

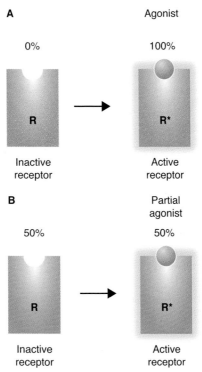

A   Agonist

FIGURE 2-4 The action of agonists **(A)**, partial agonists **(B)**, antagonists **(C)**, and inverse agonists **(D)** can be interpreted as changing the balance between the active and inactive forms of the receptor. In this case, in the absence of agonist, the receptor is in the activated state 20% of the time. This percentage changes based on the nature of the ligand bound to the receptor.

μ opioid receptor activates an inhibitory G protein that decreases adenylyl cyclase activity).
   2. The protein's response to binding of the drug is responsible for the drug effect.

IV. **Pharmacokinetics is the quantitative study of the absorption, distribution, metabolism, and excretion of injected and inhaled drugs and their metabolites (what the body does to a drug).**
   A. Pharmacokinetics determines the concentration of a drug in the plasma or at the site of drug effect.

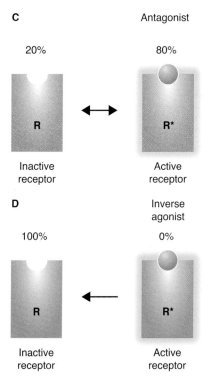

FIGURE 2-4 *(Continued).*

B. Pharmacokinetic variability is a significant component of patient-to-patient variability in drug response and may result from genetic modifications in metabolism; interactions with other drugs; or disease in the liver, kidneys, or other organs of metabolism.

C. Absorption, metabolism, distribution, and elimination are processes that are fundamental to all drugs (can be described in basic physiologic terms or using mathematical models).

1. Physiology can be used to predict how changes in organ function will affect the disposition of drugs.

2. Mathematical models can be used to calculate the concentration of drug in the blood or tissue following any arbitrary dose, at any arbitrary time.

V. **Distribution**

A. When drugs are administered, they mix with body tissues and are immediately diluted from the concentrated injectate in the syringe to the more dilute concentration measured in the plasma or tissue. This initial distribution (within 1 minute) after bolus injection is considered mixing within the "central compartment" (Fig. 2-5).

B. It may take hours or even days for the drug to fully mix with all bodily tissues because some tissues have very low perfusion.

C. Many anesthetic drugs are highly fat soluble and poorly soluble in water.

   1. High fat solubility means that the molecule will have a large volume of distribution because it will be preferentially taken up by fat, diluting the concentration in the plasma.

   2. The extreme example of this is propofol, which is almost inseparable from fat.

D. Following bolus injection, drug primarily goes to the tissues that receive the bulk of arterial blood flow: the brain, heart, kidneys, and liver. These tissues are often called *the vessel rich group*.

   1. The rapid blood flow ensures that the concentration in these highly perfused tissues rises rapidly to equilibrate with arterial blood.

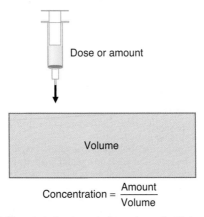

$$\text{Concentration} = \frac{\text{Amount}}{\text{Volume}}$$

FIGURE 2-5 The central volume is the volume that intravenously injected drug initially mixes into.

2. For highly fat-soluble drugs, the capacity of the fat to hold the drug greatly exceeds the capacity of highly perfused tissues.
   a. With time (initially, the fat compartment is almost invisible because fat blood flow is low), the fat gradually absorbs more and more drug, sequestering it away from the highly perfused tissues.
   b. This redistribution of drug from the highly perfused tissue to the fat accounts for a substantial part of the offset of drug effect following a bolus of an intravenous anesthetic or fat-soluble opioid (fentanyl).

VI. **Protein Binding**
   A. Most drugs are bound to some extent to plasma proteins, primarily albumin (acidic drugs) and α_1-acid glycoprotein and lipoproteins (basic drugs).
   B. Protein binding effects both the distribution of drugs (only the free or unbound fraction is readily cross cell membranes) and the apparent potency of drugs (it is the free fraction that determines the concentration of bound drug on the receptor).
      1. The extent of protein binding parallels the lipid solubility of the drug.
      2. For intravenous anesthetic drugs, the number of available protein binding sites in the plasma vastly exceeds the number of sites actually bound. As a result, the fraction bound is not dependent on the concentration of the anesthetic and only dependent on the protein concentration.
      3. Age, hepatic disease, renal failure, and pregnancy can all result in decreased plasma protein concentration.
         a. Alterations in protein binding are important only for drugs that are highly protein bound (>90%).
         b. For such drugs, the free fraction changes inversely proportionally with a change in protein concentration. If the free fraction is 2% in the normal state, then in a patient with 50% decrease in plasma proteins, the free fraction will increase to 4%, a 100% increase.
   C. Theoretically, an increase in free fraction of a drug may increase the pharmacologic effect of the drug, but in practice, it is far from certain that there will be any change in pharmacologic effect at all.

VII. **Metabolism converts pharmacologically active, lipid-soluble drugs into water-soluble and usually inactive metabolites; exceptions are metabolism to active compounds as for diazepam and opioids (morphine-6-glucuronide is more potent than morphine; codeine is a prodrug metabolized to morphine).**

A. **Pathways of Metabolism.** The four basic pathways of metabolism are (a) oxidation, (b) reduction, (c) hydrolysis, and (d) conjugation.

   1. Phase I reactions include oxidation, reduction, and hydrolysis, which increase the drug's polarity and prepare it for phase II reactions.
   2. Phase II reactions are conjugation reactions that covalently link the drug or metabolites with a highly polar molecule (carbohydrate or an amino acid) that renders the conjugate more water soluble for subsequent excretion.
   3. Hepatic microsomal enzymes (hepatic smooth endoplasmic reticulum but also present in kidneys and gastrointestinal tract) are responsible for the metabolism of most drugs.

B. **Phase I enzymes** responsible for phase I reactions include cytochrome P-450 enzymes (predominantly hepatic microsomal enzymes), noncytochrome P-450 enzymes, and flavin-containing monooxygenase enzymes.

   1. The cytochrome P-450 enzyme system is a large family of membrane-bound proteins.
   2. Drugs can alter the activity of these enzymes through induction and inhibition (phenobarbital induces microsomal enzymes and thus can render drugs less effective through increased metabolism).
   3. **Oxidation.** Cytochrome P-450 enzymes are crucial for oxidation reactions. Examples of oxidative metabolism of drugs catalyzed by cytochrome P-450 enzymes include hydroxylation, deamination, desulfuration, dealkylation, and dehalogenation.
   4. **Reduction.** Cytochrome P-450 enzymes are also essential for reduction reactions. Under conditions of low oxygen partial pressures, cytochrome P-450 enzymes transfer electrons directly to a substrate such as halothane rather than to oxygen.
   5. **Conjugation** with glucuronic acid involves cytochrome P-450 enzymes. The resulting water-soluble glucuronide conjugates are then excreted in bile and urine.
   6. **Hydrolysis.** Enzymes responsible for hydrolysis of drugs, usually at an ester bond, do not involve the cytochrome P-450 enzyme system. Hydrolysis often occurs outside of the liver (remifentanil, succinylcholine, esmolol, and

the ester local anesthetics are cleared in the plasma and tissues via ester hydrolysis).

C. **Phase II enzymes** include glucuronosyltransferases, glutathione-S-transferases, N-acetyl-transferases, and sulfotransferases.

    1. Glucuronidation is an important metabolic pathway for several drugs used during anesthesia, including propofol, morphine (yielding morphine-3-glucuronide and the pharmacologically active morphine-6-glucuronide), and midazolam (yielding the pharmacologically active 1-hydroxymidazolam).

    2. Glutathione-S-transferase (GST) enzymes are primarily a defensive system for detoxification and protection against oxidative stress.

VIII. **Hepatic Clearance**

A. Although the metabolic capacity of the body is large, it is not possible that metabolism is *always* proportional to drug concentration, because the liver does not have infinite metabolic capacity.

B. The rate at which drug flows *out* of the liver must be the rate at which drug flows *into* the liver, minus the rate at which the liver metabolizes drug (Figs. 2-6 and 2-7).

C. To understand hepatic clearance, one must understand the relationship between hepatic metabolism and drug concentration.

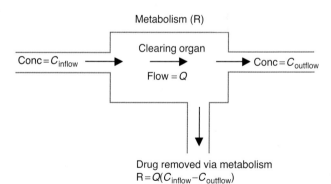

FIGURE 2-6 The relationship between drug rate of metabolism can be computed as the rate of liver blood flow times the difference between the inflowing and outflowing drug concentrations. This is a common approach to analyzing metabolism or tissue uptake across an organ in mass-balance pharmacokinetic studies.

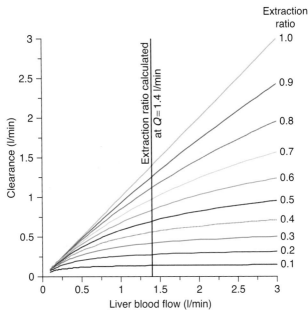

FIGURE 2-7 The relationship between liver blood flow (Q), clearance, and extraction ratio. For drugs with a high extraction ratio, clearance is nearly identical to liver blood flow. For drugs with a low extraction ratio, changes in liver blood flow have almost no effect on clearance.

IX. Renal Clearance

    A. Renal excretion of drugs involves (a) glomerular filtration, (b) active tubular secretion, and (c) passive tubular reabsorption (most prominent for lipid-soluble drugs).

        1. A highly lipid-soluble drug, such as thiopental, is almost completely reabsorbed such that little or no unchanged drug is excreted in the urine.

        2. Conversely, production of less lipid-soluble metabolites limits renal tubule reabsorption and facilitates excretion in the urine.

    B. The rate of reabsorption from renal tubules is influenced by factors such as pH and rate of renal tubular urine flow.

X. **Absorption is not particularly relevant for most anesthetic drugs.**

XI. **Ionization.** Most drugs are weak acids or bases that are present in solutions in ionized and nonionized form (Table 2-1). A high degree of ionization thus impairs absorption of drug from the gastrointestinal tract, limits access to drug-metabolizing enzymes in the hepatocytes, and facilitates excretion of unchanged drug because reabsorption across the renal tubular epithelium is unlikely.

A. **Determinants of Degree of Ionization**

1. The degree of drug ionization is a function of its dissociation constant (pK) and the pH of the surrounding fluid.

2. When the pK and the pH are identical, 50% of the drug exists in both the ionized and nonionized form. Small changes in pH can result in large changes in the extent of ionization, especially if the pH and pK values are similar.

   a. Acidic drugs, such as barbiturates, tend to be highly ionized at an alkaline pH.

   b. Basic drugs, such as opioids and local anesthetics, are highly ionized at an acid pH.

B. **Ion Trapping**

1. Because it is the nonionized drug that equilibrates across lipid membranes, a concentration difference of total drug can develop on two sides of a membrane that separates fluids with different pH.

2. Systemic administration of a weak base, such as an opioid, can result in accumulation of ionized drug (ion trapping) in the acid environment of the stomach.

3. A similar phenomenon occurs in the transfer of basic drugs, such as local anesthetics, across the placenta from mother to fetus because the fetal pH is lower than maternal pH. The lipid-soluble, nonionized fraction of local anesthetic crosses the placenta and is converted

Table 2-1		
Characteristics of Nonionized and Ionized Drug Molecules		
	Nonionized	Ionized
Pharmacologic effect	Active	Inactive
Solubility	Lipids	Water
Cross lipid barriers (gastrointestinal tract, blood–brain barrier, placenta)	Yes	No
Renal excretion	No	Yes
Hepatic metabolism	Yes	No

to the poorly lipid-soluble ionized fraction in the more acidic environment of the fetus. The ionized fraction in the fetus cannot easily cross the placenta to the maternal circulation and thus is effectively trapped in the fetus.

   a. At the same time, conversion of the nonionized to ionized fraction maintains a gradient for continued passage of local anesthetic into the fetus.

   b. The resulting accumulation of local anesthetic in the fetus is accentuated by the acidosis that accompanies fetal distress.

XII. **Route of Administration and Systemic Absorption of Drugs.** The systemic absorption rate of a drug determines the magnitude of the drug effect and duration of action. Changes in the systemic absorption rate may necessitate an adjustment in the dose or time interval between repeated drug doses. Systemic absorption, regardless of the route of drug administration, depends on the drug's solubility.

   A. **Oral Administration**

      1. Disadvantages of the oral route include (a) emesis caused by irritation of the gastrointestinal mucosa by the drug, (b) destruction of the drug by digestive enzymes or acidic gastric fluid, (c) irregularities in absorption in the presence of food or other drugs, and (d) metabolism in the gastrointestinal tract before absorption can occur.

      2. The principal site of drug absorption after oral administration is the small intestine due to the large surface area of this portion of the gastrointestinal tract.

      3. **First-pass hepatic effect** is when drugs are absorbed from the gastrointestinal tract and enter the portal venous blood and thus pass through the liver before entering the systemic circulation for delivery to tissue receptors. For drugs that undergo extensive hepatic extraction and metabolism (propranolol, lidocaine), it is the reason for large differences in the pharmacologic effect between oral and intravenous doses.

      4. **Oral Transmucosal Administration**. The sublingual or buccal route of administration permits a rapid onset of drug effect because this blood bypasses the liver and thus prevents the first-pass hepatic effect on the initial plasma concentration of drug.

   B. **Transdermal administration** of drugs provides sustained therapeutic plasma concentrations of the drug and decreases the likelihood of loss of therapeutic efficacy due to peaks and valleys associated with conventional intermittent drug injections.

XIII. **Pharmacokinetic Models.** A consideration of the derivation of these models allows consideration of their representative parts.

    A. **Zero- and First-Order Processes**. Individual consumption of oxygen and production of carbon dioxide occur at a constant rate. The rate of change (dx/dt) for a zero-order process is $\dfrac{dx}{dt} = k$

    B. **Physiologic Pharmacokinetic Models**. If the goal is to determine how to give drugs in order to obtain therapeutic plasma drug concentrations, then all that is needed is to mathematically relate dose to plasma concentration. For this purpose, compartment models are usually adequate.

       1. **Compartmental Pharmacokinetic Models**

          a. The "one compartment model" contains a single volume and a single clearance (Fig. 2-8A).

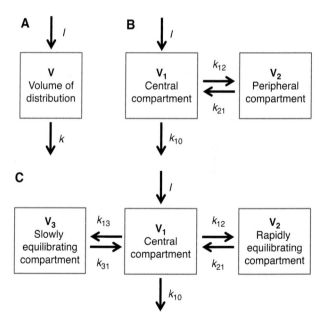

FIGURE 2-8 Standard one- **(A)**, two- **(B)**, and three-compartment **(C)** mammillary pharmacokinetic models. *I* represents any input into the system (bolus or infusion). The volumes are represented by *V* and the rate constants by *k*. The subscripts on rate constants indicate the direction of flow, noted as $k_{from\ to}$.

   b. For anesthetic drugs, the model resemble several buckets connected by pipes (two or three compartment models) (Fig. 2-8B,C).
   c. The sum of the all volumes is the volume of distribution at steady state (Vd_{ss}).
   d. The clearance leaving the central compartment for the outside is the "systemic" clearance, and the clearances between the central compartment and the peripheral compartments are the "intercompartmental" clearances.
   e. Other than clearance, none of the parameters of compartment models readily translates into any anatomic structure or physiologic process (Fig. 2-9A,B).
2. When drugs are given intravenously, every molecule reaches the systemic circulation (when given by other routes, the drug must first reach the systemic circulation).

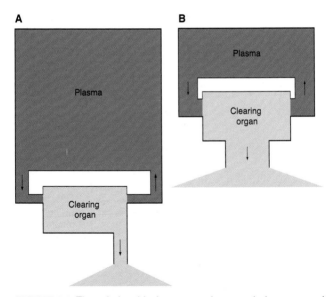

FIGURE 2-9 The relationship between volume and clearance and half-life can be envisioned by considering two settings: a big volume and a small clearance **(A)** and a small volume with a big clearance **(B)**. Drug will be eliminated faster in the latter case.

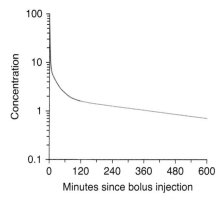

FIGURE 2-10 Typical time course of plasma concentration following bolus injection of an intravenous drug, with a rapid phase *(red)*, an intermediate phase *(blue)*, and a slow log-linear phase *(green)*. The simulation was performed with the pharmacokinetics of fentanyl. (Reused from Scott JC, Stanski DR. Decreased fentanyl and alfentanil dose requirements with age. A simultaneous pharmacokinetic and pharmacodynamic evaluation. *J Pharmacol Exp Ther.* 1987;240: 159–166.)

3. The plasma concentrations over time following an intravenous bolus resemble the curve in Figure 2-10. This curve has the characteristics common to most drugs when given by intravenous bolus (concentrations continuously decrease over time and the rate of decline is initially steep but becomes less steep over time).

4. Many anesthetic drugs appear to have three distinct phases (Fig. 2-10).

   a. There is a "rapid distribution" phase that begins immediately after bolus injection. Very rapid movement of the drug from the plasma to the rapidly equilibrating tissues characterizes this phase.

   b. Often, there is a second "slow distribution" phase that is characterized by movement of drug into more slowly equilibrating tissues and return of drug to the plasma from the most rapidly equilibrating tissues.

   c. The distinguishing characteristic of the terminal elimination phase is that the plasma concentration is lower than the tissue concentrations, and the relative proportion of drug in the plasma and peripheral volumes of distribution remains constant. During this "terminal phase," drug returns from the rapid and slow distribution volumes to the plasma and is permanently removed from plasma by metabolism or excretion.

C. **The Time Course of Drug Effect**. The plasma is not the site of drug effect for anesthetic drugs. There is a time lag between plasma drug concentration and effect-site drug concentration (Figs. 2-11 to 2-13).

D. **Dose Calculations**
   1. **Bolus Dosing**. Conventional approaches to calculate a bolus dose are designed to produce a specific plasma concentration. This makes little sense because the plasma is not the site of drug effect. By knowing the k_{e0} (the rate constant for elimination of drug from the effect site) of an intravenous anesthetic, one can design a dosing regimen that yields the desired concentration *at the site of drug effect* (avoids an overdose) (Table 2-2).
   2. **Maintenance Infusion Rate**. The best approach is through the use of target-controlled drug delivery. With target-controlled drug delivery, the user sets the desired plasma or effect-site concentration. Based on the drug's pharmacokinetics and the mathematical relationship between patient covariates (weight, age, gender) and individual pharmacokinetic parameters, the computer calculates the dose of drug necessary to rapidly achieve and then maintain any desired concentration (Fig. 2-14).
   3. **Context-sensitive half-time** is the time for the plasma concentration to decrease by 50% from an infusion that maintains a constant concentration. The context-sensitive half-time increases with longer infusion durations because it takes longer for the concentrations to fall if drug has accumulated in peripheral tissues (Figs. 2-15 and 2-16). Context-sensitive half-time and effect-site decrement times are more useful than elimination half-time in characterizing the clinical responses to drugs.

XIV. **Pharmacodynamics is the study of the intrinsic sensitivity or responsiveness of the body to a drug and the mechanisms by which these effects occur (what the drug does to the body).**
   A. Structure–activity relationships link the actions of drugs to their chemical structures and facilitate the design of drugs with more desirable pharmacologic properties.
      1. The intrinsic sensitivity is determined by measuring plasma concentrations of a drug required to evoke specific pharmacologic responses.

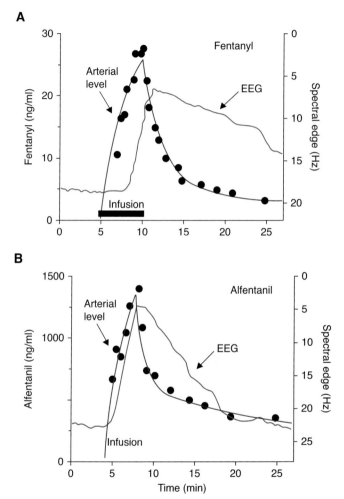

FIGURE 2-11 Fentanyl and alfentanil arterial concentrations *(circles)* and electroencephalographic (EEG) response *(irregular line)* to an intravenous infusion. Alfentanil shows a less time lag between the rise and fall of arterial concentration and the rise and fall of EEG response than fentanyl because it equilibrates with the brain more quickly.

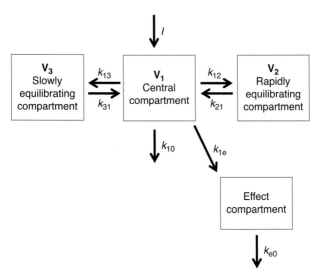

FIGURE 2-12 The three compartment model from an added effect site to account for the equilibration delay between the plasma concentration and the observed drug effect. The effect site has a negligible volume. As a result, the only parameter that affects the delay is k_{e0}.

    2. The intrinsic sensitivity to drugs varies among patients and within patients over time with aging. As a result, at similar plasma concentrations of a drug, some patients show a therapeutic response, others show no response, and, in others, toxicity develops.

B. **Concentration versus Response Relationships**. The most fundamental relationship in pharmacology is the concentration (or dose) versus response curve (Fig. 2-17). This is the time-independent relationship between exposure to the drug (x-axis) and the measured effect (y-axis).

C. **Potency and Efficacy**

    1. Clinicians often use potency to refer to the relative dose of two drugs, such as the relative potency of fentanyl and morphine (the problem with this definition is that when drugs have very different time courses, the

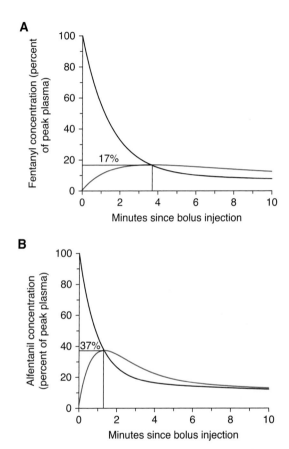

FIGURE 2-13 Plasma *(black line)* and effect-site *(red line)* concentrations following a bolus dose of fentanyl **(A)** or alfentanil **(B)**.

relative potency varies depending on the time of the measurement).
a. From a pharmacologic perspective, potency is more logically described in terms of the concentration versus response relationship (a drug with a left-shifted concentration vs. response curve [lower C_{50}]

Table 2-2

The Time to Peak Effect and t ½ k_{e0} following a Bolus Dose

Drug	Time to Peak Drug Effect (min)	t ½ k_{e0} (min)[a]
Fentanyl	3.6	4.7
Alfentanil	1.4	0.9
Sufentanil	5.6	3.0
Remifentanil	1.6	1.3
Propofol	2.2	2.4
Thiopental	1.6	1.5
Midazolam	2.8	4.0
Etomidate	2.0	1.5

[a] t ½ k_{e0} = 0.693 / k_{e0}, the effect site half-life, where k_{e0} is the rate constant for elimination of drug from the site of drug effect and t ½ k_{e0} is the time required for the concentration at the site of drug effect to fall to half of its value.

Reused from Glass PSA, Shafer S, Reves JG. Intravenous drug delivery systems. In: Miller RD, Eriksson LI, Fleisher LA, et al, eds. *Miller's Anesthesia*. 7th ed. Philadelphia, PA: Churchill Livingstone; 2010, with permission.

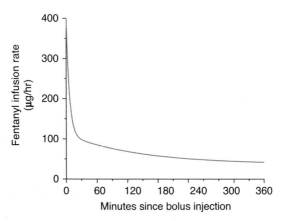

FIGURE 2-14 Fentanyl infusion rate to maintain a plasma concentration of 1 μg/hr. The rate starts off quite high because fentanyl is avidly taken up by body fat. The necessary infusion rate decreases as the fat equilibrates with the plasma.

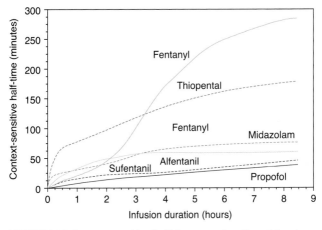

FIGURE 2-15 Context-sensitive half-times as a function of the duration of intravenous drug infusion for each fentanyl, alfentanil, sufentanil, propofol, midazolam, and thiopental. (From Hughes MA, Glass PSA, Jacobs JR. Context-sensitive half-time in multicompartment pharmacokinetic models for intravenous anesthetic drugs. *Anesthesiology*. 1992;76:334–341, with permission.)

is considered more potent, whereas a drug with a right-shifted dose vs. response curve is less potent) (Fig. 2-18).

  b. To be precise, potency should be defined in terms of a specific drug effect (50% of maximal effect of a full agonist).
2. Efficacy is a measure of the intrinsic ability of a drug to produce a given physiologic or clinical effect (Fig. 2-19).
3. Efficacy refers to the position of the concentration versus response curve in the *y*-axis, whereas potency refers to relative drug concentration for a particular response on the *y*-axis.
D. **Effective Dose and Lethal Dose**. The ED_{50} is the dose of a drug required to produce a specific desired effect in 50% of individuals receiving the drug. The LD_{50} is the dose of a drug required to produce death in 50% of patients (or, more often, animals) receiving the drug. The therapeutic index is the ratio between the LD_{50} and the ED_{50} (LD_{50}/ED_{50}) (Fig. 2-20).

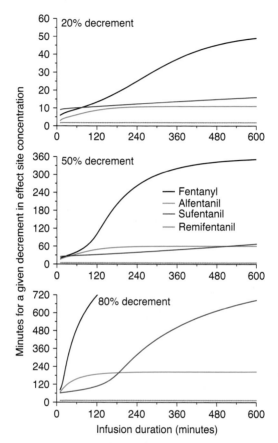

FIGURE 2-16 Effect-site decrement times. The 20%, 50%, and 80% decrement times for fentanyl *(black)*, alfentanil *(green)*, sufentanil *(red)*, and remifentanil *(blue)*. When there is substantial plasma effect-site disequilibrium, the effect-site decrement time will provide a better estimate of the time required for recover than the context-sensitive half-time.

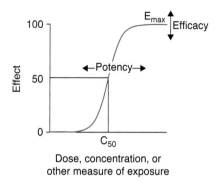

FIGURE 2-17 Drug exposure (dose, concentration, etc.) versus drug effect relationship. Potency refers to the position of the curve along the *x*-axis. Efficacy refers to the position of the maximum effect on the *y*-axis.

XV. **Drug Interactions**
   A. **Actions at Different Receptors**
      1. Opioids potently reduce the minimum alveolar concentration of inhaled anesthetics required to suppress movement to noxious stimulation (Figs. 2-21 and 2-22). Even with huge doses of opioids, some hypnotic

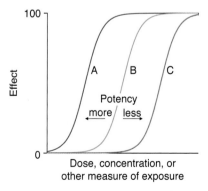

FIGURE 2-18 Dose versus response relationship for three drugs with potency. Drug A is the most potent, and drug C is the least potent.

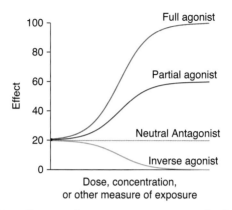

FIGURE 2-19 Concentration versus response curves for drugs with differing efficacies. Although the C_{50} of each curve is the same, the partial agonist is less potent than the full agonist because of the decreased efficacy.

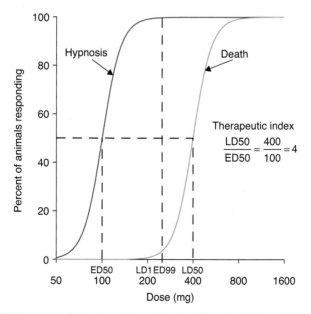

FIGURE 2-20 Analysis to determine the LD_{50}, the LD_{99}, and the therapeutic index of a drug.

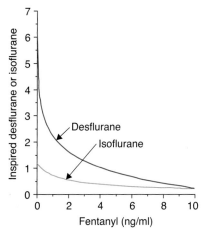

FIGURE 2-21 Interaction between fentanyl and isoflurane or desflurane on the minimum alveolar concentration required to suppress movement to noxious stimulation.

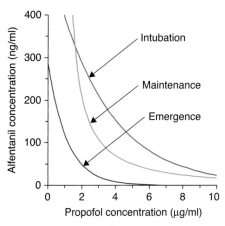

FIGURE 2-22 Interaction of propofol with alfentanil on the concentration required to suppress response to intubation, maintain nonresponsiveness during surgery, and then awaken from anesthesia.

component must be added to the anesthetic to prevent movement.

2. The interaction between pairs of intravenous drugs and intravenous drugs and inhaled anesthetics is typically synergistic.

XVI. **Stereochemistry is the study of how molecules are structured in three dimensions.**
   A. Chirality is the structural basis of *enantiomerism*. Enantiomers (substances of opposite shape) are pairs of molecules existing in two forms that are mirror images of one another (right and left hand) but cannot be superimposed.
      1. A pair of enantiomers is distinguished by the direction in which, when dissolved in solution, they rotate polarized light, either clockwise (dextrorotatory, d [+]) or counterclockwise (levorotatory, l [−]).
      2. These observed signs of rotation, d(+) and l(−), are often confused with the designations D and L used in protein and carbohydrate chemistry.
      3. The characteristic of rotation of polarized light is the origin of the term *optical isomers*. When the two enantiomers are present in equal proportions (50:50), they are referred to as a *racemic mixture*.
      4. The most applicable and unambiguous convention for designating isomers is the *sinister (S)* and *rectus (R)* classification that specifies the absolute configuration in the name of the compound.
   B. Molecular interactions that are the mechanistic foundation of pharmacokinetics and pharmacodynamics are stereoselective (relative difference between enantiomers) or stereospecific (absolute difference between enantiomers). The "lock and key" hypothesis of enzyme substrate activity emphasizes that biologic systems are inherently stereospecific.
      1. The pharmacologic extension of this concept is that drugs can be expected to interact with other biologic components in a geometrically specific way.
      2. Pharmacologically, not all enantiomers are created equal. Enantiomers can exhibit differences in absorption, distribution, clearance, potency, and toxicity (drug interactions). Enantiomers can even antagonize the effects of one another.
   C. The administration of a racemic drug mixture may in fact represent pharmacologically two different drugs with distinct pharmacokinetic and pharmacodynamic properties.
      1. The two enantiomers of the racemic mixture may have different rates of absorption, metabolism, and excretion

as well as different affinities for receptor binding sites. Although only one enantiomer is therapeutically active, it is possible that the other enantiomer contributes to side effects.

2. The therapeutically inactive isomer in a racemic mixture should be regarded as an impurity.

D. Studies on racemic mixtures may be scientifically flawed if the enantiomers have different pharmacokinetics or pharmacodynamics. An estimated one-third of drugs in clinical use are administered as racemic mixtures. Enantiomer-specific drug studies are likely to become more common in the future.

E. **Clinical Aspects of Chirality**
1. The majority of inhaled anesthetics are chiral (exception is sevoflurane). Most evidence suggests that enantiomer-selective effects for volatile anesthetics are relatively weak in contrast to much stronger evidence for specific drug-receptor interactions for intravenous anesthetics.
2. Local anesthetics, including mepivacaine, prilocaine, and bupivacaine, have a center of molecular asymmetry.
   a. In addition to pharmacokinetic differences, the cardiac toxicity of bupivacaine is thought to be predominantly due to the *R*-bupivacaine isomer.
   b. Ropivacaine is the S-enantiomer of a bupivacaine homolog that has decreased cardiac toxicity.
3. The S (+) enantiomer of ketamine is more potent than the R (−) form and is also less likely to produce emergence delirium.

F. **Individual Variability**
1. After administration of identical doses, some patients may have clinically significant adverse effects, whereas others may exhibit no therapeutic response. Some of this diversity of response can be ascribed to differences in the rate of drug metabolism, particularly by the cytochrome P-450 family of enzymes (Table 2-3).
2. The incorporation of pharmacogenetics into clinical medicine may become useful in predicting patient responses to drugs.
3. In clinical practice, the impact of interpatient variability may be masked by the administration of high doses of a drug (administration of 2 to 3 × ED_{95} of a nondepolarizing neuromuscular blocking drug).
4. It is common practice in anesthesia to administer drugs in proportion to body weight, although pharmacokinetic and pharmacodynamic principles may not support this practice.

Table 2-3

Events Responsible for Variations in Drug Responses between Individuals

Pharmacokinetics
  Bioavailability
  Renal function
  Hepatic function
  Cardiac function
  Patient age
Pharmacodynamics
  Enzyme activity
  Genetic differences
  Drug interactions

5. In attempts to minimize interindividual variability, computerized infusion systems (target-controlled infusion systems) have been developed to deliver intravenous drugs.

G. **Elderly Patients**
  1. In elderly patients, variations in drug response most likely reflect (a) decreased cardiac output, (b) increased fat content, (c) decreased protein binding, and (d) decreased renal function.
  2. Aging does not seem to be accompanied by changes in receptor responsiveness.

H. **Enzyme Activity.** Alterations in enzyme activity as reflected by enzyme induction may be responsible for variations in drug responses among individuals.

I. **Genetic Disorders**
  1. Variations in drug responses among individuals are due, in part, to genetic differences that may also affect receptor sensitivity. Genetic variations in metabolic pathways (rapid vs. slow acetylators) may have important clinical implications.
  2. Examples of diseases that are unmasked by drugs include (a) atypical cholinesterase enzyme revealed by prolonged neuromuscular blockade after administration of succinylcholine or mivacurium and (b) malignant hyperthermia triggered by succinylcholine or volatile anesthetics.

J. A drug interaction occurs when a drug alters the intensity of pharmacologic effects of another drug given concurrently. Drug interactions may reflect alterations in pharmacokinetics (increased metabolism of neuromuscular blocking drugs in patients receiving anticonvulsants chronically) or pharmacodynamics (decrease in volatile anesthetic requirements produced by opioids).

1. The net result of a drug interaction may be enhanced or diminished effects of one or both drugs, leading to desired or undesired effects.
2. The potential for drug interactions in the perioperative period is great considering the large number of drugs from different chemical classes that are likely to be part of anesthesia management.

CHAPTER 3

Neurophysiology

The most amazing aspect of the daily miracle of anesthesia is turning off consciousness to permit surgery to proceed and then fully restoring consciousness in a controlled manner. Recent advances in neurophysiology are providing insight into how drugs interact with receptors throughout the nervous system to mediate anesthesia and analgesia.

I. How Nerves Work
   A. **Neurons** are the basic elements of all rapid signal processing within the body. A neuron consists of a cell body, also called the *soma*, dendrites, and the nerve fiber, also called the *axon* (Figs. 3-1 and 3-2).
   B. **Classification of Afferent Nerve Fibers**
      1. Nerve fibers are called *afferent* if they transmit impulses from peripheral receptors to the central nervous system (CNS) and efferent if they transmit impulses from the CNS to the periphery. Afferent nerve fibers are classified as A, B, and C on the basis of fiber diameter and velocity of conduction of nerve impulses (Table 3-1).
      2. Myelin that surrounds type A and B nerve fibers acts as an insulator that prevents flow of ions across nerve membranes. Type C fibers are unmyelinated. The myelin sheath is interrupted approximately every 1 to 2 mm by the nodes of Ranvier (see Fig. 3-1).
      3. This successive excitation of nodes of Ranvier by an action potential that jumps between successive nodes is termed *saltatory conduction*. Saltatory conduction allows for a 10-fold increase in the velocity of nerve transmission.
   C. **Evaluation of Peripheral Nerve Function**
      1. Nerve conduction studies are useful in the localization and assessment of peripheral nerve dysfunction.

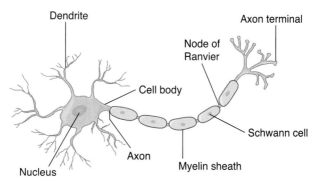

FIGURE 3-1 Anatomy of a neuron.

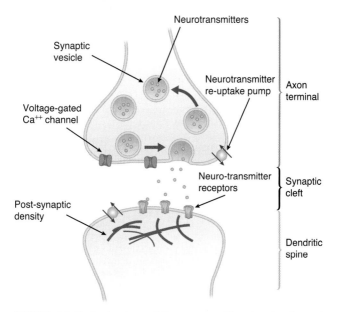

FIGURE 3-2 Basic structure of the synapse. The signal arrives at the axon terminal, where it causes the release of neurotransmitters into the synapse. These cross the synaptic cleft, where they may or may not result in a propagation of the signal. Many synapses simply render the postsynaptic cell excited or inhibited without actually triggering an action potential.

Table 3-1

Classification of Peripheral Nerve Fibers

	Myelinated	Fiber Diameter (mm)	Conduction Velocity (m/s)	Function	Sensitivity to Local Anesthetic (Subarachnoid, Procaine, %)
A-α	Yes	12–20	70–120	Innervation of skeletal muscles Proprioception	1
A-β	Yes	5–12	30–70	Touch Pressure	1
A-γ	Yes	3–6	15–30	Skeletal muscle tone	1
A-δ	Yes	2–5	12–30	Fast pain Touch Temperature	0.5
B	Yes	3	3–15	Preganglionic autonomic fibers	0.25
C	No	0.4–1.2	0.5–2.0	Slow pain Touch Temperature Postganglionic sympathetic fibers	0.5

2. Electromyographic testing is helpful in determining the etiology of neurologic dysfunction that may occur after surgery.

D. **Action Potential**

1. Electrical potentials exist across nearly all cell membranes, reflecting principally the difference in transmembrane concentrations of sodium and potassium ions.

2. The resulting voltage difference across the cell membrane is called the *resting membrane potential*. The cytoplasm is electrically negative (typically −60 to −80 mV) relative to the extracellular fluid (Fig. 3-3).

3. An action potential is the rapid change in transmembrane potential due to the opening of sodium channels (*depolarization*) and rapid influx of sodium ions down

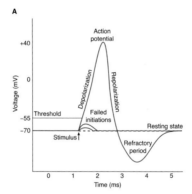

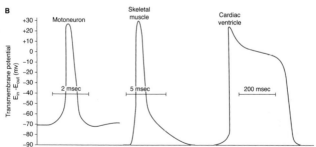

FIGURE 3-3 **A.** The elements of the action potential. **B.** The transmembrane potential and duration of the action potential varies with the tissue site. (From Berne RM, Levy MN, Koeppen B, et al. *Physiology.* 5th ed. St. Louis, MO: Mosby; 2004, with permission.)

the concentration gradient, reversing the net negative charge within the cell. The membrane resting potential is restored by the closing of the sodium channels and the opening of potassium channels (*repolarization*) after the action potential has passed.

E. **Propagation of action potentials** along the entire length of a nerve axon is the basis of rapid signal transmission along nerve cells. The size and shape of the action potential varies among excitable tissues (see Fig. 3-3).

F. **Abnormal Action Potentials**

1. A deficiency of calcium ions in the extracellular fluid (hypocalcemia) prevents the sodium channels from closing between action potentials (tetany).

2. Low potassium ion concentrations in extracellular fluid increase the negativity of the resting membrane potential, resulting in hyperpolarization and decreased cell membrane excitability.

3. Local anesthetics decrease permeability of nerve cell membranes to sodium ions, preventing achievement of a threshold potential that is necessary for generation of an action potential.

G. **Neurotransmitters and Receptors**

1. Neurotransmitters are chemical mediators that are released into the synaptic cleft in response to the arrival of an action potential at the nerve ending. Neurotransmitter release is voltage dependent and requires the influx of calcium ions into the presynaptic terminals (see Fig. 3-2).

2. Neurotransmitters may be excitatory or inhibitory, depending on the ion selectivity of the protein receptor (Table 3-2).

Table 3-2

Chemicals that Act at Synapses as Neurotransmitters

Glutamate	Gastrin
Acetylcholine	γ-Aminobutyric acid
Norepinephrine	Dopamine
Glycine	Epinephrine
Endorphins	Substance P
Serotonin	Vasopressin
Histamine	Prolactin
Oxytocin	Vasoactive intestinal peptide
Cholecystokinin	Glucagon

3. Volatile anesthetics produce a broad spectrum of actions, as reflected by their ability to modify both inhibitory and excitatory neurotransmission at presynaptic and postsynaptic loci within the CNS. The precise mechanism of these effects remains uncertain. It is likely that volatile anesthetics interact with multiple neurotransmitter systems by a variety of mechanisms.

H. **G Protein–coupled Receptors** (Fig. 3-4). The recognition site faces the exterior of the cell membrane to facilitate access of water-soluble endogenous ligands and exogenous drugs, whereas the catalytic site faces the interior of the cell.

1. G_α proteins can either be stimulatory, promoting a specific enzymatic reaction within the cell, or inhibitory, depressing a specific enzymatic reaction.

a. β-adrenergic receptors couple with stimulatory $G_{\alpha s}$ proteins and increase the activity of adenylyl cyclase.

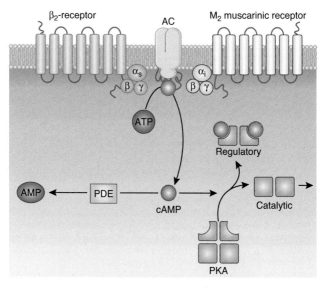

FIGURE 3-4 Schematic diagram showing G protein–coupled receptors, the β_2 adrenergic receptor, which upregulates adenylyl cyclase, and the M_2 muscarinic receptor, which downregulates adenylyl cyclase (AC). The effects of these G protein–coupled receptors are then mediated through the intercellular concentration of cyclic AMP. (Modified from Pierre S, Eschenhagen T, Geisslinger G, et al. Capturing adenylyl cyclases as potential drug targets. *Nat Rev Drug Discov.* 2009;8:321–335.)

      b. Opioid receptors are associated with inhibitory $G_{\alpha i}$ proteins that decrease the activity of adenylyl cyclase.

      c. By regulating the level of activity of adenylyl cyclase, the β-adrenergic and opioid receptors modulate the internal level of cyclic adenosine monophosphate (cAMP), which functions as an intercellular second messenger (see Fig. 3-4).

  2. Many hormones and drugs act through G protein–coupled receptors, including catecholamines, opioids, anticholinergics, and antihistamines.

      a. **Dopamine** represents more than 50% of the CNS content of catecholamines, with high concentrations in the basal ganglia. Dopamine can be either inhibitory or excitatory, depending on the specific dopaminergic receptor that it activates. Dopamine is important to the reward centers of the brain and plays a key role in addiction and drugs.

      b. **Norepinephrine** is present in large amounts in the reticular activating system and the hypothalamus, where it plays a key role in natural sleep and analgesia.

      c. **Substance P** is an excitatory neurotransmitter co-released by terminals of pain fibers that synapse in the substantia gelatinosa of the spinal cord.

      d. Endorphins are endogenous opioid peptide agonists (act through the μ opioid receptor, the same receptor responsible for the effects of administered opioids).

I. **Ion Channels**. There are three basic types of ion channels: (a) ligand-gated ion channels ionotropic receptors, (b) voltage-sensitive ion channels, and (c) ion channels that respond to other types of gating.

  1. **Ligand-gated ion channels** are complexes of protein subunits that act as switchable portals for ions (involved principally with fast synaptic transmission between excitable cells).

      a. **Excitatory ligand-gated ion channels** cause the inside of the cell to become less negative typically by facilitating the influx of cations into the cell (acetylcholine, glutamate, serotonin).

      b. **Inhibitory ligand-gated ion channels** cause the inside of the cell to become less negative, typically by facilitating the flux of chloride into the cell. Potassium channels that facilitate the efflux of potassium ions are also inhibitory (γ-amino butyric acid [GABA]), glycine).

  2. **Voltage-gated ion channels** are complexes of protein subunits that act as switchable portals sensitive

to membrane potential through which ions can pass through the cell membrane (open and close in response to changes in voltage across cell membranes).

a. Voltage-gated sodium channels are the site of local anesthetic action (local anesthetics block neural conduction by blocking passage of sodium through the voltage-gated sodium channel).

b. The human *ether-a-go-go* related gene (hERG) potassium channel is sensitive to many drugs and is responsible for sudden death from drugs that predispose the patient to *torsades de pointes* (inhibition of the hERG potassium channel is the reason for the black box warning on droperidol).

J. **Receptor Concentration**
   1. Receptors in cell membranes are not static components of cells.
   2. Excess circulating concentrations of ligand often results in a decrease in the density of the target receptors in cell membranes (excessive circulating norepinephrine in patients with pheochromocytoma leads to downregulation of β-adrenergic receptors).

K. **The Synapse**
   1. **Structure**
      a. The synapse functions as a diode that transmits an action potential from the presynaptic membrane to the postsynaptic membrane across the synaptic cleft (Fig. 3-5).
      b. Calcium triggers the fusion of the vesicle to the cell membrane and the release of the neurotransmitter into the synaptic cleft through exocytosis, resulting in the extrusion of the contents of the synaptic vesicles.
   2. **Synaptic Modulation**. The resting transmembrane potential of neurons in the CNS is about −70 mV, less than the −90 mV in large peripheral nerve fibers and skeletal muscles.
   3. **Synaptic delay** reflects the time for release of the neurotransmitter from the synaptic varicosity, diffusion of the neurotransmitter to the postsynaptic receptor, and the subsequent change in permeability of the postsynaptic membrane to various ions.
   4. **Synaptic fatigue** is a decrease in the number of discharges by the postsynaptic membrane when excitatory synapses are repetitively and rapidly stimulated (decreases excessive excitability of the brain as may accompany a seizure, thus acting as a protective mechanism against excessive neuronal activity).

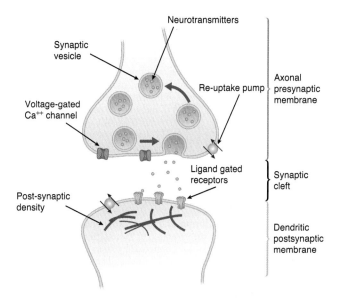

FIGURE 3-5 Structure of the synapse. Axons typically have many synapses, not just the single synapse implied by the conventional typical rendition below. The presynaptic membrane encloses the synaptic vesicles that contain the neurotransmitters, the reuptake pump that removes the neurotransmitter following synaptic transmission, and the voltage-gated calcium channel that responds to the incoming action potential. The ligand-gated receptors in the postsynaptic membrane trigger an efferent action potential. The postsynaptic density contains multiple proteins and receptors and appears responsible for organizing the structure of the receptors on the synapse.

       a. The mechanism of synaptic fatigue is presumed to be exhaustion of the stores of neurotransmitter in the synaptic vesicles.

       b. Synaptic fatigue is unmasked at the neuromuscular junction in myasthenia gravis when the enormous reserve for neuromuscular transmission is limited by either pre- or postsynaptic autoimmune damage.

    5. **Factors that Influence Neuron Responsiveness.** Neurons are highly sensitive to changes in the pH of the surrounding interstitial fluids (alkalosis enhances neuron excitability and acidosis depresses neuron excitability).

II. **Central Nervous System**. The brain, brainstem, and spinal cord constitute the central nervous system (CNS) (Fig. 3-6).

A. **Cerebral Hemispheres**. The two cerebral hemispheres, known as the *cerebral cortex*, constitute the largest division of the human brain. Regions of the cerebral cortex are classified as *sensory, motor, visual, auditory,* and *olfactory,* depending on the type of information that is processed. *Frontal, temporal, parietal,* and *occipital* designate anatomic positions of the cerebral cortex (Fig. 3-7).

B. **Anatomy of the Cerebral Cortex**
1. **Topographic Areas**. The area of the cerebral cortex to which the peripheral sensory signals are projected from the thalamus is designated the *somesthetic cortex* (see Fig. 3-7). The motor cortex is organized into topographic areas corresponding to different regions of the skeletal muscles.
2. **Corpus Callosum**. The two hemispheres of the cerebral cortex, with the exception of the anterior portions of the temporal lobes, are connected by fibers in the corpus callosum. The corpus callosum and anterior commissure make information processed or stored in one hemisphere available to the other hemisphere.

C. **Dominant versus Nondominant Hemisphere**. Language function and interpretation is typically localized in the dominant cerebral hemisphere, whereas spatiotemporal relationships (ability to recognize faces) are localized in the nondominant hemisphere. Destruction of the dominant

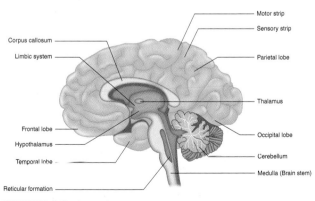

FIGURE 3-6 Brain anatomy.

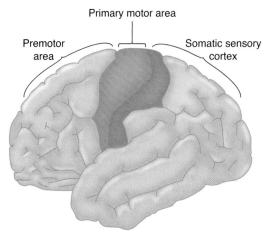

FIGURE 3-7 The sensorimotor cortex consists of the motor cortex, pyramidal (Betz) cells, and somatic sensory cortex.

cerebral hemisphere in adults results in loss of nearly all intellectual function.

D. **Memory**. The cerebral cortex, especially the temporal lobes, serves as a storage site for information that is often characterized as memory.

1. **Short-Term Memory**. The favored explanation for short-term memory is posttetanic potentiation (tetanic stimulation of a synapse for a few seconds causes increased excitability of the synapse that lasts for seconds to hours).

2. **Long-Term Memory**. Long-term memory depends on stable synaptic changes that are induced by experience. The stability of this system is evidenced by total inactivation of the brain by hypothermia or anesthesia without detectable significant loss of long-term memory.

   a. Long-term memory is thought to rely on long term synaptic potentiation mediated by structural changes.

   b. The mechanism often involves increased expression of N-methyl-D-aspartate (NMDA) receptors and voltage-gated calcium channels in the postsynaptic neuron.

E. **Postoperative cognitive dysfunction** (impaired memory) persisting after months has been described in 10% of elderly patients receiving general anesthesia without known arterial hypoxemia or systemic hypotension.

F. **Awareness and Recall During Anesthesia**
   1. The incidence of awareness with recall (conscious memory) following general anesthesia has been estimated at between 1 and 5 in 1,000 general anesthetics, depending on the risk group.
   2. Although the incidence of conscious recall of intraoperative events is rare and the development of posttraumatic stress disorder is even more uncommon, the fact that approximately 20 million general anesthetics are administered annually in the United States would correspond to 26,000 cases of awareness (0.13% of approximately 20 million) each year.
   3. The use of neuromuscular blockade is a risk factor for awareness under general anesthesia, particularly, awareness that is associated with memories of pain and complicated by posttraumatic stress disorder.
   4. Many cases of conscious awareness during surgery can be attributed to intentionally or unintentionally low concentrations of administered anesthetic.
   5. **Recognizing Awareness**. Despite a variety of monitoring methods, awareness may be difficult to recognize in real time. Indicators of awareness (heart rate, blood pressure, and skeletal muscle movement) are often masked by anesthetic and adjuvant drugs (β-adrenergic blockers) and/or neuromuscular-blocking drugs. Several different monitors based on analysis of electroencephalogram and somatosensory evoked potentials (SSEP) patterns have been introduced in hopes of addressing this issue.

G. **Brainstem**. Homeostatic life-sustaining processes are controlled subconsciously in the brainstem (control of systemic blood pressure and breathing in the medulla).

H. **Limbic System and Hypothalamus**. Behavior associated with emotions is primarily a function of structures known as the *limbic system* (hippocampus, basal ganglia) located in the basal regions of the brain.

I. **Basal Ganglia**
   1. Many of the impulses from basal ganglia are inhibitory, mediated by dopamine and GABA. The balance between agonist and antagonist skeletal muscle contractions is an important role of the basal ganglia.
   2. Whenever destruction of the basal ganglia occurs, there is associated skeletal muscle rigidity.

J. **Reticular activating system** is a polysynaptic pathway (excitatory and inhibitory) that is intimately concerned with electrical activity of the cerebral cortex. The reticular activating system determines the overall level of CNS activity, including nuclei important in determining wakefulness and sleep.

  1. **Slow-Wave Sleep**. During slow-wave sleep, sympathetic nervous system activity decreases, parasympathetic nervous system activity increases, and skeletal muscle tone is greatly decreased. As a result, there is a 10% to 30% decrease in systemic blood pressure, heart rate, breathing frequency, and basal metabolic rate.

  2. This form of sleep is characterized by active dreaming, irregular heart rate and breathing, and a desynchronized pattern of low-voltage β-waves on the EEG similar to those that occur during wakefulness (but not aware). Despite the inhibition of skeletal muscle activity, the eyes exhibit rapid movements (desynchronized sleep is also referred to as *paradoxical sleep* or *rapid eye movement* [REM] *sleep*).

K. **Cerebellum** operates subconsciously to monitor and elicit corrective responses in motor activity caused by stimulation of other parts of the brain and spinal cord. The cerebellum is important in the maintenance of equilibrium and postural adjustments.

  1. **Dysfunction of the Cerebellum**

    a. In the absence of cerebellar function, a person cannot predict prospectively how far movements will go (results in overshoot of the intended mark referred to as past pointing).

    b. In the presence of cerebellar disease, a person is unable to activate antagonist skeletal muscles that prevent a certain portion of the body from moving unexpectedly in an unwanted direction.

L. **Spinal cord** extends from the medulla oblongata to the lower border of the first and, occasionally, the second lumbar vertebra. Below the spinal cord, the vertebral canal is filled by the roots of the lumbar and sacral nerves, which are collectively known as the *cauda equina*.

  1. **Gray matter** of the spinal cord functions as the initial processor of incoming sensory signals from peripheral somatic receptors and as a relay station to send these signals to the brain. Anatomically, the gray matter of the spinal cord is divided into anterior, lateral, and dorsal horns consisting of nine separate laminae that are H-shaped when viewed in cross-section (Fig. 3-8).

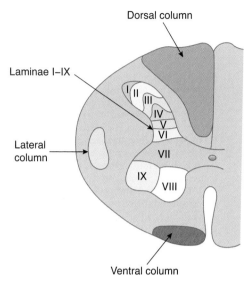

Dorsal column

Laminae I–IX

Lateral column

Ventral column

FIGURE 3-8 Schematic diagram of a cross-section of the spinal cord depicting anatomic laminae I to IX of the spinal cord gray matter and the ascending dorsal, lateral, and ventral sensory columns of the spinal cord white matter.

2. White matter of the spinal cord is formed by the axons that make up their respective ascending and descending tracts. This area of the spinal cord is divided into dorsal, lateral, and ventral columns (see Fig. 3-8).

3. **Pyramidal and Extrapyramidal Tracts**. A major pathway for transmission of motor signals from the cerebral cortex to the anterior motor neurons of the spinal cord is through the pyramidal (corticospinal) tracts (Fig. 3-9).

4. **Spinal Nerve**

   a. A pair of spinal nerves arises from each of 31 segments of the spinal cord. Spinal nerves are made up of fibers of the ventral (anterior) and dorsal (posterior) roots.

   b. Each spinal nerve innervates a segmental area of skin designated as *dermatome* and an area of skeletal muscle known as a *myotome*. A dermatome map is useful in determining the level of spinal cord injury or level of sensory anesthesia produced by a neuraxial anesthetic (Fig. 3-10).

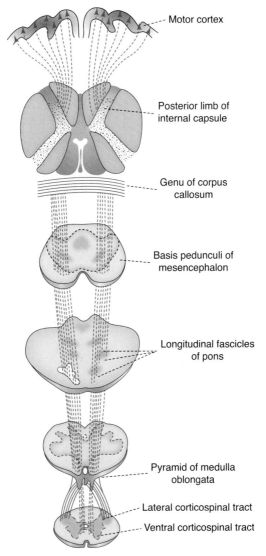

Motor cortex

Posterior limb of internal capsule

Genu of corpus callosum

Basis pedunculi of mesencephalon

Longitudinal fascicles of pons

Pyramid of medulla oblongata

Lateral corticospinal tract

Ventral corticospinal tract

FIGURE 3-9 The pyramidal tracts are major pathways for transmission of motor signals from the cerebral cortex to the spinal cord.

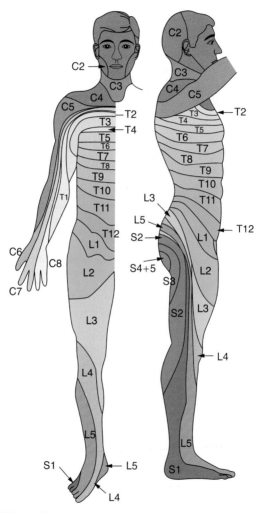

FIGURE 3-10 Dermatome map that may be used to evaluate the level of sensory anesthesia produced by regional anesthesia.

    5. **Spinal shock** is a manifestation of the abrupt loss of spinal cord reflexes that immediately follows transection of the spinal cord.

       a. The immediate manifestations of spinal shock are hypotension due to loss of vasoconstrictor tone and absence of all skeletal muscle reflexes.

       b. Within a few days to weeks, spinal cord neurons gradually regain their intrinsic excitability (bladder and colon evacuation).

M. **Imaging of the Nervous System**

    1. Computed tomography (CT) and, subsequently, magnetic resonance imaging (MRI) provide high-resolution images of brain tissue and clear discrimination between gray and white matter.

    2. Positron emission tomography (PET) and single photon emission computed tomography (SPECT) permit imaging of both structure and functional characteristics (blood flow, metabolism, and concentrations of neurochemicals and receptors) of the brain.

    3. Comparative studies indicate that MRI is superior to CT in evaluating most cerebral parenchymal lesions because of better special discrimination.

    4. CT is useful in visualizing intracranial blood that may be present in patients with subdural hematomas or cerebral hemorrhage.

N. **Cerebral blood flow** averages 50 mL/100 g/min of brain tissue.

    1. $Paco_2$ and Pao_2 influence cerebral blood flow, whereas sympathetic and parasympathetic nerves play little or no role in the regulation of cerebral blood flow (Fig. 3-11).

    2. **Autoregulation**. Cerebral blood flow is closely autoregulated between a mean arterial pressure of about 60 and 140 mm Hg (see Fig. 3-11). Autoregulation of cerebral blood flow is attenuated or abolished by hypercapnia, arterial hypoxemia, volatile anesthetics, and the area surrounding an acute cerebral infarction.

O. **Electroencephalogram (EEG)**. There is a direct relationship between the degree of cerebral activity and the frequency of brain waves.

    1. **Classification of Brain Waves**. Brain waves are classified as alpha, beta, theta, and delta waves, depending on their frequency and amplitude (Fig. 3-12).

    2. **Clinical Uses**. The EEG is useful in diagnosing different types of epilepsy and for determining the focus in the brain causing seizures.

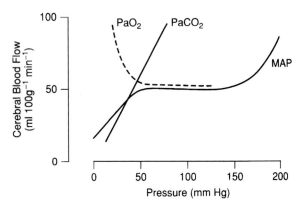

FIGURE 3-11 Cerebral blood flow is influenced by Pa_{O_2}, Pa_{CO_2}, and mean arterial pressure (MAP).

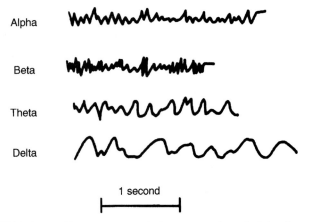

FIGURE 3-12 The electroencephalogram consists of alpha, beta, theta, and delta waves.

P. **Evoked potentials** are the electrophysiologic responses of the CNS to sensory, motor, auditory, or visual stimulation. The waveforms resulting from sensory stimulation reflect transmission of impulses through specific sensory pathways.
   1. **Somatosensory evoked potentials (SSEP)** are produced by application of a low-voltage electrical current that stimulates a peripheral nerve such as the median nerve at the wrist or the posterior tibial nerve at the ankle. The resulting evoked potentials reflect the integrity of sensory neural pathways from the peripheral nerve to the somatosensory cortex.
   2. **Visual evoked potentials** may be useful to monitor the visual pathways during β-transsphenoidal or anterior fossa neurosurgical procedures. Volatile anesthetics produce dose-dependent depression of visual evoked potentials, especially above concentrations equivalent to about 0.8 minimum alveolar concentration (MAC).
Q. **Cerebrospinal fluid (CSF)** is present in the (a) ventricles of the brain, (b) cisterns around the brain, and (c) subarachnoid space around the brain and spinal cord (Fig. 3-13).

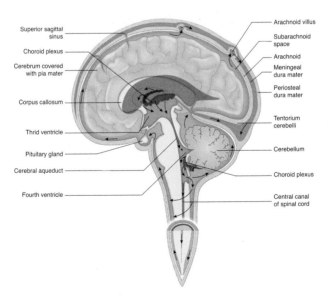

FIGURE 3-13 Cerebral spinal fluid fluxes in and out of the ventricles with the cardiac cycle.

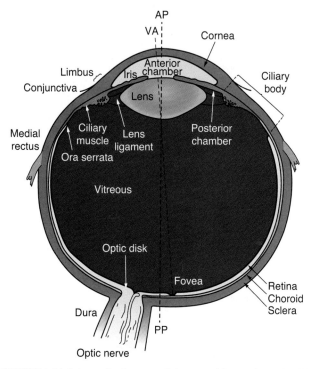

FIGURE 3-14 Schematic diagram of the eye. *AP*, anterior pole; *PP*, posterior pole; *VA*, visual axis.

R. **Intracranial pressure** (ICP) is less than 15 mm Hg. This pressure is regulated by the rate of CSF formation and resistance to CSF reabsorption through arachnoid villi as determined by venous pressure.

S. **Blood–brain barrier** reflects the impermeability of capillaries in the CNS to circulating substances such as electrolytes and exogenous drugs or toxins.

T. **Vision**. The eye is optically equivalent to a photographic camera in that it contains a lens system, a variable aperture system (pupil), and light sensitive surface (retina) (Fig. 3-14).

1. **Ischemic optic neuropathy** (ION) results from infarction of the optic nerve and is the most frequently

reported cause of vision loss following general anesthesia. Posterior ION has been reported after diverse surgical procedures (prolonged spinal fusion surgery, cardiac operations requiring cardiopulmonary bypass, radical neck surgery), and its etiology appears to be multifactorial.

2. **Other Causes of Postoperative Blindness**
   a. Cortical blindness is characterized by loss of visual sensation with retention of pupillary reaction to light and normal funduscopic examination results.
   b. Central retinal artery occlusion presents as painless, monocular blindness. Ophthalmoscopic examination of the eyes with retinal artery occlusion shows a pale edematous retina.

U. **Nausea and Vomiting**. Nausea is the conscious recognition of excitation of an area in the medulla that is associated with the vomiting (emetic) center (Fig. 3-15).

1. The medullary vomiting center is located close to the fourth cerebral ventricle and receives afferents from the (a) chemoreceptor trigger zone, (b) cerebral cortex, (c) labyrinthovestibular center, and (d) neurovegetative system.

2. The chemoreceptor trigger zone includes receptors for serotonin, dopamine, histamine, and opioids. Stimulation of the chemoreceptor trigger zone located on the floor of the fourth cerebral ventricle initiates vomiting independent of the vomiting center. The chemoreceptor trigger zone is not protected by the blood–brain barrier, and thus, this zone can be activated by chemical stimuli received through the systemic circulation as well as the CSF.

III. **Peripheral nervous system is composed of the sensory and motor nerves that connect the CNS to the tissues and organs (Fig. 3-16).**

A. **Pathways for Peripheral Sensory Impulses**. The peripheral nerves extend from the dendrite in the periphery to the dorsal root ganglion, where the cell body is located, and from there to the spinal cord by way of the dorsal root (Fig. 3-17).

B. **Pathways for Peripheral Motor Responses**. Anterior motor neurons in the anterior horns of the spinal cord gray matter give rise to A-α fibers that leave the spinal cord by way of anterior nerve roots and innervate skeletal muscles.

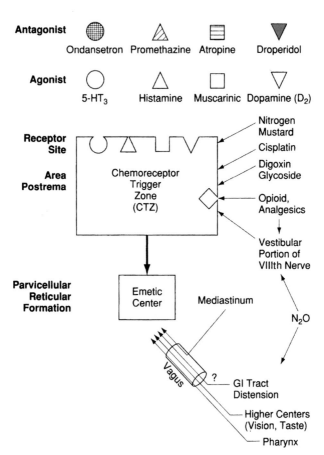

FIGURE 3-15 The chemoreceptor trigger zone and emetic center respond to a variety of stimuli resulting in nausea and vomiting. *5-HT₃*, 5-hydroxytryptamine; *GI*, gastrointestinal. (From Watcha MR, White PF. Postoperative nausea and vomiting. Its etiology, treatment, and prevention. *Anesthesiology*. 1992;77:162–184, with permission.)

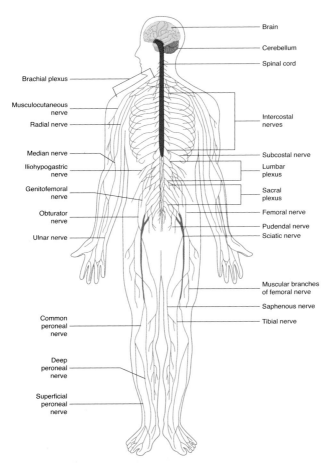

FIGURE 3-16 The peripheral nervous system connects the body tissues to the spinal cord and central nervous system.

1. Transection of the brainstem at the level of the pons (isolates the spinal cord from the rest of the brain) results in spasticity known as *decerebrate rigidity.*
2. The motor system is often divided into upper and lower motor neurons.
   a. Lower motor neurons originate in the spinal cord and directly innervate skeletal muscles. A lower motor

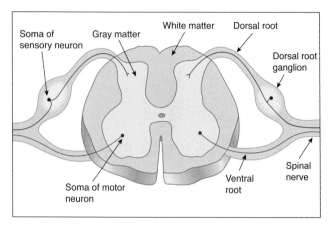

FIGURE 3-17 Cross-section of the spinal cord, showing the dorsal (posterior) and ventral (anterior) roots. The cell body of peripheral sensory nerves is in the dorsal root ganglion. The cell body of motor nerves is in the anterior horn.

neuron lesion is associated with flaccid paralysis, atrophy of skeletal muscles, and absence of stretch reflex responses.
  b. Spastic paralysis with accentuated stretch reflexes is due to destruction of upper motor neurons in the brain. Upper motor neurons originate in the cerebral cortex or brainstem, and traverse down the anterior and lateral corticospinal paths until they connect with the lower motor neuron in the ventral horn of the spinal cord.

IV. **Autonomic nervous system controls visceral functions of the body. In addition, the autonomic nervous system modulates systemic blood pressure, gastrointestinal motility and secretion, urinary bladder emptying, sweating, and body temperature maintenance. The ANS is divided into the sympathetic, parasympathetic, and enteric nervous systems (Table 3-3).**
  A. **Anatomy of the Sympathetic Nervous System**
    1. Nerves of the sympathetic nervous system arise from the thoracolumbar (T1–L2) segments of the spinal cord (Fig. 3-18).
    2. Each nerve of the sympathetic nervous system consists of a preganglionic neuron and a postganglionic neuron (Fig. 3-19).

Table 3-3

Responses Evoked by Autonomic Nervous System Stimulation

	Sympathetic Nervous System Stimulation	Parasympathetic Nervous System Stimulation
Heart		
Sinoatrial node	Increase heart rate	Decrease heart rate
Atrioventricular node	Increase conduction velocity	Decrease conduction velocity
His-Purkinje system	Increase automaticity, conduction velocity	Minimal effect
Ventricles	Increase contractility, conduction velocity Automaticity	Minimal effects, slight decrease in contractility (?)
Bronchial smooth muscle	Relaxation	Contraction
Gastrointestinal tract		
Motility	Decrease	Increase
Secretion	Decrease	Increase
Sphincters	Contraction	Relaxation
Gallbladder	Relaxation	Contraction
Urinary bladder		
Smooth muscle	Relaxation	Contraction
Sphincter	Contraction	Relaxation
Uterus	Contraction	Variable
Ureter	Contraction	Relaxation

(continued)

Table 3-3

Responses Evoked by Autonomic Nervous System Stimulation *(continued)*

	Sympathetic Nervous System Stimulation	Parasympathetic Nervous System Stimulation
Eye		
Radial muscle	Mydriasis	Miosis
Sphincter muscle		Contraction for near vision
Ciliary muscle	Relaxation for far vision	
Liver	Glycogenolysis	Glycogen synthesis
	Gluconeogenesis	
Pancreatic β-cell secretion	Decrease	
Salivary gland secretion	Increase	Marked increase
Sweat glands	Increase[a]	Increase
Apocrine glands	Increase	
Arterioles		
Coronary	Constriction (α)	Relaxation (?)
	Relaxation (β)	
Skin and mucosa	Constriction	Relaxation
Skeletal muscle	Constriction (α)	Relaxation
	Relaxation (β)	
Pulmonary	Constriction	Relaxation

[a]Postganglionic sympathetic fibers to sweat glands are cholinergic.

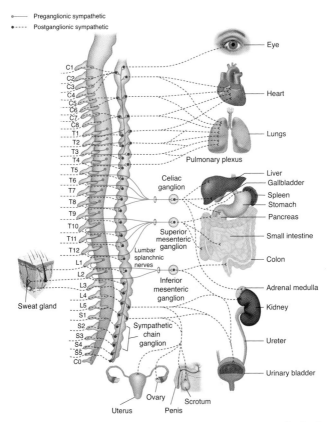

● —— Preganglionic sympathetic
● ---- Postganglionic sympathetic

FIGURE 3-18 Anatomy of the sympathetic nervous system. *Dashed lines* represent postganglionic fibers in gray rami leading to spinal nerves for subsequent distribution to blood vessels and sweat glands.

B. **Anatomy of the Parasympathetic Nervous System**
1. Nerves of the parasympathetic nervous system leave the CNS through cranial nerves III, V, VII, IX, and X (vagus) and from the sacral portions of the spinal cord (Fig. 3-20).
2. In contrast to the sympathetic nervous system, preganglionic fibers of the parasympathetic nervous system

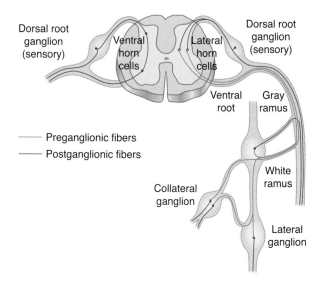

FIGURE 3-19 Anatomy of a sympathetic nervous system nerve. Preganglionic fibers pass through the white ramus to a paravertebral ganglia, where they may synapse, course up the sympathetic chain to synapse at another level, or exit the chain without synapsing to pass to an outlying collateral ganglion.

pass uninterrupted to ganglia near or in the innervated organ (see Fig. 3-20).

C. **Physiology of the Autonomic Nervous System**. Postganglionic fibers of the sympathetic nervous system secrete norepinephrine as the neurotransmitter (Fig. 3-21).

D. **Acetylcholine as a Neurotransmitter**. Acetylcholine is synthesized in the cytoplasm of varicosities of the preganglionic and postganglionic parasympathetic nerve endings.

E. **Interactions of Neurotransmitters with Receptors**. Norepinephrine and acetylcholine, acting as neurotransmitters, interact with receptors (protein macromolecules) in lipid cell membranes (Table 3-4).

1. **Norepinephrine Receptors**. The pharmacologic effects of catecholamines led to the original concept of α- and β-adrenergic receptors. Subdivision of these receptors into α_1, α_2, β_1 (cardiac), and β_2 (noncardiac) allows an

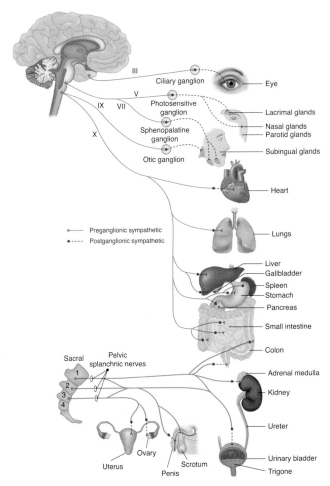

FIGURE 3-20 Anatomy of the parasympathetic nervous system.

understanding of drugs that act as either agonists or antagonists at these sites (Table 3-5).

2. **Acetylcholine Receptors**. Cholinergic receptors are classified as *nicotinic* and *muscarinic*. The links between stimulus and response are different in nicotinic and

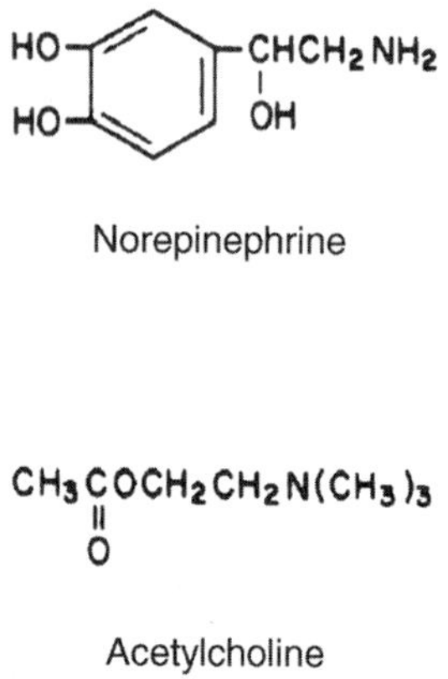

Norepinephrine

Acetylcholine

FIGURE 3-21 Neurotransmitters of the autonomic nervous system.

muscarinic receptors (see Table 3-5). Nicotinic receptors are ligand-gated receptors, whereas muscarinic receptors are G protein linked.

F. **Determination of Autonomic Nervous System Function**
1. Autonomic dysfunction associated with aging and diabetes mellitus may increase operative risk and can be associated with increased morbidity and mortality.
2. Diagnosis of autonomic neuropathy in patients with diabetes mellitus is facilitated by tests of cardiovascular function (Table 3-6).
3. **Aging and Autonomic Nervous System Dysfunction**. Common clinical manifestations of autonomic nervous system dysfunction in elderly patients are orthostatic hypotension, postprandial hypotension, hypothermia, and heat stroke. These responses reflect limited ability of elderly patients to adapt to stresses with vasoconstriction and vasodilation as mediated by the autonomic nervous system.
4. **Diabetic autonomic neuropathy** is present in 20% to 40% of insulin-dependent diabetic patients.
   a. When impotence or diarrhea is the sole manifestation of autonomic neuropathy, there is little impact on survival.
   b. The 5-year mortality rates may exceed 50% when postural hypotension or gastroparesis is present.

(Text continues on page 77.)

Table 3-4

Classification and Characterization of Adrenergic and Cholinergic Receptors

Classification	Molecular Pharmacology	Signal Transduction	Effectors
Adrenergic Receptors			
α_1	α_{1A1D}	G_{q11}	Activates phospholipase C
	α_{1B}	G_{q11}	Activates phospholipase C
	α_{1C}	G_{q11}	Activates phospholipase C
α_2	α_{2A}	G_i and G_o	Inhibits adenylate cyclase, calcium and potassium ion channels
	α_{2B}	G_i and G_o	Inhibits adenylate cyclase, calcium and potassium ion channels
	α_{2C}	G_i and G_o	Inhibits adenylate cyclase, calcium and potassium ion channels
β_1	β_1'	G_s	Stimulates adenylate cyclase and calcium ion channels
β_2	β_2'	G_s	Stimulates adenylate cyclase and calcium ion channels
β_3	β_3'	G_s	Stimulates adenylate cyclase and calcium ion channels

(continued)

Table 3-4

Classification and Characterization of Adrenergic and Cholinergic Receptors *(continued)*

Classification	Molecular Pharmacology	Signal Transduction	Effectors
Cholinergic Receptors			
Nicotinic	Autonomic ganglia	Ion channels	
	Neuromuscular junction		
	Central nervous system		
Muscarinic	M_1	G_q	Phospholipase activation
	M_3	G_q	Phospholipase activation
	M_5	G_q	Phospholipase activation
	M_2	G_i and G_o	Inhibits adenylate cyclase
	M_4	G_i and G_o	Inhibits adenylate cyclase

Table 3-5

Mechanism of Action of Drugs that Act on the Autonomic Nervous System

Mechanism	Site	Drug
Inhibition of neurotransmitter synthesis	Central SNS	α-Methyldopa
False neurotransmitter	Central SNS	α-Methyldopa
Inhibition of uptake of neurotransmitter	Central noradrenergic synapses	Tricyclic antidepressants, cocaine
Displacement of neurotransmitter from storage sites	Central SNS	Amphetamine
	PNS	Carbachol
Prevention of neurotransmitter release	SNS	Bretylium
	PNS	Botulinum toxin
Mimic action of neurotransmitter at receptor	SNS	
	α_1	Phenylephrine, methoxamine
	α_2	Clonidine dexmedetomidine
	β_1	Dobutamine
	β_2	Terbutaline, albuterol

(continued)

Table 3-5

Mechanism of Action of Drugs that Act on the Autonomic Nervous System *(continued)*

Mechanism	Site	Drug
Inhibition of action of neurotransmitter on postsynaptic receptor	SNS	
	α_1	Prazosin
	α_2	Yohimbine
	α_1 and α_2	Phentolamine
	β_1	Metoprolol, esmolol
	β_1 and β_2	Propranolol
	PNS	
	M_1	Pirenzepine
	M_1, M_2	Atropine
	N_1	Hexamethonium
	N_2	d-Tubocurarine
Inhibition of metabolism of neuro-transmitter	SNS	Monoamine oxidase inhibitors
	PNS	Neostigmine, pyridostigmine, edrophonium

PNS, parasympathetic nervous system; SNS, sympathetic nervous system.

Table 3-6

Clinical Assessment of Autonomic Nervous System Function

Clinical Observation	Method of Measurement	Normal Value
Parasympathetic Nervous System		
Heart rate response to Valsalva	Patient blows into a mouthpiece maintaining a pressure of 40 mm Hg for 15 seconds.	Ratio >1.21
	The Valsalva ratio is the ratio of the longest R-R interval on the electrocardiogram immediately after release to the shortest R-R interval during the maneuver.	
Heart rate response to standing	Heart rate is measured as the patient changes from the supine to standing position (increase maximal around 15th beat after standing and slowing maximal around 30th beat).	Ratio >1.04
	The response to standing is expressed as the "30:15" ratio and is the ratio of the longest R-R interval (around 30th beat) to the shortest R-R interval (around 15th beat).	
Heart response to deep breathing	Patient takes six deep breaths in 1 minute.	Mean difference >15 bpm
	The maximum and minimum heart rates during each cycle are measured and the mean of the differences (maximum heart rate − minimum heart rate) during three successive breathing cycles is taken as the maximum–minimum heart rate.	

(continued)

Table 3-6

Clinical Assessment of Autonomic Nervous System Function *(continued)*

Clinical Observation	Method of Measurement	Normal Value
Sympathetic Nervous System		
Blood pressure response to standing	The patient changes from the supine to standing position and the standing systolic blood pressure is subtracted from the supine systolic blood pressure.	Difference <10 mm Hg
Blood pressure response to sustained handgrip	The patient maintains a handgrip of 30% of maximum squeeze for up to 5 minutes. The blood pressure is measured every minute and the initial diastolic blood pressure is subtracted from the diastolic blood pressure just prior to release.	Difference >16 mm Hg

    c. Anesthetic risk is increased in diabetic patients with autonomic neuropathy associated with gastroparesis (aspiration hazard), postural hypotension (hemodynamic instability), and is a marker for vasculopathy in other organs including the heart.

  5. **Chronic Sympathetic Nervous System Stimulation** (pheochromocytoma)

    a. Physiologic responses and surgical stress that lead to sustained autonomic nervous system hyperactivity can result in metabolic and endocrine responses.

    b. Interventions that attenuate stress responses during the entire perioperative period (continuous epidural infusions of local anesthetics, perioperative administration of β-adrenergic blocking drugs, α-$_2$ agonists) may decrease perioperative morbidity and mortality. Inhaled anesthetics and adjuvants that block the stress response may also be beneficial in long-term outcomes following surgery.

  6. **Denervation hypersensitivity** is the increased responsiveness (decreased threshold) of the innervated organ to norepinephrine or epinephrine that develops during the first week or so after acute interruption of autonomic nervous system innervation.

V. **Thermoregulation. Both heat generation and heat loss are adjusted in order to regulate body temperature within narrow limits (36°C to 37.5°C), with circadian fluctuations being lowest in the morning and highest in the evening. This is consistent with a 10% to 15% decrease in basal metabolic rate during physiologic sleep.**

  A. **Regulation of Body Temperature**. Body temperature is regulated by feedback mechanisms predominantly mediated by the preoptic nucleus of the anterior hypothalamus.

    1. **Causes of Increased Body Temperature** (Table 3-7)

    2. **Perioperative Temperature Changes**. Anesthesia and surgery in a cool environment makes perioperative hypothermia a likely occurrence (Table 3-8).

    3. **Sequence of Temperature Changes during Anesthesia**

      a. Under general anesthesia, tonic vasoconstriction is attenuated and heat contained in the core compartment will move to the periphery, thus allowing the core temperature to decrease toward the anesthetic-induced lowered threshold for vasoconstriction. This core to peripheral heat redistribution is responsible for the

Table 3-7

Causes of Hyperthermia

Disorders associated with excessive heat production
    Malignant hyperthermia
    Neuroleptic malignant syndrome
    Thyrotoxicosis
    Delirium tremens
    Pheochromocytoma
    Salicylate intoxication
    Drug abuse (cocaine, amphetamine, MDMA)
    Status epilepticus
    Exertional hyperthermia
Disorders associated with decreased heat loss
    Autonomic nervous system dysfunction
    Anticholinergics
    Drug abuse (cocaine)
    Dehydration
    Occlusive dressings
    Heat stroke
Disorders associated with dysfunction of the hypothalamus
    Trauma
    Tumors
    Idiopathic hypothalamic dysfunction
    Cerebrovascular accidents
    Encephalitis
    Neuroleptic malignant syndrome

MDMA, 3,4-methylenedioxymethamphetamine.

Table 3-8

Events that Contribute to Decreases in Body Temperature During Surgery

Resetting of the hypothalamic thermostat
Ambient temperature <21°C
Administration of unwarmed intravenous fluids
Drug-induced vasodilation
Basal metabolic rate decreased
Attenuated shivering response
Core compartment exposed to ambient temperature
Heat required to humidify inhaled dry gases

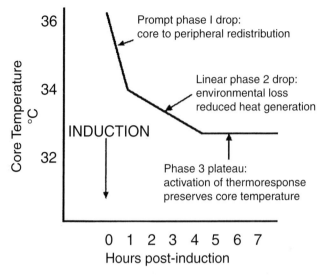

FIGURE 3-22 Graphic representation of the typical triphasic core temperature pattern that occurs after induction of anesthesia. Note that the phase 3 plateau may not occur, particularly during regional anesthesia or during combined regional and general anesthesia. Although core temperature is preserved during the phase 3 plateau, heat will continue to be lost to the environment from the peripheral compartment.

1°C to 5°C decrease in core temperature that occurs during the first hour of general anesthesia (Fig. 3-22).
b. Protection from heat loss early in a surgical procedure is important to reduce the temperature gradient from the environment to the peripheral compartment because significant heat energy has been shunted to the periphery.
c. After the first hour of general anesthesia, the core temperature usually decreases at a slower rate. This decrease is nearly linear and occurs because continuing heat loss to the environment exceeds the metabolic production of heat.
d. After 3 to 5 hours of anesthesia, the core temperature often stops decreasing (see Fig. 3-22). This type of thermal steady state is especially likely in patients who are well insulated or effectively warmed.

B. **Beneficial Effects of Perioperative Hypothermia**. Oxygen consumption is decreased by approximately 5% to 7% per degree Celsius of cooling. Thus, even moderate decreases in core temperature of 1°C to 3°C below normal provide substantial protection against cerebral ischemia and arterial hypoxemia.

C. **Adverse Consequences of Perioperative Hypothermia** (Table 3-9)

D. **Perioperative Temperature Measurement**. It is recommended that intraoperative core temperature be maintained at greater than or equal to 36°C. Measuring the temperature of the lower 25% of the esophagus (about 24 cm beyond the corniculate cartilages or site of the loudest heart sounds heard through an esophageal stethoscope) gives a reliable approximation of blood and cerebral temperature.

E. **Prevention of Perioperative Hypothermia**
  1. Passive or active airway heating and humidification contribute little to perioperative thermal management in adults because less than 10% of metabolic heat is lost via ventilation.
  2. The administration of unwarmed fluids can markedly decrease body temperature. Warming fluids to near 37°C is useful for preventing hypothermia, especially if large volumes of fluid are being infused.

Table 3-9

Immediate Adverse Consequences of Perioperative Hypothermia

Adverse Outcome	Mechanism
Increased operative blood loss	Coagulopathy and platelet dysfunction
Increased morbid cardiac events	Increased myocardial work load
Dysrhythmias and myocardial ischemia	Increased sympathetic activity
Wound infection	Sympathetic mediated cutaneous vasoconstriction
Delayed wound healing	
Delayed anesthetic emergence	Decreased drug metabolism and increased volatile agent solubility, decreased MAC
Delayed recovery room discharge	Postanesthetic shivering, delayed recovery

3. Covering the skin with surgical drapes or blankets can decrease cutaneous heat loss. A single layer of insulator decreases heat loss by approximately 30%, but additional layers do not proportionately increase the benefit.

4. Active warming is needed to prevent intraoperative hypothermia. Forced air warming is probably the most effective method available, although any method or combination of methods that maintains core body temperature near 36°C is acceptable (Fig. 3-23).

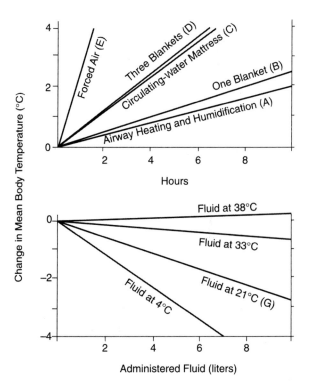

FIGURE 3-23 The effects of different warming techniques on mean body temperature plotted according to the elapsed hours of treatment **(top)** and changes in mean body temperature according to the volume of fluid administered **(bottom)**. (From Sessler DI. Mild perioperative hypothermia. *N Engl J Med*. 1997;336:1630–1637, with permission.)

CHAPTER 4

Inhaled Anesthetics

I. **History**
   A. The discovery of the anesthetic properties of nitrous oxide, diethyl ether, and chloroform in the 1840s was followed by a hiatus of about 80 years before other inhaled anesthetics were introduced (Fig. 4-1).
      1. Recognition that replacing a hydrogen atom with a fluorine atom decreased flammability led to the introduction, in 1951, of the first halogenated hydrocarbon anesthetic, fluroxene.
      2. Halothane was synthesized in 1951 and introduced for clinical use in 1956. However, the tendency for alkane derivatives such as halothane to enhance the arrhythmogenic effects of epinephrine led to the search for new inhaled anesthetics derived from ethers.
      3. Methoxyflurane was introduced into clinical practice in 1960. Although methoxyflurane did not enhance the arrhythmogenic effects of epinephrine, its high solubility in blood and lipids resulted in a prolonged induction and slow recovery from anesthesia.
      4. Enflurane, the next methyl ethyl ether derivative, was introduced for clinical use in 1973. This anesthetic, in contrast to halothane, does not enhance the arrhythmogenic effects of epinephrine or cause hepatotoxicity.
   B. In search of a drug with fewer side effects, isoflurane, a structural isomer of enflurane, was introduced in 1981. This drug was resistant to metabolism, making organ toxicity unlikely after its administration.

II. **Inhaled Anesthetics for the Present and Future**
   A. The search for even more pharmacologically "perfect" inhaled anesthetics did not end with the introduction and widespread use of isoflurane.
   B. Desflurane, a totally fluorinated methyl ethyl ether, was introduced in 1992 and was followed in 1994 by the totally

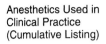

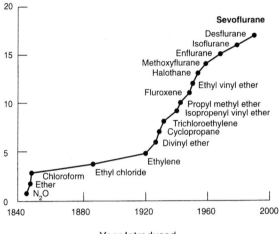

FIGURE 4-1 Inhaled anesthetics introduced into clinical practice beginning with the successful use of nitrous oxide in 1844 for dental anesthesia followed by recognition of the anesthetic properties of ether in 1846 and of chloroform in 1847. Modern anesthetics, beginning with halothane, differ from prior anesthetics in being fluorinated and nonflammable. (Modified from Eger EI. *Desflurane [Suprane]: A Compendium and Reference.* Nutley, NJ: Anaquest; 1993:1–119, with permission.)

fluorinated methyl isopropyl ether, sevoflurane. The low solubility of these volatile anesthetics in blood facilitated rapid induction of anesthesia, precise control of end-tidal anesthetic concentrations during maintenance of anesthesia, and prompt recovery at the end of anesthesia independent of the duration of administration (important for ambulatory surgery).

C. **Cost Considerations**. The costs of new inhaled anesthetics can be decreased by using low, fresh gas flow rates. Less soluble anesthetics are more suitable for use with low gas flow rates because their poor solubility permits better control of the delivered concentration.

III. **Current Clinically Useful Inhaled Anesthetics (Table 4-1) (Fig. 4-2)**

A. **Nitrous oxide** is a low-molecular-weight, odorless to sweet-smelling, nonflammable gas of low potency and poor blood solubility (blood:gas partition coefficient 0.46) that is most commonly administered in combination with opioids or volatile anesthetics to produce general anesthesia.

1. Although nitrous oxide is nonflammable, it will support combustion.

2. Its poor blood solubility permits rapid achievement of an alveolar and brain partial pressure of the drug (analgesic effects of nitrous oxide are prominent but short-lived) (Fig. 4-3).

3. The benefits of nitrous oxide must be balanced against its possible adverse effects (high-volume absorption of nitrous oxide in gas containing spaces, potential increase in the risk of postoperative nausea and vomiting, its ability to inactivate vitamin B_{12}).

B. **Halothane**, with its intermediate solubility in blood combined with a high potency, permits intermediate onset and recovery from anesthesia when administered alone or in combination with nitrous oxide or injected drugs such as opioids.

C. **Enflurane**, with its intermediate solubility in blood combined with a high potency, permits intermediate onset and recovery from anesthesia when administered alone or in combination with nitrous oxide or injected drugs such as opioids. Enflurane decreases the threshold for seizures (used for procedures in which a low threshold for seizure generation is desirable such as electroconvulsive therapy).

D. **Isoflurane**, with its intermediate solubility in blood combined with a high potency, permits intermediate onset and recovery from anesthesia using isoflurane alone or in combination with nitrous oxide or injected drugs such as opioids.

1. Although isoflurane is an isomer of enflurane, their manufacturing processes are not similar. The subsequent purification of isoflurane by distillation is complex and expensive.

2. Isoflurane is characterized by extreme physical stability.

E. **Desflurane** is a fluorinated methyl ethyl ether that differs from isoflurane only by substitution of a fluorine atom for the chlorine atom found on the α-ethyl component of isoflurane.

1. Fluorination rather than chlorination increases vapor pressure (decreases intermolecular attraction), enhances molecular stability, and decreases potency.

Table 4-1

Physical and Chemical Properties of Inhaled Anesthetics

	Nitrous Oxide	Halothane	Enflurane	Isoflurane	Desflurane	Sevoflurane
Molecular weight	44	197	184	184	168	200
Boiling point (°C)	Gas	50.2	56.5	48.5	22.8	58.5
Vapor pressure (mm Hg; 20°C)		244	172	240	669	170
Odor	Sweet	Organic	Ethereal	Ethereal	Ethereal	Ethereal
Preservative necessary	No	Yes	No	No	No	No
Stability in soda lime (40°C)	Yes	No	Yes	Yes	Yes	No
Blood:gas partition coefficient	0.46	2.54	1.90	1.46	0.42	0.69
MAC (37°C, 30 to 55 years old, P_{BRAIN} 760 mm Hg) (%)	104	0.75	1.63	1.17	6.6	1.80

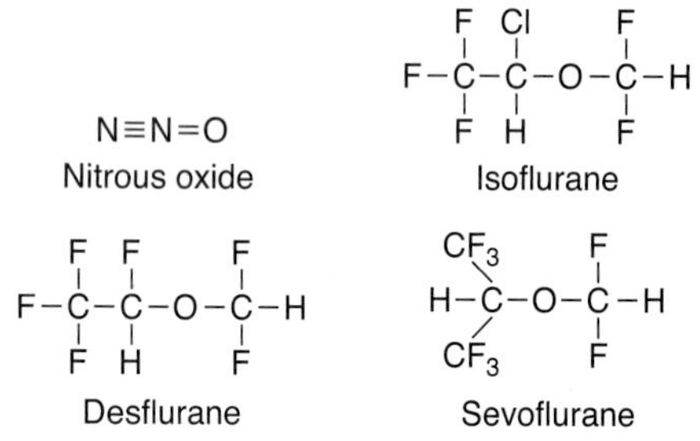

FIGURE 4-2 Inhaled anesthetics.

2. The vapor pressure of desflurane exceeds that of isoflurane by a factor of three such that desflurane would boil at normal operating room temperatures (requires a heated and pressurized vaporizer for delivery).

3. Unlike halothane and sevoflurane, desflurane is pungent, making it unlikely that inhalation induction of anesthesia will be feasible or pleasant for the patient.

4. Carbon monoxide results from degradation of desflurane by the strong base present in desiccated carbon dioxide absorbents.

5. Solubility characteristics (blood:gas partition coefficient 0.45) and potency (MAC 6.6%) permit rapid achievement of an alveolar partial pressure necessary for anesthesia followed by prompt awakening when desflurane is discontinued.

F. **Sevoflurane** is fluorinated methyl isopropyl ether.

1. The vapor pressure of sevoflurane resembles that of halothane and isoflurane, permitting delivery of this anesthetic via a conventional unheated vaporizer.

2. The solubility of sevoflurane (blood:gas partition coefficient 0.69) resembles that of desflurane, ensuring prompt induction of anesthesia and recovery after discontinuation of the anesthetic.

3. Sevoflurane is nonpungent, has minimal odor, produces bronchodilation similar in degree to isoflurane, and causes the least degree of airway irritation among the currently available volatile anesthetics (like halothane is acceptable for inhalation induction of anesthesia).

4. Sevoflurane may be 100-fold more vulnerable to metabolism than desflurane, with an estimated 3% to 5% of the dose undergoing biodegradation (fluoride).

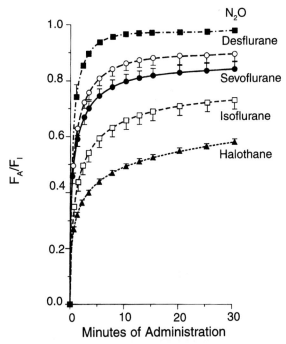

FIGURE 4-3 The pharmacokinetics of inhaled anesthetics during the induction of anesthesia is defined as the ratio of the end-tidal anesthetic concentration (F_A) to the inspired anesthetic concentration (F_I). Consistent with their relative blood:gas partition coefficients, the F_A/F_I of poorly soluble anesthetics (nitrous oxide, desflurane, sevoflurane) increases more rapidly than that of anesthetics with greater solubility in blood. A decrease in the rate of change in the F_A/F_I after 5 to 15 minutes (three time constants) reflects decreased tissue uptake of the anesthetic as the vessel-rich group tissues become saturated. (Data are mean ± SD.) (From Yasuda N, Lockhart SH, Eger EI II, et al. Comparison of kinetics of sevoflurane and isoflurane in humans. *Anesth Analg.* 1991;72:316–324, with permission.)

    5. Sevoflurane is the least likely volatile anesthetic to form carbon monoxide on exposure to carbon dioxide absorbents.

  G. **Xenon** is an inert gas with many of the characteristics considered important for an ideal inhaled anesthetic (nonexplosive, nonpungent, odorless).

IV. **Pharmacokinetics of inhaled anesthetics** describes their
(a) absorption (uptake) from alveoli into pulmonary capillary blood, (b) distribution in the body, (c) metabolism, and
(d) elimination, principally via the lungs. A series of partial
pressure gradients beginning at the anesthetic machine
serve to propel the inhaled anesthetic across various barriers
(alveoli, capillaries, cell membranes) to their sites of action
in the central nervous system. The brain and all other tissues
equilibrate with the partial pressures of inhaled anesthetics
delivered to them by arterial blood (Pa).

A. **Determinants of Alveolar Partial Pressure**. The Pa and
ultimately the P_{BRAIN} of inhaled anesthetics are determined
by input (delivery) into alveoli minus uptake (loss) of the
drug from alveoli into arterial blood (Table 4-2).

1. **Inhaled Partial Pressure (PI)**. A high PI delivered from
the anesthetic machine is required during initial administration of the anesthetic.

   a. A high initial input offsets the impact of uptake,
   accelerating induction of anesthesia as reflected by
   the rate of rise in the Pa and thus the P_{BRAIN}.

   b. With time, as uptake into the blood decreases, the
   PI should be decreased to match the decreased

Table 4-2

**Factors Determining Partial Pressure Gradients
Necessary for Establishment of Anesthesia**

**Transfer of inhaled anesthetic from anesthetic machine to
alveoli (anesthetic input)**
Inspired partial pressure
Alveolar ventilation
Characteristics of anesthetic breathing system
Functional residual capacity
**Transfer of inhaled anesthetic from alveoli to arterial blood
(anesthetic loss)**
Blood:gas partition coefficient
Cardiac output
Alveolar-to-venous partial pressure difference
**Transfer of inhaled anesthetic from arterial blood to
brain (anesthetic loss)**
Brain:blood partition coefficient
Cerebral blood flow
Arterial-to-venous partial pressure difference

anesthetic uptake and therefore maintain a constant and optimal P_{BRAIN}.

2. **Concentration Effect.** The impact of PI on the rate of rise of the Pa of an inhaled anesthetic is known as the *concentration effect* (Fig. 4-4).

3. **Second gas effect** reflects the ability of high-volume uptake of one gas (first gas) to accelerate the rate of increase of the Pa of a concurrently administered "companion" gas (second gas) (Fig. 4-5).

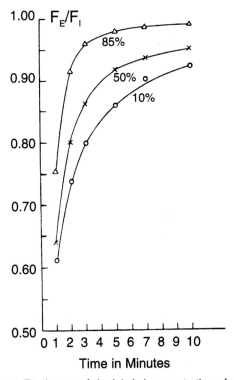

FIGURE 4-4 The impact of the inhaled concentration of an anesthetic on the rate at which the alveolar concentration increases toward the inspired (F_E/F_I) is known as the concentration effect. (From Eger EI. Effect of inspired anesthetic concentration on the rate of rise of alveolar concentration. *Anesthesiology.* 1963;24:153–157, with permission.)

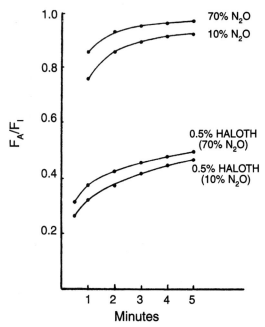

FIGURE 4-5 The second gas effect is the accelerated increase in the alveolar concentration of a second gas, halothane (HALOTH), toward the inspired (F_A/F_I) in the presence of a high inhaled concentration of the first gas (N_2O). (From Epstein RM, Rackow H, Salanitre E, et al. Influence of the concentration effect on the uptake of anesthetic mixtures: the second gas effect. *Anesthesiology.* 1964; 25:364–371, with permission.)

4. **Spontaneous versus Mechanical Ventilation.** Inhaled anesthetics influence their own uptake by virtue of dose-dependent depressant effects on alveolar ventilation. This, in effect, is a negative-feedback protective mechanism that prevents establishment of an excessive depth of anesthesia (delivery of anesthesia is decreased when ventilation is decreased) when a high PI is administered during spontaneous breathing (Fig. 4-6).

5. **Impact of Solubility.** The impact of changes in alveolar ventilation on the rate of increase in the Pa toward the PI depends on the solubility of the anesthetic in blood. For example, changes in alveolar ventilation influence

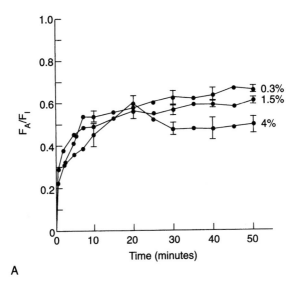

A

FIGURE 4-6 Effect of the mode of ventilation on the rate of increase of the alveolar concentration (F_A) of halothane toward the inspired concentration (F_I) as determined in an animal model. Negative-feedback inhibition of spontaneous ventilation **(A)** limits the F_A/F_I to 0.6 for all the inspired concentrations of halothane. The positive-feedback effect of controlled ventilation **(B)** results in ratios of the F_A/F_I that approach 1.0 and excessive depressant effects of halothane on the cardiovascular system at the higher inspired concentrations of the anesthetic. (Data are mean ± SD.) (From Gibbons RT, Steffey EP, Eger EI II. The effect of spontaneous versus controlled ventilation on the rate of rise in the alveolar halothane concentration in dogs. *Anesth Analg.* 1977;56:32–37, with permission.)

the rate of increase of the Pa of a soluble anesthetic (halothane, isoflurane) more than a poorly soluble anesthetic (nitrous oxide, desflurane, sevoflurane). Indeed, the rate of increase in the Pa of nitrous oxide is rapid regardless of the alveolar ventilation.

6. **Anesthetic Breathing System.** Characteristics of the anesthetic breathing system that influence the rate of increase of the Pa are the (a) volume of the external breathing system, (b) solubility of the inhaled anesthetics in the rubber or plastic components of the breathing system, and (c) gas inflow from the anesthetic machine.

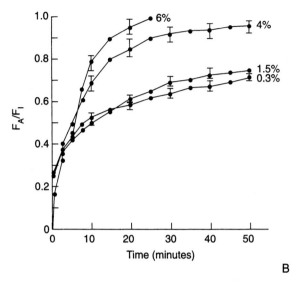

B

FIGURE 4-6 *(Continued).*

B. **Solubility**. The solubility of the inhaled anesthetics in blood and tissues is denoted by the partition coefficient (Table 4-3). A partition coefficient is a distribution ratio describing how the inhaled anesthetic distributes itself between two phases at equilibrium (partial pressures equal in both phases).

1. **Blood:Gas Partition Coefficients**. The rate of increase of the Pa toward the PI (maintained constant by mechanical ventilation of the lungs) is inversely related to the solubility of the anesthetic in blood (see Fig. 4-3).
2. **Tissue:blood partition coefficients** determine uptake of anesthetic into tissues and the time necessary for equilibration of tissues with the Pa.
   a. The time for equilibration can be estimated by calculating a time constant (amount of inhaled anesthetic that can be dissolved in the tissue divided by tissue blood flow) for each tissue.
   b. One time constant on an exponential curve represents 63% equilibration. Three time constants are equivalent to 95% equilibration. For volatile anesthetics, equilibration between the Pa and P$_{BRAIN}$ depends

Table 4-3

Comparative Solubilities of Inhaled Anesthetics

	Blood:Gas Partition Coefficient	Brain:Blood Partition Coefficient	Muscle:Blood Partition Coefficient	Fat:Blood Partition Coefficient	Oil:Gas Partition Coefficient
Soluble					
Methoxyflurane	12	2	1.3	48.8	970
Intermediately soluble					
Halothane	2.54	1.9	3.4	51.1	224
Enflurane	1.90	1.5	1.7	36.2	98
Isoflurane	1.46	1.6	2.9	44.9	98
Poorly soluble					
Nitrous oxide	0.46	1.1	1.2	2.3	1.4
Desflurane	0.42	1.3	2.0	27.2	18.7
Sevoflurane	0.69	1.7	3.1	47.5	55
Xenon	0.115				

Source: Data from Eger EI. *Desflurane (Suprane): A Compendium and Reference.* Nutley, NJ: Anaquest; 1993:1–119; and Yasuda N, Targ AC, Eger EI. Solubility of I-653, sevoflurane, isoflurane, and halothane in human tissues. *Anesth Analg.* 1989;69:370–373.

on the anesthetic's blood solubility and requires 5 to 15 minutes (three time constants).

3. **Nitrous Oxide Transfer to Closed Gas Spaces.** The blood:gas partition coefficient of nitrous oxide (0.46) is about 34 times greater than that of nitrogen (0.014). This differential solubility means that nitrous oxide can leave the blood to enter an air-filled cavity 34 times more rapidly than nitrogen can leave the cavity to enter blood.

   a. As a result of this preferential transfer of nitrous oxide, the volume or pressure of an air-filled cavity increases.

   b. Passage of nitrous oxide into an air-filled cavity surrounded by a compliant wall (intestinal gas, pneumothorax, pulmonary blebs, air bubbles) causes the gas space to expand (Fig. 4-7). Conversely, passage of nitrous oxide into an air-filled cavity surrounded by a noncompliant wall (middle ear, cerebral ventricles, supratentorial space) causes an increase in intracavitary pressure.

C. **Cardiac Output.** Cardiac output (pulmonary blood flow) influences uptake and therefore Pa by carrying away either more or less anesthetic from the alveoli. An increased cardiac output results in more rapid uptake, so the rate of

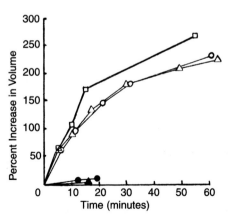

FIGURE 4-7 Inhalation of 75% nitrous oxide rapidly increases the volume of a pneumothorax *(open symbols)*. Inhalation of oxygen *(solid symbols)* does not alter the volume of the pneumothorax. (From Eger EI II, Saidman LJ. Hazards of nitrous oxide anesthesia in bowel obstruction and pneumothorax. *Anesthesiology.* 1965;26: 61–66, with permission.)

increase in the Pa and thus the induction of anesthesia is slowed. A decreased cardiac output speeds the rate of increase of the Pa because there is less uptake to oppose input.

1. Conceptually, a change in cardiac output is analogous to the effect of a change in solubility.
2. As with alveolar ventilation, changes in cardiac output mostly influence the rate of increase of the Pa of a soluble anesthetic. Conversely, the rate of increase of the Pa of a poorly soluble anesthetic, such as nitrous oxide, is rapid regardless of physiologic deviations of the cardiac output around its normal value (Fig. 4-8).

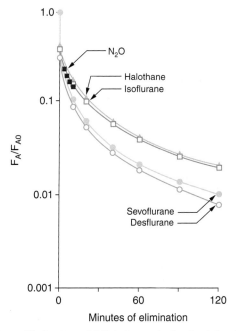

FIGURE 4-8 Elimination of inhaled anesthetics is defined as the ratio of the end-tidal anesthetic concentration (F_A) to the F_A immediately before the beginning of elimination (F_{AO}). The rate of decrease (awakening from anesthesia) in the F_A/F_{AO} is most rapid with the anesthetics that are least soluble in blood (nitrous oxide, desflurane, sevoflurane). (From Yasuda N, Lockhart SH, Eger El II, et al. Comparison of kinetics of sevoflurane and isoflurane in humans. *Anesth Analg.* 1991;72:316–324, with permission.)

Table 4-4		
Body Tissue Composition		
	Body Mass (% of 70-kg Adult)	**Blood Flow (% of Cardiac Output)**
Vessel-rich group	10	75
Muscle group	50	19
Fat group	20	6
Vessel-poor group	20	<1

D. **Alveolar-to-Venous Partial Pressure Differences** (Table 4-4)
E. **Recovery from Anesthesia** (Fig. 4-8)
   1. **Context-Sensitive Half-Time**. The pharmacokinetics of the elimination of inhaled anesthetics depends on the length of administration and the blood-gas solubility of the inhaled anesthetic.
   2. **Diffusion hypoxia** occurs when inhalation of nitrous oxide is discontinued abruptly, leading to a reversal of partial pressure gradients such that nitrous oxide leaves the blood to enter alveoli.

V. **Pharmacokinetics of Inhaled Anesthetics**
   A. **Minimum alveolar concentration** (**MAC**) of an inhaled anesthetic is defined as that concentration at 1 atmosphere that prevents skeletal muscle movement in response to a supramaximal painful stimulus (surgical skin incision) in 50% of patients.
      1. Immobility produced by inhaled anesthetics as measured by MAC is mediated principally by effects of these drugs on the spinal cord and only a minor component of immobility results from cerebral effects (Fig. 4-9).
      2. MAC is among the most useful concepts in anesthetic pharmacology because it establishes a common measure of potency (partial pressure at steady state) for inhaled anesthetics.
      3. **Factors that Alter MAC** (Table 4-5)
   B. **Mechanisms of Anesthetic Action**
      1. **Meyer-Overton Theory (Critical Volume Hypothesis)**
         a. Correlation between the lipid solubility of inhaled anesthetics (oil:gas partition coefficient) and anesthetic potency has historically been presumed to be

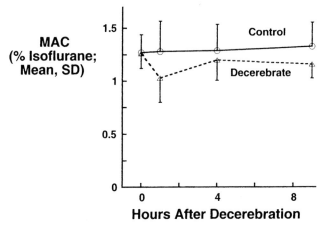

FIGURE 4-9 Decerebration does not change the minimum alveolar anesthetic concentration of isoflurane in rats confirming that the effects of volatile anesthetics on the spinal cord determine MAC. (From Rampil IJ, Mason P, Singh H. Anesthetic potency [MAC] is independent of forebrain structures in the rat. *Anesthesiology*. 1993;78:707–712, with permission.)

evidence that inhaled anesthetics act by disrupting the structure or dynamic properties of the lipid portions of nerve membranes.

b. The most compelling evidence against the Meyer-Overton theory of anesthesia is the fact that effects of inhaled anesthetics on the fluidity of lipid bilayers is implausibly small and can generally be mimicked by temperature changes of 1°C. Furthermore, not all lipid-soluble drugs are anesthetics, and, in fact, some are convulsants.

2. **Stereoselectivity**. The most definitive evidence that general anesthetics act by binding directly to proteins and not a lipid bilayer comes from observations of stereoselectivity.

C. **Mechanism of Anesthesia-Induced Unconsciousness**. A comprehensive explanation of the mechanism by which volatile anesthetics cause loss of consciousness (suppression of awareness) is not known. There is evidence that loss of consciousness (hypnosis), amnesia, and the response to skin incision (immobility as defined by MAC) are not a single continuum of increasing anesthetic depth but rather separate phenomena.

Table 4-5

Impact of Physiologic and Pharmacologic Factors on Minimum Alveolar Concentration

Increases in MAC
Hyperthermia
Excess pheomelanin production (red hair)
Drug-induced increases in central nervous system catecholamine levels
Cyclosporine
Hypernatremia
Decreases in MAC
Hypothermia
Increasing age
Preoperative medication
Drug-induced decreases in central nervous system catecholamine levels
α-2 agonists
Acute alcohol ingestion
Pregnancy
Postpartum (returns to normal in 24–72 hours)
Lithium
Lidocaine
Neuraxial opioids (?)
Ketanserin
Pao_2 <38 mm Hg
Blood pressure <40 mm Hg
Cardiopulmonary bypass
Hyponatremia
No change in MAC
Anesthetic metabolism
Chronic alcohol abuse
Gender
Duration of anesthesia (?)
$Paco_2$ 15–95 mm Hg
Pao_2 >38 mm Hg
Blood pressure >40 mm Hg
Hyperkalemia or hypokalemia
Thyroid gland dysfunction

MAC, minimum alveolar concentration.

VI. **Comparative Pharmacology of Gaseous Anesthetic Drugs.**
Inhaled anesthetics evoke different pharmacologic effects at
comparable percentages of MAC concentrations, emphasizing that dose–response curves for these drugs are not
necessarily parallel (Table 4-6). Desflurane and sevoflurane
provide a specific advantage over other currently available
potent inhaled anesthetics in that their lower blood and tissue solubility permit more precise control over the induction
of anesthesia and a more rapid recovery when the drug is
discontinued.

A. **Central Nervous System Effects**

1. Mental impairment is not detectable in volunteers
   breathing 1,600 ppm (0.16%) nitrous oxide (unlikely
   that impairment of mental function in the personnel
   who work in the operating room using modern anesthetic scavenging techniques can result from inhaling
   trace concentrations of anesthetics).

2. Cerebral metabolic oxygen requirements are decreased
   in parallel with drug-induced decreases in cerebral
   activity.

3. Drug-induced increases in cerebral blood flow (CBF)
   may increase intracranial pressure in patients with
   space-occupying lesions.

   a. Desflurane and isoflurane are similar in terms of
      increases in CBF and the preservation of reactivity to
      carbon dioxide (Fig. 4-10).

Table 4-6

**Variables that Influence Pharmacologic Effects of
Inhaled Anesthetics**

Anesthetic concentration
Rate of increase in anesthetic concentration
Spontaneous versus controlled ventilation
Variations from normocapnia
Surgical stimulation
Patient age
Coexisting disease
Concomitant drug therapy
Intravascular fluid volume
Preoperative medication
Injected drugs to induce and/or maintain anesthesia or skeletal
    muscle relaxation
Alterations in body temperature

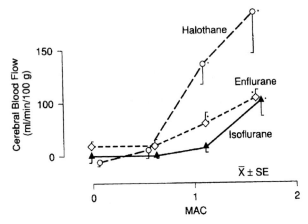

FIGURE 4-10 Cerebral blood flow measured in the presence of normocapnia and in the absence of surgical stimulation. *P <0.05. (From Eger EI. *Isoflurane [Forane]: A Compendium and Reference.* 2nd ed. Madison, WI: Ohio Medical Products; 1985:1–110, with permission; and from Eger EI II. Pharmacology of isoflurane. *Br J Anaesth.* 1984;56:71S–99S, with permission.)

      b. Anesthetic-induced increases in CBF occur within minutes of initiating administration of the inhaled drug and whether blood pressure is unchanged or decreased, emphasizing the cerebral vasodilating effects of these drugs.

   4. **Seizure Activity**. Enflurane (not desflurane or sevoflurane) can produce fast frequency and high voltage on the electroencephalograph that often progresses to spike-wave activity that is indistinguishable from changes that accompany a seizure.

   5. **Evoked Potentials**. Volatile anesthetics cause dose-related decreases in the amplitude and increases in the latency of the cortical component of median nerve somatosensory evoked potentials, visual evoked potentials, and auditory evoked potentials.

   6. **Intracranial Pressure (ICP)**. Inhaled anesthetics produce increases in ICP that parallel increases in CBF produced by these drugs. Patients with space-occupying intracranial lesions are most vulnerable to these drug-induced increases in ICP.

  B. **Circulatory Effects**. Inhaled anesthetics produce dose-dependent and drug-specific circulatory effects. The circulatory effects of desflurane and sevoflurane parallel many of the characteristics of older inhaled anesthetics with desflurane most closely resembling isoflurane, whereas sevoflurane has characteristics of both isoflurane and halothane.

1. **Mean Arterial Pressure** (Figs. 4-11 and 4-12)
2. **Heart Rate** (Fig. 4-13). A small dose of opioid (morphine in the preoperative medication or fentanyl intravenously immediately before induction of anesthesia) can prevent the heart rate increase associated with isoflurane and presumably the other volatile anesthetics.
3. **Cardiac Output and Stroke Volume** (Fig. 4-14)
4. **Systemic Vascular Resistance**. Isoflurane, desflurane, and sevoflurane, but not halothane, decrease systemic vascular resistance when administered to healthy human volunteers (Fig. 4-15).
5. **Duration of Administration**. Administration of a volatile anesthetic for 5 hours or longer is accompanied by recovery from the cardiovascular depressant effects of these drugs (compared with measurements at 1 hour, the same MAC concentration after 5 hours is associated with a return of cardiac output toward predrug levels) (Figs. 4-16 and 4-17).

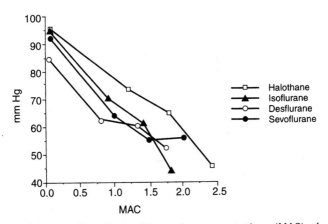

FIGURE 4-11 The effects of increasing concentrations (MAC) of halothane, isoflurane, desflurane, and sevoflurane on mean arterial pressure (mm Hg) when administered to healthy volunteers. (From Cahalan MK. Hemodynamic effects of inhaled anesthetics [review courses]. Cleveland, OH: International Anesthesia Research Society; 1996:14–18, with permission.)

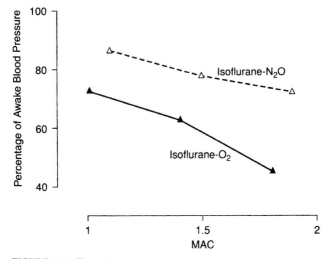

FIGURE 4-12 The substitution of nitrous oxide for a portion of iso-flurane produces less decrease in blood pressure than the same dose of volatile anesthetic alone. (From Eger EI. *Isoflurane [Forane]: A Compendium and Reference.* 2nd ed. Madison, WI: Ohio Medical Products; 1985:1–110, with permission.)

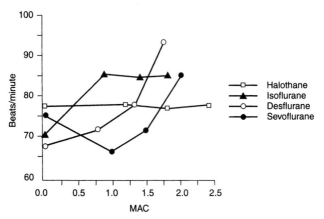

FIGURE 4-13 The effects of increasing concentrations (MAC) of hal-othane, isoflurane, desflurane, and sevoflurane on heart rate (beats/minute) when administered to healthy volunteers. (From Cahalan MK. Hemodynamic effects of inhaled anesthetics [review courses]. Cleveland, OH: International Anesthesia Research Society; 1996:14–18, with permission.)

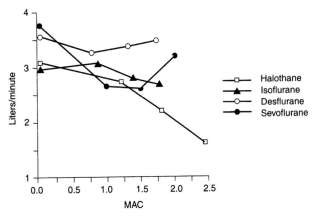

FIGURE 4-14 The effects of increasing concentrations (MAC) of halothane, isoflurane, desflurane, and sevoflurane on cardiac index (L/min) when administered to healthy volunteers. (From Cahalan MK. Hemodynamic effects of inhaled anesthetics [review courses]. Cleveland, OH: International Anesthesia Research Society; 1996:14–18, with permission.)

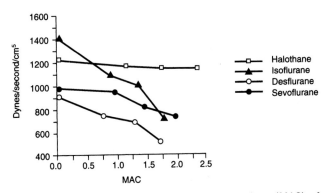

FIGURE 4-15 The effects of increasing concentrations (MAC) of halothane, isoflurane, desflurane, and sevoflurane on systemic vascular resistance (dynes/second/cm^5) when administered to healthy volunteers. (From Cahalan MK. Hemodynamic effects of inhaled anesthetics [review courses]. Cleveland, OH: International Anesthesia Research Society; 1996:14–18, with permission.)

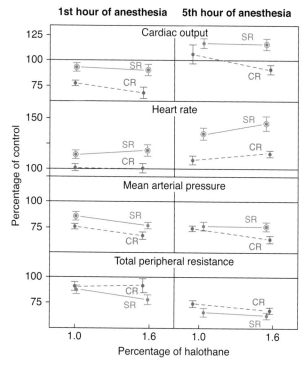

FIGURE 4-16 Comparison of circulatory effects of halothane during spontaneous breathing *(SR)* and controlled ventilation of the lungs *(CR)* after 1 and 5 hours of administration of halothane. (From Bahlman SH, Eger EI II, Halsey MJ, et al. The cardiovascular effects of halothane in man during spontaneous ventilation. *Anesthesiology.* 1972;36:494–502, with permission.)

6. **Cardiac Dysrhythmias**. The ability of volatile anesthetics to decrease the dose of epinephrine necessary to evoke ventricular cardiac dysrhythmias is greatest with the alkane derivative halothane and minimal to nonexistent with the ether derivatives isoflurane, desflurane, and sevoflurane (Figs. 4-18 to 4-20).

7. **Spontaneous Breathing**. Circulatory effects produced by volatile anesthetics during spontaneous breathing are different from those observed during normocapnia and

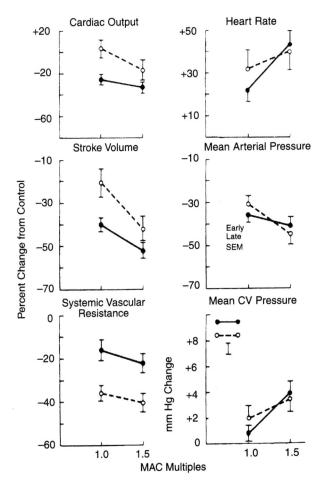

FIGURE 4-17 Comparison of circulatory effects of enflurane after 1 hour *(solid line)* and 6 hours *(broken line)* of administration during controlled ventilation of the lungs to maintain normocapnia. *CV,* cardiovascular. (From Calverley RK, Smith NT, Prys-Roberts C, et al. Cardiovascular effects of enflurane anesthesia during controlled ventilation in man. *Anesth Analg.* 1978;57:619–628, with permission.)

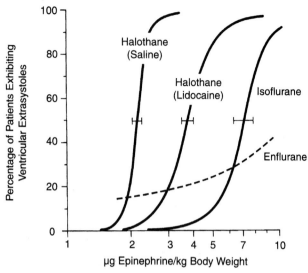

FIGURE 4-18 Percentage of patients developing ventricular cardiac dysrhythmias (three or more premature ventricular contractions [PVCs]) with increasing doses of submucosal epinephrine injected during administration of 1.25 MAC of halothane, isoflurane, or enflurane. (From Johnston PR, Eger EI II, Wilson C. A comparative interaction of epinephrine with enflurane, isoflurane, and halothane in man. *Anesth Analg.* 1976;55:709–712, with permission.)

    controlled ventilation of the lungs (reflects the impact of sympathetic nervous system stimulation due to accumulation of carbon dioxide [respiratory acidosis] and improved venous return during spontaneous breathing).

8. **Coronary Blood Flow.** Volatile anesthetics induce coronary vasodilation.

9. **Preexisting Diseases and Drug Therapy**

    a. Volatile anesthetics decrease myocardial contractility of normal and failing cardiac muscle by similar amounts, but the significance is greater in diseased cardiac muscle because contractility is decreased even before administration of depressant anesthetics.

    b. Valvular heart disease may influence the significance of anesthetic-induced circulatory effects (peripheral vasodilation produced by isoflurane and presumably also desflurane and sevoflurane is undesirable in patients with aortic stenosis but may be beneficial by

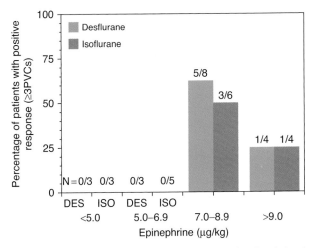

FIGURE 4-19 Responses to submucosally injected epinephrine in patients receiving desflurane (DES) or isoflurane (ISO) anesthesia. *PVCs*, premature ventricular contractions. (Modified from Moore MA, Weiskopf RB, Eger EI II, et al. Arrhythmogenic doses of epinephrine are similar during desflurane or isoflurane anesthesia in humans. *Anesthesiology.* 1993;79:943–947, with permission.)

    providing afterload reduction in those with mitral or aortic regurgitation).

   c. Prior drug therapy that alters sympathetic nervous system activity (antihypertensives, β-adrenergic antagonists) may influence the magnitude of circulatory effects produced by volatile anesthetics.

C. **Ventilation Effects.** Inhaled anesthetics produce dose-dependent and drug-specific effects on the (a) pattern of breathing, (b) ventilatory response to carbon dioxide, (c) ventilatory response to arterial hypoxemia, and (d) airway resistance. The Pao_2 predictably declines during administration of inhaled anesthetics in the absence of supplemental oxygen.

  1. **Patterns of Breathing**

   a. Inhaled anesthetics, except for isoflurane, produce dose-dependent increases in the frequency of breathing (isoflurane increases the frequency of breathing similarly to other inhaled anesthetics up to a dose of 1 MAC but at a concentration of >1 MAC does

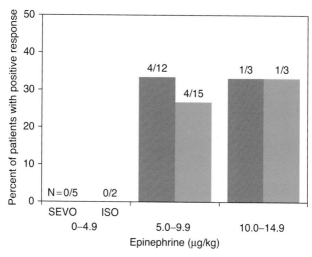

FIGURE 4-20 Responses to submucosally injected epinephrine in patients receiving sevoflurane (SEVO) or isoflurane (ISO) anesthesia. (Modified from Navarro R, Weiskopf RB, Moore MA, et al. Humans anesthetized with sevoflurane or isoflurane have similar arrhythmic response to epinephrine. *Anesthesiology*. 1994;80:545–549, with permission.)

not produce a further increase in the frequency of breathing).

   b. Tidal volume is decreased in association with anesthetic-induced increases in the frequency of breathing.

   c. The net effect of these changes is a rapid and shallow pattern of breathing during general anesthesia. The increase in frequency of breathing is insufficient to offset decreases in tidal volume, leading to decreases in minute ventilation and increases in Pa_{CO_2}.

2. **Ventilatory Response to Carbon Dioxide**. Volatile anesthetics produce dose-dependent depression of ventilation characterized by decreases in the ventilatory response to carbon dioxide and increases in the Pa_{CO_2} (Fig. 4-21).

3. **Surgical stimulation** increases minute ventilation by about 40% because of increases in tidal volume and frequency of breathing. The Pa_{CO_2}, however, decreases only

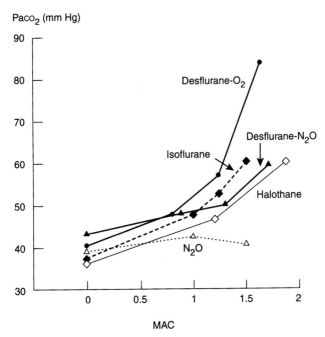

FIGURE 4-21 Inhaled anesthetics produce drug-specific and dose-dependent increases in Paco₂. (From Eger EI. *Desflurane [Suprane]: A Compendium and Reference*. Nutley, NJ: Anaquest; 1993:1–119, with permission.)

about 10% (4 to 6 mm Hg) despite the larger increase in minute ventilation (see Fig. 4-22).
   a. The reason for this discrepancy is speculated to be an increased production of carbon dioxide resulting from activation of the sympathetic nervous system in response to painful surgical stimulation.
   b. Increased production of carbon dioxide is presumed to offset the impact of increased minute ventilation on Paco₂.
4. **Management of Ventilatory Depression**
   a. The predictable ventilatory depressant effects of volatile anesthetics are most often managed by institution of mechanical (controlled) ventilation of the patient's lungs (inherent ventilatory depressant

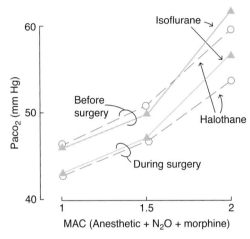

FIGURE 4-22 Impact of surgical stimulation on the resting $Paco_2$ (mm Hg) during administration of isoflurane or halothane. (From Eger EI. *Isoflurane [Forane]: A Compendium and Reference*. 2nd ed. Madison, WI: Ohio Medical Products; 1985:1–110, with permission.)

        effects of volatile anesthetics facilitate the initiation of controlled ventilation).

    b. Assisted ventilation of the lungs is a questionably effective method for offsetting the ventilatory depressant effects of volatile anesthetics (apneic threshold [maximal $Paco_2$ that does not initiate spontaneous breathing] is only 3 to 5 mm Hg lower than the $Paco_2$ present during spontaneous breathing).

  5. **Ventilatory Response to Hypoxemia.** All inhaled anesthetics, including nitrous oxide, profoundly depress the ventilatory response to hypoxemia that is normally mediated by the carotid bodies.

  6. **Airway Resistance and Irritability** (Fig. 4-23)

D. **Hepatic Effects**

  1. **Hepatic blood flow** during administration of desflurane and sevoflurane is maintained similar to isoflurane (Fig. 4-24). Maintenance of hepatic oxygen delivery relative to demand during exposure to anesthetics is uniquely important in view of the evidence that hepatocyte hypoxia is a significant mechanism in the multifactorial etiology of postoperative hepatic dysfunction.

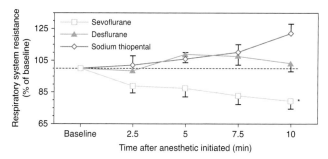

FIGURE 4-23 Changes in respiratory system resistance as a percentage of the thiopental baseline recorded after tracheal intubation but before the addition of sevoflurane or desflurane to the inhaled gases or beginning the infusion of thiopental. Airway resistance responses to sevoflurane were significantly different from desflurane and thiopental. *$P < 0.05$ (Modified from Goff MJ, Arain SR, Ficke DJ, et al. Absence of bronchodilation during desflurane anesthesia. *Anesthesiology*. 2000;93:404–408, with permission.)

2. **Drug Clearance**. Volatile anesthetics may interfere with clearance of drugs from the plasma as a result of decreases in hepatic blood flow or inhibition of drug-metabolizing enzymes.

3. **Liver Function Tests**. Transient increases in the plasma alanine aminotransferase activity follow administration of enflurane and desflurane, but not isoflurane administration, to human volunteers (Fig. 4-25).

4. **Hepatotoxicity**. Postoperative liver dysfunction has been associated with most volatile anesthetics, with halothane receiving the most attention (Fig. 4-26).

E. **Renal Effects**. Volatile anesthetics produce similar dose-related decreases in renal blood flow, glomerular filtration rate, and urine output (most likely reflect the effects of volatile anesthetics on systemic blood pressure and cardiac output). Preoperative hydration attenuates or abolishes many of the changes in renal function associated with volatile anesthetics.

1. **Fluoride-induced nephrotoxicity**. All volatile anesthetics introduced since methoxyflurane undergo significantly less metabolism, and their decreased solubility compared with methoxyflurane means that substantial amounts of the anesthetic are exhaled and thus are not available for hepatic metabolism to fluoride.

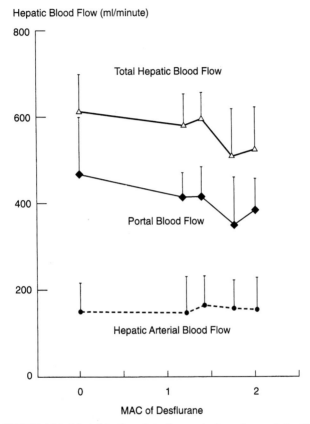

Hepatic Blood Flow (ml/minute)

FIGURE 4-24 Administration of desflurane to dogs does not significantly alter hepatic perfusion. (Mean ± SD.) (Modified from Eger EI. *Desflurane [Suprane]: A Compendium and Reference.* Nutley, NJ: Anaquest; 1993:1–119, with permission.)

2. **Vinyl Halide Nephrotoxicity.** Carbon dioxide absorbents containing potassium and sodium hydroxide react with sevoflurane (degradation product produced in greatest amounts). Compound A is a dose-dependent nephrotoxin in rats. The amount of compound A produced under clinical conditions has consistently been far below those concentrations associated with nephrotoxicity in animals.

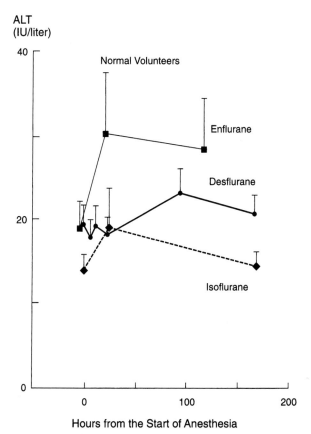

FIGURE 4-25 Plasma alanine aminotransferase (ALT) levels do not change significantly when enflurane, desflurane, or isoflurane are administered to healthy volunteers. (Mean ± SD.) (Modified from Eger EI. *Desflurane [Suprane]: A Compendium and Reference.* Nutley, NJ: Anaquest; 1993:1–119, with permission.)

F. **Skeletal Muscle Effects**
1. **Neuromuscular Junction**. Volatile anesthetics produce dose-dependent enhancement of the effects of neuromuscular-blocking drugs, with the effects of enflurane, isoflurane, desflurane, and sevoflurane being similar and greater than halothane.

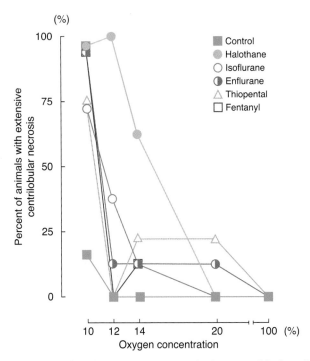

FIGURE 4-26 Hepatic damage may occur in the rat model after administration of inhaled or injected drugs when the inhaled oxygen concentration is 10%. Conversely, hepatic damage occurs after administration of halothane, but not enflurane or isoflurane, when the inhaled concentration of oxygen is 12% or 14%. (From Shingu K, Eger EI, Johnson BH, et al. Effect of oxygen concentration, hyperthermia, and choice of vendor on anesthetic-induced hepatic injury in rats. *Anesth Analg*. 1983;62:146–150, with permission.)

2. **Malignant Hyperthermia**. All volatile anesthetics including desflurane and sevoflurane can trigger malignant hyperthermia in genetically susceptible patients even in the absence of concomitant administration of succinylcholine.

G. **Obstetric Effects**. Volatile anesthetics produce similar and dose-dependent decreases in uterine smooth muscle contractility and blood (Fig. 4-27).

H. **Resistance to Infection**. Many normal functions of the immune system are depressed after patient exposure to

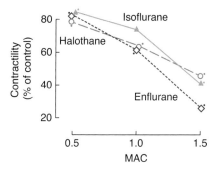

FIGURE 4-27 Impact of volatile anesthetics on contractility of uterine smooth muscle strips studied in vitro. *$P > .05$. (From Eger EI. *Isoflurane [Forane]: A Compendium and Reference.* Madison, WI: Ohio Medical Products; 1985:1–110, with permission.)

the combination of anesthesia (likely the result of surgical trauma and the subsequent endocrine and inflammatory responses).

I. **Peripheral Neuropathy**. Humans who chronically inhale nitrous oxide for nonmedical purposes may develop a neuropathy characterized by sensorimotor polyneuropathy that is often combined with signs of posterior lateral spinal cord degeneration resembling pernicious anemia (ability of nitrous oxide to oxidize irreversibly the cobalt atom of vitamin B_{12} such that activity of vitamin B_{12}–dependent enzymes is decreased).

VII. Metabolism of inhaled anesthetics is very small but intermediary metabolites, end-metabolites, or breakdown products from exposure to carbon dioxide absorbents may be toxic to the kidneys, liver, or reproductive organs (Table 4-7).

A. **Determinants of Metabolism**. The magnitude of metabolism of inhaled anesthetics is determined by the (a) chemical structure, (b) hepatic enzyme activity, (c) blood concentration of the anesthetic, and (d) genetic factors (Fig. 4-28).

1. **Chemical Structure**. The ether bond and carbon-halogen bond are the sites in the anesthetic molecule most susceptible to oxidative metabolism.

2. **Hepatic Enzyme Activity**. The activity of hepatic cytochrome P-450 enzymes responsible for metabolism of volatile anesthetics may be increased by a variety of drugs, including the anesthetics themselves.

Table 4-7

Metabolism of Volatile Anesthetics as Assessed by Metabolite Recovery versus Mass Balance Studies

	Magnitude of Metabolism	
Anesthetic	Metabolite Recovery (%)	Mass Balance (%)
Nitrous oxide	0.004	
Halothane	15–20	46.1
Enflurane	3	8.5
Isoflurane	0.2	0[a]
Desflurane	0.02	
Sevoflurane	5	

[a]Metabolism of isoflurane assumed to be zero for this calculation.
Source: Data adapted from Carpenter RL, Eger EI, Johnson BH, et al. The extent of metabolism of inhaled anesthetics in humans. *Anesthesiology*. 1986;65:201–205.

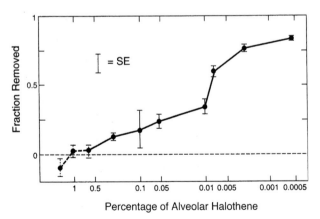

FIGURE 4-28 Fraction of halothane removed during passage through the liver at progressively decreasing alveolar concentrations. (From Sawyer DC, Eger EI II, Bahlam SH, et al. Concentration dependence of hepatic halothane metabolism. *Anesthesiology*. 1971;34:230–235, with permission.)

B. **Metabolism of Specific Inhaled Anesthetics**
   1. **Nitrous oxide**. An estimated 0.004% of an absorbed dose of nitrous oxide undergoes reductive metabolism to nitrogen in the gastrointestinal tract. There is no evidence that nitrous oxide undergoes oxidative metabolism in the liver.
   2. **Enflurane**. An estimated 3% of absorbed enflurane undergoes oxidative metabolism by cytochrome P-450 enzymes to form inorganic fluoride and organic fluoride compounds (see Table 4-7).
   3. **Isoflurane**. An estimated 0.2% of absorbed isoflurane undergoes oxidative metabolism by cytochrome P-450 enzymes (see Table 4-7).
   4. **Desflurane**. An estimated 0.02% of absorbed desflurane undergoes oxidative metabolism by cytochrome P-450 enzymes (see Table 4-7).
   5. **Carbon monoxide toxicity** reflects the degradation of volatile anesthetics that contain a CHF_2 moiety (desflurane, enflurane, and isoflurane) by the strong bases present in desiccated carbon dioxide absorbents.
      a. Desflurane produces the highest carbon monoxide concentration (package insert for desflurane describes this risk) followed by enflurane and isoflurane.
      b. Sevoflurane do not possess a vinyl group and thus carbon monoxide production on exposure to carbon dioxide absorbents has been considered unlikely. Nevertheless, carbon monoxide formation is a risk of sevoflurane administration in the presence of desiccated carbon dioxide absorbent especially when an exothermic reaction between the volatile anesthetic and desiccated absorbent occurs.
   6. **Intraoperative detection** of carbon monoxide is difficult because pulse oximetry cannot differentiate between carboxyhemoglobin and oxyhemoglobin.
      a. Moderately decreased pulse oximetry readings despite adequate arterial partial pressures of oxygen (especially during the first case of the day, "Monday morning phenomena") should suggest the possibility of carbon monoxide exposure and the need to measure carboxyhemoglobin.
      b. Delayed neurophysiologic sequelae due to carbon monoxide poisoning (cognitive defects, personality changes, gait disturbances) may occur as late as 3 to 21 days after anesthesia.

7. **Sevoflurane**. An estimated 5% of absorbed sevoflurane undergoes oxidative metabolism by cytochrome P-450 enzymes to form organic and inorganic fluoride metabolites (see Table 4-7).

   a. Peak plasma fluoride concentrations are higher after administration of sevoflurane than after comparable doses of enflurane, but the duration of exposure of renal tubules to fluoride that results from sevoflurane metabolism is limited because of the rapid pulmonary elimination of this poorly blood-soluble anesthetic.

   b. Hepatic production of fluoride from sevoflurane may be less of a nephrotoxic risk than is intrarenal production of fluoride from enflurane.

CHAPTER 5

Intravenous Sedatives and Hypnotics

I. **Overview.** No other class of pharmacologic agents is more central to the practice of anesthesiology than the intravenous sedatives and hypnotics (anxiolysis, light and deep sedation, general anesthesia). *Sedative* refers to a drug that induces a state of calm or sleep, whereas *hypnotic* refers to drug that induces hypnosis or sleep. There is significant overlap in the two terms and often refer to all of these drugs as *sedative-hypnotics*. Depending on the specific agent, the dose, and the rate of administration, many sedative-hypnotics can be used to allay anxiety with minimal sedation, produce varying degrees of sedation, or rapidly induce the state of drug-induced unconsciousness (general anesthesia).

II. **γ-Aminobutyric Acid Agonists.** Propofol is chemically distinct from all other drugs that act as intravenous (IV) sedative-hypnotics. Administration of propofol, 1.5 to 2.5 mg/kg IV (equivalent to thiopental, 4 to 5 mg/kg IV, or methohexital, 1.5 mg/kg IV) as a rapid IV injection (<15 seconds), produces unconsciousness within about 30 seconds. Awakening is more rapid and complete than that after induction of anesthesia with all other drugs used for rapid IV induction of anesthesia. The more rapid return of consciousness with minimal residual central nervous system (CNS) effects is one of the most important advantages of propofol compared with alternative drugs administered for the same purpose.

   A. **Commercial Preparations**

   1. Propofol is an insoluble drug that requires a lipid vehicle for emulsification. Current formulations of propofol use soybean oil as the oil phase and egg lecithin as the emulsifying agent that is composed of long chain triglycerides. This formulation supports bacterial growth and causes increased plasma triglyceride concentrations when prolonged IV infusions are used.

   2. Diprivan and generic propofol differ with respect to the preservatives used.

3. Mixing of propofol with any other drug is not recommended as this may result in coalescence of oil droplets which may pose the risk of pulmonary embolism.

4. A low-lipid emulsion of propofol (Ampofol) does not require a preservative or microbial growth retardant.

5. An alternative to emulsion formulations of propofol and associated side effects (pain on injection, risk of infection, hypertriglyceridemia, pulmonary embolism) is creation of a prodrug (Aquavan). Compared with propofol, this prodrug has a slower onset, larger volume of distribution, and higher potency.

B. **Mechanism of Action**. Propofol is presumed to exert its sedative-hypnotic effects through a γ-aminobutyric acid-A ($GABA_A$) receptor interaction (GABA is the principal inhibitory neurotransmitter in the brain).

C. **Pharmacokinetics**

1. Clearance of propofol from the plasma exceeds hepatic blood flow, emphasizing that tissue uptake (possibly into the lungs), as well as hepatic oxidative metabolism by cytochrome P450, is important in removal of this drug from the plasma (Table 5-1).

2. The context-sensitive half-time of propofol is only minimally influenced by the duration of the infusion (when used as a sedative for prolonged intensive care unit [ICU] care, the context sensitive half-time is highly relevant).

3. Despite the rapid clearance of propofol by metabolism, there is no evidence of impaired elimination in patients with cirrhosis of the liver.

D. **Clinical Uses**

1. **Induction of Anesthesia**. The induction dose of propofol in healthy adults is 1.5 to 2.5 mg/kg IV (elderly patients require a 25% to 50% lower induction dose). Complete awakening without residual CNS effects is characteristic of propofol.

2. **Intravenous Sedation**

   a. The short context-sensitive half-time of propofol, combined with the short effect-site equilibration time, make this a readily titratable drug for production of IV sedation. Prompt recovery without residual sedation and low incidence of nausea and vomiting make propofol particularly well suited to ambulatory conscious sedation techniques. The typical conscious sedation dose of 25 to 100 μg/kg/minute IV produces minimal analgesic and amnestic effects. In selected

Table 5-1

Comparative Characteristics of Common Induction Drugs

	Elimination Half-Time (h)	Volume of Distribution (L/kg)	Clearance (mL/kg/min)	Systemic Blood Pressure	Heart Rate
Propofol	0.5–1.5	3.5–4.5	30–60	Decreased	Decreased
Etomidate	2–5	2.2–4.5	10–20	No change to decreased	No change
Ketamine	2–3	2.5–3.5	16–18	Increased	Increased

      patients, midazolam or an opioid may be added to propofol for continuous IV sedation.

    b. Propofol has emerged as the agent of choice for sedation for brief gastrointestinal endoscopy procedures. SEDASYS is a computer-assisted delivery system to provide sedation for upper endoscopy and colonoscopy.

    c. Increasing metabolic acidosis, lipemic plasma, bradycardia, and progressive myocardial failure has been described.

  3. **Maintenance of Anesthesia**. The typical dose of propofol for maintenance of anesthesia is 100 to 300 μg/kg/minute IV, often in combination with a short-acting opioid. General anesthesia that includes propofol is typically associated with minimal postoperative nausea and vomiting, and awakening is prompt, with minimal residual sedative effects.

E. **Nonhypnotic Therapeutic Applications**

  1. **Antiemetic Effects**. The incidence of postoperative nausea and vomiting is decreased when propofol is administered, regardless of the anesthetic technique. When administered to induce and maintain anesthesia, it is more effective than ondansetron in preventing postoperative nausea and vomiting. Subhypnotic doses of propofol that are effective as an antiemetic do not inhibit gastric emptying and propofol is not considered a prokinetic drug.

  2. **Antipruritic Effects**. Propofol, 10 mg IV, is effective in the treatment of pruritus associated with neuraxial opioids or cholestasis.

  3. **Anticonvulsant Activity**. Propofol possesses antiepileptic properties, presumably reflecting GABA-mediated presynaptic and postsynaptic inhibition of chloride ion channels (doses >1 mg/kg IV decreases seizure duration 35% to 45% in patients undergoing electroconvulsive therapy).

  4. **Attenuation of Bronchoconstriction**. Propofol decreases the prevalence of wheezing after induction of anesthesia and tracheal intubation in healthy and asthmatic patients (Fig. 5-1). However, a formulation of propofol that uses metabisulfite as a preservative may cause bronchoconstriction in asthmatic patients.

F. **Effects on Organ Systems**

  1. **Central Nervous System**

    a. Propofol decreases cerebral metabolic rate for oxygen ($CMRO_2$), cerebral blood flow, and intracranial pressure (ICP).

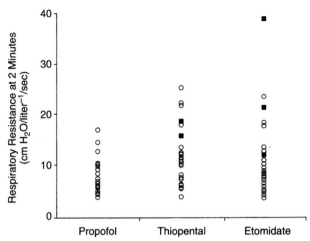

FIGURE 5-1 Respiratory resistance after tracheal intubation is less after induction of anesthesia with propofol than after induction of anesthesia with thiopental or etomidate. The solid squares represent four patients in whom audible wheezing was present. (From Eames WO, Rooke GA, Sai-Chuen R, et al. Comparison of the effects of etomidate, propofol, and thiopental on respiratory resistance after tracheal intubation. *Anesthesiology.* 1996;84:1307–1311, with permission.)

    b. Cortical somatosensory evoked potentials as used for monitoring spinal cord function are not significantly modified in the presence of propofol alone but the addition of nitrous oxide or a volatile anesthetic results in decreased amplitude.

    c. Development of tolerance to drugs that depress the CNS is a common finding, occurring with repeated exposure to opioids, sedative-hypnotic drugs, ketamine, and nitrous oxide (tolerance to propofol does not develop in children undergoing repeated exposure to the drug during radiation therapy).

2. **Cardiovascular System**

    a. Propofol produces decreases in systemic blood pressure (Fig. 5-2). The relaxation of vascular smooth muscle produced by propofol is primarily due to inhibition of sympathetic vasoconstrictor nerve activity.

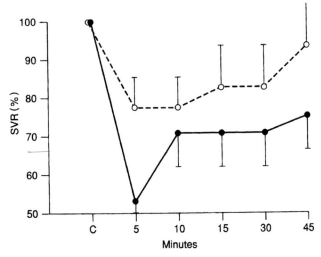

FIGURE 5-2 Comparative changes (expressed in % changes [mean ± SD]) from control values (C) in systemic vascular resistance (SVR) in the 45 minutes after the administration of thiopental, 5 mg/kg IV *(open circles)*, or propofol, 2.5 mg/kg IV *(solid circles)*. (From Rouby JJ, Andreev A, Leger P, et al. Peripheral vascular effects of thiopental and propofol in humans with artificial hearts. *Anesthesiology.* 1991;75:32–42, with permission.)

b. The blood pressure effects of propofol may be exaggerated in hypovolemic patients, elderly patients, and patients with compromised left ventricular function. Adequate hydration before rapid IV administration of propofol is recommended to minimize the blood pressure reduction.

c. **Bradycardia-Related Death**. Profound bradycardia and asystole after administration of propofol have been described in healthy adult patients, despite prophylactic anticholinergics (risk of bradycardia-related death during propofol anesthesia has been estimated to be 1.4 in 100,000). Treatment of propofol-induced bradycardia may require treatment with a direct β-agonist such as isoproterenol.

3. **Lungs**. Propofol produces dose-dependent depression of ventilation, with apnea occurring in 25% to 35% of patients after induction of anesthesia with propofol.

Opioids administered with the preoperative medication enhance ventilatory depressant.

4. **Hepatic and Renal Function**. Propofol does not normally affect hepatic or renal function as reflected by measurements of liver transaminase enzymes or creatinine concentrations.

   a. Prolonged infusions of propofol may also result in excretion of green urine, reflecting the presence of phenols in the urine (does not alter renal function).

   b. Urinary uric acid excretion is increased after administration of propofol and may manifest as cloudy urine when the uric acid crystallizes in the urine under conditions of low pH and temperature (not considered to be detrimental).

5. **Intraocular Pressure**. Propofol is associated with significant decreases in intraocular pressure that occur immediately after induction of anesthesia and are sustained during tracheal intubation.

6. **Coagulation**. Propofol inhibits platelet aggregation that is induced by proinflammatory lipid mediators including thromboxane A_2 and platelet-activating factor.

7. **Allergic Reactions**. Patients who develop evidence of anaphylaxis on first exposure to propofol may have been previously sensitized to the diisopropyl radical, which is present in many dermatologic preparations. Anaphylaxis to propofol during the first exposure to this drug has been observed, especially in patients with a history of other drug allergies, often to neuromuscular blocking drugs.

8. **Lactic acidosis** ("propofol infusion syndrome") has been described in pediatric and adult patients receiving prolonged high-dose infusions of propofol (>75 µg/kg/minute) for longer than 24 hours.

   a. The mechanism for sporadic propofol-induced metabolic acidosis is unclear but may reflect poisoning (cytopathic hypoxia) of the electron transport chain and impaired oxidation of long chain fatty acids by propofol or a propofol metabolite in uniquely susceptible patients (mimics the mitochondrial myopathies).

   b. The differential diagnosis when propofol-induced lactic acidosis is suspected includes hyperchloremic metabolic acidosis associated with large volume infusions of 0.9% saline and metabolic acidosis associated with excessive generation of organic acids, such as lactate and ketones (diabetic acidosis, release of a tourniquet). Measurement of the anion gap and individual measurements of anions and organic acids will differentiate hyperchloremic metabolic acidosis from lactic acidosis.

9. **Proconvulsant Activity**. The majority of reported propofol-induced "seizures" during induction of anesthesia or emergence from anesthesia reflect spontaneous excitatory movements of subcortical origin (not thought to be due to cortical epileptic activity). There appears to be no reason to avoid propofol for sedation, induction, and maintenance of anesthesia in patients with known seizures.

10. **Abuse Potential**. Intense dreaming activity, amorous behavior, and hallucinations have been reported during recovery from and low-dose infusions of propofol. Addiction has been described.

11. **Bacterial Growth**
    a. Propofol strongly supports the growth of *Escherichia coli* and *Pseudomonas aeruginosa*. Postoperative surgical infections manifesting as temperature elevations have been attributed to extrinsic contamination of propofol. For this reason, it is recommended that (a) an aseptic technique is used in handling propofol as reflected by disinfecting the ampule neck surface or vial rubber stopper with 70% isopropyl alcohol; (b) the contents of the ampule containing propofol should be withdrawn into a sterile syringe immediately after opening and administered promptly; and (c) the contents of an opened ampule must be discarded if they are not used within 6 hours.
    b. Despite these concerns, there is evidence that when propofol is aseptically drawn into an uncapped syringe, it will remain sterile at room temperature for several days.

12. **Antioxidant Properties**. Propofol has potent antioxidant properties that resemble those of the endogenous antioxidant vitamin E (neuroprotective effect of propofol).

13. **Pain on injection** is the most commonly reported adverse event associated with propofol administration to awake patients. Preceding the propofol with 1% lidocaine or prior administration of a potent short-acting opioid decreases the incidence of discomfort experienced by the patient.

14. **Miscellaneous Effects**
    a. Propofol does not trigger malignant hyperthermia.
    b. Secretion of cortisol is not influenced by propofol.

III. **Etomidate is a carboxylated imidazole–containing compound that is chemically unrelated to any other drug used for the IV induction of anesthesia.**
A. **Commercial Preparation**
   1. The original formulation of etomidate (high incidence of pain during IV injection) has been changed to a fat emulsion which has virtually abolished pain on injection and venous irritation, whereas the incidence of myoclonus remains unchanged.
   2. An oral formulation of etomidate for transmucosal delivery has been shown to produce dose-dependent sedation. Administration through the oral mucosa results in direct systemic absorption while bypassing hepatic metabolism (higher blood concentrations are achieved more rapidly compared with drug that is administered by mouth).
B. **Mechanism of Action**. The anesthetic effect of etomidate resides predominantly in the $R(+)$ isomer, which is approximately five times as potent as the $S(-)$ isomer. Stereoselectivity of etomidate supports the concept that $GABA_A$ receptors are the site of action of etomidate.
C. **Pharmacokinetics Uptake** (see Table 5-1). Prompt awakening after a single dose of etomidate principally reflects the redistribution of the drug from brain to inactive tissue sites. Rapid metabolism is also likely to contribute to prompt recovery.
D. **Metabolism**. Etomidate is rapidly metabolized by hydrolysis of the ethyl ester side chain to its carboxylic acid ester, resulting in a water-soluble, pharmacologically inactive compound.
E. **Clinical Uses**
   1. Etomidate may be viewed as an alternative to propofol or barbiturates for the IV induction of anesthesia, especially in the presence of an unstable cardiovascular system. After a standard induction dose of 0.2 to 0.4 mg/kg IV, the onset of unconsciousness occurs within one arm-to-brain circulation time.
   2. Involuntary myoclonic movements are common during the induction period as a result of alteration in the balance of inhibitory and excitatory influences on the thalamocortical tract (frequency of this myoclonic-like activity can be attenuated by prior administration of an opioid).

3. The principal limiting factor in the clinical use of etomidate for induction of anesthesia is the ability of this drug to transiently depress adrenocortical function.

F. **Side Effects**

1. **Central Nervous System**

   a. Etomidate is a potent direct cerebral vasoconstrictor that decreases cerebral blood flow and $CMRO_2$ 35% to 45% (previously increased ICP is lowered by etomidate). Suppression of adrenocortical function limits the clinical usefulness for long-term treatment of intracranial hypertension.

   b. Etomidate may activate seizure foci, manifesting as fast activity on the electroencephalogram (EEG) (use with caution in patients with focal epilepsy). This characteristic may be used to facilitate localization of seizure foci in patients undergoing cortical resection of epileptogenic tissue. Etomidate also possesses anticonvulsant properties and has been used to terminate status epilepticus.

   c. Etomidate has been observed to augment the amplitude of somatosensory evoked potentials, making monitoring of these responses more reliable.

2. **Cardiovascular System**

   a. Cardiovascular stability is characteristic of induction of anesthesia with 0.3 mg/kg IV of etomidate (minimal changes in heart rate, stroke volume, or cardiac output, whereas mean arterial blood pressure may decrease up to 15% because of decreases in systemic vascular resistance).

   b. Etomidate has been proposed for induction of anesthesia in patients with little or no cardiac reserve. Etomidate may differ from most other IV anesthetics in that depressive effects on myocardial contractility are minimal at concentrations needed for the production of anesthesia.

3. **Ventilation**. The depressant effects of etomidate on ventilation seem to be less than those of barbiturates, although apnea may occasionally accompany a rapid IV injection of the drug. In the majority of patients, etomidate-induced decreases in tidal volume are offset by compensatory increases in the frequency of breathing.

4. **Pain on injection** and venous irritation has been virtually eliminated with use of etomidate in a lipid emulsion vehicle rather than propylene glycol.

5. **Myoclonus**

   a. Commonly administered IV anesthetics can cause excitatory effects that may manifest as spontaneous movements, such as myoclonus, dystonia, and tremor. These spontaneous movements, particularly myoclonus, occur in 50% to 80% of patients receiving etomidate in the absence of premedication. Prior administration of an opioid (fentanyl, 1 to 2 μg/kg IV) or a benzodiazepine may decrease the incidence of myoclonus associated with administration of etomidate.

   b. The mechanism of etomidate-induced myoclonus appears to be disinhibition of subcortical structures that normally suppress extrapyramidal motor activity.

6. **Adrenocortical Suppression**

   a. Etomidate causes adrenocortical suppression by producing a dose-dependent inhibition of the conversion of cholesterol to cortisol (Fig. 5-3). The specific enzyme inhibited by etomidate appears to

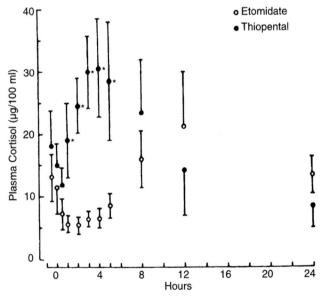

FIGURE 5-3 Etomidate, but not thiopental, is associated with decreases in the plasma concentrations of cortisol. *$P < .05$ compared with thiopental; mean ± SD. (From Fragen RJ, Shanks CA, Molteni A, et al. Effects of etomidate on hormonal responses to surgical stress. *Anesthesiology.* 1984;61:652–656, with permission.)

be 11-β-hydroxylase (enzyme inhibition lasts 4 to 8 hours after an induction dose of etomidate).

    b. Conceivably, patients experiencing sepsis or hemorrhage and who might require an intact cortisol response would be at a disadvantage should etomidate be administered.

    c. Conversely, suppression of adrenocortical function could be considered desirable from the standpoint of "stress-free" anesthesia.

  7. **Allergic reactions** following administration of etomidate is very low.

IV. Benzodiazepines (Table 5-2). Midazolam is the most commonly used benzodiazepine in the perioperative period. The longer context-sensitive half-time of lorazepam makes this drug an attractive choice to facilitate sedation of patients in critical care environments. Benzodiazepines are unique in the availability of a specific pharmacologic antagonist, *flumazenil*.

  A. **Mechanism of Action**. Benzodiazepines appear to produce all their pharmacologic effects by facilitating the actions of GABA (do not activate the $GABA_A$ receptors but rather enhance the affinity of the receptors for GABA) (Fig. 5-4).

Table 5-2

Pharmacologic Effects of Benzodiazepine

Anxiolysis	
Sedation	Treat acute insomnia
Anticonvulsant actions	
Spinal cord–mediated muscle relaxation	Not adequate for surgical procedures
	No influence on required dose of neuromuscular blocking drugs
Anterograde amnesia (acquisition or encoding of new information)	Amnestic potency is greater than sedative effect.
	Stored information (retrograde amnesia is not altered)
Low tendency to produce tolerance, abuse, or addiction	

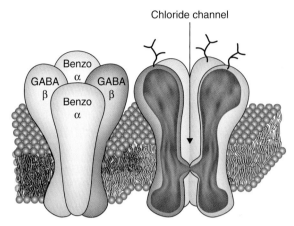

FIGURE 5-4 Model of the γ-aminobutyric acid (GABA) receptor forming a chloride channel. Benzodiazepines (benzo) attach selectively to α subunits and are presumed to facilitate the action of the inhibitory neurotransmitter GABA on α subunits. (From Mohler H, Richards JG. The benzodiazepine receptor: a pharmacologic control element of brain function. *Eur J Anesthesiol Suppl.* 1988;2:15–24, with permission.)

B. **Side Effects**
1. Fatigue and drowsiness are the most common side effects in patients treated chronically with benzodiazepines.
2. Although effects on ventilation seem to be absent, it may be prudent to avoid these drugs in patients with chronic lung disease characterized by hypoventilation and/or decreased arterial oxygenation as they may interact with other medications to have adverse effects.
3. Decreased motor coordination and impairment of cognitive function may occur, especially when benzodiazepines are used in combination with other CNS depressant drugs.
4. Acute administration of benzodiazepines may produce transient anterograde amnesia, especially if there is concomitant ingestion of alcohol.

C. **Drug Interactions**
1. Benzodiazepines exert synergistic sedative effects with other CNS depressants including alcohol, inhaled and injected anesthetics, opioids, and α₂ agonists.

2. Anesthetic requirements for inhaled and injected anesthetics are decreased by benzodiazepines.

3. Although benzodiazepines, especially midazolam, potentiate the ventilatory depressant effects of opioids, the analgesic actions of opioids are reduced by benzodiazepines.

D. **Midazolam** has replaced diazepam for use in preoperative medication and conscious sedation. The amnestic effects of midazolam are more potent than its sedative effects (patients may be awake but remain amnestic for events and conversations such as postoperative instructions for several hours).

1. **Pharmacokinetics** (Table 5-3)
   a. Midazolam undergoes rapid absorption from the gastrointestinal tract and prompt passage across the blood–brain barrier.
   b. Despite this prompt passage into the brain, midazolam is considered to have a slow effect-site equilibration time (0.9 to 5.6 minutes) compared with other drugs such as propofol and thiopental. In this regard, IV doses of midazolam should be sufficiently spaced to permit the peak clinical effect to be appreciated before a repeat dose is considered.
   c. The short duration of action of a single dose of midazolam is due to its lipid solubility, leading to rapid redistribution from the brain to inactive tissue sites as well as rapid hepatic clearance.

2. **Metabolism**. Midazolam is rapidly metabolized by hepatic and small intestine cytochrome P450 (CYP3A4) enzymes to active and inactive metabolites (Fig. 5-5). The principal metabolite of midazolam, 1-hydroxymidazolam, has approximately half the activity of the parent compound.

3. **Effects on Organ Systems**
   a. **Central Nervous System**. Midazolam, like other benzodiazepines, produces decreases in $CMRO_2$ and cerebral blood flow analogous to barbiturates and propofol. Induction of anesthesia with midazolam does not prevent increases in ICP associated with direct laryngoscopy for tracheal intubation. Paradoxical excitement occurs in less than 1% of all patients receiving midazolam and is effectively treated with a specific benzodiazepine antagonist, flumazenil.
   b. **Ventilation**. Midazolam produces dose-dependent decreases in ventilation (patients with chronic obstructive pulmonary disease experience even greater

Table 5-3

Comparative Pharmacology of Benzodiazepines

	Equivalent Dose (mg)	Volume of Distribution (L/kg)	Protein Binding (%)	Clearance (mL/kg/min)	Elimination Half-Time (h)
Midazolam	0.15–0.3	1.0–1.5	96–98	6–8	1–4
Diazepam	0.3–0.5	1.0–1.5	96–98	0.2–0.5	1–37
Lorazepam	0.05	0.8–1.3	96–98	0.7–1.0	10–20

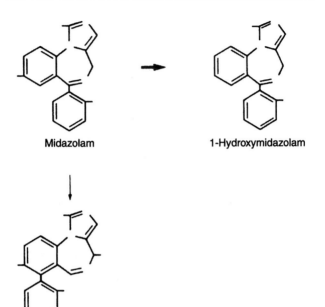

Midazolam → **1-Hydroxymidazolam**

4-Hydroxymidazolam

FIGURE 5-5 The principal metabolite of midazolam is 1-hydroxy-midazolam. A lesser amount of midazolam is metabolized to 4-hydroxymidazolam. (From Reves JG, Fragen RJ, Vinik HR, et al. Midazolam: pharmacology and uses. *Anesthesiology*. 1985;62: 310–324, with permission.)

midazolam-induced depression of ventilation). Transient apnea may occur after rapid injection of large doses of midazolam (>0.15 mg/kg IV), especially in the presence of preoperative medication that includes an opioid.

c. **Cardiovascular System**. Cardiac output is not altered by midazolam, suggesting that blood pressure changes are due to decreases in systemic vascular resistance.

4. **Clinical Uses**

a. **Preoperative Medication**. Midazolam is the most commonly used oral preoperative medication for children. Oral midazolam syrup (2 mg/mL) is effective for producing sedation and anxiolysis at a dose of 0.25 mg/kg with minimal effects on ventilation and oxygen saturation. Midazolam, 0.5 mg/kg administered orally 30 minutes before induction of anesthesia, provides reliable sedation and anxiolysis in children without producing delayed awakening.

b. **Intravenous Sedation**. Midazolam in doses of 1.0 to 2.5 mg IV (onset within 30 to 60 seconds, time to peak effect 3 to 5 minutes, duration of sedation 15 to 80 minutes) is effective for sedation during regional anesthesia as well as for brief therapeutic procedures. The most significant side effect of midazolam when used for sedation is depression of ventilation. Midazolam-induced depression of ventilation is exaggerated (synergistic effects) in the presence of opioids and other CNS depressant drugs. Increasing age greatly increases pharmacodynamic variability and is associated with generally increased sensitivity to the hypnotic effects of midazolam.

c. **Induction of Anesthesia**. Anesthesia can be induced by administration of midazolam, 0.1 to 0.2 mg/kg IV, over 30 to 60 seconds. Onset of unconsciousness (synergistic interaction) is facilitated when a small dose of opioid (fentanyl, 50 to 100 μg IV or its equivalent) precedes the injection of midazolam by 1 to 3 minutes. In healthy patients receiving small doses of benzodiazepines, the cardiovascular depression associated with these drugs is minimal. When significant cardiovascular responses occur, it is most likely a reflection of benzodiazepine-induced peripheral vasodilation.

d. **Maintenance of Anesthesia**. Midazolam may be administered to supplement opioids, propofol, and/or inhaled anesthetics during maintenance of anesthesia (anesthetic requirements for volatile anesthetics are decreased in a dose-dependent manner by midazolam).

e. **Postoperative Sedation**. Long-term IV administration of midazolam (loading dose 0.5 to 4 mg IV and maintenance dose 1 to 7 mg per hour IV) to produce sedation in intubated patients results in relative saturation of peripheral tissues with midazolam and clearance from the systemic circulation becomes less dependent on redistribution into peripheral tissues and more dependent on hepatic metabolism. The concomitant administration of analgesic doses of opioids greatly decreases the needed dose of midazolam and results in a more rapid recovery from sedation following discontinuation of the IV infusion of midazolam. Emergence time from midazolam infusion is increased in elderly patients, obese patients, and in the presence of severe liver disease.

f. **Paradoxical vocal cord motion** is a cause of nonorganic upper airway obstruction and stridor that may manifest postoperatively (midazolam 0.5 to 1 mg IV may be an effective treatment).

E. **Diazepam** is a highly lipid-soluble benzodiazepine with a more prolonged duration of action compared with midazolam. Because of the beneficial aspects of midazolam pharmacology, parenteral diazepam is seldom used as part of current anesthetic regimens (see Table 5-3).

F. **Lorazepam** is a more potent sedative and amnesic than midazolam and diazepam, whereas its effects on ventilation, the cardiovascular system, and skeletal muscles resemble those of other benzodiazepines.

G. **Oxazepam** is a pharmacologically active metabolite of diazepam (duration of action is slightly shorter than that of diazepam because oxazepam is converted to pharmacologically inactive metabolites).

H. **Alprazolam** has significant anxiety-reducing effects in patients with primary anxiety and panic attacks (may be an alternative to midazolam for preoperative medication).

I. **Clonazepam** is a highly lipid-soluble benzodiazepine that is well absorbed after oral administration and is particularly effective in the control and prevention of seizures, especially myoclonic and infantile spasms.

J. **Flurazepam** is used exclusively to treat insomnia (30 mg orally to adults produces a hypnotic effect in 15 to 25 minutes and lasts 7 to 8 hours).

K. **Temazepam** is an orally active benzodiazepine administered exclusively for the treatment of insomnia. Despite the relatively long elimination half-time, temazepam, as used to treat insomnia, is unlikely to be accompanied by residual drowsiness the following morning.

L. **Triazolam** is an orally absorbed benzodiazepine that is effective in the treatment of insomnia. Marked anterograde amnesia has developed when this drug has been self-administered in attempts to facilitate sleep when traveling through several time zones.

M. **Flumazenil** is a specific and exclusive benzodiazepine antagonist with a high affinity for benzodiazepine receptors, where it exerts minimal agonist activity (prevents or reverses, in a dose-dependent manner, all the agonist effects of benzodiazepines).

1. **Dose and Administration**
   a. The dose of flumazenil should be titrated individually to obtain the desired level of consciousness. The recommended initial dose is 0.2 mg IV (8 to 15 µg/kg IV), which typically reverses the CNS effects of benzodiazepine agonists within about 2 minutes. If required, further doses of 0.1 mg IV (to a total of 1 mg IV) may be administered at 60-second intervals.
   b. The duration of action of flumazenil is 30 to 60 minutes, and supplemental doses of the antagonist may be needed to maintain the desired level of consciousness. An alternative to repeated doses of flumazenil to maintain wakefulness is a continuous low-dose infusion of flumazenil, 0.1 to 0.4 mg per hour.
   c. The administration of flumazenil to patients being treated with antiepileptic drugs for control of seizure activity is not recommended as it could precipitate acute withdrawal seizures.

2. **Side Effects**. Flumazenil-induced antagonism of excess benzodiazepine agonist effects is not followed by acute anxiety, hypertension, tachycardia, or neuroendocrine evidence of a stress response in postoperative patients.

V. **Short-Acting Nonbenzodiazepine Benzodiazepines.** Zaleplon, zolpidem, and eszopiclone have selectivity for certain subunits of GABA receptors, resulting in a clinical profile for treatment of sleeping disorders that is more efficacious with fewer side effects than occur with conventional benzodiazepines. Zaleplon (10 mg orally) has a rapid elimination so there are few residual side effects after taking a single dose at bedtime.

VI. **Barbiturates.** The introduction of thiopental in 1934 revolutionized the practice of anesthesia by making it possible to induce general anesthesia in seconds, avoiding a slow, often unpleasant, more dangerous induction with diethyl ether. Today, thiopental and other barbiturate sedative-hypnotics that were imported from overseas are no longer available as these companies have ceased exporting barbiturates to the

United States in order to protest their use as a part of the lethal injection "cocktail" for capital punishment.

VII. **Non–γ-Aminobutyric Acid Sedatives and Hypnotics**
   A. **Ketamine** is a phencyclidine derivative that produces "dissociative anesthesia," which is characterized by evidence on the EEG of dissociation between the thalamocortical and limbic systems (resembles a cataleptic state in which the eyes remain open with a slow nystagmic gaze, the patient is noncommunicative, although wakefulness may appear to be present). Varying degrees of hypertonus and purposeful skeletal muscle movements often occur independently of surgical stimulation. The patient is amnesic, and analgesia is intense. The frequency of emergence delirium limits the clinical usefulness of ketamine as a sole agent. Ketamine is a drug with significant abuse potential.
      1. **Structure–Activity Relationships**
         a. The presence of an asymmetric carbon atom results in the existence of two optical isomers of ketamine. The racemic form of ketamine has been the most frequently used preparation although $S(+)$-ketamine is clinically available (produces more intense analgesia, more rapid metabolism and thus recovery, less salivation, and a lower incidence of emergence reactions than $R[-]$-ketamine).
         b. Both isomers of ketamine appear to inhibit uptake of catecholamines back into postganglionic sympathetic nerve endings (cocaine-like effect).
      2. **Mechanism of Action.** Ketamine is known to interact with multiple CNS receptors (N-methyl-D-aspartate [NMDA], opioid receptors, monoaminergic receptors, muscarinic receptors) but clear association between receptor interaction and specific behavior has not been established.
      3. **Pharmacokinetics** (see Table 5-1). Peak plasma concentrations of ketamine occur within 1 minute after IV administration and within 5 minutes after intramuscular (IM) injection. The extreme lipid solubility of ketamine ensures its rapid transfer across the blood–brain barrier (ketamine-induced increases in cerebral blood flow could facilitate delivery of drug).
      4. **Metabolism**
         a. An important pathway of metabolism is demethylation of ketamine by cytochrome P450 enzymes to form norketamine (this active metabolite may

contribute to prolonged effects of ketamine especially with repeated doses or a continuous IV infusion).

b. Tolerance may occur in burn patients receiving more than two short-interval exposures to ketamine. Development of tolerance is also consistent with reports of ketamine dependence.

5. **Clinical Uses**. Ketamine is a unique drug evoking intense analgesia at subanesthetic doses and producing prompt induction of anesthesia when administered IV at higher doses. Inclusion of an antisialagogue in the preoperative medication is often recommended to decrease the likelihood of coughing and laryngospasm due to ketamine-induced salivary secretions.

a. **Analgesia**. Intense analgesia can be achieved with subanesthetic doses of ketamine, 0.2 to 0.5 mg/kg IV. Analgesia is thought to be greater for somatic than for visceral pain. The analgesic effects of ketamine are likely due to its activity in the thalamic and limbic systems, which are responsible for the interpretation of painful signals.

b. **Induction of anesthesia** is produced by administration of ketamine, 1 to 2 mg/kg IV or 4 to 8 mg/kg IM. Consciousness is lost in 30 to 60 seconds after IV administration and in 2 to 4 minutes after IM injection. Unconsciousness is associated with maintenance of normal or only slightly depressed pharyngeal and laryngeal reflexes. Return of consciousness usually occurs in 10 to 20 minutes after an injected induction dose of ketamine. Because of its rapid onset of action, ketamine has been used as an IM induction drug in children and difficult-to-manage mentally challenged patients regardless of age. Due to its intense analgesic activity, ketamine has been used extensively for burn dressing changes, débridements, and skin grafting procedures. Induction of anesthesia in acutely hypovolemic patients is often accomplished with ketamine, taking advantage of the drug's cardiovascular-stimulating effects (may become a myocardial depressant if endogenous catecholamine stores are depleted and sympathetic nervous system compensatory responses are impaired). Nystagmus associated with administration of ketamine may be undesirable in operations or examinations of the eye performed under anesthesia. Ketamine has been administered safely to patients with malignant hyperthermia.

c. **Reversal of Opioid Tolerance**. Subanesthetic doses of ketamine are effective in preventing and reversing morphine-induced tolerance (believed to involve interaction between NMDA receptors, the nitric oxide pathway, and μ-opioid receptors).

6. **Side Effects**. Ketamine is unique among injected anesthetics in its ability to stimulate the cardiovascular system and produce emergence delirium.

a. **Central Nervous System**. Ketamine is traditionally considered to increase cerebral blood flow and $CMRO_2$, although there is also evidence suggesting that this may not be a valid generalization.

b. **Cardiovascular System**. Ketamine produces cardiovascular effects that resemble sympathetic nervous system stimulation (Table 5-4). Critically ill patients occasionally respond to ketamine with unexpected decreases in systemic blood pressure and cardiac output, which reflect depletion of endogenous

Table 5-4

Circulatory Effects of Ketamine

	Control	Ketamine (2 mg/kg IV)	Percent Change
Heart rate (beats/min)	74	98	+33
Mean arterial pressure (mm Hg)	93	119	+28
Stroke volume index (mL/m²)	43	44	
Systemic vascular resistance (units)	16.2	15.9	
Right atrial pressure (mm Hg)	7.0	8.9	
Left ventricular end diastolic pressure (mm Hg)	13.0	13.1	
Pulmonary artery pressure (mm Hg)	17.0	24.5	+44
Minute work index (kg/min/m²)	5.4	8.9	+40
Tension-time index (mm Hg/s)	2,700	4,600	+68

catecholamine stores and exhaustion of sympathetic
nervous system compensatory mechanisms, leading
to an unmasking of ketamine's direct myocardial
depressant effects.

c. **Ventilation and Airway**. Ketamine does not produce
significant depression of ventilation. Upper airway
skeletal muscle tone is well maintained, and upper
airway reflexes remain relatively intact after administration of ketamine. Despite continued presence of
upper airway reflexes, ketamine anesthesia does not
negate the need for protection of the lungs against aspiration by placement of a cuffed tube in the patient's
trachea. Salivary and tracheobronchial mucous gland
secretions are increased by IM or IV administration
of ketamine, leading to the frequent recommendation
that an antisialagogue be included in the preoperative
medication when use of this drug is anticipated.

d. **Bronchomotor Tone**. Ketamine has bronchodilatory
activity and has been used in subanesthetic doses to
treat bronchospasm in the operating room and ICU.

e. **Allergic Reactions**. Ketamine does not evoke the
release of histamine and rarely, if ever, causes allergic
reactions.

7. **Emergence Delirium (Psychedelic Effects)**. Emergence
from ketamine anesthesia in the postoperative period
may be associated with visual, auditory, propriocep-
tive, and confusional illusions, which may progress to
delirium. Cortical blindness may be transiently present.
Dreams and hallucinations can occur up to 24 hours
after administration of ketamine.

a. **Incidence**. The observed incidence of emergence
delirium after ketamine ranges from 5% to 30%
and is partially dose dependent. Factors associated
with an increased incidence of emergence delirium
include (a) age older than 15 years, (b) female gender,
(c) doses of ketamine of greater than 2 mg/kg IV,
and (d) a history of personality problems or frequent
dreaming.

b. **Prevention**. Benzodiazepines have proved the most
effective in prevention of this phenomenon, with
midazolam being more effective than diazepam. A
common approach is to administer the benzodiazepine IV about 5 minutes before induction of anesthesia with ketamine. The inclusion of atropine in the
preoperative medication may increase the incidence

of emergence delirium. Despite contrary opinions, there is no evidence that permitting patients to awaken from ketamine anesthesia in quiet areas alters the incidence of emergence delirium.

8. **Drug Interactions**

   a. The importance of an intact and normally functioning CNS in determining the cardiovascular effects of ketamine is emphasized by hemodynamic depression rather than stimulation that occurs when ketamine is administered in the presence of inhaled anesthetics.

   b. Ketamine-induced enhancement of nondepolarizing neuromuscular blocking drugs may reflect interference by ketamine with calcium ion binding or its transport.

B. **Dextromethorphan** is a low-affinity NMDA antagonist that is a common ingredient in over-the-counter cough suppressants. Unlike codeine, this drug rarely produces sedation or gastrointestinal disturbances. Its euphoric effects lead to a significant abuse potential.

C. **Dexmedetomidine** is a highly selective, specific, and potent α_2-adrenergic agonist (1,620:1 α_2 to α_1). One of the highest densities of α_2 receptors is present in the pontine locus ceruleus, an important source of sympathetic nervous system innervation of the forebrain and a vital modulator of vigilance (sedative effects evoked by dexmedetomidine most likely reflect inhibition of this nucleus).

1. **Clinical Uses**. As with clonidine, pretreatment with dexmedetomidine attenuates hemodynamic responses to tracheal intubation, decreases plasma catecholamine concentrations during anesthesia, decreases perioperative requirements for inhaled anesthetics and opioids, and increases the likelihood of hypotension. Despite marked dose-dependent analgesia and sedation produced by this drug, there is only mild depression of ventilation. Dexmedetomidine markedly increases the range of temperatures not triggering thermoregulatory defenses. For this reason, dexmedetomidine, like clonidine, is likely to promote perioperative hypothermia and also prove to be an effective treatment for nonthermally induced shivering. Severe bradycardia may follow the administration of dexmedetomidine.

2. **Postoperative Sedation**. Dexmedetomidine (0.2 to 0.7 µg/kg/hour IV) is useful for sedation of postoperative critical care patients in an ICU environment, particularly when mechanical ventilation via a tracheal tube is necessary.

VIII. **Scopolamine readily crosses the blood–brain barrier, where it binds muscarinic cholinergic receptors (Table 5-5).**
   A. **Clinical Uses**
      1. **Sedation**
         a. Scopolamine is the only anticholinergic drug used primarily for sedation (0.3 to 0.5 mg IM or IV). Scopolamine also greatly enhances the sedative effects of concomitantly administered drugs, especially opioids and benzodiazepines (combination of IM morphine and scopolamine was once a very popular form of preoperative sedation).
         b. Occasionally, CNS effects of anticholinergic drugs, especially scopolamine, cause symptoms ranging from restlessness to somnolence. These symptoms are more likely to occur in elderly patients and should be considered as a possible explanation for delayed awakening from anesthesia or agitation in the early postoperative period. Physostigmine (2 mg IV) is effective in reversing restlessness or somnolence due to CNS effects of tertiary amine anticholinergic drugs.
      2. **Antisialagogue Effect**. Scopolamine is a potent antisialagogue selected and is selected when both an antisialagogue effect and sedation are desired results of preoperative medication.
   B. **Side Effects**
      1. **Mydriasis and Cycloplegia**
         a. Patients with glaucoma and parturients require special considerations in using anticholinergic drugs for preoperative medication (mydriatic effects of scopolamine are greater than those of atropine, suggesting caution in the administration of scopolamine to patients with glaucoma).
         b. Mydriasis produced by an anticholinergic drug is completely offset by topical placement on the cornea of an anticholinesterase drug such as pilocarpine.
      2. **Central Anticholinergic Syndrome**
         a. Scopolamine and, to a lesser extent, atropine can enter the CNS and produce symptoms characterized as the central anticholinergic syndrome (symptoms range from restlessness and hallucinations to somnolence and unconsciousness).
         b. Physostigmine, a lipid-soluble tertiary amine anticholinesterase drug administered in doses of 15 to 60 µg/kg IV, is a specific treatment for the central

Table 5-5

Comparative Effects of Anticholinergic Drugs

	Sedation	Antisialagogue	Increase Heart Rate	Decrease Gastric Hydrogen Ion Secretion	Relax Smooth Muscle
Atropine	+	+	+++	+	++
Scopolamine	+++	+++	+	++	+
Glycopyrrolate	0	++	++	+	++

	Mydriasis, Cycloplegia	Prevent Motion-Induced Nausea			Alter Fetal Heart Rate
Atropine	+	+			0
Scopolamine	+++	+++			?
Glycopyrrolate	0	0			0

0, none; +, mild; ++, moderate; +++, marked.

anticholinergic syndrome. Treatment may need to be repeated every 1 to 2 hours.

C. **Overdose**

1. Deliberate or accidental overdose with an anticholinergic drug produces a rapid onset of symptoms characteristic of muscarinic cholinergic receptor blockade (mouth becomes dry, swallowing and talking is difficult, vision is blurred, photophobia is present, and tachycardia is prominent). The skin is dry and flushed, and a rash may appear especially over the face, neck, and upper chest (blush area). Even therapeutic doses of anticholinergic drugs sometimes may selectively dilate cutaneous vessels in the blush area. Body temperature is likely to be increased by anticholinergic drugs, especially when the environmental temperature is also increased.

2. Fatal events due to an overdose of an anticholinergic drug include seizures, coma, and medullary ventilatory center paralysis.

CHAPTER 6

Pain Physiology

The definition of pain as proposed by the International Association for the Study of Pain emphasizes the complex nature of pain as a physical, emotional, and psychological condition. Failure to appreciate the complex factors that affect the experience of pain and reliance entirely on physical examination findings and laboratory tests may lead to misunderstanding and inadequate treatment of pain. The nociceptive system is highly complex and adaptable. Sensitivity of most of its components can be reset by a variety of physiologic and pathologic conditions.

I. Societal Impact of Pain
   A. It is estimated that chronic pain may affect as many as 40% of the adult population (prevalence of low back pain ranges from 8% to 37%).
   B. The costs to society related to chronic pain are immense, with an estimated annual cost attributed to back pain, migraine headache, and arthritis of $40 billion, excluding the costs of surgical procedures to treat pain and lost workdays.

II. Neurobiology of Pain. The experience of pain involves a series of complex neurophysiologic processes, collectively termed *nociception*, with four distinct components: transduction, transmission, modulation, and perception (Table 6-1).

III. Peripheral Nerve Physiology of Pain
   A. **Nociceptors (pain receptors)** are a specialized class of primary afferents that respond to intense, noxious stimuli in skin, muscles, joints, viscera, and vasculature.
      1. Nociceptors are inactive until they are stimulated by sufficient energy to reach the stimulus (resting) threshold.
      2. Specific types of nociceptors react to different types of stimuli (Table 6-2).

Table 6-1

Components of Pain

Transduction	Process by which a noxious stimulus (heat, cold, mechanical distortion) is converted to an electrical impulse in sensory nerve endings
Transmission	Conduction of electrical impulses to the CNS
Modulation	Process of altering pain transmission (inhibitory and excitatory mechanisms)
Perception	Likely mediated through the thalamus

CNS, central nervous system.

B. **Sensitization of nociceptors** refers to the increased responsiveness of peripheral neurons responsible for pain transmission to heat, cold, mechanical, or chemical stimulation (attributable to the release of inflammatory mediators and adaptation of signaling pathways).
  1. Chronic pain occurs if the conditions associated with inflammation do not resolve, resulting in sensitization of peripheral and central pain signaling pathway and increased pain sensations to normally painful stimuli (*hyperalgesia*) and the perception of pain sensations in response to normally nonpainful stimuli (*allodynia*).
  2. Numerous endogenous chemicals, neurotransmitters, and peptides (such as substance P) can directly activate nociceptors, whereas others (serotonin, histamine) may activate the inflammatory cells which, in turn, release cytokines (Fig. 6-1).

Table 6-2

Response of Nociceptors Do Different Types of Stimuli

Type of Nociceptor	Stimuli Evoking a Response
Unmyelinated C fiber afferents (conduction velocity <2 m/s)	Burning pain from heat and sustained pressure
Type 1 myelinated A fiber afferents (conduction velocity >2 m/s)	Heat, mechanical, and chemical stimuli
Type II myelinated (conduction velocity about 15 m/s)	Heat

C. Primary Hyperalgesia and Secondary Hyperalgesia

1. Tissue injury and inflammation may activate a cascade of events leading to enhanced pain in response to a given noxious stimulus (*hyperalgesia*).
2. Hyperalgesia at the original site of injury is termed *primary hyperalgesia*, and hyperalgesia in the uninjured skin surrounding the injury is termed *secondary hyperalgesia*.

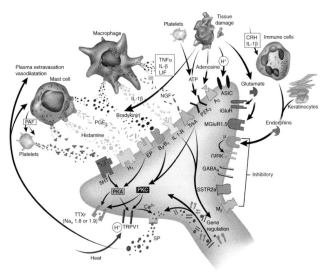

FIGURE 6-1 Cellular mechanism underlying nociceptor sensitization induced by peripheral inflammation. Activated immune cells (macrophages, mast cells, and other immune cells) and injured cells release numerous chemicals, which may directly or indirectly sensitize the peripheral nerve terminals. A_2, adenosine A_2 receptor; ASIC, acid-sensing ion channel; B_2/B_1, bradykinin receptor B_2/B_1; CRH, corticotropin-releasing hormone; EP, E-prostanoid receptor; GIRK, G protein–coupled inward rectifying potassium channel; H_1, histamine H_1 receptor; iGluR, ionotropic glutamate receptor; IL-1β, interleukin-1β; mGluR, metabotropic glutamate receptor; NGF, nerve growth factor; $P2X_3$, purinergic receptor P2X ligand-gated ion channel 3; PAF, platelet-activating factor; PGE_2, prostaglandin E_2; PKA, protein kinase A; PKC, protein kinase C; SP, substance P; SSTR2A, somatostatin receptor 2A; TNF-α, tumor necrosis factor α; TrkA, tyrosine kinase receptor A; TRPV1, transient receptor potential vanilloid receptor 1; TTXr, tetrodotoxin-resistant sodium channel; μ, mu-opioid receptor; M_2, muscarinic receptor; 5HT, serotonin; LIF, leukemia inhibitory factor.

IV. **Central Nervous System Physiology. Pain transmission from peripheral nociceptors to the spinal cord and higher structures of the CNS is a dynamic process involving several pathways, numerous receptors, neurotransmitters, and secondary messengers (Fig. 6-2).**
   A. **Dorsal Horn: The Relay Center for Nociception**
      1. Afferent fibers from peripheral nociceptors enter the spinal cord in the dorsal root, ascend or descend several segments in Lissauer's tract, and synapse with the dorsal horn neurons for the primary integration of peripheral nociceptive information.
      2. The central terminals of primary afferents occupy highly ordered spatial locations in the dorsal horn. The dorsal horn consists of six laminae (Fig. 6-3).
   B. **Gate theory** proposes that painful information is projected to the supraspinal brain regions if the gate is open, whereas painful stimulus is not felt if the gate is closed by the simultaneous inhibitory impulses (Fig. 6-4).
   C. **Central Sensitization of Dorsal Horn Neurons**
      1. Peripheral inflammation and nerve injury could alter the synaptic efficacy and induce central sensitization in the dorsal horn neurons and is considered a fundamental mechanism underlying the induction and maintenance of chronic pain.
      2. One form of central sensitization is windup of dorsal horn neurons, an activity-dependent progressive increase in the response of neurons over the course of a train of inputs.
      3. The second form of central sensitization is a heterosynaptic, activity-dependent plasticity that outlasts the initiating stimulus for tens of minutes (Fig. 6-5).
   D. **Ascending Pathway for Pain Transmission**
      1. Ascending pathways (spinothalamic tract, spinohypothalamic tract) from the spinal cord to sites in the brainstem and thalamus are important for the perception and integration of nociceptive information.
      2. The spinothalamic tract is the most closely associated with pain, temperature, and itch sensation.
   E. **Supraspinal Modulation of Nociception**
      1. Several brain areas have been identified that are critically involved in the formation of emotional aspects of pain and the central modulation of pain perception.
      2. Anesthetized humans, without conscious awareness of pain, still exhibit significant pain-evoked cerebellar activation, suggesting that pain-evoked cerebellar activity may be more important in regulation of afferent nociceptive activity than in the perception of pain.

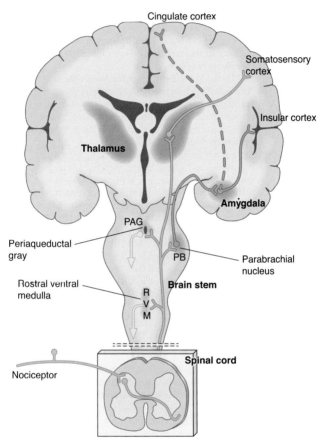

FIGURE 6-2 The projection pathway for the transmission of pain information to the brain. Primary afferent nociceptors convey noxious information to projection neurons within the dorsal horn of the spinal cord. A subset of these projection neurons transmit information to the somatosensory cortex via the thalamus, providing information about the location and intensity of the painful stimulus. Other projection neurons engage the cingulate and insular cortices via connections in the brainstem (parabrachial nucleus) and amygdala, contributing to the affective component of the pain experience. This ascending information also accesses neurons of the rostral ventral medulla and midbrain periaqueductal gray to engage descending feedback systems that modulate the transmission of nociceptive information through the spinal cord.

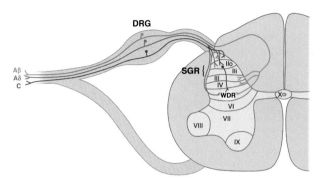

FIGURE 6-3 Schematic representation of the spinal projections of primary afferent fibers. In general, unmyelinated C fibers synapse with the interneurons in laminae I (marginal layer) and II (substantia gelatinosa of Rolando *[SGR]*). Cutaneous A-δ fibers usually project to laminae I, II, V, and A-β fibers primarily terminate in laminae III–V in dorsal horn. Large-diameter myelinated fibers innervating muscles, joint, and viscera may also terminate in laminae I, IV–VII, and the ventral horn. Second-order wide dynamic range *(WDR)* neurons are located in lamina V and receive input from nociceptive and nonnociceptive neurons.

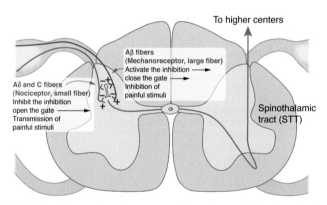

FIGURE 6-4 Illustration of gate theory for pain modulation in spinal dorsal horn. Lightly rubbing the skin of a painful, injured area seems to somehow relieve the pain. Large-diameter myelinated afferents (Aβ) conveying pressure and touch information have "faster" conduction speed than A-δ fibers or C fibers conveying painful information to the dorsal horn. Thus, the application of light peripheral mechanical stimuli resulting in excitation of A-β fibers can activate the inhibitory interneurons in the dorsal horn and thus close the "gate" to the simultaneous incoming pain signals carried by A-δ fibers and C fibers. Although the gate control theory is overly simplistic, it remains a valid conceptual framework for understanding pain and pain-related experiences.

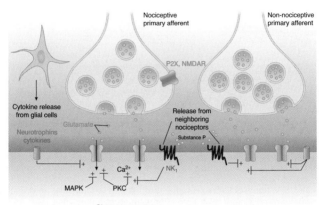

Glutamate receptors

FIGURE 6-5 The synaptic mechanism underlying peripheral, nociceptive, stimuli-induced, and persistent heterosynaptic potentiation of dorsal horn neurons. Transmitters and mediators released from primary afferents and surrounding microglial cells, including substance P, neurotrophins, and cytokines may act at a distance on dorsal horn neurons to produce long-lasting heterosynaptic potentiation of glutamatergic transmission. Note that both inputs from nociceptors and nonnociceptors may be potentiated. *MAPK*, mitogen-activated protein kinase; *P2X*, purinoceptor; *PKC*, protein kinase C; *NK1*, neurokinin 1 (substance P receptor).

F. **Descending Pathways for Pain Modulation**. Evidence demonstrates that descending pathways originating from certain supraspinal regions may concurrently promote and suppress nociceptive transmission through the dorsal horn (Fig. 6-6).

V. **Transition from Acute Pain to Chronic Pain**
   A. Acute pain and the accompanying sensitization that accompany any injury do not typically persist after the initial injury has healed. In contrast, chronic pain is persistent pain that persists after all tissue healing appears to be complete and extends beyond the expected period of healing.
   B. There is no clear delineation between when acute ends and chronic pain begins. Two common and practical cutoff points are often used, 3 months and 6 months after initial injury, because the likelihood that the pain will resolve diminishes with time and the likelihood that chronic pain will persist rises.

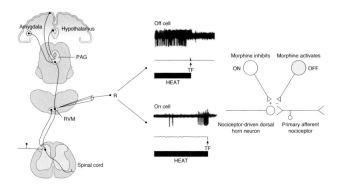

FIGURE 6-6 Properties of proposed medullary pain-modulating neurons. Single-unit extracellular recordings were performed by microelectrodes placed in the rostral ventromedial medulla (RVM) while peripheral noxious stimuli (heat) were applied. As shown by the oscilloscope sweeps, the firing of the off-cell pauses just prior to the tail flick reflex (indicating pain sensation) in response to noxious heat, whereas the typical on-cell firing occurs before the tail flick. The right diagram illustrates that both on and off cells project to the spinal cord, where they exert bidirectional control over nociceptive dorsal horn neurons.

   C. Sensitization of peripheral and central nocisponsive neurons underlies the neurobiologic basis of the transition from acute pain to chronic pain (an individual's psychologic response after injury also important).

VI. Psychobiology of Pain
   A. Discomfort, fear of pain, and anxiety are the most common psychological responses observed in the patients with pain.
   B. Affective qualities of pain are transmitted and processed via the same pathways as those for the painful sensory transmission.

VII. Some Specific Types of Pain
   A. **Neuropathic pain** is pain that persists after tissue injury has healed and is characterized by reduced sensory and nociceptive thresholds (allodynia and hyperalgesia).
      1. Cancer patients are at increased risk of neuropathic pain caused by radiotherapy or a variety of chemotherapeutic agents.

2. Current treatments (opioids, gabapentin, amitriptyline, medicinal cannabis) for neuropathic pain are only modestly effective.

3. The pathophysiologic processes that lead to neuropathic pain has the hallmarks of a neuroinflammatory response following innate immune system activation.

B. **Visceral pain** is diffuse and poorly localized (somatic pain localized and characterized by distinct sensations), typically referred to somatic sites (muscle and skin), and it is usually associated with stronger emotional and autonomic reactions.

1. Among all tissues in the body, the viscera are unique in that each organ receives innervation from two sets of nerves, either vagal and spinal nerves or pelvic and spinal nerves, and the visceral afferent innervation is sparse relative to somatic innervation.

2. The vagus afferent innervation plays an important role in the prominent autonomic and emotional reactions in visceral diseases associated with pain (Fig. 6-7).

C. **Complex regional pain syndrome (CRPS)** are defined as "a variety of painful conditions following injury, which appears regionally having a distal predominance of abnormal findings, exceeding in both magnitude and duration the expected clinical course of the inciting event often resulting in significant impairment of motor function, and showing variable progression over time."

1. Two forms of CRPS are type I (reflex sympathetic dystrophy, absence of major nerve injury) and type II (causalgia, presence of a major identifiable nerve injury).

2. The incidence of CRPS I is 1% to 2% after fractures, 12% after brain lesions, and 5% after myocardial infarction, and the incidence of CRPS II in peripheral nerve injury varies from 2% to 14%.

3. The mechanism underlying the pathogenesis of CRPS remains unclear, although it is recognized that CRPS is a neurologic disease, including the autonomic, sensory, and motor systems as well as cortical areas involved in the processing of cognitive and affective information, and the inflammatory component appears to be particularly important in the acute phase of the disease.

4. Effective, evidence-based treatment regimens for CRPS are lacking.

D. **Pain in Neonate and Infant**. Accumulating evidence overrides the outdated thought that young children do not feel pain due to the immaturity of the peripheral and central

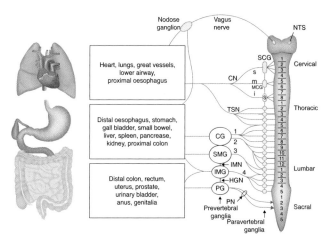

FIGURE 6-7 Visceral innervation. The vagus nerve, with cell bodies in the nodose ganglion and central terminals in the nucleus tractus solitarii *(NTS)*, innervates organs in the thoracic and abdominal cavities. Afferent nerves with terminals in the spinal cord innervate the same thoracic and abdominal organs as well as those in the pelvic floor. Visceral spinal afferents pass through pre- and/or paravertebral ganglia en route to the spinal cord; their cell bodies are located in dorsal root ganglia (not illustrated). Prevertebral ganglia: *CG*, coeliac ganglion; *SMG* and *IMG*, superior and inferior mesenteric ganglia, respectively; and *PG*, pelvic ganglion. Paravertebral ganglia: *SCG* and *MCG*, superior and middle cervical ganglia, respectively; and *S*, stellate ganglion. Nerves: *CN*, cardiac nerves (s, m, and i, superior, middle, and inferior, respectively); *TSN*, thoracic splanchnic nerves; *1, 2, 3* and *4*, greater, lesser, least, and lumbar splanchnic nerves, respectively; *IMN*, intermesenteric nerve; *HGN*, hypogastric nerve; and *PN*, pelvic nerve.

nervous systems (emphasizes the importance of optimal pain management in this age group).

VIII. **Embryologic Origin and Localization of Pain**

    A. The position in the spinal cord to which visceral afferent fibers pass for each organ depends on the segment (dermatome) of the body from which the organ developed embryologically (explains the phenomenon pain that is referred to a site distant from the tissue causing the pain) (Fig. 6-8).

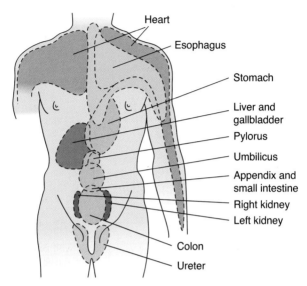

FIGURE 6-8 Surface area of referred pain from different visceral organs.

B. The heart originates in the neck and upper thorax such that visceral afferents enter the spinal cord at C3–C5. As a result, the pain of myocardial ischemia is referred to the neck and arm. The gallbladder originates from the 9th thoracic segment, so visceral afferents from the gallbladder enter the spinal cord at T9.

CHAPTER 7

Opioid Agonists and Antagonists

I. **Introduction**
   A. Opioids remain the mainstay of modern perioperative care and pain management. The modern word "opium" is derived from the Greek word *opion* ("poppy juice").
      1. Drugs derived from opium are referred to as *opiates* (morphine is the best-known opiate).
      2. The term *narcotic* is derived from the Greek word for stupor and traditionally has been used to refer to potent morphine-like analgesics with the potential to produce physical dependence.
   B. The development of synthetic drugs with morphine-like properties has led to the use of the term *opioid* to refer to all exogenous substances, natural and synthetic, that bind specifically to any of several subpopulations of opioid receptors and produce at least some agonist (morphine-like) effects (Table 7-1).

II. **Chemical Structure of Opium Alkaloids.** The active components of opium can be divided into two distinct chemical classes: phenanthrenes and benzylisoquinolines. The principal phenanthrene alkaloids present in opium are morphine, codeine, and thebaine (Fig. 7-1).
   A. **Semisynthetic Opioids.** Simple modification of the morphine molecule yields many derivative compounds with differing properties. Substitution of a methyl group for the hydroxyl group on carbon 3 results in methylmorphine (codeine) and substitution of acetyl groups on carbons 3 and 6 results in diacetylmorphine (heroin).
   B. **Synthetic Opioids.** Synthetic opioids contain the phenanthrene nucleus of morphine but are manufactured by synthesis rather than chemical modification of morphine.
      1. **Fentanyl,** sufentanil, alfentanil, and remifentanil are synthetic opioids that are widely used to supplement general anesthesia or as primary anesthetic drugs in very high doses (Fig. 7-2).

Table 7-1

Classification of Opioid Agonists and Antagonists

Agonists	Agonists–Antagonists	Antagonists
Morphine	Pentazocine	Naloxone
Morphine-6-glucuronide	Butorphanol	Naltrexone
Meperidine	Nalbuphine	Nalmefene
Sufentanil	Buprenorphine	
Fentanyl	Nalorphine	
Alfentanil	Bremazocine	
Remifentanil	Dezocine	
Codeine	Meptazinol	
Hydromorphone		
Oxymorphone		
Oxycodone		
Hydrocodone		
Propoxyphene		
Methadone		
Tramadol		
Heroin		

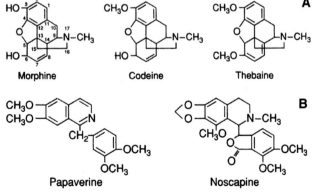

FIGURE 7-1 Chemical structures of opium alkaloids. Phenanthrene **(A)** and benzylisoquinoline **(B)** alkaloids.

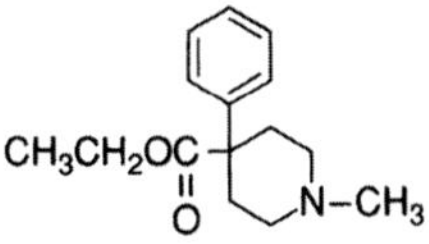

Meperidine

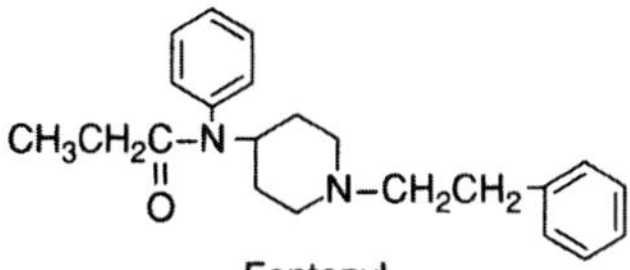

Fentanyl

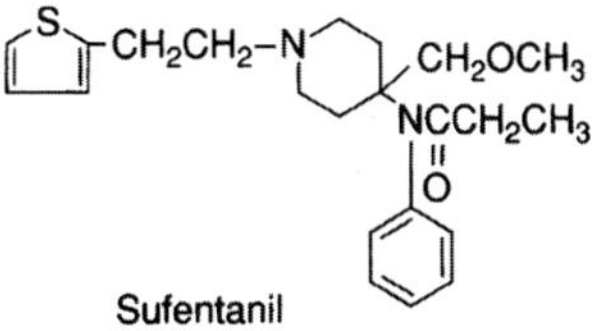

Sufentanil

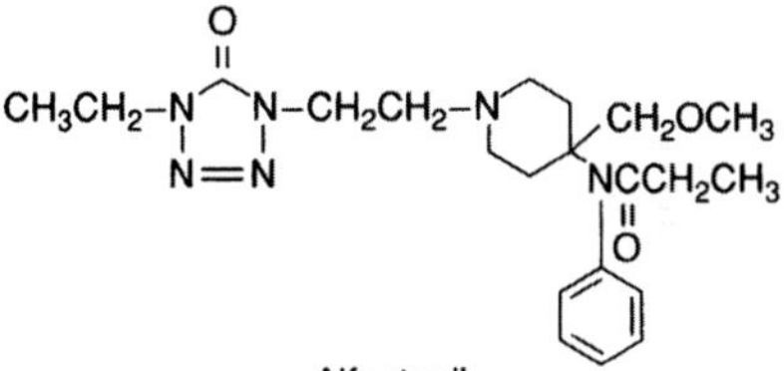

Alfentanil

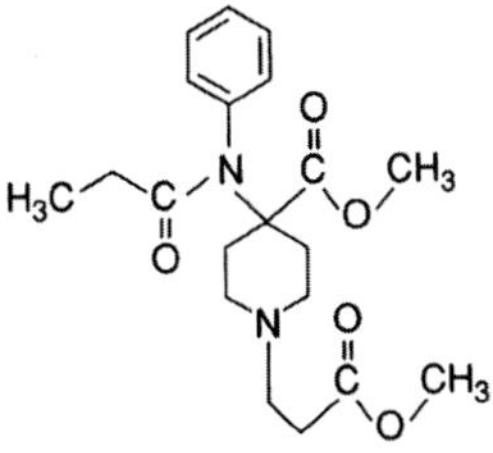

Remifentanil

FIGURE 7-2 Synthetic opioid agonists.

2. The major pharmacodynamic differences between these drugs are potency and rate of equilibration between the plasma and the site of drug effect (biophase).

III. Mechanism of Action
   A. Opioids act as agonists at specific opioid receptors at presynaptic and postsynaptic sites in the central nervous system (mainly the brainstem and spinal cord) as well as in the periphery.
   B. These opioid receptors normally are activated by three endogenous peptide opioid receptor ligands known as *enkephalins*, *endorphins*, and *dynorphins*. (Opioids mimic the actions of these endogenous ligands by binding to opioid receptors, resulting in activation of pain-modulating [antinociceptive] systems.)
      1. The principal effect of opioid receptor activation is a decrease in neurotransmission that occurs largely by presynaptic inhibition of neurotransmitter release (acetylcholine, dopamine, norepinephrine, substance P).
      2. The intracellular biochemical events initiated by occupation of opioid receptors with an opioid agonist are characterized by increased potassium conductance (leading to hyperpolarization), calcium channel inactivation, or both, which produce an immediate decrease in neurotransmitter release.

IV. Opioid Receptors (Table 7-2)
   A. μ Receptors are principally responsible for supraspinal and spinal analgesia.
   B. Respiratory depression characteristic of μ receptor activation is less prominent with κ receptor activation, although dysphoria and diuresis may accompany activation of these receptors.
      1. κ Receptor–mediated analgesia may be less effective for high-intensity painful stimulation than μ opioid–mediated.
      2. Opioid agonist–antagonists often act principally on κ receptors.

V. Common Opioid Side Effects. All opioids possess similar side effects that vary only in degree.
   A. Cardiovascular System
      1. Morphine, even in large doses, given to supine and normovolemic patients is unlikely to cause direct myocardial depression or hypotension.
         a. The same patients changing from a supine to a standing position, however, may manifest orthostatic hypotension and syncope, presumably reflecting morphine-induced impairment of compensatory sympathetic nervous system responses.

Table 7-2

Classification of Opioid Receptors

	Mu$_1$[a]	Mu$_2$[a]	Kappa	Delta
Effect	Analgesia (supraspinal, spinal)	Analgesia (spinal)	Analgesia (supraspinal, spinal)	Analgesia (supraspinal, spinal)
	Euphoria	Depression of ventilation	Dysphoria, sedation	Depression of ventilation
	Low abuse potential	Physical dependence	Low abuse potential	Physical dependence
	Miosis		Miosis	
		Constipation (marked)		Constipation (minimal)
	Bradycardia			
	Hypothermia			
	Urinary retention		Diuresis	Urinary retention
Agonists	Endorphins[b]	Endorphins[b]	Dynorphins	Enkephalins
	Morphine	Morphine		
	Synthetic opioids	Synthetic opioids		
Antagonists	Naloxone	Naloxone	Naloxone	Naloxone
	Naltrexone	Naltrexone	Naltrexone	Naltrexone
	Nalmefene	Nalmefene	Nalmefene	Nalmefene

[a]The existence of specific mu$_1$ and mu$_2$ receptors is not supported based on cloning studies of μ receptors.
[b]μ Receptors seem to be a universal site of action for all endogenous opioid receptors.
Adapted from Atcheson R, Lambert DG. Update on opioid receptors. *Br J Anaesth.* 1994;73:132–134.

    b. Morphine can also evoke decreases in systemic blood pressure due to drug-induced bradycardia (stimulation of the vagal nuclei in the medulla, direct depressant effect on the sinoatrial node) or histamine release (not all patients respond to morphine infusion with the release of histamine, emphasizing the individual variability). In contrast to morphine, the infusion of fentanyl does not cause release of histamine in any patient.

  2. Morphine does not sensitize the heart to catecholamines or otherwise predispose to cardiac dysrhythmias as long as hypercarbia or arterial hypoxemia does not result from ventilatory depression.

  3. During anesthesia, opioids are commonly administered with inhaled or intravenous anesthetics to ensure amnesia.

    a. The combination of an opioid agonist such as morphine or fentanyl with nitrous oxide results in cardiovascular depression (decreased cardiac output and systemic blood pressure plus increased cardiac filling pressures), which does not occur when either drug is administered alone.

    b. Decreases in systemic vascular resistance and systemic blood pressure may accompany the combination of an opioid and a benzodiazepine, whereas these effects do not accompany the administration of either drug alone.

  4. Opioids have been increasingly recognized as playing a role in protecting the myocardium from ischemia.

B. **Ventilation**

  1. All opioid agonists produce dose-dependent and gender-specific depression of ventilation, primarily through an agonist effect at mu_2 receptors, leading to a direct depressant effect on brainstem ventilation centers. Because analgesic and ventilatory effects of opioids occur by similar mechanisms, it is assumed that equianalgesic doses of all opioids will produce some degree of ventilatory depression and reversal of ventilatory depression with an opioid antagonist always involves some reversal of analgesia.

    a. Opioid-induced depression of ventilation is characterized by decreased responsiveness of these ventilation centers to carbon dioxide as reflected by an increase in the resting $Paco_2$ and displacement of the carbon dioxide response curve to the right.

    b. Death from an opioid overdose is almost invariably due to depression of ventilation.

2. Clinically, depression of ventilation produced by opioids manifests as a decreased frequency of breathing that is often accompanied by a compensatory increase in tidal volume (incompleteness of this compensatory increase in tidal volume is evidenced by predictable increases in the $Paco_2$).

C. **Central Nervous System**

1. In the absence of hypoventilation, opioids decrease cerebral blood flow and possibly intracranial pressure (ICP) (use with caution in patients with head injury).

2. **Rigidity**. Rapid intravenous (IV) administration of large doses of an opioid (particularly fentanyl and its derivatives as used in cardiac surgery) can lead to generalized skeletal muscle rigidity.

3. **Sedation**. Postoperative titration of morphine frequently induces sedation that precedes the onset of analgesia. The usual recommendation for morphine titration includes a short interval between boluses (5 to 7 minutes) to allow evaluation of its clinical effect.

4. **Nausea and Vomiting**. Opioid-induced nausea and vomiting are caused by direct stimulation of the chemoreceptor trigger zone in the floor of the fourth ventricle. Morphine may also cause nausea and vomiting by increasing gastrointestinal secretions and delaying passage of intestinal contents toward the colon.

5. **Placental Transfer**. Opioids are readily transported across the placenta (depression of the neonate can occur).

6. **Overdose**

a. The principal manifestation of opioid overdose is depression of ventilation, manifesting as a slow breathing frequency, which may progress to apnea (triad of miosis, hypoventilation, and coma should suggest overdose with an opioid).

b. Treatment of opioid overdose is mechanical ventilation of the patient's lungs with oxygen and administration of an opioid antagonist such as naloxone (may precipitate acute withdrawal in dependent patients).

7. **Pharmacodynamic tolerance and physical dependence** with repeated opioid administration are characteristics of all opioid agonists and are among the major limitations of their clinical use.

a. Physical dependence on morphine usually requires about 25 days to develop.

b. When physical dependence is established, discontinuation of the opioid agonist produces a typical withdrawal abstinence syndrome (Table 7-3).

Table 7-3			
Time Course of Opioid Withdrawal			
Opioid	**Onset**	**Peak Intensity**	**Duration**
Meperidine	2–6 h	6–12 h	4–5 days
Fentanyl	2–6 h	6–12 h	4–5 days
Morphine	6–18 h	36–72 h	7–10 days
Heroin	6–18 h	36–72 h	7–10 days
Methadone	24–48 h	3–21 days	6–7 weeks

Adapted from Mitra S, Sinatra RS. Perioperative management of acute pain in the opioid-dependent patient. *Anesthesiology.* 2004;101:212–227.

VI. **Opioid Agonists (see Table 7-1).** The most notable feature of the clinical use of opioids is the extraordinary variation in dose requirements for effective treatment of pain.

A. **Morphine** is the prototype opioid agonist to which all other opioids are compared, producing analgesia, euphoria, sedation, nausea, and pruritus (especially in the cutaneous areas around the nose) (see Fig. 7-1). The cause of pain persists, but even low doses of morphine increase the threshold to pain and modify the perception of noxious stimulation such that it is no longer experienced as pain (continuous, dull pain is relieved by morphine more effectively than is sharp, intermittent pain). In contrast to nonopioid analgesics, morphine is effective against pain arising from the viscera. Analgesia is most prominent when morphine is administered before the painful stimulus occurs (in the absence of pain, however, morphine may produce dysphoria rather than euphoria).

1. **Pharmacokinetics**

   a. Morphine is well absorbed after intramuscular (IM) administration, with onset of effect in 15 to 30 minutes, a peak effect in 45 to 90 minutes and a clinical duration about 4 hours.

   b. Morphine is usually administered IV in the perioperative period, thus eliminating the unpredictable influence of drug absorption. The peak effect (equilibration time between the blood and brain) after IV administration of morphine is delayed compared with opioids such as fentanyl and alfentanil, requiring about 15 to 30 minutes (Table 7-4).

Table 7-4

Pharmacokinetics of Opioid Agonists

	pK	Percent Nonionized (pH 7.4)	Protein Binding (%)	Clearance (mL/min)	Volume of Distribution (L)	Partition Coefficient	Elimination Half-Time (h)	Context Sensitive Half-Time: 4-Hour Infusion (min)	Effect-Site (Blood–Brain) Equilibration Time (min)
Morphine	7.9	23	35	1,050	224	1	1.7–3.3		
Meperidine	8.5	7	70	1,020	305	32	3–5		
Fentanyl	8.4	8.5	84	1,530	335	955	3.1–6.6	260	6.8
Sufentanil	8.0	20	93	900	123	1,727	2.2–4.6	30	6.2
Alfentanil	6.5	89	92	238	27	129	1.4–1.5	60	1.4
Remifentanil	7.3	58	66–93	4,000	30		0.17–0.33	4	1.1

    c. Only a small amount of administered morphine gains access to the central nervous system (CNS) (estimated that <0.1% of morphine that is administered IV has entered the CNS at the time of peak plasma concentrations).

  2. **Metabolism** of morphine is primarily through conjugation with glucuronic acid in hepatic and extrahepatic sites, especially the kidneys (about 75% to 85% of a dose of morphine appears as morphine-3-glucuronide [pharmacologically inactive], and 5% to 10% as morphine-6-glucuronide [pharmacologically active with an analgesic potency 650-fold higher than morphine]).

  3. **Elimination Half-Time** (see Table 7-4). The decrease in the plasma concentration of morphine after initial distribution of the drug is principally due to metabolism because only a small amount of unchanged opioid is excreted in the urine. Concentrations of morphine in the colostrum of parturients receiving patient-controlled analgesia with morphine are low and it is unlikely that significant amounts of drug will be transferred to the breast-fed neonate.

B. **Meperidine** is a synthetic opioid agonist at μ and κ opioid receptors (analogues of meperidine include fentanyl, sufentanil, alfentanil, and remifentanil). Meperidine shares several structural features that are present in local anesthetics and structurally is similar to atropine (possesses a mild atropine-like antispasmodic effect on smooth muscle).

  1. **Pharmacokinetics**. Meperidine is about one-tenth as potent as morphine producing equivalent sedation, euphoria, nausea, vomiting, and depression of ventilation with a duration of action of 2 to 4 hours.

  2. **Metabolism** is extensive, with about 90% of the drug initially undergoing demethylation to normeperidine and hydrolysis to meperidinic acid. Normeperidine (one-half as active as an analgesic) subsequently undergoes hydrolysis to normeperidinic acid. Normeperidine toxicity manifesting as myoclonus and seizures is most likely during prolonged administration (3 days) of meperidine as during patient-controlled analgesia, especially in the presence of impaired renal function.

  3. **Elimination half-time** of meperidine is 3 to 5 hours (see Table 7-4).

  4. **Clinical Uses**

    a. The clinical use of meperidine has declined greatly in recent years patient-controlled analgesia with meperidine cannot be recommended because of possible normeperidine toxicity.

    b. Meperidine may be effective in suppressing postoperative shivering that may result in detrimental increases in metabolic oxygen consumption (antishivering effects may reflect stimulation of κ receptors)

  5. **Side effects** of meperidine generally resemble those described for morphine, but meperidine, in contrast to morphine, rarely causes bradycardia but instead may increase heart rate, reflecting its modest atropine-like qualities. Large doses of meperidine result in decreases in myocardial contractility, which, among opioids, is unique for this drug.

C. **Fentanyl** is a phenylpiperidine-derivative synthetic opioid agonist that is structurally related to meperidine. As an analgesic, fentanyl is 75 to 125 times more potent than morphine.

  1. **Pharmacokinetics**

    a. A single dose of fentanyl administered IV has a more rapid onset and shorter duration of action than morphine. Despite the clinical impression that fentanyl produces a rapid onset, there is a distinct time lag between the peak plasma fentanyl concentration and peak slowing on the electroencephalogram (EEG) (reflects the effect-site equilibration time between blood and the brain for fentanyl, which is 6.4 minutes). The greater potency and more rapid onset of action reflect the across the blood–brain barrier.

    b. The lungs also serve as a large inactive storage site, with an estimated 75% of the initial fentanyl dose undergoing first-pass pulmonary uptake. (This nonrespiratory function of the lungs limits the initial amount of drug that reaches the systemic circulation and may play an important role in determining the pharmacokinetic profile of fentanyl.)

  2. **Metabolism**. Fentanyl is extensively metabolized by *N*-demethylation and the pharmacologic activity of fentanyl metabolites is believed to be minimal.

  3. **Elimination Half-Time**

    a. Despite the clinical impression that fentanyl has a short duration of action, its elimination half-time is longer than that for morphine (see Table 7-4). This longer elimination half-time reflects a larger volume of distribution (Vd) of fentanyl due to its greater lipid solubility and thus more rapid passage into highly vascular tissues compared with the less lipid-soluble morphine (more than 80% of the injected dose leaves the plasma in <5 minutes).

b. The plasma concentrations of fentanyl are maintained by slow reuptake from inactive tissue sites, which accounts for persistent drug effects that parallel the prolonged elimination half-time.

c. A prolonged elimination half-time for fentanyl in elderly patients is due to decreased clearance of the opioid because Vd is not changed in comparison with younger adults.

4. **Context-Sensitive Half-Time.** As the duration of continuous infusion of fentanyl increases beyond about 2 hours, the context-sensitive half-time of this opioid becomes greater than sufentanil (Fig. 7-3). This reflects saturation of inactive tissue sites with fentanyl during prolonged infusions and return of the opioid from peripheral compartments to the plasma. This tissue reservoir of fentanyl replaces fentanyl eliminated by hepatic metabolism so as to slow the rate of decrease in the plasma concentration of fentanyl when the infusion is discontinued.

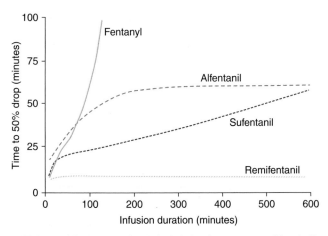

FIGURE 7-3 Computer simulation–derived context-sensitive half-times (time necessary for the plasma concentration to decrease 50% after discontinuation of the infusion) as a function of the duration of the IV infusion. (From Egan TD, Lemmens HJM, Fiset P, et al. The pharmacokinetics of the new short-acting opioid remifentanil [GI87084B] in healthy adult male volunteers. *Anesthesiology.* 1993;79:881–892, with permission.)

Table 7-5

Clinical Uses of Fentanyl

Analgesia (1–2 μg/kg IV)
Adjuvant to inhaled anesthetics to blunt the response to direct
    laryngoscopy or sudden changes in the level of surgical stimu-
    lation (2–20 μg/kg IV) (consider effect-site equilibration time)
Decrease doses of inhaled anesthetics needed to blunt sym-
    pathetic nervous system responses to surgical stimulation
    (1.5–3 μg/kg IV 5 min before induction of anesthesia)
Produce surgical anesthesia (50–150 μg/kg IV)
Analgesia for early labor (25 μg intrathecal)
Preoperative medication (transmucosal)
Postoperative analgesia (transdermal patch)

---

5. **Clinical Uses** (Table 7-5)
6. **Side effects** of fentanyl resemble those of morphine
    (persistent or recurrent depression of ventilation).
    a. **Cardiovascular Effects.** Unlike morphine, fentanyl,
        even in large doses (50 μg/kg IV), does not evoke the
        release of histamine. Bradycardia is more promi-
        nent with fentanyl than morphine and may lead to
        occasional decreases in blood pressure and cardiac
        output.
    b. **Seizure Activity.** In the absence of EEG evidence of
        seizure activity, it is difficult to distinguish opioid-in-
        duced skeletal muscle rigidity or myoclonus from
        seizure activity.
    c. **Intracranial Pressure.** Administration of fentanyl
        and sufentanil to head injury patients has been asso-
        ciated with modest increases (6 to 9 mm Hg) in ICP
        despite maintenance of an unchanged $Paco_2$.
7. **Drug Interactions**
    a. Analgesic concentrations of fentanyl greatly
        potentiate the effects of benzodiazepines (marked
        synergism with respect to hypnosis and depression of
        ventilation).
    b. In clinical practice, the advantage of synergy between
        opioids and benzodiazepines for the maintenance
        of patient comfort is carefully weighed against the
        disadvantages of the potentially adverse depressant
        effects of this combination.

D. **Sufentanil** is a thienyl analogue of fentanyl with an analgesic potency of sufentanil that is 5 to 10 times that of fentanyl.

1. **Pharmacokinetics**
   a. The elimination half-time of sufentanil is intermediate between that of fentanyl and alfentanil (see Table 7-4).
   b. A high tissue affinity is consistent with the lipophilic nature of sufentanil, which permits rapid penetration of the blood–brain barrier and onset of CNS effects (effect-site equilibration time of 6.2 minutes is similar to that of 6.8 minutes for fentanyl).
   c. A rapid redistribution to inactive tissue sites terminates the effect of small doses, but a cumulative drug effect can accompany large or repeated doses of sufentanil.

2. **Metabolism.** Sufentanil is rapidly metabolized by N-dealkylation and the products are pharmacologically inactive, whereas desmethyl sufentanil has about 10% of the activity of sufentanil.

3. **Context-sensitive half-time** of sufentanil is less than that for alfentanil for continuous infusions of up to 8 hours in duration (see Fig. 7-3).
   a. After termination of a sufentanil infusion, the decrease in the plasma drug concentration is accelerated by metabolism and by continued redistribution of sufentanil into peripheral tissue compartments.
   b. Compared with alfentanil, sufentanil may have a more favorable recovery profile when used over a longer period of time. Conversely, alfentanil has a pharmacokinetic advantage for the treatment of discrete and transient noxious stimuli because its short effect-site equilibration time allows rapid access of the drug to the brain and facilitates titration.

4. **Clinical Uses**
   a. A single dose of sufentanil, 0.1 to 0.4 µg/kg IV, produces a longer period of analgesia and less depression of ventilation than does a comparable dose of fentanyl (1 to 4 µg/kg IV).
   b. Compared with large doses of morphine or fentanyl, sufentanil, 18.9 µg/kg IV, results in more rapid induction of anesthesia, earlier emergence from anesthesia, and earlier tracheal extubation.
   c. Bradycardia produced by sufentanil may be sufficient to decrease cardiac output.

E. **Alfentanil** is an analogue of fentanyl that is less potent
(one-fifth to one-tenth) and has one-third the duration of
action of fentanyl (see Fig. 7-2). A unique advantage of alfentanil compared with fentanyl and sufentanil is the more
rapid onset of action (rapid effect-site equilibration) after
the IV administration of alfentanil.

   1. **Pharmacokinetics**
      a. Alfentanil has a short elimination half-time com-
         pared with fentanyl and sufentanil (see Table 7-4).
      b. Despite its lesser lipid solubility, penetration of the
         blood–brain barrier by alfentanil is rapid because of
         its large nonionized fraction at physiologic pH.

   2. **Metabolism**
      a. The efficiency of hepatic metabolism is emphasized
         by clearance of about 96% of alfentanil from the
         plasma within 60 minutes of its administration.
      b. Attempts to develop reliable infusion regimens to
         attain and maintain specific plasma concentra-
         tions of alfentanil have been confounded by the
         10-fold interindividual variability in alfentanil
         pharmacokinetics.
      c. Alfentanil clearance is markedly influenced by
         CYP3A activity.

   3. **Context-Sensitive Half-Time**
      a. The context-sensitive half-time of alfentanil is actu-
         ally longer than that of sufentanil for infusions up to
         8 hours in duration (see Fig. 7-3).
      b. Despite the short elimination half-time of alfentanil,
         it may not necessarily be a superior choice to sufenta-
         nil for ambulatory sedation techniques.

   4. **Clinical Uses**
      a. Alfentanil has a rapid onset and offset of intense an-
         algesia, reflecting its very prompt effect-site equilibra-
         tion. This characteristic of alfentanil used to provide
         analgesia (15 μg/kg IV, about 90 seconds before) is
         acute but transient (laryngoscopy and tracheal intu-
         bation, performance of a retrobulbar block).
      b. Alfentanil, compared with equipotent doses of
         fentanyl and sufentanil, is associated with a lower
         incidence of postoperative nausea and vomiting in
         outpatients.

F. **Remifentanil** is a selective μ opioid agonist with an analgesic potency similar to that of fentanyl (15 to 20 times
as potent as alfentanil) and a blood–brain equilibration
(effect-site equilibration) time similar to that of alfentanil

(Table 7-4). Although chemically related to the fentanyl family of short-acting phenylpiperidine derivatives, remifentanil is structurally unique because of its ester linkage structure that renders it susceptible to hydrolysis by nonspecific plasma and tissue esterases to inactive metabolites. This unique pathway of metabolism leads to (a) brief action, (b) precise and rapidly titratable effect due to its rapid onset and offset, (c) lack of accumulation, and (d) rapid recovery after discontinuation of its administration.

1. **Pharmacokinetics** of remifentanil are characterized by small Vd, rapid clearance, and low interindividual variability compared to other IV anesthetic drugs (means that remifentanil will accumulate less than other opioids) (see Table 7-4).

   a. Because of its rapid systemic clearance, remifentanil provides pharmacokinetic advantages in clinical situations requiring predictable termination of drug effect.

   b. The combination of rapid clearance and small Vd produces a drug with a uniquely transient effect (context-sensitive half-time of the remifentanil plasma concentration is nearly independent of the infusion duration) (see Fig. 7-3).

2. **Metabolism**. Remifentanil is unique among the opioids in undergoing metabolism by nonspecific plasma and tissue esterases to inactive metabolites.

   a. Remifentanil does not appear to be a substrate for butyrylcholinesterases (pseudocholinesterase), and thus its clearance should not be affected by cholinesterase deficiency or anticholinergics.

   b. It is likely that remifentanil's pharmacokinetics will be unchanged by renal or hepatic failure because esterase metabolism is usually preserved in these states.

3. **Elimination Half-Time**. An estimated 99.8% of remifentanil is eliminated during the distribution (0.9 minute) and elimination (6.3 minutes) half-time.

4. **Context-sensitive half-time** for remifentanil is independent of the duration of infusion and is estimated to be about 4 minutes (rapid clearance is responsible for the lack of accumulation even during prolonged periods of infusion) (see Table 7-4) (Fig. 7-4).

5. **Clinical uses** of remifentanil reflect the unique pharmacokinetics of this drug, which allows rapid onset of drug effect, precise titration to the desired effect, the

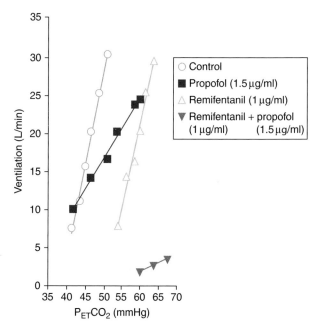

FIGURE 7-4 Ventilatory response curves from one individual. The combined administration of remifentanil and propofol decreased the slope of the carbon dioxide response curve and caused a rightward shift. (From Niewenhuijs DJ, Olofsen E, Romberd RR, et al. Response surface modeling of remifentanil-propofol interaction on cardiorespiratory control and bispectral index. *Anesthesiology.* 2003;98:312–322, with permission.)

ability to maintain a sufficient effect-site concentration to suppress the stress response, and rapid recovery from the drug's effects.
a. Anesthesia can be induced with remifentanil, 1 μg/kg IV, administered over 60 to 90 seconds.
b. Remifentanil, 0.05 to 0.10 μg/kg/min in combination with midazolam, 2 mg IV, provides effective sedation and analgesia during monitored anesthesia care in otherwise healthy adult patients (midazolam also produces a dose-dependent potentiation of remifentanil's depressant effect on breathing rate).

6. **Side Effects**
   a. The advantage of remifentanil possessing a short recovery period may be considered a disadvantage if the infusion is stopped suddenly, whether it be deliberate or accidental (it is important to administer a longer acting opioid for postoperative analgesia).
   b. Nausea and vomiting, depression of ventilation, and mild decreases in systemic blood pressure and heart rate may accompany the administration of remifentanil.
7. **Hyperalgesia.** Postoperative analgesic requirements in patients receiving relatively large doses of remifentanil intraoperatively are often surprisingly high, suggesting remifentanil may be associated with acute opioid tolerance (Fig. 7-5).

G. **Codeine** is the result of the substitution of a methyl group for the hydroxyl group on the number 3 carbon of morphine (see Fig. 7-1). The presence of this methyl group limits first-pass hepatic metabolism and accounts for the efficacy of codeine when administered orally. About 10% of administered codeine is demethylated in the liver to morphine, which may be responsible for the analgesic effect of

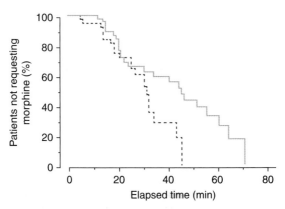

FIGURE 7-5 Cumulative curves for patients who did not request an additional morphine injection following discontinuation of remifentanil *(dashed line)* or desflurane *(solid line)*. (From Guignard B, Bossard AE, Coste C, et al. Acute opioid tolerance: intraoperative remifentanil increases postoperative pain and morphine requirement. *Anesthesiology.* 2000;93:409–417, with permission.)

codeine, although codeine-6-glucuronide may also exert an analgesic effect.

1. Codeine is effective at suppressing cough at oral doses of 15.
2. Maximal analgesia, equivalent to that produced by 650 mg of aspirin, occurs with 60 mg of codeine. When administered IM, 120 mg of codeine is equivalent in analgesic effect to 10 mg of morphine.
3. Most often, codeine is included in medications as an antitussive or is combined with nonopioid analgesics for the treatment of mild to moderate pain.

H. **Hydromorphone** is a derivative of morphine that is about five times as potent as morphine but has a slightly shorter duration of action. Hydromorphone is an effective alternative to morphine in the treatment of opioid-responsive moderate to severe pain.

I. **Oxymorphone** is about 10 times as potent as morphine and seems to cause more nausea and vomiting. The potential for physical dependence is great.

J. **Oxycodone** is commonly used orally for treating acute pain (about twice as potent as oral morphine and has a similar duration of analgesic action). Abuse potential is but new, abuse-resistant formulations that are not easily solubilized for IV injection are now widely marketed.

K. **Hydrocodone** is a commonly used oral opioid for treating acute pain and is similar in potency to oral morphine and has a similar duration of analgesic action (high abuse potential).

L. **Methadone** is a synthetic opioid agonist that produces analgesia in the setting of chronic pain syndromes and is highly effective by the oral route. The efficient oral absorption, prompt onset of action, and prolonged duration of action of methadone render this an attractive drug for suppression of withdrawal symptoms in physically dependent persons such as heroin addicts.

M. **Tramadol** is a centrally acting analgesic that is 5 to 10 times less potent than morphine in volunteers; naloxone antagonized only an estimated 30% of the effect of tramadol.

N. **Heroin** (diacetylmorphine) is a synthetic opioid produced by acetylation of morphine. When administered parenterally, there is rapid penetration of heroin into the brain (reflects lipid solubility), where it is hydrolyzed to the active metabolites monoacetylmorphine and morphine. Compared with morphine, parenteral heroin has a (a) more rapid onset, (b) less opioid-induced nausea, and (c) greater potential for physical dependency.

VII. Opioid Agonist–Antagonists (Fig. 7-6). These drugs bind to μ receptors, where they produce limited responses (partial agonists) or no effect (competitive antagonists). Antagonist properties of these drugs can attenuate the efficacy of subsequently administered opioid agonists. The side effects are similar to those of opioid agonists, and, in addition, these drugs may cause dysphoric reactions. The advantages of opioid agonist–antagonists are the ability to produce analgesia with limited depression of ventilation and a low potential to produce physical dependence. In general, agonist–antagonist drugs should be reserved for patients who are unable to tolerate a pure agonist.

  A. **Pentazocine** possesses opioid agonist actions (antagonized by naloxone) as well as weak antagonist actions (sufficient to precipitate withdrawal symptoms when administered

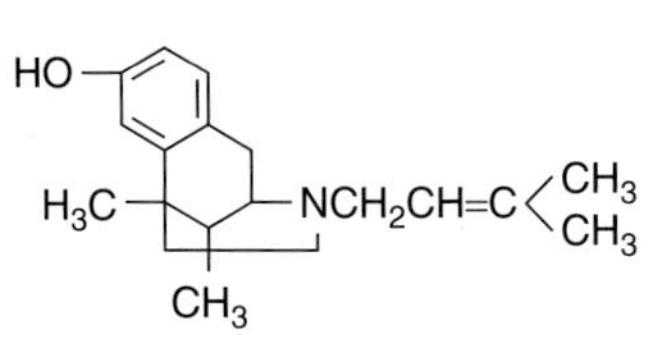

Pentazocine

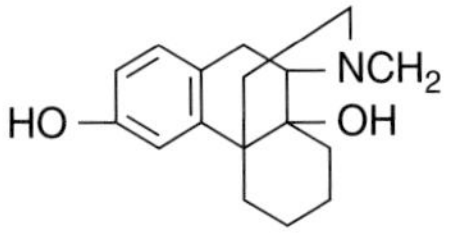

Butorphanol

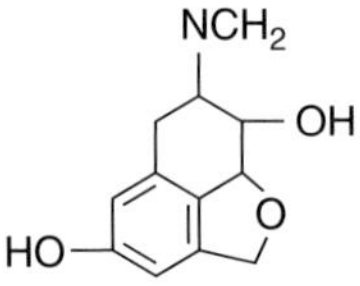

Nalbuphine

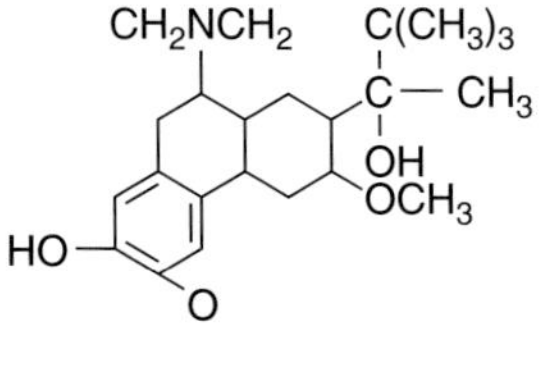

Buprenorphine

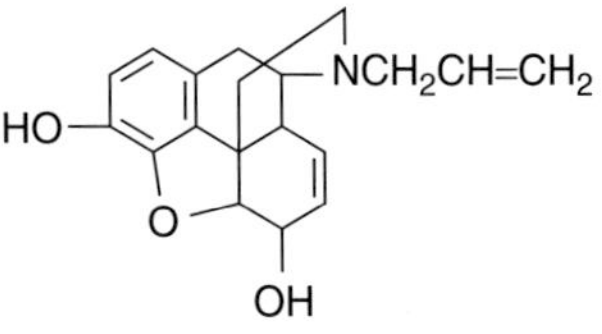

Nalorphine

FIGURE 7-6 Opioid agonist–antagonists.

to patients who have been receiving opioids on a regular basis).

1. **Pharmacokinetics** is well absorbed after oral or parenteral administration. First-pass hepatic metabolism is extensive, with only about 20% of an oral dose entering the circulation.

2. **Clinical Uses**
   a. Pentazocine, 10 to 30 mg IV or 50 mg orally, is used most often for the relief of moderate pain. An oral dose of 50 mg is equivalent in analgesic potency to 60 mg of codeine.
   b. Pentazocine is useful for treatment of chronic pain when there is a high risk of physical dependence.

3. **Side Effects**
   a. The most common side effect of pentazocine is sedation.
   b. Nausea and vomiting are less common than with morphine.
   c. Dysphoria, including fear of impending death, is associated with high doses.
   d. Pentazocine, 20 to 30 mg IM, produces analgesia, sedation, and depression of ventilation similar to 10 mg of morphine.

B. **Butorphanol**
   1. Compared with pentazocine, butorphanol's agonist effects are about 20 times greater, whereas its antagonist actions are 10 to 30 times greater.
   2. Butorphanol is rapidly and almost completely absorbed after IM injection.
   3. In postoperative patients, 2 to 3 mg IM produces analgesia and depression of ventilation similar to 10 mg of morphine.
   4. **Side Effects.** Common side effects of butorphanol include sedation, nausea, and diaphoresis. Dysphoria is infrequent after administration of butorphanol.

VIII. **Opioid Antagonists (Fig. 7-7). Minor changes in the structure of an opioid agonist can convert the drug into an opioid antagonist at one or more of the opioid receptor sites. Naloxone, naltrexone, and nalmefene are pure μ opioid receptor antagonists with no agonist activity.**

A. **Naloxone** is a nonselective antagonist at all three opioid (1 to 4 μg/kg IV reverses opioid-induced analgesia and depression of ventilation). The short duration of action of naloxone (30 to 45 minutes) is presumed to be due to its rapid removal from the brain (emphasizes that

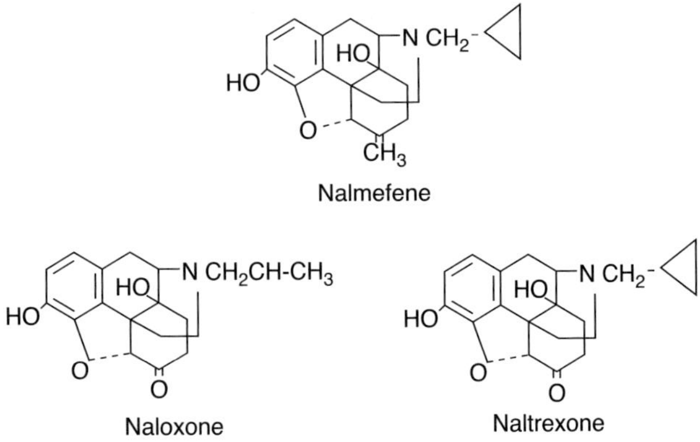

FIGURE 7-7 Opioid antagonists.

supplemental doses of naloxone will likely be necessary for sustained antagonism of opioid agonists). In this regard, a continuous infusion of naloxone, 5 μg/kg/hour, prevents depression of ventilation without altering analgesia produced by neuraxial opioids (190).

1. **Side Effects**
   a. Antagonism of opioid-induced depression of ventilation is accompanied by an inevitable reversal of analgesia. It may be possible, however, to titrate the dose of naloxone such that depression of ventilation is partially but acceptably antagonized to also maintain partial analgesia.
   b. Nausea and vomiting appear to be closely related to the dose and speed of injection of naloxone.
   c. Cardiovascular stimulation reflected as increased sympathetic nervous system activity may manifest as tachycardia, hypertension, pulmonary edema, and cardiac dysrhythmia. Even ventricular fibrillation has occurred after the IV administration of naloxone and the associated sudden increase in sympathetic nervous system activity.

2. **Antagonism of General Anesthesia**. A role of endorphins in the production of general anesthesia is not supported by data demonstrating a failure of naloxone to alter anesthetic requirements (minimum alveolar concentration [MAC]) in animals.

B. **Naltrexone**, in contrast to naloxone, is highly effective orally, producing sustained antagonism of the effects of opioid agonists for as long as 24 hours.

IX. **Opioid Allergy.** Although many patients claim "allergies" to opioids, true opioid allergy is rare. More often, predictable side effects of opioids such as localized histamine release, orthostatic hypotension, nausea, and vomiting are misinterpreted as an allergic reaction.

X. **Anesthetic Requirements.** The contribution of opioids to total anesthetic requirements can be estimated by determining the decrease in MAC of a volatile anesthetic in the presence of opioids.

XI. **Patient-Controlled Analgesia.** As an alternative to intermittent bolus dosing of medication, patients may be provided with a mechanism to address their own analgesic requirements (patient-controlled analgesia [PCA]). Rather than wide swings between inadequate analgesia and oversedation, the PCA regimen is designed to allow patients to self-titrate their dosing to optimize their pain management (Table 7-6 and Fig. 7-8).

XII. **Neuraxial Opioids.** Placement of opioids in the epidural or subarachnoid space to manage acute or chronic pain is based on the knowledge that opioid receptors (principally μ receptors) are present in the substantia gelatinosa of the spinal cord.
   A. **Pharmacokinetics**
      1. Opioids placed in the epidural space may undergo uptake into epidural fat, systemic absorption, or diffusion across the dura into the cerebrospinal fluid (CSF). Epidural administration of opioids produces considerable CSF concentrations of drug.
      2. Epidural administration of morphine, fentanyl, and sufentanil produces opioid blood concentrations that are similar to those produced by an intramuscular injection of an equivalent dose.
      3. Cephalad movement of opioids in the CSF principally depends on lipid solubility. (Lipid-soluble opioids such as fentanyl and sufentanil are limited in their cephalad migration by uptake into the spinal cord, whereas less lipid-soluble morphine remains in the CSF for transfer to more cephalad locations.)

Table 7-6

Suggested Starting Intravenous Patient-Controlled Analgesia Opioid Regimens

Drug	Basal Rate[a]	Bolus Dose	Bolus Interval (min)
Morphine	0–2 mg/h	1–2 mg	6–10
Hydromorphone	0–0.4 mg/h	0.2–0.4 mg	6–10
Fentanyl	0–60 µg/h	20–50 µg	5–10

[a]Basal infusions are not typically recommended for opioid-naive patients.

B. **Side Effects**

1. **Pruritus** induced by neuraxial opioids is likely due to cephalad migration of the opioid in CSF and subsequent interaction with opioid receptors in the trigeminal nucleus.

2. **Urinary Retention**. In humans, epidural morphine causes marked detrusor muscle relaxation within 15 minutes of injection that persists for up to 16 hours; it is readily reversed *with naloxone*.

3. **Depression of ventilation** is the most serious side effect of neuraxial (may occur within minutes of administration or may be delayed for hours). The incidence of ventilatory depression requiring intervention after conventional doses of neuraxial opioids is about 1%, which is the same as that after conventional doses of IV or IM opioids.

   a. Early depression of ventilation occurs within 2 hours of neuraxial injection of the opioid, whereas delayed depression of ventilation occurs more than 2 hours after neuraxial opioid administration and reflects cephalad migration of the opioid in the CSF and subsequent interaction with opioid receptors located in the ventral medulla.

   b. Factors that increase the risk of delayed depression of ventilation, especially concomitant use of any IV opioid or sedative, must be considered in determining the dose of neuraxial opioid (see Table 7-3).

   c. Pulse oximetry reliably detects opioid-induced arterial hypoxemia, and supplemental oxygen (2 L/min) is an effective treatment. The most reliable clinical sign of depression of ventilation is a depressed level of consciousness, possibly caused by hypercarbia.

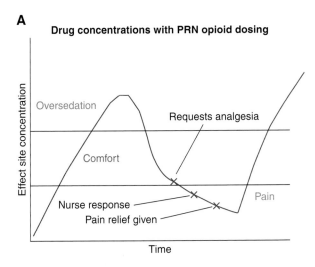

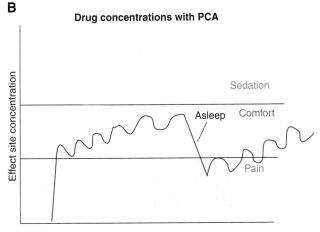

FIGURE 7-8 Effect-site concentrations with traditional versus patient-controlled opioid dosing. After achieving effective concentrations, PCA allows patients to self-titrate opioid dosing to maintain effective analgesia. *PRN*, as needed.

4. **Sedation** after administration of neuraxial opioids appears to be dose related and occurs with all opioids but is most commonly associated with the use of sufentanil. When sedation occurs with neuraxial opioids, depression of ventilation must be considered.
5. **Central Nervous System Excitation**
   a. Tonic skeletal muscle rigidity resembling seizure activity is a well-known side effect of large IV doses of opioids, but this response is rarely observed after neuraxial administration.
   b. Cephalad migration of the opioid in CSF and subsequent interaction with nonopioid receptors in the brainstem or basal ganglia is the most likely explanation for opioid-induced CNS excitation.
6. **Viral Reactivation**. A link exists between the use of epidural morphine in obstetric patients and reactivation of herpes simplex labialis virus.

CHAPTER 8

Centrally Acting Nonopioid Analgesics

I. **Introduction**

   A. Opioid analgesics are widely used drugs for the management of both acute and chronic pain. Side effects of opioids may limit their use and concerns over drug dependence; misuse and abuse sets boundaries on their use.

   B. Nonopioid centrally administered analgesics relieve pain by mechanisms unrelated to opioid receptors; they do not cause respiratory depression, physical dependence, or abuse and are not regulated under the Controlled Substances Act.

   C. In order to minimize the adverse effects of opioid analgesic medications, anesthesiologists and surgeons are increasingly turning to nonopioid analgesic techniques (multimodal analgesia) as adjuvants for managing pain during the perioperative period.

   D. Neuraxial drug administration is a group of techniques that deliver drugs in close proximity to the spinal cord (intrathecally into the cerebrospinal fluid [CSF] or epidurally into the fatty tissues surrounding the dura) by injection or infusion (bypasses the blood–brain barrier, resulting in much higher CSF concentrations while using reduced amounts of medication to achieve equipotent doses).

II. **α_2-Adrenergic Agonists. Epidural or intrathecal administration of α_2-adrenergic agonists provides analgesia by activating α_2-adrenergic receptors (G protein–coupled inhibitory receptors) on the sympathetic preganglionic neurons that mediate a reduction in norepinephrine (NE) release (overall effect is sympatholysis, resulting in analgesia, hypotension, bradycardia, and sedation).**

   A. **Clonidine** acts as a selective partial α_2-receptor agonist.

      1. Neuraxial clonidine (epidural 75 to 150 μg, intrathecal 30 to 60 μg) is an effective analgesic for chronic cancer and noncancer pain as well as for postoperative pain.

      2. Neuraxially administered opioids and α_2 agonists exhibit synergism (addition of clonidine to opioids for

postoperative analgesia as a continuous epidural infusion reduces opioid requirements by 20% to 60%).
   3. Clonidine is a useful adjunct for labor epidural analgesia.
   4. Neuraxial clonidine is indicated for the treatment of intractable pain in cancer patients unresponsive to maximum doses of opioids.
   B. **Dexmedetomidine** has a higher affinity for α_2 receptors than clonidine, produces spinal analgesia as efficiently as clonidine, and is associated with a fewer hemodynamic and systemic side effects.
      1. A dose of 3 μg of intrathecal dexmedetomidine is equipotent to 30 μg of clonidine.
      2. Epidural dexmedetomidine exhibits synergism with local anesthetics, increasing the density of motor block, prolonging the duration of both sensory and motor block, and improving postoperative analgesia.

III. **Neostigmine acts by inhibiting acetylcholinesterase and preventing the breakdown of acetylcholine. Antinociceptive effects are independent of opioid and α_2-receptor systems and are primarily due to stimulation of muscarinic (but not nicotinic) cholinergic receptors.**

IV. Ketamine
   A. Anesthetic and subanesthetic doses of ketamine have analgesic properties as a result of noncompetitive antagonism of N-methyl-D-aspartate (NMDA) receptors.
   B. Neuraxial ketamine must be administered in a preservative-free solution (preservative benzalkonium chloride is neurotoxic).
      1. Combination of epidural ketamine with local anesthetic and/or opioid infusions results in improved analgesia without significantly increasing adverse effects.
      2. Adding low-dose ketamine to a multimodal epidural analgesia regimen provides better postoperative analgesia and reduces morphine consumption in thoracic, upper abdominal, and lower abdominal surgeries.
      3. Ketamine has also shown efficacy in the management of neuropathic pain, and it is believed to work through one or more of these mechanisms. In high doses, ketamine may have additional minor analgesic effects by modulating descending inhibitory pathways through inhibition of reuptake of neurotransmitters.
      4. The advantage of intrathecal ketamine is the lack of cardiovascular effects and respiratory depression. The main

drawbacks of intrathecal ketamine are the frequency of psychomimetic reactions, inadequate motor blockade, and short duration of action.

V. **Midazolam**
   A. Intrathecal midazolam (neurotoxicity a risk) produces analgesia by acting on γ-aminobutyric acid ($GABA_A$) receptors and reducing spinal cord excitability.
   B. Midazolam added to fentanyl–ropivacaine epidural analgesia was associated with a significant reduction in the incidence of postoperative nausea and vomiting (mechanism of antiemetic action unknown) compared with fentanyl–ropivacaine alone.

VI. **Droperidol**
   A. Epidural droperidol is effective for reducing pruritus and postoperative nausea and vomiting.
   B. Long-term administration of intrathecal droperidol is an excellent antiemetic in patients with nonmalignant pain.

VII. **Conclusion**
   A. Neuraxial drug administration via the intrathecal and epidural route remains an important treatment option for the provision of anesthesia as well as analgesia in acute, cancer, and chronic pain.
   B. Additional dose-effect studies are needed for most agents to strengthen our understanding of the safety profile of these drugs when administered neuraxially before they become a part of routine clinical practice.

CHAPTER 9

Peripherally Acting Analgesics

I. **Introduction**
  A. Peripheral analgesics act at the sensory input level by blocking transmission of the impulse to the brain and their common feature was believed to be their site of action within the damaged tissues, and hence they were termed "peripheral analgesics." Experimental and clinical studies support the possibility of central site of action of many of these agents.
  B. Peripheral administration of drugs can potentially optimize drug concentrations at the site of the origin of pain while leading to lower systemic levels and fewer adverse systemic effects and fewer drug interactions.
  C. Nociceptive, inflammatory, and neuropathic pain all depend to some degree on the peripheral activation of primary sensory afferent neurons. Inhibiting the actions of inflammatory mediators (prostanoids, bradykinin, adenosine triphosphate [ATP], histamine, serotonin) represents a strategy for the development of analgesics.
  D. Combinations of agents that act via different mechanisms may be particularly useful.

II. **Nonsteroidal antiinflammatory drugs (NSAIDs) are among the most commonly prescribed drugs in the world (includes aspirin and several other selective and nonselective cyclooxygenase inhibitors with common analgesic, antiinflammatory, and antipyretic properties).**
  A. NSAIDs inhibit the biosynthesis of prostaglandins by preventing the substrate arachidonic acid from binding to the cyclooxygenase (COX) enzyme active site (Fig. 9-1). The COX enzyme exists as COX-1 and COX-2 isoenzymes.
    1. COX-1 is constitutively expressed and catalyzes the production of prostaglandins that are involved in numerous physiologic functions (maintenance of normal renal function in the kidneys, mucosal protection in

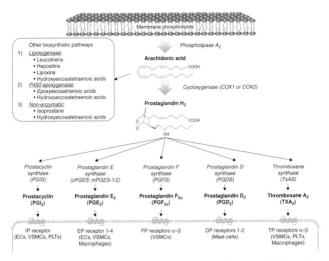

FIGURE 9-1 The cyclooxygenases pathway. *ECs*, endothelial cells; *EP*, PGE$_2$ receptor; *DP*, PGD$_2$ receptor; *FP*, PGF$_{2\alpha}$ receptor; *IP*, prostacyclin receptor; *PLTs*, platelets; *TP*, thromboxane receptor; and *VSMCs*, vascular smooth muscle cells. (Reproduced from Cipollone F, Santovito D. EP receptors and coxibs: seeing the light at the end of the tunnel. *Circ Res.* 2013;113:91–93.)

the gastrointestinal tract, production of proaggregatory thromboxane A$_2$ in the platelets).

2. COX-2 expression can be induced by inflammatory mediators in many tissues and has a role in the mediation of pain, inflammation, and fever.

   a. COX-2 selective inhibitors (known as the "coxibs") have less gastrointestinal toxicity than nonselective NSAIDs. However, increased cardiovascular risk has been associated with the use of this class of drugs (celecoxib is the only COX-2 selective inhibitor available for clinical use).

   b. Coxibs may be a safer alternative to NSAIDs (platelet dysfunction and gastrointestinal toxicity in the perioperative settings); benefits include improved quality of analgesia, reduced incidence of gastrointestinal side effects *versus* conventional NSAIDs, and no platelet inhibition.

III. **NSAIDS belong to a number of chemical families including acetic acids, oxicams, propionic acids, salicylates, fenamates, furanones, and coxibs (Table 9-1). All NSAIDs are weakly acidic chemical compounds and share similarities in pharmacokinetic properties. Gastrointestinal absorption of NSAIDs occurs rapidly, usually within 15 to 30 minutes. The liver metabolizes most NSAIDs, with subsequent excretion into urine or bile (reduced renal function prolongs NSAID half-life and the dose should be lowered proportionally in patients with impaired kidney function, and moderate to severe liver disease impairs NSAID metabolism, increasing the potential for toxicity).**

A. **Side Effects of NSAIDs** (Table 9-2)

1. **Platelet Function.** NSAIDs and aspirin inhibit the activity of COX-1 (thromboxane production), but the COX-2 specific inhibitors have no effect on COX-1 and thus no effect on platelet function.

2. **Gastrointestinal Side Effects.** NSAIDs are associated with a spectrum of upper gastrointestinal complications, ranging from endoscopic ulcers in 10% to 30% of patients to serious ulcer complications in 1% to 2% of patients, including perforation and bleeding (patients with gastrointestinal risk factors should be treated with COX-2 selective agents or nonselective NSAIDs with gastrointestinal protective cotherapy).

3. **Cardiovascular Side Effects.** NSAIDs are associated with an increased risk of cardiovascular adverse events (myocardial infarction, heart failure, hypertension). COX inhibition is likely to disturb the balance between COX-2–mediated production of proaggregatory thromboxane in platelets and antiaggregatory prostaglandin I_2 in endothelial cells.

a. A meta-analysis of randomized trials on nonselective NSAIDs found that high-dose ibuprofen and high-dose diclofenac were associated with a moderately increased risk of vascular events compared with placebo, similar to that observed with COX-2–selective agents.

b. The risks associated with naproxen, although they cannot be completely excluded, appeared to be substantially lower.

4. **Renal Side Effects.** The effects of the NSAIDs on renal function include changes in the excretion of sodium, changes in tubular function, potential for interstitial nephritis, and reversible renal failure due to alterations in filtration rate and renal plasma flow (prostaglandins

Table 9-1

Characteristics of Commonly Prescribed Nonsteroidal Antiinflammatory Drugs

	Dose[a]		Pharmacokinetics	
Generic Name (Trade Name)	Available Dosages (mg)	Common Dosing Intervals	Drug Metabolism	Elimination Half-Life (h)
Nonselective NSAIDs				
Acetic Acid Group				
Diclofenac DR (*Voltaren*)	25 50 75	BID-TID QD-BID	Oxidation	1–2
Diclofenac XR (*Voltaren XR*)	100			
Etodolac (*Lodine*)	200 300 400	BID-TID QD	Oxidation, conjugation	7
Etodolac XL (*Lodine XL*)	500 400 500 600			
Ketorolac IM, IV injection (*generic*)	30	QD-QID	Conjugation	2.5–8.5

Table 9-1

Characteristics of Commonly Prescribed Nonsteroidal Antiinflammatory Drugs *(continued)*

Generic Name (Trade Name)	Dose[a] Available Dosages (mg)	Dose[a] Common Dosing Intervals	Pharmacokinetics Drug Metabolism	Pharmacokinetics Elimination Half-Life (h)
Indomethacin *(Indocin)*	25 50	BID-TID QD-BID	Oxidation, conjugation	4.5–6
Indomethacin SR *(Indocin SR)*	75			
Nabumetone *(Relafen)*	500 750	QD-BID	Oxidation	22–30
Sulindac *(Clinoril)*	150 200	BID	Oxidation, reduction	16
Tolmetin *(Tolectin)*	400 600	TID	Conjugation	5
Oxicam Group				
Meloxicam *(Mobic)*	7.5 15	QD	Oxidation	13–20
Piroxicam *(Feldene)*	10 20	QD	Oxidation	30–86

Table 9-1

Characteristics of Commonly Prescribed Nonsteroidal Antiinflammatory Drugs *(continued)*

Generic Name (Trade Name)	Dose*a*		Pharmacokinetics	
	Available Dosages (mg)	Common Dosing Intervals	Drug Metabolism	Elimination Half-Life (h)
Propionic Acid Group				
Fenoprofen (*Nalfon*)	200 300	TID-QID	Glucuronidation	3
Flurbiprofen (*Ocufen*)	50 100	BID-QID	Oxidation	3–6
Ibuprofen (*Motrin*)	400 600 800	TID-QID	Oxidation	2–2.5
Ketoprofen	50 75	TID-QID QD	Conjugation	2–4 3–7
Ketoprofen CR	100 150 200			
Naproxen (*Naprosyn*)	250 375	BID QD	Conjugation, oxidation	12–15

(continued)

Table 9-1

Characteristics of Commonly Prescribed Nonsteroidal Antiinflammatory Drugs (continued)

Generic Name (Trade Name)	Dose[a] Available Dosages (mg)	Dose[a] Common Dosing Intervals	Pharmacokinetics Drug Metabolism	Pharmacokinetics Elimination Half-Life (h)
(Naprelan)	500 375 500			
Oxaprozin (Daypro)	600	QD-BID	Oxidation, conjugation	50–60
Salicylate				
Aspirin	81	QD	Hydrolysis, conjugation, glucuronidation	0.25–0.5
(Ecotrin, Ascriptin)	325	BID-QID		
Choline magnesium	500	BID-TID		
	500			
Trisalicylate	750		Conjugation	2–12
(Trilisate)	1000			
Cyclooxygenase-2 Agents				
Coxib Group				
Celecoxib	100	QD-BID	Conjugation	11–16
(Celebrex)	200			

[a]A dosage range exists for each NSAID that must be individualized depending on patient characteristics and disease mechanism.
Reproduced from Vincent JL, Abraham E, Moore FA, et al. *Textbook of Critical Care*, 6th ed. Philadelphia, PA: Elsevier Saunders; 2011:1346–1353.

Table 9-2

Adverse Effects of Nonsteroidal Antiinflammatory Drugs

System	Adverse Effects
Cardiovascular	Hypertension, can exacerbate or induce heart failure, thrombotic events, possible increased risk of thrombotic/cardiovascular events with long-term use (use with caution in patients with preexisting disease; more likely with COX-2 inhibitors)
Respiratory	Nasal polyps, rhinitis, dyspnea, bronchospasm, angioedema, may exacerbate asthma
Hepatic	Hepatitis
Gastrointestinal	Gastropathy (can be asymptomatic), gastric bleeding, esophageal disease, pancreatitis
Hematologic	Increased intraoperative bleeding due to platelet inhibition/dysfunction (coxibs do not affect platelet function), will potentiate anticoagulation effect
Dermatologic	Urticaria, erythema multiforme, rash
Genitourinary	Renal insufficiency (use with caution in patients with preexisting renal disease), sodium/fluid retention, papillary necrosis, interstitial nephritis
Central nervous system	Headache, aseptic meningitis, hearing disturbances
Skeletal	Potential to inhibit bone growth/healing/formation
Pharmacologic interactions	NSAIDs displace albumin-bound drugs and can potentiate their effects (e.g., warfarin)

and prostacyclins are important for maintenance of intrarenal blood flow and tubular transport). Avoiding perioperative use of NSAIDs in patients with hypovolemia from any cause is an important means of minimizing renal injury.

5. **Pulmonary Side Effects**
   a. Many adverse reactions attributed to NSAIDs are due to inhibition of prostaglandin synthesis in local

tissues (patients with allergic rhinitis, nasal polyposis, and asthma are at increased risk for anaphylaxis).

b. The use of selective COX-2 inhibitors as an alternative to aspirin and other NSAIDs has been suggested for patients with aspirin-exacerbated respiratory disease.

6. **Hypersensitivity reactions** to NSAIDs rarely occur, and they are more common in individuals with nasal polyps or asthma.

B. **Drug–drug interactions** with NSAID therapy may result from their pharmacodynamic or pharmacokinetic interactions.

1. Nonselective NSAIDs affect other antiplatelet agents *via* additive inhibition of platelet aggregation (result is an increased bleeding risk with the concomitant use of NSAIDs and other antiplatelet agents).

2. NSAIDs decrease lithium clearance and increase serum lithium concentrations by inhibiting renal prostaglandin production and altering intrarenal blood flow.

3. Concurrent administration of digoxin and NSAIDs can decrease renal clearance of digoxin, increase plasma drug concentration, and potentiate digoxin toxicity.

4. NSAIDs interact with anticonvulsant agents (phenytoin and valproic acid) by displacing the anticonvulsants from their protein-binding sites, which increases the free drug concentration.

IV. **Acetaminophen (Tylenol) is a popular antipyretic and analgesic (little, if any, antiinflammatory action) found in many over-the-counter and prescription products.**

A. Acetaminophen is the leading cause of acute liver failure in the United States, and nearly half of acetaminophen-associated cases are due to unintentional overdose.

1. Damage to the liver results from one of acetaminophen's metabolites, N-acetyl-p-benzoquinoneimine (NAPQI). NAPQI leads to liver failure by depleting the liver's natural antioxidant glutathione and directly damaging liver cells, leading to liver failure.

2. Treatment is aimed at removing the paracetamol from the body and replacing glutathione. Acetylcysteine is administered as an antidote and acts as a precursor for glutathione and can neutralize NAPQI directly.

B. Oral acetaminophen has excellent bioavailability. The conventional oral dose of acetaminophen is 325 to 650 mg every 4 to 6 hours; total daily doses should not exceed 4,000 mg.

    C. Acetaminophen is the first-line analgesic in osteoarthritis and particularly valuable for patients in whom aspirin is not recommended.

    D. An intravenous (IV) preparation of acetaminophen is currently available for clinical use.

V. **Acetylsalicylic acid (Aspirin) is the oldest and most widely used medicinal compound in the world, acting as a general analgesic by blocking the action of the COX enzymes and thus prevents the production of prostaglandins (effectively treats headaches, back and muscle pain). Aspirin irreversibly inactivates COX, leading to prolonged inhibition of platelet aggregation.**

    A. **Overdose**

        1. The mechanism of NSAID toxicity in overdose is related to both their acidic nature and their inhibition of prostaglandin production.

        2. Symptoms include nausea, vomiting, abdominal pain, tinnitus, hearing impairment, and central nervous system (CNS) depression (see Table 9-2). With higher dose aspirin ingestion, metabolic acidosis, renal failure, CNS changes (agitation, confusion, coma), and hyperventilation with respiratory alkalosis due to stimulation of the respiratory center occurs. The presence of acidemia permits more salicylic acid to cross the blood–brain barrier.

        3. Management should be directed at symptomatic support (no antidote available), prevention of further absorption, and correction of acid–base imbalance.

            a. Appropriate hydration and activated charcoal should be considered within 1 hour after ingestion.

            b. Urine alkalinization increases salicylate elimination.

VI. **Steroids (Tables 9-3 and 9-4)**

    A. Glucocorticoids have the most powerful antiinflammatory characteristics of all steroids. The primary corticosteroid is hydrocortisone, which is the standard against which the pharmacologic properties of various synthetic corticosteroids are judged. Many synthetic agents that are more potent, have longer durations of action, have greater antiinflammatory activity, and generate fewer unwanted mineralocorticoid side effects than hydrocortisone have been developed.

    B. Mineralocorticoids are adrenal cortical steroid hormones that have a greater effect on water and electrolyte balance. The main endogenous hormone is aldosterone.

Table 9-3

Comparative Pharmacology of Endogenous and Synthetic Corticosteroids

	Antiinflammatory Potency	Sodium Retaining Potency	Equivalent Dose (mg)	Elimination Half-Time (h)	Duration of Action (h)	Route of Administration
Cortisol	1	1	20	1.5–3.0	8–12	Oral, topical, IV, IM, IA
Cortisone	0.8	0.8	25	0.5	8–36	Oral, topical, IV, IM, IA
Prednisolone	4	0.8	5	2–4	12–36	Oral, topical, IV, IM, IA
Prednisone	4	0.8	5	2–4	12–36	Oral
Methylpredniso-lone	5	0.5	4	2–4	12–36	Oral, topical, IV, IM, IA, epidural
Betamethasone	25	0	0.75	5	36–54	Oral, topical, IV, IM, IA
Dexamethasone	25	0	0.75	3.5–5.0	36–54	Oral, topical, IV, IM, IA
Triamcinolone	5	0	4	3.5	12–36	Oral, topical, IV, IM, epidural
Fludrocortisone	10	250	2	—	24	Oral, topical, IV, IM
Aldosterone	0	3,000				

IV, intravenous; IM, intramuscular; IA, intraarticular.

Table 9-4

Potential Side Effects Associated with Corticosteroid Therapy

Dermatologic and Soft Tissue
  Skin thinning and purpura
  Cushingoid appearance
  Alopecia
  Acne
  Hirsutism
  Striae
  Hypertrichosis
Eye
  Posterior subcapsular cataract
  Elevated intraocular pressure/glaucoma
  Exophthalmos
Cardiovascular
  Hypertension
  Perturbations of serum lipoproteins
  Premature atherosclerotic disease
  Arrhythmias with pulse infusions
Gastrointestinal
  Gastritis
  Peptic ulcer disease
  Pancreatitis
  Steatohepatitis
  Visceral perforation

Renal
  Hypokalemia
  Fluid volume shifts
Genitourinary and reproductive
  Amenorrhea/infertility
  Intrauterine growth retardation
Bone
  Osteoporosis
  Avascular necrosis
Muscle
  Myopathy
Neuropsychiatric
  Euphoria
  Dysphoria/depression
  Insomnia/akathisia
  Psychosis
  Pseudo tumor cerebri
Endocrine
  Diabetes mellitus
  Hypothalamic-pituitary–adrenal insufficiency
Infectious disease
  Heightened risk of typical infections
  Opportunistic infections
  Herpes zoster

From Saag KG, Furst D. Major side effects of glucocorticoids. In: Bose BD, ed. *UpToDate*. Waltham, MA: UpToDate; 2004, with permission.

C. There is evidence supporting the use of corticosteroids in multimodal analgesia protocols to contribute to the postoperative recovery of the patient by minimizing opioid doses and, therefore, side effects.

D. Dexamethasone has been found to prolong local anesthetic block duration.

E. Epidural injection of corticosteroids has been used to treat back pain (mainly due to nerve root irritation). The only proven efficacy of epidural steroid injections is their ability to speed resolution of leg pain ("sciatica") in patients with acute intervertebral disc herniation and associated radicular pain.

VII. **Systemic Local Anesthetics**
A. Lidocaine produces analgesia by suppressing the activity of sodium channels in neurons that respond to noxious stimuli, thereby preventing nerve conduction and pain transmission.
B. **Topical application of 5% lidocaine** has been used in postherpetic neuralgia.

VIII. **Ketamine. There has been a renewed interest in the use of subanesthetic doses of ketamine as an adjunct to provide postoperative pain relief in opioid-dependent patients. The usefulness of low-dose ketamine in the perioperative management of the opioid-tolerant patient is in need of further study.**

IX. **Dexmedetomidine's proanesthetic and proanalgesic effects at 0.5 to 2 μg/kg given intravenously stem mainly from its ability to blunt the central sympathetic response by an, as yet, unknown mechanism. Dexmedetomidine, when used as an adjunct, can reduce postoperative morphine consumption in various surgical settings.**

X. **Clonidine in low doses has proved to be a useful adjunct analgesic when given neuraxially and in combination with peripheral nerve blocks.**

XI. **Opioids are potent centrally acting analgesics (injected locally into soft tissues or joints produce potent analgesic effects that are mediated by peripheral opioid receptors, occurring in the absence of central analgesic activity).**

CHAPTER 10

Local Anesthetics

I. Introduction

A. Local anesthetics are used to provide analgesia and anesthesia for various surgical and nonsurgical procedures (acute and chronic pain management, reduce perioperative stress, improve perioperative outcomes, treat dysrhythmias).

B. Local anesthetics produce reversible conduction blockade of impulses along central and peripheral nerve pathways. With progressive increases in concentrations of local anesthetics, the transmission of autonomic, somatic sensory, and somatic motor impulses is interrupted, producing autonomic nervous system blockade, sensory anesthesia, and skeletal muscle paralysis in the area innervated by the affected nerve.

II. Molecular Structure

A. Local anesthetics consist of a lipophilic and a hydrophilic portion separated by a connecting hydrocarbon chain (Fig. 10-1). In almost all instances, an ester (–CO–) or an amide (–NHC–) bond links the hydrocarbon chain to the lipophilic aromatic ring.

B. The nature of the connecting hydrocarbon chain is the basis for classifying drugs that produce conduction blockade of nerve impulses as *ester* local anesthetics or *amide* local anesthetics (Fig. 10-2). The important differences between ester and amide local anesthetics relate to the site of metabolism and the potential to produce allergic reactions.

III. Structure-Activity Relationships

A. Modifying the chemical structure of a local anesthetic alters its pharmacologic effects (Table 10-1).

1. Substituting a butyl group for the amine group on the benzene ring of procaine results in tetracaine. Compared with procaine, tetracaine is more lipid soluble, is 10 times more potent, and has a longer duration of action corresponding to a 4- to 5-fold decrease in the rate of metabolism.

199

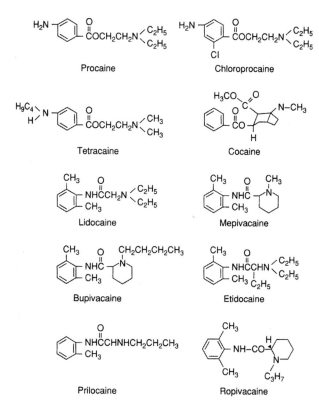

FIGURE 10-1 Local anesthetics consist of a lipophilic and hydrophilic portion separated by a connecting hydrocarbon chain.

FIGURE 10-2 Ester and amide local anesthetics. Mepivacaine, bupivacaine, and ropivacaine are chiral drugs because the molecules possess an asymmetric carbon atom.

Table 10-1

Comparative Pharmacology of Local Anesthetics

Classification	Potency	Onset	Duration after Infiltration (min)	Maximum Single Dose for Infiltration (mg)	Toxic Plasma Concentration (µg/mL)	pK	Protein Binding (%)
Esters							
Procaine	1	Slow	45–60	500		8.9	6
Chloroprocaine	4	Rapid	30–45	600		8.7	
Tetracaine	16	Slow	60–180	100 (topical)		8.5	76
Amides							
Lidocaine	1	Rapid	60–120	300	>5	7.9	70
Prilocaine	1	Slow	60–120	400	>5	7.9	55
Mepivacaine	1	Slow	90–180	300	>5	7.6	77
Bupivacaine	4	Slow	240–480	175	>3	8.1	95
Levobupivacaine	4	Slow	240–480	175		8.1	>97
Ropivacaine	4	Slow	240–480	200	>4	8.1	94

(continued)

Table 10-1

Comparative Pharmacology of Local Anesthetics *(continued)*

Classification	Fraction Nonionized (%) at pH 7.4	Fraction Nonionized (%) at pH 7.6	Lipid Solubility	Volume of Distribution (L)	Clearance (L/min)	Elimination Half-Time (min)
Esters						
Procaine	3	5	0.6	65		9
Chloroprocaine	5	7		35		7
Tetracaine	7	11	80			
Amides						
Lidocaine	25	33	2.9	91	0.95	96
Prilocaine	24	33	0.9	191	9.78	96
Mepivacaine	39	50	1	84		114
Bupivacaine	17	24	28	73	0.47	210
Levobupivacaine	17	24		55		156
Ropivacaine	17	24		59	0.44	108

Adapted from Denson DD. Physiology and pharmacology of local anesthetics. In: Sinatra RS. *Acute pain: Mechanisms and management.* St. Louis, MO: Mosby; 1992:124; and Burm AG, van der Meer AD, van Kleef JW, et al. Pharmacokinetics of the enantiomers of bupivacaine following intravenous administration of the racemate. *Br J Clin Pharmacol.* 1994;38:125–129.

2. Halogenation of procaine to chloroprocaine results in a 3- to 4-fold increase in the hydrolysis rate of chloroprocaine by plasma cholinesterase. This rapid hydrolysis rate of chloroprocaine limits the duration of action and systemic toxicity of this local anesthetic.

B. Mepivacaine, bupivacaine, and ropivacaine are characterized as pipecoloxylidides (see Fig. 10-2).

1. Addition of a butyl group to the piperidine nitrogen of mepivacaine results in bupivacaine, which is 35 times more lipid soluble and has a potency and duration of action three to four times that of mepivacaine.

2. Ropivacaine structurally resembles bupivacaine and mepivacaine, with a propyl group on the piperidine nitrogen atom of the molecule.

IV. **Racemic Mixtures or Pure Isomers.** The pipecoloxylidide local anesthetics (mepivacaine, bupivacaine, ropivacaine, levobupivacaine) are chiral drugs because their molecules possess an asymmetric carbon atom (see Fig. 10-2). As such, these drugs may have a left- (S) or right- (R) handed configuration.

A. The S enantiomers of bupivacaine and mepivacaine appear to be less toxic than the commercially available racemic mixtures of these local anesthetics.

B. In contrast to mepivacaine and bupivacaine, ropivacaine and levobupivacaine have been developed as a pure S enantiomers (less neurotoxicity and cardiotoxicity than the R enantiomers).

V. **Liposomal Local Anesthetics.** Drugs such as lidocaine, tetracaine, and bupivacaine have been incorporated into liposomes to prolong the duration of action (hemorrhoidectomy, bunionectomy) and decrease toxicity.

VI. **Mechanism of Action.** Local anesthetics prevent transmission of nerve impulses (conduction blockade) by inhibiting passage of sodium ions through ion-selective sodium channels (a specific receptor for local anesthetic molecules) in nerve membranes (Fig. 10-3). Failure of sodium ion channel permeability to increase slows the rate of depolarization such that threshold potential is not reached and thus an action potential is not propagated (see Fig. 10-3).

A. **Sodium Channels.** The sodium channel is a dynamic transmembrane protein consisting of the large sodium-conducting pore (α subunit) and varying numbers of adjacent smaller β subunits.

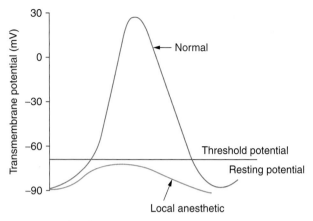

FIGURE 10-3 Local anesthetics slow the rate of depolarization of the nerve action potential such that the threshold potential is not reached. As a result, an action potential cannot be propagated in the presence of local anesthetic and conduction blockade results.

B. **Frequency-Dependent Blockade**
 1. Sodium ion channels tend to recover from local anesthetic–induced conduction blockade between action potentials and to develop additional conduction blockade each time sodium channels open during an action potential (frequency-dependent blockade).
 2. Local anesthetic molecules can gain access to receptors only when sodium channels are in activated-open states and local anesthetic binds more strongly to inactivated state. For this reason, selective conduction blockade of nerve fibers by local anesthetics may be related to the nerve's characteristic frequencies of activity as well as to its anatomic properties such as diameter.
C. **Other Site of Action Targets**. In addition to sodium ion channels, local anesthetics block voltage-dependent potassium ion channels.
D. **Minimum effective concentration** of local anesthetic necessary to produce conduction blockade of nerve impulses is termed the C_m (analogous to the minimum alveolar concentration [MAC] for inhaled anesthetics).
 1. Each local anesthetic has a unique C_m, reflecting differing potencies of each drug.

2. The C_m of motor fibers is approximately twice that of sensory fibers; thus, sensory anesthesia may not always be accompanied by skeletal muscle paralysis.

3. Despite an unchanged C_m, less local anesthetic is needed for subarachnoid anesthesia than for epidural anesthesia, reflecting greater access of local anesthetics to unprotected nerves in the subarachnoid space.

E. **Differential conduction blockade** is illustrated by selective blockade of preganglionic sympathetic nervous system B fibers using low concentrations of local anesthetics. Slightly higher concentrations of local anesthetics interrupt conduction in small C fibers and small- and medium-sized A fibers, with loss of sensation for pain and temperature. Nevertheless, touch, proprioception, and motor function are still present such that the patient will sense pressure but not pain with surgical stimulation (may be misinterpreted as failure of the local anesthetic).

F. **Changes during Pregnancy.** Increased sensitivity (more rapid onset of conduction blockade) may be present during pregnancy.

VII. **Pharmacokinetics (see Table 10-1)**

A. Local anesthetics are weak bases that have pK values somewhat above physiologic pH (<50% of the local anesthetic exists in a lipid-soluble nonionized form at physiologic pH). Local anesthetics with pKs nearest to physiologic pH have the most rapid onset of action, reflecting the presence of an optimal ratio of ionized to nonionized drug fraction.

B. Intrinsic vasodilator activity will also influence apparent potency and duration of action (enhanced vasodilator action of lidocaine compared with mepivacaine results in the greater systemic absorption and shorter duration of action of lidocaine).

C. **Absorption and Distribution**

1. Absorption of a local anesthetic from its site of injection into the systemic circulation is influenced by the site of injection and dosage, use of epinephrine, and pharmacologic characteristics of the drug (Fig. 10-4).

2. The ultimate plasma concentration of a local anesthetic is determined by the rate of tissue distribution and the rate of clearance of the drug.

D. **Lung Extraction**

1. The lungs are capable of extracting local anesthetics (lidocaine, bupivacaine, prilocaine) from the circulation.

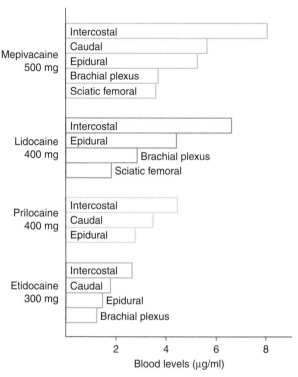

FIGURE 10-4 Peak plasma concentrations of local anesthetic are influenced by the site of injection for accomplishment of regional anesthesia. (From Covino BG, Vassallo HL. *Local anesthetics: Mechanisms of action and clinical use*. New York, NY: Grune & Stratton; 1976, with permission.)

2. This pulmonary extraction will limit the concentration of drug that reaches the systemic circulation for distribution to the coronary and cerebral circulations.

E. **Placental Transfer**

1. There may be clinically significant transplacental transfer of local anesthetics between the mother and fetus.

2. Bupivacaine, which is highly protein bound (approximately 95%), has an umbilical vein–maternal arterial concentration ratio of about 0.32 compared with a ratio of 0.73 for lidocaine (approximately 70% protein bound).

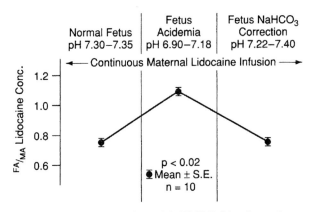

FIGURE 10-5 Fetal–maternal arterial (FA/MA) lidocaine ratios are greater during acidemia compared with a normal pH. (From Biehl D, Shnider SM, Levinson G, et al. Placental transfer of lidocaine: effects of fetal acidosis. *Anesthesiology.* 1978;48:409–412, with permission.)

    3. Acidosis in the fetus, which may occur during prolonged labor, can result in accumulation of local anesthetic molecules in the fetus (ion trapping) (Fig. 10-5).

F. **Renal Elimination and Clearance**

    1. The poor water solubility of local anesthetics usually limits renal excretion of unchanged drug to less than 5% (exception is cocaine, of which 10% to 12% of unchanged drug can be recovered in urine).

    2. Water-soluble metabolites of local anesthetics, such as para-aminobenzoic acid resulting from metabolism of ester local anesthetics, are readily excreted in urine.

VIII. **Metabolism of Amide Local Anesthetics.** Amide local anesthetics undergo varying rates of metabolism by microsomal enzymes located primarily in the liver. Prilocaine undergoes the most rapid metabolism; lidocaine and mepivacaine are intermediate; and etidocaine, bupivacaine, and ropivacaine undergo the slowest metabolism among the amide local anesthetics. Compared with that of ester local anesthetics, the metabolism of amide local anesthetics is more complex and slower. This slower metabolism means that sustained increases of the plasma concentrations of amide local anesthetics, and thus systemic toxicity, are more likely than with ester local anesthetics. Furthermore, cumulative drug effects of amide local anesthetics are more likely than with ester local anesthetics.

A. **Lidocaine**
   1. The principal metabolic pathway of lidocaine is oxidative dealkylation in the liver to monoethylglycinexylidide (approximately 80% of the activity of lidocaine for protecting against cardiac dysrhythmias) followed by hydrolysis of this metabolite to xylidide.
   2. Xylidide has only approximately 10% of the cardiac antidysrhythmic activity of lidocaine.

B. **Prilocaine** is an amide local anesthetic that is metabolized to orthotoluidine (an oxidizing compound capable of converting hemoglobin to its oxidized form, methemoglobin, resulting in a potentially life-threatening complication, methemoglobinemia).
   1. Methemoglobinemia is readily reversed by the administration of methylene blue, 1 to 2 mg/kg intravenously (IV), over 5 minutes (total dose should not exceed 7 to 8 mg/kg).
   2. Prilocaine causes less vasodilation than other local anesthetics and thus can be utilized without epinephrine added to the local anesthetic solution.

C. **Mepivacaine**
   1. Mepivacaine has pharmacologic properties similar to those of lidocaine, although the duration of action of mepivacaine is somewhat longer.
   2. In contrast to lidocaine, mepivacaine lacks vasodilator activity (an alternate selection when addition of epinephrine to the local anesthetic solution is not recommended).

D. **Bupivacaine**
   1. Possible pathways for metabolism of bupivacaine include aromatic hydroxylation, N-dealkylation, amide hydrolysis, and conjugation.
   2. α_1-Acid glycoprotein is the most important plasma protein binding site of bupivacaine, and its concentration is increased in many clinical situations, including postoperative trauma.

E. **Ropivacaine** is metabolized to 2,6-pipecoloxylidide and 3-hydroxyropivacaine by hepatic cytochrome P-450 enzymes (both metabolites have significantly less local anesthetic potency than ropivacaine).
   1. Because only a very small fraction of ropivacaine is excreted unchanged in the urine (about 1%) when the

liver is functioning normally, dosage adjustments based on renal function do not seem necessary.

2. Overall, clearance of ropivacaine is higher than that determined for bupivacaine (may offer an advantage over bupivacaine in terms of systemic toxicity).

3. Ropivacaine is highly bound to α_1-acid glycoprotein.

F. Dibucaine is an amide local anesthetic known for its ability to inhibit the activity of normal butyrylcholinesterase (plasma cholinesterase) by more than 70%, compared with only approximately 20% inhibition of the activity of atypical enzyme. Laboratory evaluation of patients suspected of having atypical pseudocholinesterase is facilitated by measurement of the degree of enzyme suppression by dibucaine, a test termed the *dibucaine number*.

IX. **Metabolism of Ester Local Anesthetics.** Ester local anesthetics undergo hydrolysis by cholinesterase enzyme (exception is cocaine), principally in the plasma and to a lesser extent in the liver. The rate of hydrolysis varies, with chloroprocaine being most rapid, procaine being intermediate, and tetracaine being the slowest. The resulting metabolites are pharmacologically inactive, although para-aminobenzoic acid may be an antigen responsible for subsequent allergic reactions. Systemic toxicity is inversely proportional to the rate of hydrolysis; thus, tetracaine is more likely than chloroprocaine to result in excessive plasma concentrations. Because cerebrospinal fluid contains little to no cholinesterase enzyme, anesthesia produced by subarachnoid placement of tetracaine will persist until the drug has been absorbed into the systemic circulation. Patients with atypical plasma cholinesterase may be at increased risk for developing excess systemic concentrations of an ester local anesthetic due to absent or limited plasma hydrolysis.

A. **Procaine** is hydrolyzed to para-aminobenzoic acid, which is excreted unchanged in urine.

B. **Chloroprocaine**

1. Addition of a chlorine atom to the benzene ring of procaine to form chloroprocaine increases by 3.5 times the rate of hydrolysis of the local anesthetic by plasma cholinesterase.

2. Resulting pharmacologically inactive metabolites of chloroprocaine are 2-chloro-aminobenzoic acid and 2-diethylaminoethanol.

C. **Tetracaine** undergoes hydrolysis by plasma cholinesterase, but the rate is slower than for procaine.

D. **Benzocaine** is unique among clinically useful local anesthetics because it is a weak acid (pK$_a$ 3.5), so that it exists predominantly in the nonionized form at physiologic pH.
  1. Benzocaine is ideally suited for topical anesthesia of mucous membranes prior to tracheal intubation, endoscopy, transesophageal echocardiography, and bronchoscopy.
  2. Methemoglobinemia is a rare but potentially life-threatening complication following topical application of benzocaine, especially when the dose exceeds 200 to 300 mg.

E. **Cocaine** is metabolized by plasma and liver cholinesterases to water-soluble metabolites that are excreted in urine. Plasma cholinesterase activity is decreased in parturients, neonates, the elderly, and patients with severe underlying hepatic disease.
  1. Cocaine may be present in urine for 24 to 36 hours, depending on the route of administration and cholinesterase activity.
  2. Assays for the metabolites of cocaine in urine are useful markers of cocaine use or absorption.

X. **Alkalinization of local anesthetic solutions shortens the onset of neural blockade, enhances the depth of sensory and motor blockade, and increases the spread of epidural blockade (adding sodium bicarbonate will speed the onset of peripheral nerve block and epidural block by 3 to 5 minutes).**

XI. Use of Vasoconstrictors
  A. The duration of action of a local anesthetic is proportional to the time the drug is in contact with nerve fibers (epinephrine [1:200,000 or 5 μg/mL] added to local anesthetic solutions produces vasoconstriction, which limits systemic absorption and maintains the drug concentration in the vicinity of the nerve fibers to be anesthetized) (Fig. 10-6).
  B. Most local anesthetics, with the exception of ropivacaine, possess intrinsic vasodilator properties, and it is possible that epinephrine-induced vasoconstriction will slow clearance from the injection site, thus prolonging the time the drug is in contact with nerve fibers.
  C. The impact of adding epinephrine to the local anesthetic solution is influenced by the specific local anesthetic selected and the level of sensory blockade required if a spinal or epidural anesthetic is chosen.
    1. The impact of epinephrine in prolonging the duration of conduction blockade and decreasing systemic absorp-

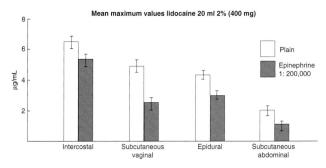

FIGURE 10-6 Addition of epinephrine to the solution containing lidocaine or prilocaine decreases systemic absorption of the local anesthetic by about one-third. (From Scott DB, Jebson PJR, Braid B, et al. Factors affecting plasma levels of lidocaine and prilocaine. *Br J Anaesth.* 1972;44:1040–1049, with permission.)

tion of bupivacaine and etidocaine is less than that observed with lidocaine, presumably because the greater lipid solubility of bupivacaine and etidocaine causes them to bind avidly to tissues.

2. The duration of sensory anesthesia in the lower extremities, but not the abdominal region, is extended when epinephrine (0.2 mg) or phenylephrine (2 mg) is added to local anesthetic solutions of bupivacaine or lidocaine placed into the subarachnoid space.

3. Vasoconstrictors prolong the effect of tetracaine for spinal anesthesia.

4. Decreased systemic absorption of local anesthetic due to vasoconstriction produced by epinephrine increases the likelihood that the rate of metabolism will match that of absorption, thus decreasing the possibility of systemic toxicity.

5. Whenever local anesthetic solutions containing epinephrine are administered in the presence of inhaled anesthetics, the possibility of enhanced cardiac irritability should be considered.

6. Systemic absorption of epinephrine may accentuate systemic hypertension in vulnerable patients.

XII. **Adverse Effects of Local Anesthetics**

A. **Allergic reactions** to local anesthetics are rare despite the frequent use of these drugs (estimated that <1% of all adverse reactions to local anesthetics are due to an allergic mechanism and instead are manifestations of excess plasma concentrations of the local anesthetic). Esters of local anesthetics that produce metabolites related to para-aminobenzoic acid are more likely than amide local anesthetics, which are not metabolized to para-aminobenzoic acid, to evoke an allergic reaction. An allergic reaction after the use of a local anesthetic may be due to methylparaben or similar substances used as preservatives in commercial preparations of ester and amide local anesthetics. These preservatives are structurally similar to para-aminobenzoic acid (as a result, an allergic reaction may reflect prior stimulation of antibody production by the preservative and not a reaction to the local anesthetic).

1. **Cross-sensitivity** between local anesthetics reflects the common metabolite para-aminobenzoic acid (a patient with a known allergy to an ester local anesthetic can receive an amide local anesthetic without an increased risk of an allergic reaction). An ester local anesthetic can be administered to a patient with a known allergy to an amide local anesthetic. It is important that the "safe" local anesthetic be preservative-free.

2. **Documentation of allergy** to a local anesthetic is based on the clinical history and perhaps the use of intradermal testing (requires injection of preservative-free preparations of local anesthetic solutions).

   a. The occurrence of rash, urticaria, and laryngeal edema, with or without hypotension and bronchospasm, is highly suggestive of a local anesthetic–induced allergic reaction.

   b. Hypotension associated with syncope or tachycardia when an epinephrine-containing local anesthetic solution is administered suggests an accidental intravascular injection of drug.

B. **Local anesthetic systemic toxicity** (LAST) is due to an excess plasma concentration of the drug. Accidental direct intravascular injection of local anesthetic solutions during performance of peripheral nerve block anesthesia or epidural anesthesia is the most common mechanism for production of excess plasma concentrations of local anesthetics. (see Table 10-1). Addition of 5 μg of epinephrine to every milliliter of local anesthetic solution (1:200,000 dilution) decreases systemic absorption of local anesthetics by approximately one-third.

1. Local anesthetics differ with regard to their central nervous system (CNS) toxicity and cardiac toxicity.

Table 10-2	

Dose-Dependent Effects of Lidocaine

Plasma Lidocaine Concentration (μg/mL)	Effect
1–5	Analgesia
5–10	Circumoral numbness
	Tinnitus
	Skeletal muscle twitching
	Systemic hypotension
	Myocardial depression
10–15	Seizures
	Unconsciousness
15–25	Apnea
	Coma
>25	Cardiovascular depression

2. Bupivacaine is a more potent local anesthetics and generates arrhythmias at lower concentrations compared with lidocaine and mepivacaine.

C. **Central Nervous System Effects** (Table 10-2)

D. **Cardiovascular System Effects** (see Table 10-2)

1. **Selective Cardiac Toxicity**

a. Accidental IV injection of bupivacaine may result in precipitous hypotension, cardiac dysrhythmias, and atrioventricular heart block (pregnancy may increase sensitivity to cardiotoxic effects of bupivacaine, but not ropivacaine). Caution must be taken in the use of bupivacaine in patients who are on antidysrhythmic drugs or other cardiac medications known to depress impulse propagation. Epinephrine and phenylephrine may increase bupivacaine cardiotoxicity, reflecting bupivacaine-induced inhibition of catecholamine-stimulated production of cAMP.

b. All local anesthetics depress the maximal depolarization rate of the cardiac action potential (V_{max}) by virtue of their ability to inhibit sodium ion influx via sodium channels. Tachycardia can enhance frequency-dependent blockade of cardiac sodium channels by bupivacaine, further contributing to the selective cardiac toxicity of this local anesthetic.

XIII. **Treatment of LAST**

    A. Treatment of local anesthetic–induced seizures includes ventilation of the patient's lungs with oxygen because arterial hypoxemia and metabolic acidosis occur within seconds. IV administration of a benzodiazepine such as midazolam or diazepam is effective in suppressing local anesthetic–induced seizures.

    B. Early use of lipid emulsion for the treatment of local anesthetic toxicity is becoming standard of care (Fig. 10-7). Initial bolus of 1.5 mL/kg 20% lipid emulsion followed by 0.25 mL/kg per minute of infusion, continued for at least 10 minutes after circulatory stability is attained, is recommended.

    C. Epinephrine should be used at a lower than typical dose 10 to 100 μg during resuscitation, and vasopressin use is not recommended. Calcium channel blockers and β-blockers should be avoided.

    D. Nonresponse to treatment should prompt institution of cardiopulmonary bypass.

XIV. **Neural tissue toxicity (neurotoxicity)** from placement of local anesthetic–containing solutions into the epidural or subarachnoid space may range from patchy groin numbness and persistent isolated myotomal weakness to cauda equina syndrome. Myofascial pain may be erroneously diagnosed as transient neurologic symptoms after intrathecal placement of local anesthetics. Overall, permanent neurologic injury after regional anesthesia remains a very rare event.

    A. **Transient neurologic symptoms (TNS)** manifest as moderate to severe pain in the lower back, buttocks, and posterior thighs that appears within 6 to 36 hours after complete recovery from uneventful single-shot spinal anesthesia (relief of pain with trigger point injections and nonsteroidal antiinflammatory drugs suggests a musculoskeletal component). In TNS, the sensory and motor neurologic examination is not abnormal and full recovery from symptoms usually occurs within 1 to 7 days. The incidence of transient neurologic symptoms is greatest following the intrathecal injection of lidocaine (as high as 30%).

    B. **Cauda equina syndrome (CES)** occurs when diffuse injury across the lumbosacral plexus produces varying degrees of sensory anesthesia, bowel and bladder sphincter dysfunction, and paraplegia (has been reported after intrathecal injection of 100 mg of 5% lidocaine through a 25-gauge needle).

A. If signs and symptoms of LAST occur, prompt and effective airway management is crucial to preventing hypoxia and acidosis, which are known to potentiate LAST.

B. If seizures occur, they should be rapidly halted with benzodiazepines. If benzodiazepines are not readily available, small doses of propofol or thiopental are acceptable.

C. Although propofol can stop seizures, large doses further depress cardiac function; propofol should be avoided when there are signs of CV compromise. If seizures persist despite benzodiazepines, small doses of succinylcholine or similar neuromuscular blocker should be considered to minimize acidosis and hypoxemia.

D. If cardiac arrest occurs, we recommend standard Advanced Cardiac Life Support with the following modifications:
- If epinephrine is used, small initial doses (10–100 μg boluses in the adult) are preferred.
- Vasopressin is not recommended.
- Avoid calcium channel blockers and β-adrenergic receptor blockers.
- If ventricular arrhythmias develop, amiodarone is preferred.

E. Lipid emulsion therapy
- Consider administering at the first signs of LAST, after airway management.
- Dosing:
  • 1.5 mL/kg 20% lipid emulsion bolus
  • 0.25 mL/kg per minute of infusion, continued for at least 10 minutes after circulatory stability is attained
  • If circulatory stability is not attained, consider rebolus and increasing infusion to 0.5 mL/kg per minute.
  • Approximately 10 mL/kg lipid emulsion for 30 minutes is recommended as the upper limit for initial dosing

F. Propofol is not a substitute for lipid emulsion.

G. Failure to respond to lipid emulsion and vasopressor therapy should prompt institution of cardiopulmonary bypass (CPB). Because there can be considerable lag in beginning CPB, it is reasonable to notify the closest facility capable of providing it when CV compromise is first identified during an episode of LAST.

FIGURE 10-7 American Society of Regional Anesthesia and Pain Medicine recommendations for managing LAST. CV, cardiovascular. (Redrawn from Neal JM, Bernards CM, Butterworth JF IV, et al. ASRA practice advisory on local anesthetic systemic toxicity. *Reg Anesth Pain Med.* 2010;35:152–161.)

C. **Anterior spinal artery syndrome** consists of lower extremity paresis with a variable sensory deficit that is usually diagnosed as the neural blockade resolves.

1. The etiology of this syndrome is uncertain (addition of epinephrine to local anesthetic solutions has been implicated, but spinal cord perfusion studies do not show a deleterious effect of the catecholamine).

2. Advanced age and the presence of peripheral vascular disease may predispose patients to development of anterior spinal artery syndrome.

3. It may be difficult to distinguish symptoms due to anterior spinal artery syndrome from those caused by spinal cord compression produced by an epidural abscess or hematoma.

XV. **Methemoglobinemia is a rare but potentially life-threatening complication (decreased oxygen-carrying capacity) that may follow the administration of certain drugs (prilocaine, benzocaine, nitroglycerin) or chemicals that cause oxidation of hemoglobin to methemoglobin more rapidly than methemoglobin is reduced to hemoglobin.**

A. The presence of methemoglobinemia is suggested by a difference between the calculated and measured arterial oxygen saturation. The diagnosis is confirmed by qualitative measurements of methemoglobin by co-oximetry.

B. Methemoglobinemia is readily reversed by the administration of methylene blue, 1 to 2 mg/kg IV, over 5 minutes (total dose should not exceed 7 to 8 mg/kg).

XVI. Uses of Local Anesthetics (Table 10-3)

A. **Regional anesthesia** is classified according to the following six sites of placement of the local anesthetic solution: (a) topical or surface anesthesia, (b) local infiltration, (c) peripheral nerve block, (d) IV regional anesthesia (Bier block), (e) epidural anesthesia, and (f) spinal (subarachnoid) anesthesia. Maximum doses of local anesthetics (based on body weight) as recommended for topical or peripheral nerve block anesthesia must be viewed as imprecise guidelines that often do not consider the pharmacokinetics of the drugs.

B. **Topical Anesthesia**

1. Cocaine (4% to 10%, estimated that topical cocaine anesthesia is used in >50% of rhinolaryngologic procedures performed annually in the United States), tetracaine (1% to 2%), and lidocaine (2% to 4%) are most often used.

Table 10-3

Clinical Uses of Local Anesthetics

	Clinical Use	Concentration (%)	Onset	Duration (min)	Recommended Maximum Single Dose (mg)
Lidocaine	Topical	4	Fast	30–60	300
	Infiltration	0.5–1	Fast	60–240	300 or 500 with epinephrine
	IVRA	0.25–0.5	Fast	30–60	300
	PNB	1–1.5	Fast	60–180	300 or 500 with epinephrine
	Epidural	1.5–2	Fast	60–120	300 or 500 with epinephrine
	Spinal	1.5–5	Fast	30–60	100
Mepivacaine	Infiltration	0.5–1	Fast	60–240	400 or 500 with epinephrine
	PNB	1–1.5	Fast	120–240	400 or 500 with epinephrine
	Epidural	1.5–2	Fast	60–180	400 or 500 with epinephrine
	Spinal	2–4	Fast	60–120	100
Prilocaine	Infiltration	0.5–1	Fast	60–120	600
	IVRA	0.25–0.5	Fast	30–60	600
	PNB	1.5–2	Fast	90–180	600
	Epidural	2–3	Fast	60–180	600
Bupivacaine	Infiltration	0.25	Fast	120–480	175 or 225 with epinephrine
	PNB	0.25–0.5	Slow	240–960	175 or 225 with epinephrine
	Epidural	0.5–0.75	Moderate	120–300	175 or 225 with epinephrine
	Spinal	0.5–0.75	Fast	60–240	20

(continued)

Table 10-3

Clinical Uses of Local Anesthetics (continued)

	Clinical Use	Concentration (%)	Onset	Duration (min)	Recommended Maximum Single Dose (mg)
Levobupivacaine	Infiltration	0.25	Fast	120–480	150
	PNB	0.25–0.5	Slow	840–1,020	150
	Epidural	0.5–0.75	Moderate	300–540	150
	Spinal	0.5–0.75	Fast	60–360	20
Ropivacaine	Infiltration	0.2–0.5	Fast	120–360	200
	PNB	0.5–1	Slow	300–480	250
	Epidural	0.5–1	Moderate	120–360	200
	Spinal?				
Chloroprocaine	Infiltration	1	Fast	30–60	800 or 1,000 with epinephrine
	PNB	2	Fast	30–60	800 or 1,000 with epinephrine
	Epidural	2–3	Fast	30–60	800 or 1,000 with epinephrine
	Spinal	2–3	Fast	30–60	Preservative free[a]
Procaine	Spinal	10	Fast	30–60	1,000
Tetracaine	Topical	2	Fast	30–60	20
	Spinal	0.5	Fast	120–360	20
Benzocaine	Topical	Up to 20%	Fast	30–60	200
Cocaine	Topical	4–10	Fast	30–60	150

[a] Off label use.

IVRA, intravenous regional anesthesia; PNB, peripheral nerve block.

Adapted from Covino BG, Wildsmith JAW. Clinical pharmacology of local anesthetic agents. In: Cousins MJ, Bridenbaugh PO, eds. *Neural Blockade in Clinical Anesthesia and Management of Pain*. Philadelphia, PA: Lippincott-Raven; 1998:97–128; and Foster RH, Markham A. Levobupivacaine: a review of its pharmacology and use as a local anesthetic. *Drugs*. 2000;59:551–579.

2. Nebulized lidocaine is used to produce surface anesthesia of the upper and lower respiratory tract before fiberoptic laryngoscopy and/or bronchoscopy and as a treatment for patients experiencing intractable coughing.

3. **Eutectic Mixture of Local Anesthetics**

   a. A 5% lidocaine–prilocaine cream (2.5% lidocaine and 2.5% prilocaine) allows the use of high concentrations of the anesthetic bases without concern about local irritation, uneven absorption, or systemic toxicity (combination of local anesthetics is considered a eutectic mixture of local anesthetics [EMLA]).

   b. EMLA cream is not recommended for use on mucous membranes because of the faster absorption of lidocaine and prilocaine than through intact skin. EMLA cream is not recommended for skin wounds, and the risk of wound infection may be increased.

   c. Patients being treated with certain antidysrhythmic drugs (mexiletine) may experience additive and potentially synergistic effects when exposed to EMLA cream.

C. **Local infiltration** anesthesia involves extravascular placement of local anesthetic (most often lidocaine) in the area to be anesthetized.

   1. The duration of infiltration anesthesia can be approximately doubled by adding 1:200,000 epinephrine to the local anesthetic solution.

   2. Epinephrine-containing solutions, however, should not be injected intracutaneously or into tissues supplied by end-arteries (fingers, ears, and nose) because resulting vasoconstriction can produce ischemia and may result in tissue necrosis.

D. **Peripheral nerve block anesthesia** is achieved by injection of local anesthetic solutions into tissues surrounding individual peripheral nerves or nerve plexuses such as the brachial plexus.

   1. Duration of peripheral nerve block anesthesia depends on the dose of local anesthetic, its lipid solubility, its degree of protein binding, and concomitant use of a vasoconstrictor such as epinephrine.

   2. The duration of action is prolonged more safely by epinephrine than by increasing the dose of local anesthetic, which also increases the likelihood of systemic toxicity.

   3. **Continuous peripheral nerve blocks**. The modern practice of regional anesthesia has moved toward

ultrasound (US)-guided peripheral nerve blocks and using perineural catheters for continuous infusions (use of US guidance increases the chances for successful block) (Table 10-4).

4. **Intravenous Regional Anesthesia (Bier Block).** The IV injection of a local anesthetic solution into an extremity isolated from the rest of the systemic circulation by a tourniquet produces a rapid onset of anesthesia and skeletal muscle relaxation (ester and amide local anesthetics produce satisfactory effects when used for IV regional anesthesia; lidocaine is the most frequently selected amide local anesthetic).

E. **Epidural Anesthesia**

1. Local anesthetic solutions placed in the epidural or sacral caudal space produce epidural anesthesia (local anesthetic diffuses across the dura to act on nerve roots and the spinal cord and local anesthetic also diffuses into the paravertebral area through the intervertebral foramina, producing multiple paravertebral nerve blocks). These slow diffusion processes account for the 15- to 30-minute delay in onset of sensory anesthesia after placement of local anesthetic solutions in the epidural space.

2. Lidocaine is commonly used for epidural anesthesia because of its good diffusion through tissues. Despite a reasonable safety profile, bupivacaine is being replaced by levobupivacaine and ropivacaine, as these local anesthetics are associated with less risk for cardiac and central nervous system toxicity and are also less likely to result in unwanted postoperative motor blockade.

3. In contrast to spinal anesthesia, during epidural anesthesia, there often is not a zone of differential sympathetic nervous system blockade, and the zone of differential motor blockade may average up to four rather than two segments below the sensory level. Another difference from spinal anesthesia is the larger dose required to produce epidural anesthesia, leading to substantial systemic absorption of the local anesthetic.

4. Addition of opioids to local anesthetic solutions placed in the epidural or intrathecal space results in improved analgesia.

F. **Spinal Anesthesia**

1. Local anesthetic solutions placed into lumbar cerebrospinal fluid act on superficial layers of the spinal

Table 10-4

Dosage Chart for Common Continuous Nerve Blocks

Block Type	Local Anesthetic	Continuous Rate (mL/hr)	Bolus Dose (mL)	Lock out Interval (min)	Number of Doses per Hour
Interscalene	0.25 % Bupivacaine or 0.2 % ropivacaine	8	12	60	1
Supraclavicular	0.25 % Bupivacaine or 0.2 % ropivacaine	8	12	60	1
Popliteal	0.25 % Bupivacaine or 0.2 % ropivacaine	8	12	60	1
Femoral[a]	0.12 % Bupivacaine or 0.1 % ropivacaine	8	0	—	—

[a]Lower concentration used for femoral block to reduce the chances of motor blockade and to prevent falls.

cord, but the principal site of action is the preganglionic fibers as they leave the spinal cord in the anterior rami.

2. Dosages of local anesthetics used for spinal anesthesia vary according to the (a) height of the patient, which determines the volume of the subarachnoid space, (b) segmental level of anesthesia desired, and (c) duration of anesthesia desired.

   a. The total dose of local anesthetic administered for spinal anesthesia is more important than the concentration of drug or the volume of the solution injected.

   b. Tetracaine, lidocaine, bupivacaine, ropivacaine, and levobupivacaine are the local anesthetics most likely to be administered for spinal anesthesia.

3. **Physiologic Effects**. The goal of spinal anesthesia is to provide sensory anesthesia and skeletal muscle relaxation. It is the accompanying level of sympathetic nervous system blockade that produces physiologic alterations.

4. **Cardiac arrest** may accompany hypotension and bradycardia associated with spinal anesthesia.

   a. Risk factors for hypotension include sensory anesthesia above T5 and baseline systolic blood pressure of less than 120 mm Hg.

   b. Risk factors for bradycardia include sensory anesthesia above T5, baseline heart rate less than 60 beats/minute, prolonged P-R interval on the electrocardiogram, and concomitant treatment with β-blocking drugs.

5. **Apnea** that occurs with an excessive level of spinal anesthesia probably reflects ischemic paralysis of the medullary ventilatory centers due to profound hypotension and associated decreases in cerebral blood flow. Rarely is the cause of apnea due to phrenic nerve paralysis.

6. **Analgesia**. Continuous low-dose infusion of lidocaine to maintain a plasma concentration of 1 to 2 μg/mL decreases the severity of postoperative pain and decreases requirements for opioids without producing systemic toxicity.

7. **Suppression of Ventricular Cardiac Dysrhythmias**. In addition to suppressing ventricular cardiac dysrhythmias, the IV administration of lidocaine may increase the defibrillation threshold.

XVII. **Tumescent Liposuction**
   A. The "tumescent" technique for liposuction is carried out via the subcutaneous infiltration of large volumes (5 or more liters) of solution containing highly diluted lidocaine (0.05% to 0.10%) with epinephrine (1:100,000).
   B. Slow and sustained release of lidocaine into the circulation is associated with plasma concentrations less than 1.5 μg/mL that peak 12 to 14 hours after injection and then decline gradually over the next 6 to 14 hours.
   C. When highly diluted lidocaine solutions are administered for tumescent liposuction, the dose of lidocaine may range from 35 to 55 mg/kg ("mega-dose lidocaine").
   D. Causes of death may include lidocaine toxicity or local anesthetic–induced depression of cardiac conduction and contractility. Overall complication rate in a nationwide quality improvement study was 0.7% in which 0.57% were minor complications and 0.14% were major complications.

XVIII. **Cocaine Toxicity. Cocaine produces sympathetic nervous system stimulation by blocking the presynaptic uptake of norepinephrine and dopamine, thus increasing their postsynaptic concentrations. Because of this blocking effect, dopamine remains at high concentrations in the synapse and continues to affect adjacent neurons, producing the characteristic cocaine "high."**
   A. **Pharmacokinetics**. The maximum physiologic effects of intranasal cocaine occur within 15 to 40 minutes, and the maximum subjective effects occur within 10 to 20 minutes. The duration of effects is approximately 60 minutes or longer after peak effects.
   B. **Adverse Physiologic Effects**
      1. Cocaine is known to cause coronary vasospasm, myocardial ischemia, myocardial infarction, and ventricular cardiac dysrhythmias, including ventricular fibrillation.
      2. Cocaine may produce hyperpyrexia, which could contribute to seizures.
   C. **Treatment**
      1. Nitroglycerin has been used to treat cocaine-induced myocardial ischemia.
      2. Although esmolol has been recommended to treat tachycardia due to cocaine overdose, there is also evidence that β-adrenergic blockade accentuates coronary artery vasospasm in the setting of acute cocaine overdose.
         a. Whether β-adrenergic blockade is harmful for coronary vasospasm in the setting of chronic cocaine

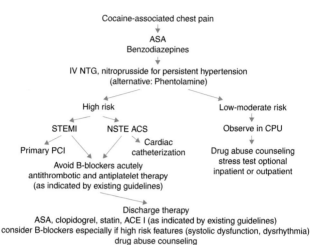

FIGURE 10-8 Therapeutic and diagnostic recommendations in cocaine-associated chest pain. ASA, acetylsalicylic acid; IV NTG, intravenous nitroglycerin; STEMI, ST-segment elevation myocardial infarction; NSTE ACS, Non–ST-segment elevation acute coronary syndrome; PCI, percutaneous coronary intervention; CPU, chest pain unit; ACE, angiotensin-converting enzyme.

use is not known, but administration of β-blocking drugs in the presence of catecholamine-induced hypertension and tachycardia has been associated with profound cardiovascular collapse and cardiac arrest that is unresponsive to aggressive cardiopulmonary resuscitation.

b. In this situation, administration of a vasodilating drug such as nitroprusside may be the safest intervention.

3. The American Heart Association has published a statement for management of cocaine-associated chest pain and myocardial infarction (Fig. 10-8).

CHAPTER 11

Neuromuscular Physiology

I. **Introduction.** The neuromuscular junction is a synapse that develops between a motor neuron and a muscle fiber and is made up of several components: the presynaptic nerve terminal, the postsynaptic muscle membrane, and the intervening cleft (or gap).

II. **Muscle Types**
   A. Muscle is generally classified as skeletal, smooth, or cardiac. Skeletal muscle is responsible for voluntary actions, whereas smooth muscle and cardiac muscle subserve functions related to the cardiovascular, respiratory, gastrointestinal, and genitourinary systems.
   B. Muscle composes 45% to 50% of total body mass, with skeletal muscles accounting for approximately 40% of body mass.

III. **Motor Units.** Vertebrate skeletal muscles are innervated by large myelinated α motor neurons that originate from cell bodies located in the brainstem or ventral (anterior) horns of the spinal cord (Fig. 11-1). The myelinated nerve axon reaches the muscle through mixed peripheral nerves. Motor nerves branch in the skeletal muscle with each nerve terminal innervating a single muscle cell.

IV. **The neuromuscular junction (NMJ) or the endplate** is a highly specialized synapse at which presynaptic motor nerve endings meet the postsynaptic membranes of skeletal muscles (motor endplates) (Fig. 11-2). The NMJ is designed to transmit electrical impulses from the nerve terminal to the skeletal muscle via the chemical transmitter, acetylcholine (ACh). Structurally, the NMJ is consisted of a three components: (a) the *presynaptic* (or prejunctional) nerve terminal containing synaptic vesicles (filled with ACh) and mitochondria; (b) the *synaptic cleft* that contains basal lamina to which acetylcholinesterase enzyme responsible for hydrolysis

225

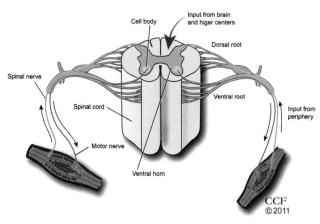

FIGURE 11-1 Schematic depiction of skeletal muscle innervation.

of free ACh is attached; and (c) the *postsynaptic* (or postjunctional) muscle membrane that opposes the nerve terminal.

A. **Presynaptic Region**
   1. **Synaptic vesicles** are specialized secretory organelles (see Fig. 11-2). Each vesicle appears to contain 5,000 to 10,000 molecules of acetylcholine. Nearly 50% of the released acetylcholine is rapidly hydrolyzed by the acetylcholinesterase during the time of diffusion across the synaptic cleft.

B. **Synaptic cleft** separates nerve and muscle fiber plasma membranes (Fig. 11-3). Acetylcholinesterase ranks as one of the highest catalytic efficiencies known (4,000 molecules of acetylcholine hydrolyzed per active site per second) at near diffusion-limited rates.

C. **The Nicotinic Acetylcholine Receptor at the Neuromuscular Junction** (Fig. 11-4).
   1. Nondepolarizing neuromuscular blocking drugs bind to one or both α subunits, but unlike acetylcholine, lack agonist activity (competitive blockade).
      a. As a result, conformational changes do not occur, and the receptor channel remains closed.
      b. Therefore, ions do not flow through these channels, and depolarization cannot occur at these sites. If enough channels remain closed, there is blockade of neuromuscular transmission.

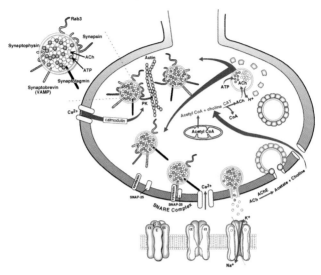

FIGURE 11-2 The synaptic vesicle exocytosis–endocytosis cycle. After an action potential and Ca^{2+} influx, phosphorylation of synapsin is activated by calcium-calmodulin activated protein kinases I and II. This results in the mobilization of synaptic vesicles (SVs) from the cytomatrix toward the plasma membrane. The formation of the SNARE complex is an essential step for the docking process. After fusion of SVs with the presynaptic plasma membrane, acetylcholine (ACh) is released into the synaptic cleft. Some of the released acetylcholine molecules bind to the nicotinic acetylcholine receptors (nAChRs) on the postsynaptic membrane while the rest is rapidly hydrolyzed by the acetylcholinesterase (AChE) present in the synaptic cleft to choline and acetate. Choline is recycled into the terminal by a high-affinity uptake system, making it available for the resynthesis of acetylcholine. Exocytosis is followed by endocytosis in a process dependent on the formation of a clathrin coat and of action of dynamin. After recovering of SV membrane, the coated vesicle uncoats and another cycle starts again. See text for details. Acetyl CoA, acetylcoenzyme A; CAT, choline acetyltransferase; PK, protein kinase. (From Naguib M, Flood P, McArdle JJ, et al. Advances in neurobiology of the neuromuscular junction: implications for the anesthesiologist. *Anesthesiology.* 2002;96:202–231.)

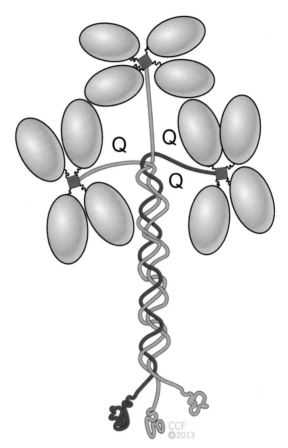

FIGURE 11-3 Structure of acetylcholinesterase.

2. SCh, which is structurally two molecules of acetylcholine bound together, is a partial agonist at nAChRs and depolarizes (opens) the ion channels. Because SCh is not hydrolyzed by acetylcholinesterase, the channel remains open for a longer period of time than would be produced by acetylcholine, resulting in a depolarizing block (sustained depolarization prevents propagation of an action potential).

α SUBUNIT

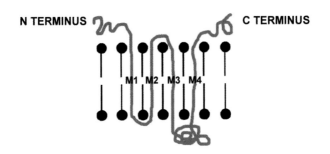

PENTAMERIC COMPLEX

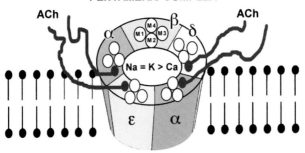

FIGURE 11-4 Subunit composition of the nicotinic acetylcholine receptor (nAChR) in the endplate surface of adult mammalian muscle. The adult AChR is an intrinsic membrane protein with five distinct subunits ($\alpha 2\beta\delta\varepsilon$). Each subunit contains four helical domains labeled M1 to M4. The M2 domain forms the channel pore. The *upper panel* shows a single α subunit with its N and C termini on the extracellular surface of the membrane lipid bilayer. Between the N and C termini, the α subunit forms four helices (M1, M2, M3, and M4), which span the membrane bilayer. The *lower panel* shows the pentameric structure of the nAChR of adult mammalian muscle. The N termini of two subunits cooperate to form two distinct binding pockets for acetylcholine. These pockets occur at the ε–α and the δ–α subunit interface. The M2 membrane spanning domain of each subunit lines the ion channel. The doubly liganded ion channel has equal permeability to Na^+ and K^+; Ca^{2+} contributes approximately 2.5% to the total permeability. (From Naguib M, Flood P, McArdle JJ, et al. Advances in neurobiology of the neuromuscular junction: implications for the anesthesiologist. *Anesthesiology.* 2002;96:202–231.)

V. **Neuromuscular Transmission and Excitation-Contraction Coupling**
   A. **Motor Nerve**. Depolarization of the motor nerve will open the voltage-gated Ca^{2+} channels that trigger both mobilization of synaptic vesicles and the fusion machinery in the nerve terminal to release acetylcholine.
   B. **Muscle**
      1. The released acetylcholine binds to α subunits of the nAChRs, causing a conformational shift in the subunits. When the channel opens, sodium ions flow down their electrochemical gradient and depolarize the muscle cell membrane at the NMJ, whereas potassium simultaneously exits.
      2. This depolarization activates voltage-gated sodium channels, which mediate the initiation and propagation of action potentials resulting in the upstroke of the action potential.
   C. **Blood Flow**. Skeletal muscle blood flow can increase more than 20 times (a greater increase than in any other tissue of the body) during strenuous exercise. The increase in cardiac output that occurs during exercise results principally from local vasodilation in active skeletal muscles and subsequent increased venous return to the heart. Among inhaled anesthetics, isoflurane is a potent vasodilator, producing marked increases in skeletal muscle blood flow.
   D. **Smooth muscle** is distinguished anatomically from skeletal and cardiac muscle.
      1. Smooth muscle contraction is controlled almost exclusively by nerve signals, and spontaneous contractions rarely occur (ciliary muscles of the eye, iris of the eye, and smooth muscles of many large blood vessels).
      2. Smooth muscle cells lack T-tubules that provide electrical links to sarcoplasmic reticulum. Calcium ion channels on the sarcoplasmic reticulum of smooth muscles includes ryanodine receptors and inositol 1,4,5-triphosphate (IP_3)-gated calcium ion channels.
      3. Visceral smooth muscle is characterized by cell membranes that contact adjacent cell membranes, forming a functional syncytium that often undergoes spontaneous contractions as a single unit in the absence of nerve stimulation (peristaltic motion in sites such as the bile ducts, ureters, and gastrointestinal tract).
      4. In addition to stimulation in the absence of extrinsic innervation, smooth muscles are unique in their sensitivity to hormones or local tissue factors (smooth muscle

spasm may persist for hours in response to norepinephrine or antidiuretic hormone, whereas local factors such
as lack of oxygen or accumulation of hydrogen ions
cause vasodilation).

E. **Mechanism of Contraction**
  1. Smooth muscles contain both actin and myosin but,
     unlike skeletal muscles, lack troponin.
  2. Most of the calcium that causes contraction of smooth
     muscles enters from extracellular fluid at the time of the
     action potential (time required for this diffusion is 200
     to 300 ms).
     a. This calcium ion pump is slow compared with the
        sarcoplasmic reticulum pump in skeletal muscles.
     b. As a result, the duration of smooth muscle contrac-
        tion is often seconds rather than milliseconds as is
        characteristic of skeletal muscles.
  3. Smooth muscles, unlike skeletal muscles, do not atrophy
     when denervated, but they do become hyperresponsive
     to the normal neurotransmitter. This denervation hyper-
     sensitivity is a general phenomenon that is largely due to
     synthesis or activation of more receptors.
  4. An NMJ similar to that present on skeletal muscles
     does not occur in smooth muscles. Instead, nerve fibers
     branch diffusely on top of a sheet of smooth muscle
     fibers without making actual contact (these nerve fibers
     secrete their neurotransmitter into an interstitial fluid
     space).
     a. Two different neurotransmitters, acetylcholine and
        norepinephrine, are secreted by the autonomic ner-
        vous system nerves that innervate smooth muscles.
     b. Acetylcholine is an excitatory neurotransmitter for
        smooth muscles at some sites and functions as an
        inhibitory neurotransmitter at other sites.
     c. Norepinephrine exerts the reverse effect of
        acetylcholine.

F. **Uterine smooth muscle** is characterized by a high degree
   of spontaneous electrical and contractile activity (unlike the
   heart, there is no pacemaker and the contraction process
   spreads from one cell to another at a rate of 1 to 3 cm/s).

CHAPTER 12

Neuromuscular Blocking Drugs and Reversal Agents

I. **Introduction.** Neuromuscular blockers are classified as (a) nondepolarizing neuromuscular blockers or (b) depolarizing neuromuscular blockers (succinylcholine).

   A. Nondepolarizing neuromuscular blockers compete with acetylcholine for the active binding sites at the postsynaptic nicotinic acetylcholine receptor and are also called **competitive antagonists**.

   B. Depolarizing neuromuscular blockers act as agonists (they are similar in structure to acetylcholine) at postsynaptic nicotinic acetylcholine receptors and cause prolonged membrane depolarization resulting in neuromuscular blockade.

II. **Principles of Action of Neuromuscular Blockers at the Neuromuscular Junction**

   A. Binding of a single molecule of a nondepolarizing neuromuscular blocker (a competitive antagonist) to one α subunit is sufficient to produce neuromuscular block. Depolarizing neuromuscular blockers, such as succinylcholine, produce prolonged depolarization of the endplate region that results in failure of action potential generation due to membrane hyperpolarization, and block ensues.

   B. Two enzymes hydrolyze choline esters: acetylcholinesterase and butyrylcholinesterase.

   1. Acetylcholinesterase (also known as "true" cholinesterase) is present at the neuromuscular junction and is responsible for the rapid hydrolysis of released acetylcholine to acetic acid and choline.

   2. Butyrylcholinesterase (also known as plasma cholinesterase or pseudocholinesterase) is synthesized in the liver. Butyrylcholinesterase catalyzes the hydrolysis of succinylcholine, which occurs mainly in the plasma.

III. **Structure of Neuromuscular Blocking Drugs**
  A. All neuromuscular blockers, being quaternary ammonium compounds, are structurally related to acetylcholine.
  B. The majority of neuromuscular blocking drugs currently available for clinical use are synthetic alkaloids.

IV. **Characteristics of Nondepolarizing and Depolarizing Neuromuscular Block.** During complete neuromuscular block, no response can be elicited by any pattern of nerve stimulation—single twitch, train-of-four (TOF) stimulation (four stimuli delivered every 0.5 second), or a tetanic stimulus. However, during partial neuromuscular block, the pattern of muscle response varies with the type of neuromuscular blocker administered and the degree of block.
  A. **Nondepolarizing neuromuscular block** is characterized by (a) decrease in twitch tension, (b) fade during repetitive stimulation (TOF or tetanic), and (c) posttetanic potentiation (Fig. 12-1).

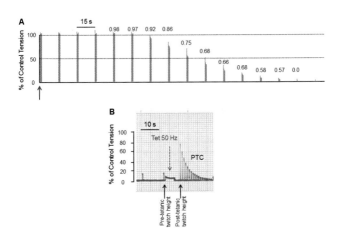

FIGURE 12-1 Acceleromyographic recording during the course of neuromuscular blockade induced by a nondepolarizing agent. **A.** Train-of-four (TOF) fade is noted during the onset of block. The *arrow* indicates the time of administration of a 2 × ED$_{95}$ dose of the nondepolarizing neuromuscular blocking drug. The values corresponding to each TOF recording is the TOF ratio. **B.** Mechanomyographic recording during partial recovery from a nondepolarizing blockade. Tetanic fade and posttetanic potentiation are present after application of a 5-second, 50-Hz tetanic (Tet) stimulation (Tet 50 Hz). PTC, posttetanic count.

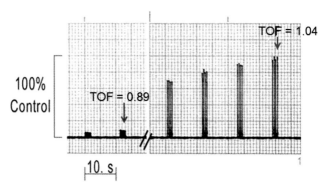

FIGURE 12-2 Mechanomyographic recording during recovery from 1.0 mg/kg succinylcholine. Note that there is no significant fade in the train-of-four (TOF) response during recovery. At 8% recovery of T1 (the first twitch in the train-of-four), the TOF ratio was 0.89, and at 96% recovery of T1, the TOF ratio was 1.04.

    B. **Depolarizing neuromuscular block** (also called *phase I block*) is often preceded by muscle fasciculation. During partial neuromuscular block, depolarizing block is characterized by (a) decrease in twitch tension, (b) no fade during repetitive stimulation (tetanic or TOF), and (c) no posttetanic potentiation (Fig. 12-2).

V. Pharmacology of Succinylcholine
    A. **Structure–Activity Relationships for Succinylcholine**
        1. Succinylcholine is a long, thin, flexible molecule composed of two molecules of acetylcholine linked through the acetate methyl groups (Fig. 12-3).
        2. Like acetylcholine, succinylcholine stimulates cholinergic receptors at the neuromuscular junction and at nicotinic (ganglionic) and muscarinic autonomic sites, opening the ionic channel in the acetylcholine receptor.
    B. **Pharmacokinetics, Pharmacodynamics, and Pharmacogenomics of Succinylcholine**
        1. Succinylcholine has an elimination half-life of 47 seconds (95% confidence interval of 24 to 70 seconds), and the dose of succinylcholine causing on average 95% suppression of twitch height (the ED_{95}) is approximately 0.3 mg/kg.
        2. The usual dose of succinylcholine required for tracheal intubation in adults is 1.0 mg/kg (results in complete

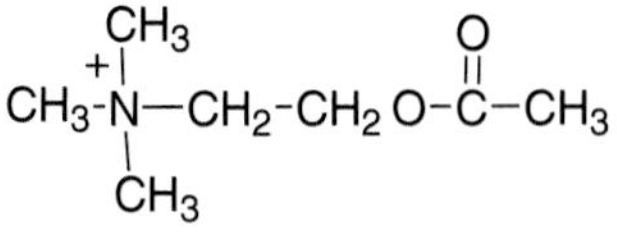

$$CH_3-\underset{\underset{CH_3}{|}}{\overset{\overset{CH_3}{\overset{+}{|}}}{N}}-CH_2-CH_2 \, O-\overset{\overset{O}{\|}}{C}-CH_3$$

Acetylcholine

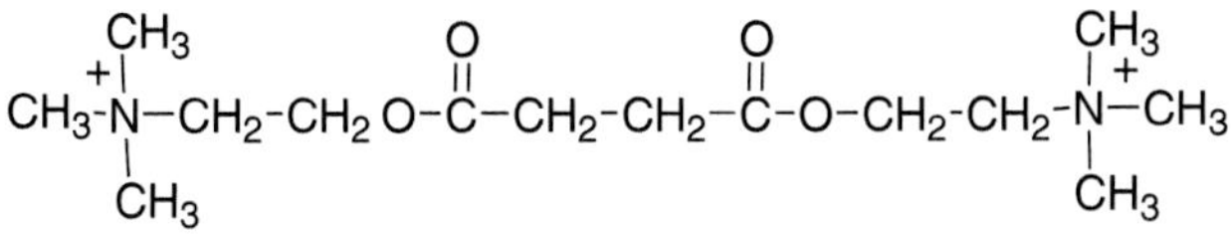

$$CH_3-\underset{\underset{CH_3}{|}}{\overset{\overset{CH_3}{\overset{+}{|}}}{N}}-CH_2-CH_2 \, O-\overset{\overset{O}{\|}}{C}-CH_2-CH_2-\overset{\overset{O}{\|}}{C}-O-CH_2-CH_2-\underset{\underset{CH_3}{|}}{\overset{\overset{CH_3}{\overset{+}{|}}}{N}}-CH_3$$

Succinylcholine

FIGURE 12-3 Structural relationship of succinylcholine, a depolarizing neuromuscular blocking agent, to acetylcholine. Succinylcholine consists of two acetylcholine molecules linked through the acetate methyl groups. Like acetylcholine, succinylcholine stimulates nicotinic receptors at the neuromuscular junction.

suppression of response to neuromuscular stimulation in approximately 60 seconds).

3. In patients with genotypically normal butyrylcholinesterase activity, time to recovery to 90% muscle strength following administration of 1 mg/kg succinylcholine ranges from 9 to 13 minutes.

4. The short duration of action of succinylcholine is due to its rapid hydrolysis by butyrylcholinesterase (plasma cholinesterase) to succinylmonocholine and choline.

   a. There is little or no butyrylcholinesterase at the neuromuscular junction.

   b. Butyrylcholinesterase influences the onset and duration of action of succinylcholine by controlling the rate at which the drug is hydrolyzed in the plasma before it reaches, and after it leaves, the neuromuscular junction.

C. **Factors Affecting Butyrylcholinesterase Activity**

   1. Butyrylcholinesterase is synthesized by the liver and found in the plasma.

   2. Butyrylcholinesterase is responsible for metabolism of succinylcholine, mivacurium, procaine, chloroprocaine,

tetracaine, cocaine, and heroin. Neuromuscular block induced by succinylcholine or mivacurium is prolonged when there is a significant reduction in the concentration or activity of butyrylcholinesterase.

3. Neostigmine (and to a lesser degree edrophonium) causes a profound decrease in butyrylcholinesterase activity. Even 30 minutes after administration of neostigmine, the butyrylcholinesterase activity remains about 50% of control values.

D. **Genetic Variants of Butyrylcholinesterase**

1. Neuromuscular block induced by succinylcholine or mivacurium can be significantly prolonged if the patient has an abnormal genetic variant of butyrylcholinesterase.

2. The dibucaine number reflects quality of cholinesterase enzyme (ability to hydrolyze succinylcholine) and not the quantity of the enzyme that is circulating in the plasma.

   a. In case of the usual butyrylcholinesterase genotype ($E_1^u E_1^u$), the dibucaine number is 70 or higher, whereas in individuals homozygous for the atypical gene ($E_1^a E_1^a$) (frequency in general population of 1 in 3,500), the dibucaine number is less than 30.

   b. In individuals with the heterozygous atypical variant ($E_1^u E_1^a$) (frequency in general population of 1 in 480), the dibucaine number is in the range of 40 to 60.

   c. In individuals with the homozygous atypical genotype ($E_1^a E_1^a$), the neuromuscular block induced by succinylcholine or mivacurium is prolonged to 4 to 8 hours, and in individuals with the heterozygous atypical genotype ($E_1^u E_1^a$), the period of neuromuscular block induced by succinylcholine or mivacurium is about 1.5 to 2 times that seen in individuals with the usual genotype ($E_1^u E_1^u$).

3. Phase II block may appear after prolonged or repeated administration of succinylcholine and has characteristics similar to nondepolarizing neuromuscular blockers (edrophonium or neostigmine do not consistently result in adequate antagonism of neuromuscular blockade). The alternative is to keep the patient adequately sedated and maintain artificial ventilation until the TOF ratio has recovered to 0.9 or more.

E. **Side Effects of Succinylcholine**

1. **Cardiovascular Effects**

   a. Sinus bradycardia, junctional rhythm, and even sinus arrest may follow administration of succinylcholine. Cardiac dysrhythmias are most likely to occur when a second dose of succinylcholine is administered approximately 5 minutes after the first dose. Atropine is effective in treating or preventing bradycardia.

b. In contrast to actions at cardiac muscarinic cholinergic receptors, the effects of succinylcholine at autonomic nervous system ganglia may produce ganglionic stimulation and associated increases in heart rate and systemic blood pressure.

2. **Hyperkalemia**

a. The administration of succinylcholine is associated with approximately 0.5 mEq/dL increase in the plasma potassium concentration in healthy individuals, which is well tolerated and generally does not cause dysrhythmias. (Patients with renal failure are no more susceptible to an exaggerated hyperkalemic response.)

b. Succinylcholine has been associated with severe hyperkalemia in patient conditions associated with up-regulation of extrajunctional acetylcholine receptors (e.g., hemiplegia or paraplegia, muscular dystrophies, Guillain-Barré syndrome, and burn).

3. **Increased Intraocular Pressure**

a. Succinylcholine usually causes an increase in intraocular pressure (peaks at 2 to 4 minutes after administration and returns to normal by 6 minutes).

b. The use of succinylcholine is not widely accepted in open eye injury (when the anterior chamber is open) even though succinylcholine has not been shown to cause adverse events.

4. **Increased Intragastric Pressure**. Administration of succinylcholine does not predispose to regurgitation in patients with an intact lower esophageal sphincter because the increase in intragastric pressure does not exceed the "barrier pressure."

5. **Increased Intracranial Pressure**. The potential for succinylcholine to increase intracranial pressure can be attenuated or prevented by pretreatment with a nondepolarizing neuromuscular blocker.

6. **Myalgias**

a. Postoperative skeletal muscle myalgia, which is particularly prominent in the skeletal muscles of the neck, back, and abdomen, can occur after administration of succinylcholine, especially to young adults undergoing minor surgical procedures that permit early ambulation. Myalgia localized to neck muscles may be perceived as pharyngitis ("sore throat") by the patient and attributed to tracheal intubation by the anesthesiologist.

   b. Muscle pain occurs more frequently in patients undergoing ambulatory surgery, especially in women, than in bedridden patients.

   c. Myalgia may best be prevented with muscle relaxants, lidocaine, or nonsteroidal antiinflammatory drugs. However, myalgias following outpatient surgery occur even in the absence of succinylcholine.

  7. **Masseter Spasm**. An increase in tone of the masseter muscle may be an early indicator of malignant hyperthermia, but it is not consistently associated with malignant hyperthermia.

VI. **Pharmacology of Nondepolarizing Neuromuscular Blockers** (Tables 12-1 to 12-3)

  A. **Benzylisoquinolinium Compounds**

    1. **Atracurium** undergoes spontaneous degradation at physiologic temperature and pH by Hofmann elimination (a chemical process), yielding laudanosine (central nervous system stimulant) and a monoquaternary acrylate as metabolites. Atracurium can also undergo ester hydrolysis. There is no evidence to suggest that prolonged

---

Table 12-1

Classification of Commonly Used and New Nondepolarizing Neuromuscular Blockers According to Duration of Action (Time to T1 = 25% of Control) after Administration of 2 × ED_{95}[a]

	Duration of Action		
	Long (>50 min)	Intermediate (20–50 min)	Short (10–20 min)
Steroidal compounds	Pancuronium	Vecuronium Rocuronium	—
Benzylisoquinolinium compounds	Tubocurarine	Atracurium Cisatracurium	Mivacurium

ED_{95} is the dose that results in 95% depression of twitch height.
[a]The majority of nondepolarizing neuromuscular blockers are bisquaternary ammonium compounds. Tubocurarine, vecuronium, and rocuronium are monoquaternary compounds.

Table 12-2

Dose-Response Relationships and Pharmacodynamic Parameters for Nondepolarizing Neuromuscular Blocking Drugs in Human Subjects[a]

	ED_{50} (mg/kg)	ED_{95} (mg/kg)	CE_{50} (ng/mL)	K_{e0} (min^{-1})	Intubating Dose (mg/kg)	Maximum Block (%)	Time to Maximum Block (min)	Clinical Duration of Response[b] (min)
Long-acting								
d-Tubocurarine	0.23	0.48	370	0.13	0.6	97	5.7	81
Pancuronium	0.036	0.067	88	—	0.08	100	2.9	86
Intermediate-acting								
Rocuronium	0.147	0.305	3510	0.405	0.6	100	1.7	36
Vecuronium	0.027	0.043	92	0.17	0.1	100	2.4	44
Atracurium	0.12	0.21	449	0.13	0.5	100	3.2	46
Cisatracurium	0.026	0.04	126–158	0.07–0.09	0.1	100	5.2	45
Short-acting								
Mivacurium	0.039	0.067	79.9	0.18	0.15	100	3.3	16.8

ED_{50} and ED_{95} are the doses of each drug that produce, respectively, 50% and 95% decrease in the force of contraction or amplitude of the electromyogram of the adductor pollicis muscle following ulnar nerve stimulation.

CE_{50} is the neuromuscular junction concentration of each drug that produces a 50% decrease in the force of contraction or amplitude of the electromyogram of the adductor pollicis muscle following ulnar nerve stimulation.

k_{e0} is the rate constant for equilibration of drug between the plasma and the neuromuscular junction.

[a]Derived using simultaneous pharmacokinetic/pharmacodynamic modeling.

[b]Time from injection of the intubating dose to recovery of twitch to 25% of control.

Table 12-3

Pharmacokinetic Parameters for Neuromuscular Blocking Drugs

	Plasma Clearance (mL/kg/min)	Volume of Distribution (mL/kg)	Elimination Half-life (min)
Short-acting			
Mivacurium isomers			
Cis-trans	106	278	2.0
Trans-trans	57	211	2.3
Cis-cis	3.8	227	68
Intermediate-acting			
Atracurium	6.1	182	21
	10.9	280	17.3
Cisatracurium	5.2	31	—
Vecuronium	3.0	194	78
	5.3	199	53
Rocuronium	2.9	207	71
Long-acting			
d-Tubocurarine	2.4	250	84
Pancuronium	1.7	261	132

administration of atracurium in the operating room or in the intensive care unit in patients with normal or impaired renal function is likely to result in concentrations of laudanosine capable of producing convulsions.

2. **Cisatracurium** is metabolized by Hofmann elimination to laudanosine and a monoquaternary alcohol metabolite, but there is no ester hydrolysis of the parent molecule.

    a. Because cisatracurium is about four to five times as potent as atracurium, about five times less laudanosine is produced, and accumulation of this metabolite is not thought to be of any consequence in clinical practice.

    b. Unlike atracurium, cisatracurium in the clinical dose range does not cause histamine release.

3. **Mivacurium** is the only currently available short-acting neuromuscular blocker in the European Union, but its use in the United States has been discontinued.

B. **Steroidal Compounds** (Fig. 12-4)

1. **Pancuronium** is a potent long-acting neuromuscular blocking drug with both vagolytic and butyrylcholin-

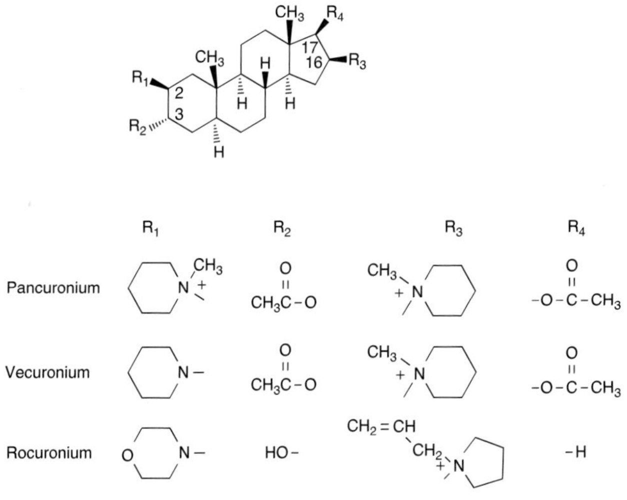

FIGURE 12-4 Chemical structures of the steroidal neuromuscular blockers pancuronium, vecuronium, and rocuronium.

esterase-inhibiting properties. About 40% to 60% of pancuronium is cleared by the kidney, 11% is excreted in the bile, and 15% to 20% is metabolized in the liver. Accumulation of the 3-OH metabolite is responsible for prolongation of the duration of block induced by pancuronium.

2. **Vecuronium** is pancuronium without the quaternizing methyl group in the 2-piperidino substitution (see Fig. 12-4). The minor molecular difference between vecuronium and pancuronium means that vecuronium is characterized by a slight decrease in potency and virtual loss of the vagolytic properties of pancuronium.

    a. The liver is the principal organ of elimination for vecuronium, renal excretion accounts for excretion of approximately 30% of the administered dose, and approximately 30% to 40% of vecuronium is cleared in the bile as parent compound.

    b. The duration of the vecuronium-induced neuromuscular block is dependent primarily on hepatic function (deacetylation) and, to a lesser extent, on renal function. The 3-OH metabolite has 80% the neuromuscular blocking potency of vecuronium (this metabolite may contribute to prolonged neuromuscular blockade).

3. **Rocuronium** is an intermediate-acting monoquaternary neuromuscular blocker with a faster onset of action than either pancuronium or vecuronium (see Fig. 12-4).

    a. Rocuronium is about six times less potent than vecuronium.

    b. Rocuronium is primarily eliminated by the liver and excreted in bile.

VII. Potency of Nondepolarizing Neuromuscular Blockers. The potency of neuromuscular blockers can be expressed as the dose of drug required to produce an effect—for example, 50% or 95% depression of twitch height (ED_{50} and ED_{95}, respectively) (see Table 12-2). It has been suggested that the ED_{50} value should be employed rather than the ED_{95} value when comparing the potency of neuromuscular blockers.

   A. **Factors that Increase the Potency of Nondepolarizing Neuromuscular Blockers**

   1. Inhalational anesthetics potentiate the neuromuscular blocking effect of nondepolarizing neuromuscular

blockers (results mainly in a decrease in the required
dosage and prolongation of both the duration of action).

    a. The magnitude of this potentiation depends on
several factors, including the duration of inhalational
anesthesia, the specific inhalational anesthetic used,
and the concentration of inhalational agent used.

    b. The rank order of potentiation is desflurane > sevo-
flurane > isoflurane > halothane > nitrous oxide–
barbiturate–opioid or propofol anesthesia.

2. Some antibiotics potentiate neuromuscular blockade.

    a. The aminoglycoside antibiotics, the polymyxins, and
lincomycin and clindamycin primarily inhibit the
prejunctional release of acetylcholine and also depress postjunctional nicotinic acetylcholine receptor
sensitivity to acetylcholine.

    b. Tetracyclines exhibit postjunctional activity only.

3. Hypothermia or magnesium sulfate potentiates the
neuromuscular blockade induced by nondepolarizing
neuromuscular blockers.

4. Some local anesthetics when given in large doses potentiate neuromuscular block (no clinically significant
potentiation occurs with smaller doses).

5. Antidysrhythmic drugs (quinidine) potentiate neuromuscular block.

B. **Factors that Decrease the Potency of Nondepolarizing
Neuromuscular Blockers**. Resistance to nondepolarizing
muscle blockers has been demonstrated in patients receiving chronic anticonvulsant therapy (attributed to increased
clearance, increased binding of the neuromuscular blockers
to α_1-acid glycoproteins, and/or upregulation of neuromuscular acetylcholine receptors).

C. **Effect of Drug Potency on Speed of Onset**

1. The speed of onset of action is inversely proportional to
the potency of nondepolarizing neuromuscular blockers
(low potency is predictive of rapid onset and high potency is predictive of slow onset).

2. The influence of potency on speed of onset is explained
by the fact that, for an equipotent dose (a dose that
results in 50% receptor occupancy), a low-potency drug
(such as rocuronium) will have a higher number of
molecules than a high-potency drug.

3. The concept of "buffered diffusion" explains the slow
recovery of long-acting neuromuscular blockers (diffusion of a neuromuscular blocker from the neuromuscular junction is impeded because it binds to extremely

high-density receptors within a restricted space represented by the neuromuscular junction).

VIII. **Adverse Effects of Neuromuscular Blockers. Neuromuscular blocking agents seem to play a prominent role in adverse reactions that occur during anesthesia.**
   A. **Autonomic Effects**
      1. Neuromuscular blocking agents interact with nicotinic and muscarinic cholinergic receptors within the sympathetic and parasympathetic nervous systems and at the nicotinic receptors of the neuromuscular junction.
      2. Pancuronium has a direct vagolytic effect and can block muscarinic receptors on sympathetic postganglionic nerve terminals, resulting in inhibition of a negative-feedback mechanism whereby excessive catecholamine release is modulated or prevented.
   B. **Histamine release** by benzylisoquinolinium compounds can cause skin flushing, decreases in blood pressure and systemic vascular resistance, and increases in pulse rate (steroidal neuromuscular blocking drugs are not associated with histamine release in typical clinical doses).
   C. **Allergic Reactions**
      1. Life-threatening anaphylactic (immune-mediated) or anaphylactoid reactions during anesthesia have been estimated to occur in 1 in 1,000 to 1 in 25,000 administrations (more frequent than allergic reactions to latex or antibiotics) and are associated with a mortality rate of about 5%.
      2. There are currently no standards regarding which diagnostic tests (skin prick test, interdermal test, or immunoglobulin E testing) should be performed to identify patients at risk.
      3. Treatment of anaphylactic reactions includes immediate administration of oxygen (100%) and intravenous epinephrine (10 to 20 μg/kg). Early tracheal intubation with a cuffed endotracheal tube should be considered in patients with rapidly developing angioedema. Fluids (crystalloid and/or colloid solutions) must be administered concurrently. The use of antihistamines and/or steroids is controversial.

IX. **Drugs for Reversal of Neuromuscular Blockade**
   A. **Acetylcholinesterase at the neuromuscular junction**. At the neuromuscular junction, acetylcholinesterase is the enzyme responsible for rapid hydrolysis of released acetylcholine.

B. **Mechanisms of Action of Acetylcholinesterase Inhibitors**
1. Recovery from muscle relaxation induced by nondepolarizing neuromuscular blockers ultimately depends on elimination of the neuromuscular blocker from the body.
2. Acetylcholinesterase inhibitors (neostigmine, edrophonium, and less commonly, pyridostigmine) are used clinically to antagonize the residual effects of neuromuscular blockers and to accelerate recovery from nondepolarizing neuromuscular blockade.
   a. In practical terms, the maximum depth of block that can be antagonized approximately corresponds to the reappearance of the fourth response to TOF stimulation.
   b. Because of their ceiling effect, the anticholinesterases cannot effectively antagonize profound or deep levels of neuromuscular blockade (administering more neostigmine at this point may worsen neuromuscular recovery).
3. Antagonism of nondepolarizing neuromuscular blockade by acetylcholinesterase inhibitors depends primarily on five factors: (a) the depth of the blockade when reversal is attempted, (b) the anticholinesterase chosen, (c) the dose administered, (d) the rate of spontaneous clear of the neuromuscular blocker from plasma, and (e) the choice and depth of anesthetic agents administered.
C. **Clinical Pharmacology**
1. **Pharmacokinetics of Acetylcholinesterase Inhibitors**. Renal failure decreases the plasma clearance of neostigmine, pyridostigmine, and edrophonium as much as, if not more than, that of the long-acting neuromuscular blockers.
2. **Side Effects of Acetylcholinesterase Inhibitors**. Inhibition of acetylcholinesterase not only increases the concentration of acetylcholine at the neuromuscular junction (nicotinic site) but also at all other synapses that use acetylcholine as a transmitter.
   a. **Cardiovascular Side Effects**. Because only the nicotinic effects of acetylcholinesterase inhibitors are desired, the muscarinic effects must be blocked by atropine or glycopyrrolate (to minimize the muscarinic cardiovascular side effects of acetylcholinesterase inhibitors, an anticholinergic agent should be coadministered with the acetylcholinesterase inhibitor). Atropine (7 to 10 μg/kg) matches the onset of action

and pharmacodynamic profile of the rapid-acting edrophonium (0.5 to 1.0 mg/kg), and glycopyrrolate (7 to 15 µg/kg) matches the slower acting neostigmine (40 to 70 µg/kg) and pyridostigmine.

b. **Pulmonary and Alimentary Side Effects**. Administration of acetylcholinesterase inhibitors is associated with bronchoconstriction, increased airway resistance, increased salivation, and increased bowel motility (muscarinic effects). Anticholinergics tend to reduce this effect. Neostigmine has been described as having antiemetic properties and as having no effect on the incidence of postoperative nausea and vomiting.

X. Monitoring of neuromuscular function after administration of a neuromuscular blocking drug allows one to administer these agents with appropriate dosing and it ensures that the patient recovers adequately from residual effects of the neuromuscular blocker.

A. Most commonly, contraction of the adductor pollicis muscle associated with stimulation of the ulnar nerve, either at the wrist or the elbow, is monitored.

B. Clinical bedside criteria for tracheal extubation (such as a 5-second head lift, or ability to generate a peak negative inspiratory force of -25 to -30 cm H_2O) are insensitive indicators of the adequacy of neuromuscular recovery. Subjective (visual or tactile) evaluation of the evoked muscular response to TOF stimulation is extremely inaccurate.

C. Depth of the blockade during maintenance of and recovery from the blockade should be monitored with repeated TOF stimuli.

1. Following administration of a nondepolarizing neuromuscular blocking agent, it is essential to ensure adequate return of normal neuromuscular function, to a TOF ratio of ≥0.9.

2. The use of an objective neuromuscular monitor can decrease the incidence of postoperative residual neuromuscular blockade.

a. Although quantitative neuromuscular function monitoring is recommended, many anesthetics are given without such monitoring.

b. Appropriate intraoperative use of a conventional nerve stimulator may decrease (but not eliminate) the incidence of postoperative residual neuromuscular blockade.

XI. **Limitations of Acetylcholinesterase Inhibitors.** Postanesthetic morbidity in the form of incomplete reversal and residual postoperative weakness is a frequent occurrence.

XII. **Sugammadex: A Novel Selective Relaxant-binding Agent**
   A. **Chemistry**. Sugammadex is a modified γ-cyclodextrin (Fig. 12-5). Their three-dimensional structures, which resemble a hollow, truncated cone or a doughnut, have a hydrophobic cavity that traps the drug into the cyclodextrin cavity (the doughnut hole), resulting in formation of a water-soluble guest-host complex.
   B. Sugammadex exerts its effect by forming very tight complexes at a 1:1 ratio with steroidal neuromuscular blocking agents (rocuronium > vecuronium >> pancuronium).
      1. Sugammadex is the first selective relaxant-binding agent (it exerts no effect on acetylcholinesterases or on any receptor system in the body, thus eliminating the need for anticholinergic drugs and their undesirable adverse effects).
      2. The unique mechanism of reversal by encapsulation is independent of the depth of neuromuscular block; thus, reversal can be accomplished even during profound neuromuscular block.
   C. **Pharmacokinetics and Metabolism**
      1. Sugammadex is biologically inactive and does not bind to plasma proteins.
      2. Approximately 75% of the dose was eliminated through the urine. The renal excretion of rocuronium is increased

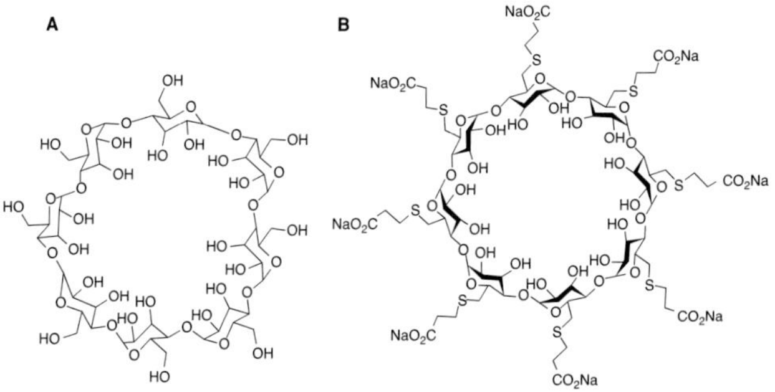

FIGURE 12-5 γ-Cyclodextrin **(A)** and sugammadex (modified γ-cyclodextrin) **(B)**.

by more than 100% after administration of 4 to 8 mg/kg of sugammadex.

3. Metabolism of sugammadex is at most very limited, and the drug is predominantly eliminated unchanged by the kidneys (should be avoided in patients with a creatinine clearance of <30 mL per minute).

D. **Pharmacodynamics**

1. Sugammadex, used in appropriate doses, is capable of reversing any depth of neuromuscular blockade (profound or shallow) induced by rocuronium or vecuronium to a TOF ratio of ≥0.9 within 3 minutes (no recurarization has been reported in human studies).

2. With profound block induced by rocuronium or vecuronium, larger doses of sugammadex (8 to 16 mg/kg) are required for adequate and rapid recovery.

3. Sugammadex is ineffective against succinylcholine and benzylisoquinolinium neuromuscular blockers such as mivacurium, atracurium, and cisatracurium because it cannot form inclusion complexes with these drugs.

E. **Safety and Tolerability**. The U.S. Food and Drug Administration has expressed concerns about the safety of sugammadex, citing its possible association with allergic reactions and bleeding, and sugammadex has not been approved for clinical use in the United States. More than 5 million doses of sugammadex have been administered worldwide.

CHAPTER 13

Antiepileptic and Other Neurologically Active Drugs

I. **Antiepileptic Drugs.** Although 10% of people will report at least one seizure in their lifetime, it is estimated that 1% to 2% of the population worldwide meets the diagnostic criteria for epilepsy (Table 13-1). The goal of pharmacologic treatment of epilepsy is to control seizures with minimal medication-related adverse effects (~70% of patients with epilepsy will become seizure-free using a single antiepileptic drug) (Tables 13-2, 13-3, and 13-4).

A. **Pharmacokinetics** (see Table 13-4)
1. All antiepileptic drugs are administered once daily or more frequently.
2. Because of their ability to induce or inhibit drug metabolism, all antiepileptic drugs (except gabapentin, levetiracetam, vigabatrin) may be associated with pharmacokinetic drug interactions in which plasma drug concentrations and resulting pharmacologic effects of concomitantly administered drugs may be altered.
3. Such drug interactions should be anticipated in all patients receiving antiepileptic drugs and subsequently receiving drugs for other purposes.

B. **Drug Interactions Related to Protein Binding**
1. Salicylates that compete for protein-binding sites of highly bound antiepileptic drugs (phenytoin, valproate, carbamazepine) can displace the bound drug and lead to increases in the plasma concentration of pharmacologically active antiepileptic drug.
2. Hypoalbuminemia, as may accompany renal or hepatic disease or malnutrition, can result in increased plasma concentrations of unbound antiepileptic drug, resulting in toxicity despite therapeutic plasma concentrations.

C. **Drug Interactions Related to Accelerated Metabolism**
1. Enzyme-inducing antiepileptic drugs that accelerate metabolism (carbamazepine, lamotrigine, oxcarbazepine, phenobarbital, phenytoin, topiramate, and primidone)

Table 13-1

Classification of Epileptic Seizures

Partial seizures (beginning locally)
    Simple partial seizures (consciousness not impaired)
    Complex partial seizures (consciousness impaired)
    Partial seizures evolving into secondary generalized seizures
Generalized seizures (convulsive or nonconvulsive)
    Absence seizures (petit mal)
    Myoclonic seizures
    Clonic seizures
    Tonic seizures
    Tonic-clonic seizures
Unclassified seizures

Adapted from Brodie MJ, Dichter MA. Antiepileptic drugs. *N Engl J Med.* 1996;334:168–175.

        may accelerate the metabolism of estrogen and progesterone and thus render oral contraceptives ineffective at usual doses.
    2. Patients being treated with antiepileptic drugs have increased dose requirements for thiopental, propofol, midazolam, opioids, and nondepolarizing neuromuscular blocking drugs.
  D. **Principles of Dosing**
    1. The initial dose is that which is high enough to expect clinical effect but low enough to avoid significant side effects (see Table 13-3).
    2. To maintain plasma drug concentrations in a therapeutic range, equal doses of the antiepileptic drug are often administered at intervals equivalent to less than one elimination half-time of the drug (see Table 13-4).
  E. **Plasma Concentrations and Laboratory Testing**. Phenytoin is the only agent for which monitoring is routinely recommended due to its nonlinear saturation dose kinetics.

II. **Mechanism of Seizure Activity.** The reason for the high frequency and synchronous firing in a seizure focus is usually unknown (possible explanations include local biochemical changes, ischemia, loss of cellular inhibitory systems, infections, and head trauma). Once initiated,

Table 13-2

Antiepileptic Drugs Used to Treat Epilepsy

Drug	Principal Mechanism of Action	Targeted Seizure	Dosage Type
Carbamazepine	Sodium ion channel blockade	Partial seizures	10–40 mg/kg/day in two to three divided doses
Ethosuximide	T-type calcium ion change	Generalized seizures	15–40 mg/kg/day in two to three divided doses
Felbamate	Sodium ion channel blockade Glutamate antagonism Calcium ion channel blockade	Partial seizures Generalized seizures	15–45 mg/kg/day in two to three divided doses
Gabapentin	Unknown (? increases GABA release)	Partial seizures Generalized seizures	10–60 mg/kg/day
Lamotrigine	Sodium ion channel blockade Calcium ion channel blockade	Partial seizures Generalized seizures	200–500 mg/day in two divided doses
Levetiracetam	Unknown (? potassium and calcium ion channel blockade)	Partial seizures Generalized seizures	1,000–3,000 mg/day in two divided doses
Oxcarbazepine	Sodium ion channel blockade	Partial seizures Generalized seizures	900–2,400 mg/day in two divided doses
Phenobarbital	Chloride ion channels	Partial seizures Generalized seizures	2–5 mg/kg/day every day or in two divided doses

(continued)

Table 13-2

Antiepileptic Drugs Used to Treat Epilepsy (continued)

Drug	Principal Mechanism of Action	Targeted Seizure	Dosage Type
Phenytoin	Sodium ion channel blockade Calcium ion channels NMDA receptors	Partial seizures Generalized seizures	3–7 mg/kg/day in three divided doses
Primidone	Chloride ion channels GABA uptake	Partial seizures Generalized seizures	500–1,500 mg/day in two to three divided doses
Tiagabine	Enhanced GABA activity Carbonic anhydrase inhibition	Partial seizures Generalized seizures	32–56 mg/kg/day in two to four divided doses
Topiramate	Sodium ion channel blockade Enhanced GABA activity Glutamate antagonism Calcium ion channel blockade	Partial seizures Generalized seizures	500–3,000 mg/day in two to four divided doses
Valproate	Sodium ion channel blockade Calcium ion channels	Partial seizures Generalized seizures	500–3,000 mg/day in two to four divided doses
Vigabatrin	GABA transaminase inhibition	Complex partial Infantile spasms	3,000 mg/day in two divided doses
Zonisamide	Sodium ion channel blockade Calcium ion channel blockade	Partial seizures Generalized seizures	200–600 mg/day in two to four divided doses

GABA, γ-aminobutyric acid; NMDA, N-methyl-D-aspartate.

Table 13-3		
Side Effects of Antiepileptic Drugs		
	Dose-Related	**Idiosyncratic**
Carbamazepine	Diplopia Vertigo Neutropenia Nausea Drowsiness Hyponatremia	Agranulocytosis Aplastic anemia Allergic dermatitis (rash) Stevens-Johnson syndrome Hepatotoxic effects Pancreatitis Teratogenicity
Ethosuximide	Nausea Anorexia Vomiting Agitation Headache Drowsiness	Agranulocytosis Aplastic anemia Allergic dermatitis (rash) Stevens-Johnson syndrome Lupus-like syndrome
Clonazepam	Sedation Vertigo Hyperactivity (children)	Allergic dermatitis (rash) Thrombocytopenia
Felbamate	Insomnia Anorexia Nausea Headache Irritability	Aplastic anemia Hepatotoxic effects
Gabapentin	Sedation Ataxia Vertigo Gastrointestinal disturbances	

Lamotrigine	Tremor
	Vertigo
	Diplopia
	Ataxia
	Headache
	Gastrointestinal
	  disturbances
		Stevens-Johnson
		  syndrome

Levetiracetam	Sedation Anxiety Headache	Allergic dermatitis (rash)
Oxcarbazepine		Allergic dermatitis (rash)

(continued)

Table 13-3

Side Effects of Antiepileptic Drugs *(continued)*

	Dose-Related	Idiosyncratic

Phenobarbital	Sedation
	Depression
	Hyperactivity
	  (children)
		Agranulocytosis
		Allergic dermatitis (rash)
		Stevens-Johnson
		  syndrome
		Arthritic changes
		Hepatotoxic effects
		Teratogenicity

Phenytoin	Nystagmus
	Ataxia
	Nausea and
	  vomiting
	Gingival
	  hyperplasia
	Depression
	Megaloblastic
	  anemia
	Drowsiness
		Agranulocytosis
		Aplastic anemia
		Allergic dermatitis (rash)
		Stevens-Johnson
		  syndrome
		Hepatotoxic effects
		Pancreatitis
		Acne
		Coarse facies
		Hirsutism
		Teratogenicity
		Dupuytren contracture

Primidone	Sedation	Rash Thrombocytopenia Agranulocytosis Lupus-like syndrome Teratogenicity
Tiagabine	Dizziness Aphasia Tremor	Allergic dermatitis (rash)
Topiramate	Sedation Ataxia Dizziness	Allergic dermatitis (rash)

Valproic acid	Tremor
	Weight gain
	Dyspepsia
	Nausea and
	  vomiting
	Alopecia
	Peripheral
	  edema
	Encephalopathy
	Teratogenicity
	Sedation
		Agranulocytosis
		Aplastic anemia
		Allergic dermatitis (rash)
		Stevens-Johnson
		  syndrome
		Hepatotoxic effects
		Pancreatitis

	Dose-Related	Idiosyncratic
Table 13-3		
Side Effects of Antiepileptic Drugs *(continued)*		
Vigabatrin	Anemia Sedation Permanent visual loss	
Zonisamide	Teratogenicity Dizziness Ataxia Nephrolithiasis Hyperactivity (children) Mania (adults)	Allergic dermatitis

Adapted in part from Brodie MJ, Dichter MA. Antiepileptic drugs. *N Engl J Med*. 1996;334:168–175; Dichter MA, Brodie MJ. New antiepileptic drugs. *N Engl J Med*. 1996;334:1583–1590.

a seizure is most likely maintained by reentry of excitatory impulses in a closed feedback pathway that may not even include the original seizure focus.

III. **Mechanism of Drug Action.** The mechanism of action of antiepileptic drugs is incompletely understood. It is commonly presumed that antiepileptic drugs control seizures by decreasing neuronal excitability or enhancing inhibition of neurotransmission.

IV. **Major Antiepileptic Drugs** (see Table 13-2)
   A. **Adverse Side Effects.** Antiepileptic drugs may potentially produce numerous and varied adverse side effects (see Table 13-3).
   B. **Maternal Epilepsy**
      1. Seizures during pregnancy can result in significant morbidity and mortality to both mother and fetus, making seizure control during this period imperative (fetal organogenesis is largely complete by 8 weeks).
      2. Significant teratogenicity may occur during this period if pregnancy is not detected early enough to permit discontinuation of potentially teratogenic medications.

Table 13-4

Pharmacokinetics of Antiepileptic Drugs

	Plasma Therapeutic Concentration (µg/mL)	Protein Binding (%)	Elimination Half-Time (h)	Route of Elimination
Carbamazepine	6–12	70–80	8–24	Hepatic metabolism (active metabolite)
Clonazepam	0.02–0.08	80–90	30–40	Hepatic metabolism
Diazepam		95	20–35	Hepatic metabolism (active metabolites)
Ethosuximide	40–100	0	20–60	Hepatic metabolism (25% excreted unchanged)
Felbamate		22–25	20–23	Renal excretion
Gabapentin	2–20	0	6	Renal excretion
Lamotrigine		54	25	Hepatic metabolism
Lorazepam		80	14	Hepatic metabolism
Oxcarbazepine		40	8–10	Renal excretion
Phenobarbital	10–40	48–54	72–144	Hepatic metabolism (25% excreted unchanged)
Phenytoin	10–20	90–93	9–40	Saturable hepatic metabolism

Table 13-4

Pharmacokinetics of Antiepileptic Drugs *(continued)*

	Plasma Therapeutic Concentration (μg/mL)	Protein Binding (%)	Elimination Half-Time (h)	Route of Elimination
Primidone	5–12	20–30	4–12	Hepatic metabolism to active metabolites of which 40% are excreted unchanged
Tiagabine		95	5–8	Hepatic metabolism
Topiramate		10	8–15	Renal excretion and hepatic metabolism
Valproic acid	50–100	88–92	7–17	Hepatic metabolism (active metabolites)
Zonisamide		50	50–70	Hepatic metabolism

Adapted in part from Brodie MJ, Dichter MA. Antiepileptic drugs. *N Engl J Med.* 1996;334:168–175; Dichter MA, Brodie MJ. New antiepileptic drugs. *N Engl J Med.* 1996;334:1583–1590.

C. **Carbamazepine** is effective for suppression of nonconvulsive and convulsive partial seizures and is useful in the management of patients with trigeminal neuralgia and glossopharyngeal neuralgia.
   1. **Pharmacokinetics** (see Table 13-4)
   2. **Side Effects** (see Table 13-3). Sedation, vertigo, diplopia, nausea, and vomiting are the most frequent side effects of this drug. Aplastic anemia, thrombocytopenia, hepatocellular and cholestatic jaundice, oliguria, hypertension, and cardiac dysrhythmias are rare but potentially life-threatening complications.
      a. In addition to inducing its own metabolism, carbamazepine can accelerate the hepatic oxidation and conjugation of other lipid-soluble drugs.
      b. The most common interaction is with oral contraceptive pills, and most women require an increase in the daily dose of estrogen.

D. **Ethosuximide** is the drug of choice for suppression of absence (petit mal) epilepsy in patients who do not also have tonic-clonic seizures.
   1. **Pharmacokinetics** (see Table 13-4)
   2. **Side Effects** (see Table 13-3). Toxicity of ethosuximide is low, manifesting most often as gastrointestinal intolerance (nausea, vomiting) and central nervous system (CNS) effects (lethargy, dizziness, ataxia, photophobia).

E. **Felbamate** is not used as a first-line drug for treatment of seizures (toxicity) but rather is reserved for patients with intractable epilepsy.
   1. **Pharmacokinetics** (see Table 13-4)
   2. **Side Effects** (see Table 13-3). Serious side effects include aplastic anemia and hepatotoxicity. Monitoring of treated patients with complete blood counts and liver function tests is indicated.

F. **Gabapentin** is an analog of γ-aminobutyric acid (GABA) that increases synaptic GABA concentrations. Gabapentin induces dose-related sedation and it has efficacy in the treatment of anxiety, panic, and major depression. Despite its multiple other uses, gabapentin has limited efficacy in the treatment of epilepsy.

G. **Lamotrigine** has a broad spectrum of activity and is effective when used alone or in combination in adults who have partial seizures or generalized seizures and in children with Lennox-Gastaut syndrome (see Table 13-3).
   1. Drugs that induce hepatic microsomal enzymes (phenobarbital, phenytoin, and carbamazepine) decrease

the elimination half-time of lamotrigine by about 50%, necessitating a higher dose.

2. Conversely, valproic acid slows the metabolism of lamotrigine and extends its elimination half-time to about 60 hours.

H. **Phenytoin** is the prototype of the hydantoins and is effective for the treatment of partial and generalized seizures. Available in oral and intravenous (IV) preparations, phenytoin may be administered acutely to achieve effective plasma concentrations within 20 minutes. This drug has a high therapeutic index, and its administration is not accompanied by excessive sedation.

1. **Mechanism of Action**. Phenytoin regulates neuronal excitability and thus the spread of seizure activity from a seizure focus by regulating sodium and possibly calcium ion transport across neuronal membranes (stabilizing effect on cell membranes is relatively selective for the cerebral cortex).

2. **Pharmacokinetics** (see Table 13-4)
   a. The initial daily adult oral dosage (intramuscular administration is not recommended) is 3 to 4 mg/kg (doses of >500 mg daily are rarely tolerated).
   b. The rate of IV administration of phenytoin should not exceed 50 mg per minute in adults and 1 to 3 mg/kg/min (or 50 mg per minute, whichever is slower) in pediatric patients because of the risk of severe hypotension and cardiac arrhythmias.

3. **Plasma Concentrations**
   a. Control of seizures is usually obtained when plasma concentrations of phenytoin are 10 to 20 μg/mL.
   b. In the control of digitalis-induced cardiac dysrhythmias, phenytoin, 0.5 to 1.0 mg/kg IV, is administered every 15 to 30 minutes until a satisfactory response is achieved or a maximum dose of 15 mg/kg is administered.

4. **Protein Binding**. Phenytoin is bound approximately 90% to plasma albumin. A greater fraction of phenytoin remains unbound in neonates, in patients with hypoalbuminemia, and in uremic patients.

5. **Metabolism** of phenytoin to inactive metabolites is by hepatic microsomal enzymes that are susceptible to stimulation or inhibition by other drugs.

6. **Side Effects** (Table 13-5)

I. **Valproic acid** is effective in the treatment of all primary generalized epilepsies and all convulsive epilepsies (acts by

Table 13-5

Side Effects of Phenytoin

CNS toxicity (nystagmus, ataxia, vertigo)
Peripheral neuropathy
Gingival hyperplasia
Fetal hydantoin syndrome
Allergic reactions
Hyperglycemia and glycosuria
Megaloblastic anemia
Hepatotoxicity (genetically susceptible persons)
Increased dose requirements for nondepolarizing neuromuscular
  blocking drugs

CNS, central nervous system.

limiting sustained repetitive neuronal firing through
voltage-dependent sodium channels).

1. **Pharmacokinetics**. After oral administration, absorption is prompt, with peak plasma concentrations of
   valproic acid occurring in 1 to 4 hours.
2. **Side Effects**
   a. At higher doses, a fine distal tremor may develop.
   b. Thrombocytopenia is seen frequently at higher
      doses. The most serious side effect of valproic acid is
      hepatotoxicity occurring in about 0.2% of children
      younger than 2 years of age being treated chronically
      with this drug (incidence decreases dramatically after
      2 years of age).
   c. Valproic acid is an enzyme inhibitor but this does not
      interfere with the action of oral contraceptives.

V. **Benzodiazepines display anxiolytic, sedative, muscle-relaxant,
   and anticonvulsant effects (benzodiazepine receptors in the
   brain are a subset of GABA$_A$ receptors).**
   A. **Clonazepam** is generally added to other drug therapy and
      is used as a first-line drug only for myoclonic seizures.
      1. **Pharmacokinetics**. Absorption of clonazepam after oral
         administration is rapid, with peak plasma concentrations
         occurring within 2 to 4 hours (see Table 13-4). IV administration of clonazepam results in rapid CNS effects.
      2. **Side Effects**
         a. Sedation is present in approximately 50% of patients
            but tends to subside with chronic administration (see
            Table 13-3).

b. Skeletal muscle incoordination and ataxia occur in approximately 30% of patients.

c. Generalized seizure activity may be precipitated if the drug is discontinued abruptly.

B. **Diazepam** is a mainstay for the treatment of status epilepticus and local anesthetic–induced seizures. The typical approach is administration of 0.1 mg/kg IV every 10 to 15 minutes until seizure activity has been suppressed or a maximum dose of 30 mg has been administered.

VI. **Status epilepticus is a medical emergency where the patient experiences prolonged or rapidly recurring convulsions for 5 minutes or more.**

A. **Treatment** begins with ensuring a patent upper airway (may require tracheal intubation) and administration of oxygen.

1. If hypoglycemia cannot be excluded, the patient is treated empirically with IV glucose (50 mL of 50% glucose for adults).

2. Drug therapy of status epilepticus is typically with a benzodiazepine such as diazepam.

VII. **Drugs Used for Treatment of Parkinson's Disease. Parkinson's disease is a chronically progressive neurodegenerative disease that results from the loss of dopaminergic neurons in the substantia nigra pars compacta region of the basal ganglia. Dopamine is thought to act principally as an inhibitory neurotransmitter and acetylcholine as an excitatory neurotransmitter within the extrapyramidal system, and a proper balance is necessary for normal function. Treatment regimens are selected based on the age of the patient as well as severity of symptoms.**

A. **Levodopa.** Because dopamine does not readily cross the blood–brain barrier, the major approaches to therapy have involved the administration of its precursor, levodopa, which crosses the blood–brain barrier and is converted to dopamine by aromatic-L-amino-acid decarboxylase. Levodopa is usually administered with a peripheral decarboxylase inhibitor so as to maximize the entrance of the precursor into the brain before it is converted to dopamine. Abrupt discontinuation of levodopa therapy may result in a precipitous return of symptoms of Parkinson's disease and has been associated with a neuroleptic malignant-like syndrome (levodopa should be continued throughout the perioperative period).

1. **Metabolism**

a. Approximately 95% of orally administered levodopa is rapidly decarboxylated to dopamine during the

Table 13-6

Side Effects of Levodopa

Nausea
Orthostatic hypotension
Cardiac dysrhythmias (propranolol effective treatment)
Abnormal involuntary movements (tolerance does not occur)
Psychiatric disturbances (avoid treatment with neuroleptic drugs)
Inhibits secretion of prolactin
Hypokalemia (aldosterone release)
False-positive test for ketoacidosis

initial passage through the liver (resulting dopamine cannot easily cross the blood–brain barrier to exert beneficial effects, whereas increased plasma concentrations of dopamine often lead to undesirable side effects).

    b. In this regard, inhibition of the peripheral activity of the decarboxylase enzyme greatly increases the fraction of administered levodopa that remains intact to cross the blood–brain barrier.

  2. **Side Effects** (Table 13-6)

VIII. Antipsychotic drugs such as butyrophenones and phenothiazines can antagonize the effects of dopamine (administration of droperidol to patients being treated with levodopa has produced severe skeletal muscle rigidity and even pulmonary edema). Metoclopramide may also interfere with dopamine activity.

  A. **Monoamine Oxidase Inhibitors**. Nonspecific monoamine oxidase inhibitors interfere with the inactivation of catecholamines, including dopamine, and can exaggerate the peripheral and CNS effects of levodopa. Hypertension and hyperthermia are side effects associated with the concurrent administration of these drugs.

  IX. Anticholinergic drugs act synergistically with levodopa to improve certain symptoms of Parkinson's disease, especially tremor.

  X. Pyridoxine, in doses as low as 5 mg as present in multivitamin preparations, can abolish the therapeutic efficacy of levodopa by enhancing the activity of pyridoxine-dependent dopa decarboxylase and thus increasing the metabolism of levodopa in the circulation before it can enter the CNS.

XI. Peripheral Decarboxylase Inhibitors
   A. Levodopa is usually administered with a peripheral carboxylase inhibitor such as carbidopa or benserazide (more levodopa escapes metabolism to dopamine in the peripheral circulation and is available to enter the CNS).
      1. Side effects related to high systemic concentrations of dopamine are decreased when levodopa is administered with a peripheral decarboxylase inhibitor.
      2. Carbidopa and benserazide do not cross the blood–brain barrier and lack pharmacologic activity when administered alone.

XII. Central Nervous System Stimulants
   A. **Doxapram** acts centrally and at peripheral chemoreceptors to augment breathing efforts (stimulus to ventilation produced by administration of doxapram, 1 mg/kg IV, is similar to a Pao_2 of 38 mm Hg).
      1. Doxapram has a large margin of safety as reflected by a 20- to 40-fold difference in the dose that stimulates ventilation and the dose that produces seizures. Nevertheless, continuous infusion (single IV dose lasts only 5 to 10 minutes) of doxapram, as is required to produce a sustained effect on ventilation, often results in evidence of subconvulsive CNS stimulation (hypertension, tachycardia, cardiac dysrhythmias, vomiting, and increased body temperature).
      2. **Clinical Uses** (Table 13-7)
   B. **Methylphenidate** is a mild CNS stimulant structurally related to amphetamine (useful in the treatment of attention

Table 13-7

Clinical Uses of Doxapram

Maintain ventilation in patients dependent on hypoxic drive
Prevent opioid-induced ventilatory depression without altering analgesia
Treat postoperative shivering
Delay or prevent need for tracheal intubation in apneic neonates

deficit hyperactivity disorder, narcolepsy). Hypertension, tachycardia, priapism, seizures, and serious cardiovascular events such as sudden cardiac death, stroke, and myocardial infarction have been described in patients treated with methylphenidate.

C. **Methylxanthines** (caffeine, theophylline, theobromine) stimulate the CNS, produce diuresis, increase myocardial contractility, and relax smooth muscle, especially those in the airways.

1. **Mechanism of Action**. The best characterized cellular action of methylxanthines is antagonism of receptor-mediated actions of adenosine thus facilitating the release of catecholamines.

2. **Clinical Uses**

   a. Methylxanthines are used as analeptics to treat primary apnea of prematurity (slowed metabolism of methylxanthines in neonates compared to adults is a consideration when using theophylline to stimulate ventilation in neonates).

   b. The administration of theophylline during maintenance of anesthesia appears to have no added bronchodilator effect over that of the volatile anesthetic alone (selective β_2-adrenergic agonists delivered by inhalation have largely replaced theophylline preparations in the treatment of bronchospasm associated with asthma).

3. **Toxicity**

   a. Theophylline plasma concentrations only slightly greater than the recommended therapeutic range can produce evidence of CNS stimulation (nervousness, tremors, seizures).

   b. Vomiting most likely reflecting CNS stimulation is common when plasma concentrations exceed 15 μg/mL.

   c. Tachycardia and cardiac dysrhythmias may appear most likely due to drug-induced release of catecholamines from the adrenal medulla.

4. **Drug Interactions**

   a. Drugs may enhance (carbamazepine, rifampin) or inhibit (cimetidine, erythromycin) the hepatic metabolism of theophylline.

   b. Larger doses of benzodiazepines may be required in the presence of theophylline.

   c. Ketamine may decrease the seizure threshold for theophylline.

        d. Theophylline can partially antagonize the effects of nondepolarizing neuromuscular blocking drugs presumably by inhibition of phosphodiesterase.

5. **Caffeine** is a methylxanthine-derived phosphodiesterase inhibitor that is present in a variety of beverages and non-prescription medications. A prominent effect of caffeine is CNS stimulation. Caffeine acts as a cerebral vasoconstrictor and may cause secretion of acidic gastric fluid.

        a. Pharmacologic uses of caffeine include administration to neonates experiencing apnea of prematurity.

        b. Treatment of postdural puncture headache has historically been treated with doses ranging from 75 to 300 mg oral caffeine.

        c. Caffeine may be included in common cold remedies in an attempt to offset the sedating effects of certain antihistamines.

D. **Almitrine** acts on the carotid body chemoreceptors to increase minute ventilation (used as a measure to improve or prevent hypoxia during one-lung ventilation techniques, especially with IV anesthesia techniques). Side effects of prolonged oral almitrine therapy include dyspnea and peripheral neuropathy which significantly limits its use.

E. **Modafinil** is a wakefulness-promoting drug approved for patients with excessive daytime sleepiness associated with narcolepsy, obstructive sleep apnea, and shiftwork sleep disorder.

XIII. **Centrally Acting Muscle Relaxants. The primary indication for centrally acting muscle relaxants is spasticity, which may accompany pathologic conditions such as stroke, cerebral palsy, multiple sclerosis, amyotrophic lateral sclerosis, and injuries to the CNS.**

A. **Baclofen** acts as an agonist at $GABA_B$ receptors in the dorsal horn of the spinal cord and is often administered for treatment of spastic hypertonia of cerebral and spinal cord origin. Use of baclofen is limited by its side effects, which include sedation, skeletal muscle weakness, and confusion.

B. **Benzodiazepines** (diazepam and clonazepam) are widely used as centrally acting skeletal muscle relaxants. Sedation may limit the efficacy of these drugs as muscle relaxants but may be useful for relief of spasms that limit sleep.

C. **Botulinum toxin** causes irreversible inhibition of presynaptic acetylcholine release. Injections are made into spastic muscles—blepharospasm, hemifacial spasm, and torticollis—thereby causing weakening of muscle tone.

D. **Cyclobenzaprine** is related structurally and pharmacologically to the tricyclic antidepressants (anticholinergic effects).

   1. The agent is commonly used in the short term (1 to 2 weeks) management of lumbar sprain-strain injuries associated with painful muscle spasm.

   2. In view of the potential adverse side effects of some tricyclic antidepressant drugs on the heart, the use of cyclobenzaprine may be questionable in patients with cardiac dysrhythmias or altered conduction of cardiac impulses.

E. **Dantrolene** exerts antispasmodic effects by inducing relaxation directly on muscle by decreasing calcium release from the sarcoplasmic reticulum. There is a potential for hepatotoxicity especially in those patients with preexisting hepatic compromise.

CHAPTER 14

Circulatory Physiology

I. Systemic circulation supplies blood to all the tissues of the body except the lungs. The fetal circulation possesses many unique features that distinguish it from the systemic circulation after birth.

II. Endothelial Function. The endothelium is not simply an inert lining layer of the circulation but is an important "organ" that is involved in many physiologic processes in health and disease (Tables 14-1 and 14-2). The healthy endothelium promotes vasodilatation and confers antithrombotic and antiadhesive properties to the vessel wall. Damage to the endothelium results in increased vascular permeability and adherence of inflammatory mediators and cells. Cardiovascular risk factors including smoking, diabetes mellitus, hyperlipidemia, obesity, and systemic hypertension are related to their adverse effects upon endothelial function.

A. **Endothelial Function and Regulation of Vascular Tone**. Endothelial synthesis and release of vasoactive mediators are important elements in the regulation of vascular tone. Under physiologic conditions, local vascular pressure and flow are the primary stimuli for endothelial vasoactive substance release. Nitric oxide and prostacyclin are powerful vasodilators released by endothelial cells and both also inhibit platelet aggregation and thrombosis.

III. Components of the Systemic Circulation. The components of the systemic circulation are the arteries, arterioles, capillaries, venules, and veins.

IV. Physical Characteristics of the Systemic Circulation. The systemic circulation contains about 80% of the blood volume,

Table 14-1

Physiologic Roles of Endothelial Function

Endothelial Function	Example
Regulation of vascular tone	Vasodilator release (nitric oxide, prostacyclin)
	Vasoconstrictor release (thromboxane A_2, leukotriene, endothelia, angiotensin-converting enzyme)
Regulation of coagulation	Procoagulant release
	Anticoagulant release
Vascular growth regulation (angiogenesis)	Growth factor synthesis and release
Lipid clearance	LDL receptor expression
	Lipoprotein lipase synthesis
Inflammatory regulation and defense	Inflammatory mediator synthesis and release
Vascular support matrix elaboration	Synthesis of collagen, laminin, fibronectin proteoglycans, proteases
Regulation of molecular transport	Transport of glucose, amino acid, and albumin

with the remainder present in the pulmonary circulation and heart (Fig. 14-1). The heart ejects blood intermittently into the aorta such that blood pressure in the aorta fluctuates between a systolic level of about 120 mm Hg and a diastolic level of about 80 mm Hg (Table 14-3) (Fig. 14-2).

Table 14-2

Pathologic Processes Associated with Endothelial Dysfunction

Systemic hypertension
Pulmonary hypertension
Atherosclerosis
Sepsis and inflammation
Multisystem organ failure
Metastatic tumor spread
Thrombotic disorders

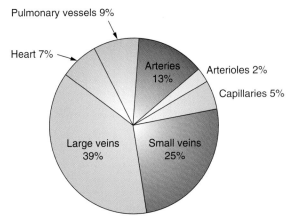

FIGURE 14-1 Distribution of blood volume in the systemic and pulmonary circulation. (From Guyton AC, Hall JE. *Textbook of Medical Physiology*. 10th ed. Philadelphia, PA: Saunders; 2000, with permission.)

Table 14-3

Normal Pressures in the Systemic Circulation

	Mean Value (mm Hg)	Range (mm Hg)
Systolic blood pressure[a]	120	90–140
Diastolic blood pressure[a]	80	70–90
Mean arterial pressure	92	77–97
Left ventricular end diastolic pressure	6	0–12
Left atrium		
a wave	10	2–12
v wave	13	6–20
Right atrium		
a wave	6	2–10
c wave	5	2–10
v wave	3	0–8

[a]Measured in the radial artery.

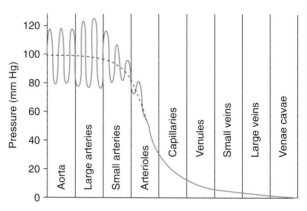

FIGURE 14-2 Systemic blood pressure decreases as blood travels from the aorta to large veins. (From Guyton AC, Hall JE. *Textbook of Medical Physiology*. 10th ed. Philadelphia, PA: Saunders; 2000, with permission.)

Standard physiologic monitors (heart rate, blood pressure, pulse oximetry, capnography) all serve as surrogate markers of organ perfusion and oxygenation.

A. **Progressive Declines in Systemic Blood Pressure**. As blood flows through the systemic circulation, perfusion pressure decreases progressively to nearly 0 mm Hg by the time blood reaches the right atrium (see Fig. 14-2). The decrease in systemic blood pressure in each portion of the systemic circulation is directly proportional to the resistance to flow in the vessels.

1. **Pulse pressure in arteries** reflects the intermittent ejection of blood into the aorta by the heart (see Table 14-3). The difference between systolic and diastolic blood pressure is the pulse pressure (Fig. 14-3).

2. **Factors That Alter Pulse Pressure**. The principal factors that alter pulse pressure in the arteries are the left ventricular stroke volume, velocity of blood flow, and compliance of the arterial tree.

3. **Transmission of the Pulse Pressure**. There is often enhancement of the pulse pressure as the pressure wave is transmitted peripherally (Fig. 14-4). Augmentation of the peripheral pulse pressure must be identified whenever systemic blood pressure measurements are made in peripheral arteries (systolic pressure in the radial artery is sometimes as much as 20% to 30% higher than

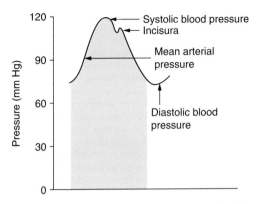

FIGURE 14-3 Schematic depiction of systemic blood pressure recorded from a large systemic artery. Mean arterial pressure is equal to the area under the blood pressure curve divided by the duration of systole.

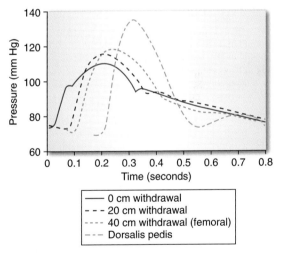

FIGURE 14-4 There is enhancement of the pulse pressure as the systemic blood pressure is transmitted peripherally. (From Guyton AC, Hall JE. *Textbook of Medical Physiology*. 10th ed. Philadelphia, PA: Saunders; 2000, with permission.)

that pressure present in the central aorta, and diastolic pressure is often decreased as much as 10% to 15%). Mean arterial pressures are similar regardless of the site of blood pressure measurement in a peripheral artery.

4. **Systemic Blood Pressure Measurement during and after Cardiopulmonary Bypass**
    a. Reversal of the usual relationship between aortic and radial artery blood pressures can occur during the late period of hypothermic cardiopulmonary bypass and in the early period after termination of cardiopulmonary bypass (Fig. 14-5).
    b. Failure to recognize this disparity may lead to an erroneous diagnosis and unnecessary treatment. Systemic blood pressure measured in the brachial artery is more accurate and reliable during the periods surrounding cardiopulmonary bypass.

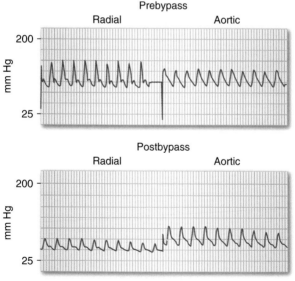

FIGURE 14-5 There may be a reversal of the usual relationship of simultaneous recordings of radial and aortic blood pressures (prebypass) in the early period after separation from cardiopulmonary bypass (postbypass). (From Stern DH, Gerson JI, Allen FB, et al. Can we trust the direct radial artery pressure immediately following cardiopulmonary bypass? *Anesthesiology*. 1985;62:557–561, with permission.)

5. **Pulsus paradoxus** is an exaggerated decrease in systolic blood pressure (>10 mm Hg) during inspiration in the presence of increased intrapericardial pressures (cardiac tamponade).

6. **Pulsus alternans** is alternating weak and strong cardiac contractions causing a similar alteration in the strength of the peripheral pulse (associated with digitalis toxicity, atrioventricular heart block, left ventricular dysfunction).

7. **Electrical alternans** is a phenomenon where the amplitude of the QRS complex changes between heart beats (cardiac tamponade, pericardial effusion).

8. **Pulse Deficit**. In the presence of atrial fibrillation or ectopic ventricular beats, two beats of the heart may occur so close together that the ventricle does not fill adequately and the second cardiac contraction ejects an insufficient volume of blood to create a peripheral pulse. In this circumstance, a second heart beat is audible with a stethoscope applied on the chest directly over the heart, but a corresponding pulsation in the radial artery cannot be palpated.

B. **Measurement of blood pressure by auscultation** uses the principle that blood flow in large arteries is laminar and not audible.

1. If blood flow is arrested by an inflated cuff and the pressure in the cuff is released slowly, audible tapping sounds (Korotkoff's sounds) can be heard when the pressure of the cuff decreases just below systolic blood pressure and blood starts flowing in the brachial artery. Diastolic blood pressure correlates with the onset of muffled auscultatory sounds. The auscultatory method for determining systolic and diastolic blood pressure usually gives values within 10% of those determined by direct measurement from the arteries.

2. The width of the blood pressure cuff will affect measurements; ideally, the width of the blood pressure cuff should be 20% to 50% greater than the diameter of the patient's extremity. If the cuff is too narrow, the blood pressure will be overestimated. If the cuff is too large, the blood pressure may be underestimated.

C. **Right atrial pressure** is regulated by a balance between venous return and the ability of the right ventricle to eject blood (normal right atrial pressure is about 5 mm Hg). Poor right ventricular contractility or any event that increases venous return (hypervolemia, venoconstriction) tends to

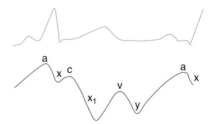

FIGURE 14-6 Simultaneous recording of the electrocardiogram *(top tracing)* and jugular venous pressure waves *(bottom tracing)*. (From Cook DJ, Simel DL. Does this patient have abnormal venous pressure? *JAMA.* 1996;275:630–634, with permission.)

increase right atrial pressure. Pressure in the right atrium is commonly designated the *central venous pressure* (CVP).

1. **Jugular venous pressure** mirrors the CVP. The normal jugular venous pressure reflects phasic changes in the right atrium and consists of three positive waves and three negative troughs (Fig. 14-6). Abnormalities of these venous waveforms may be useful in the diagnosis of various cardiac conditions (Table 14-4).

D. **Effect of Hydrostatic Pressure**

1. Pressure in veins below the heart is increased and that in veins above the heart is decreased by the effect of gravity (Fig. 14-7).

   a. As a guideline, pressure changes 0.77 mm Hg for every centimeter the vessel is above or below the heart (pressure in the veins of the feet is 90 mm Hg).

   b. Veins above the heart tend to collapse, with the exception being veins inside the skull, where they are held open by surrounding bone. As a result, negative pressure can exist in the dural sinuses and air can be entrained immediately if these sinuses are entered during surgery.

2. Hydrostatic pressure affects peripheral pressure in arteries and capillaries as well as veins (systemic blood pressure of 100 mm Hg at the level of the heart has a blood pressure of about 190 mm Hg in the feet).

E. **Venous Valves and the Pump Mechanism**. Valves in veins are arranged so that the direction of blood flow can be only toward the heart (in a standing human, the movement of the legs compresses skeletal muscles and veins so blood is directed toward the heart). If an individual stands immobile, the venous pump does not function and pressures in

Table 14-4

Abnormalities of Jugular Venous Pressure Waveforms

Waveform	Cardiac Abnormality
Absent a wave	Atrial fibrillation
	Sinus tachycardia
Flutter waves	Atrial flutter
Prominent a waves	First-degree atrioventricular heart block
Large a wave	Tricuspid stenosis
	Pulmonary hypertension
	Pulmonic stenosis
	Right atrial myxoma
Cannon a waves	Atrioventricular dissociation
	Ventricular tachycardia
Absent x wave descent	Tricuspid regurgitation
Large cv waves	Tricuspid regurgitation
	Constrictive pericarditis
Slow y wave descent	Tricuspid stenosis
	Right atrial myxoma
Rapid y wave descent	Tricuspid regurgitation
	Atrial septal defect
	Constrictive pericarditis
Absent y wave descent	Cardiac tamponade

Adapted from Cook DJ, Simel DL. Does this patient have abnormal central venous pressure? *JAMA*. 1996;275:630–634.

the veins and capillaries of the legs can increase resulting in leakage of fluid from the intravascular space (as much as 15% of the blood volume can be lost from the intravascular space in the first 15 minutes of quiet standing).

1. **Varicose Veins**
   a. Valves of the venous system can be destroyed when the veins are chronically distended by increased venous pressure as occurs during pregnancy or in an individual who stands most of the day (result is varicose veins characterized by bulbous protrusions of the veins beneath the skin of the legs).
   b. Venous and capillary pressures remain increased because of the incompetent venous pump, and this causes constant edema in the legs of these individuals. Edema interferes with diffusion of nutrients from the capillaries to tissues, so there is often skeletal muscle discomfort and the skin may ulcerate.

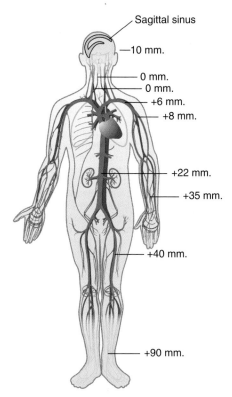

Sagittal sinus

-10 mm.

0 mm.
0 mm.
+6 mm.
+8 mm.

+22 mm.

+35 mm.

+40 mm.

+90 mm.

FIGURE 14-7 Effect of hydrostatic pressure on venous pressures throughout the body.

F. **Reference Level for Measuring Venous Pressure**
   1. Hydrostatic pressure does not alter venous or arterial pressures that are measured at the level of the tricuspid valve (considered to be the level of the tricuspid valve). External reference points for the level of the tricuspid valve in a supine individual are about one-third the distance from the anterior chest and about one-fourth the distance above the lower end of the sternum.
   2. For each centimeter below, the hydrostatic point adds 0.77 mm Hg to the measured pressure, whereas 0.77 mm Hg is subtracted for each centimeter above this point.

The potential error introduced by measuring pressures above or below the tricuspid valve is greatest with venous pressures that are normally low.

3. The reason for lack of hydrostatic effects at the tricuspid valve is the ability of the right ventricle to act as a regulator of pressure at this site.

4. A venous pressure measurement in mm Hg can be converted to cm H_2O by multiplying the pressure by 1.36, which adjusts for the density of mercury relative to water (10 mm Hg equals 13.6 cm H_2O). Conversely, dividing the CVP measurement in cm H_2O by 1.36 converts this value to an equivalent pressure in mm Hg.

G. **Blood Viscosity**

1. The percentage of blood comprising erythrocytes is the hematocrit, which to a large extent determines the viscosity of blood (Fig. 14-8). When the hematocrit increases to 60% to 70%, viscosity of blood is increased

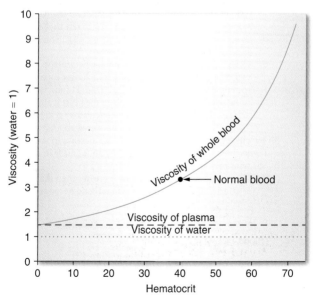

FIGURE 14-8 Hematocrit greatly influences the viscosity of blood. (From Guyton AC, Hall JE. *Textbook of Medical Physiology.* 10th ed. Philadelphia, PA: Saunders; 2000, with permission.)

about 10-fold compared with water, and flow through blood vessels is greatly decreased.

2. Plasma is considered extracellular fluid that is identical to interstitial fluid except for the greater concentrations of proteins (albumin, globulin, fibrinogen) in plasma. These greater concentrations reflect the inability of plasma proteins to pass easily through capillaries into the interstitial spaces. The presence of albumin creates colloid osmotic pressure, which prevents fluid from leaving the capillaries.

V. **Determinants of Tissue Blood Flow.** Tissue blood flow is directly proportional to the pressure difference between two points (not absolute pressure) and inversely proportional to resistance to flow through the vessel (Fig. 14-9). It is important to understand that resistance to blood flow cannot be measured but rather is a calculated value based on measurement of driving pressures and the cardiac output.

A. **Vascular Distensibility**

1. Blood vessels are distensible such that increases in systemic blood pressure cause the vascular diameter to increase, which in turn decreases resistance to blood flow. Conversely, decreases in intravascular pressure increase the resistance to blood flow.

2. Systemic blood pressure can eventually decrease to a level where intravascular pressure is no longer capable of keeping the vessel open (averages 20 mm Hg and is defined as the *critical closing pressure*). When the heart is abruptly stopped, the pressure in the entire circulatory system (mean circulatory pressure) equilibrates at about 7 mm Hg.

B. **Vascular compliance** is defined as the increase in volume (capacitance) of a vessel produced by an increase in intravascular pressure.

1. The compliance of veins is much greater than that of arteries. Enhancement of sympathetic nervous

$$\text{Blood Flow} \atop (Q) = \frac{\text{Pressure Difference Between Two Points (P)}}{\text{Resistance to Flow (R)}}$$

$$\Delta P = Q \times R$$

$$R = \Delta P / Q$$

FIGURE 14-9 The relationship between blood flow, pressure, and resistance to flow can be expressed as a variant of Ohm's law.

outflow to the blood vessels, especially the veins, decreases the dimensions to the circulatory system, and the circulation continues to function almost normally even when as much as 25% of the total blood volume has been lost.

2. *Vasoconstriction* or *vasodilation* refer to resistance changes in arterioles, whereas changes in the caliber of veins are described as *venoconstriction* or *venodilation*.

VI. **Control of Tissue Blood Flow. Control of blood flow to different tissues includes local mechanisms, autonomic nervous system responses, and release of hormones (Table 14-5).**
   A. **Local control of blood flow** is most often based on the need for delivery of oxygen or other nutrients such as glucose or fatty acids to the tissues.
   B. **Autoregulation of blood flow** is a local mechanism that controls blood flow in which a specific tissue is able to maintain a relatively constant blood flow over a wide range of mean arterial pressures. Autoregulatory responses to sudden changes in mean arterial pressure occur within 60 to 120 seconds.

Table 14-5

Tissue Blood Flow

	Approximate Blood Flow		Cardiac Output (% of Total)
	(mL/min)	(mL/100 g/min)	
Brain	750	50	15
Liver	1,450	100	29
Portal vein	1,100		
Hepatic artery	350		
Kidneys	1,000	320	20
Heart	225	75	5
Skeletal muscles (at rest)	750	4	15
Skin	400	3	8
Other tissues	425	2	8
Total	5,000		100

Adapted from Guyton AC, Hall JE. *Textbook of Medical Physiology*. 10th ed. Philadelphia, PA: Saunders; 2000.

C. **Long-Term Control of Blood Flow**
1. Long-term regulatory mechanisms that return local tissue blood flow to normal involve a change in vascularity of tissues.
2. Inadequate delivery of oxygen to a tissue is the stimulus for the development of collateral vessels. Neonates exposed to increased concentrations of oxygen can manifest cessation of new vascular growth in the retina. Subsequent removal of the neonate from a high-oxygen environment causes an overgrowth of new vessels to offset the abrupt decrease in availability of oxygen (retrolental fibroplasia).

D. **Autonomic nervous system control of blood flow** is characterized by a rapid response time (within 1 second) and an ability to regulate blood flow to certain tissues at the expense of other tissues.
1. **Mass reflex** is characterized by stimulation of all portions of the vasomotor center, resulting in generalized vasoconstriction and an increase in cardiac output in an attempt to maintain tissue blood flow.
2. **Syncope**. Emotional fainting (vasovagal syncope) may reflect profound bradycardia and skeletal muscle vasodilation such that systemic blood pressure decreases abruptly and syncope occurs. This phenomenon may occur in patients who have an intense fear of needles, resulting in syncope during placement of an intravenous catheter.

E. **Hormone Control of Blood Flow.** Vasoconstrictor hormones that may influence local tissue blood flow include epinephrine, norepinephrine, angiotensin, and arginine vasopressin (formerly known as *antidiuretic hormone*). Carbon dioxide also has an indirect vasoconstrictor effect because it stimulates the outflow of sympathetic nervous system impulses from the vasomotor center.

VII. **Regulation of Systemic Blood Pressure. Systemic blood pressure is maintained over a narrow range by reciprocal changes in cardiac output and systemic vascular resistance. Because a greater portion of the cardiac cycle is nearer the diastolic blood pressure, it follows that mean arterial pressure is not the arithmetic average of the systolic and diastolic blood pressures. Mean arterial blood pressure is the most important determinant of tissue blood flow because it is the average, tending to drive blood through the systemic circulation.**
A. **Rapid-acting mechanisms for the regulation of systemic blood pressure** involve nervous system responses as reflected by the baroreceptor reflexes, chemoreceptor reflexes,

atrial reflexes, and central nervous system ischemic reflex. These reflex mechanisms respond almost immediately to changes in systemic blood pressure.

1. **Baroreceptor Reflexes**
   a. Baroreceptors are nerve endings in the walls of large arteries in the neck and thorax, especially in the internal carotid arteries just above the carotid bifurcation and in the arch of the aorta.
   b. These nerve endings respond rapidly to changes in systemic blood pressure and are crucial for maintaining normal blood pressure when an individual changes from the supine to standing position.

2. **Chemoreceptor Reflexes**
   a. Chemoreceptors are cells that transduce chemical signals into nerve impulses. There are chemoreceptors located in the carotid bodies and aortic body. Each carotid or aortic body is supplied with an abundant blood flow through a nutrient artery so that the chemoreceptors are always exposed to oxygenated blood. When the systemic blood pressure, and thus the blood flow, decrease below a critical level, the chemoreceptors in the carotid body are stimulated by decreased availability of oxygen and also because of excess carbon dioxide and hydrogen ions that are not removed by the sluggish blood flow.
   b. Chemoreceptors do not respond strongly until systemic blood pressure decreases below 80 mm Hg.
   c. Chemoreceptors are more important in stimulating breathing when the Pao_2 decreases below 60 mm Hg (ventilatory response to arterial hypoxemia). The ventilatory response to arterial hypoxemia is inhibited by subanesthetic concentrations of most of the volatile anesthetics (0.1 minimum alveolar concentration) as well as injected drugs such as barbiturates and opioids.

3. **Central nervous system ischemic reflex** occurs when blood flow to the medullary vasomotor center is decreased to the extent that ischemia of this vital center occurs. As a result of this ischemia, there is an intense outpouring of sympathetic nervous system activity, resulting in profound increases in systemic blood pressure. The central nervous system reflex response does not become highly active until mean arterial pressure decreases to less than 50 mm Hg and reaches its greatest degree of stimulation at systemic blood pressures of 15 to 20 mm Hg.

4. **Cushing reflex** is a central nervous system ischemic reflex response that results from increased intracranial pressure. When intracranial pressure increases to equal arterial pressure, the Cushing reflex acts to increase systemic blood pressure above intracranial pressure. Cushing's triad is defined as having (a) hypertension, (b) bradycardia, and (c) irregular respirations (due to brainstem dysfunction). The latter is not often seen in this era, as most patients with severe intracranial hypertension are now mechanically ventilated.

5. **Respiratory Variations in Systemic Blood Pressure**
   a. Systemic blood pressure normally varies by 4 to 6 mm Hg in a wavelike manner during quiet spontaneous breathing. This is due to increased venous return to the right heart during inspiration, which takes a few cardiac cycles to be transmitted to the left heart.
   b. Positive pressure ventilation of the lungs produces a reversed sequence of blood pressure change because the initial positive airway pressure simultaneously pushes more blood toward the left ventricle.
   c. Continuous or beat-to-beat monitoring of the changes in arterial blood pressure, pulse pressure, and stroke volume occurring during mechanical ventilation may provide an indication of the patient's ability to respond to volume administration with an increase in cardiac output (fluid responsiveness). Respiratory variation in these parameters of more than 12% to 15% generally indicates fluid responsiveness.

6. **Heart Rate Variability**
   a. Variations in heart rate occur during normal respiration, whereby inspiration increases heart rate and expiration decreases it. Analysis of heart rate variability provides information regarding the integrity of the autonomic nervous system.
   b. Low heart rate variability can be a manifestation of disease (myocardial infarction, heart failure, neuropathy) and occurs universally following the denervation that occurs during cardiac transplantation.

B. **Moderately Rapid-Acting Mechanisms for the Regulation of Systemic Blood Pressure**. There are at least three hormonal mechanisms that provide either rapid or moderately rapid control of systemic blood pressure (catecholamine-induced vasoconstriction, renin-angiotensin–induced vasoconstriction, vasoconstriction induced by arginine vasopressin).

C. **Long-term mechanisms for the regulation of systemic blood pressure**, unlike the short-term regulatory mechanisms, have a delayed onset but do not adapt, providing a sustained regulatory effect on systemic blood pressure. The renal–body fluid system plays a predominant role in long-term control of systemic blood pressure because it controls both the cardiac output and systemic vascular resistance.

VIII. **Regulation of Cardiac Output and Venous Return. Cardiac output is the amount of blood pumped by the left ventricle into the aorta each minute (product of stroke volume and heart rate), and venous return is the amount of blood flowing from the veins into the right atrium each minute (cardiac output must equal venous return). Cardiac output for the average person weighing 70 kg and with a body surface area of 1.7 m^2 is about 5 L per minute. This value is about 10% less in women.**

A. **Determinants of Cardiac Output**

1. Venous return is the main determinant of cardiac output. Any factor that interferes with venous return can lead to decreased cardiac output. Hemorrhage decreases blood volume such that venous return decreases and cardiac output decreases. Acute venodilation, such as that produced by spinal anesthesia and accompanying sympathetic nervous system blockade, can so increase the capacitance of peripheral vessels that venous return is reduced and cardiac output declines.

2. Factors that increase cardiac output are associated with decreases in systemic vascular resistance (anemia decreases the viscosity of blood, leading to a decrease in systemic vascular resistance and increase in venous return).

3. **Ventricular function curves** (Frank-Starling curves) depict the cardiac output at different atrial (ventricular end diastolic) filling pressures (Figs. 14-10 and 14-11). Clinically, ventricular function curves are used to estimate myocardial contractility.

B. **Shock Syndromes**. Circulatory shock is characterized by inadequate tissue blood flow and oxygen delivery to cells resulting in generalized deterioration of cellular and organ function. Consciousness is likely to be lost as shock progresses. Low cardiac output greatly decreases urine output. An important feature of persistent shock is eventual progressive deterioration of the heart.

1. **Hemorrhagic Shock**. Hemorrhage is the most common cause of shock due to decreased venous return. Venoconstriction is particularly important for sustaining

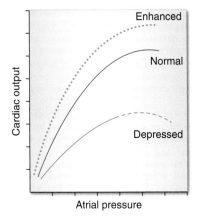

FIGURE 14-10 Ventricular function curves (Frank-Starling curves) depict the volume of forward ventricular ejection (cardiac output) at different atrial filling pressures and varying degrees of myocardial contractility.

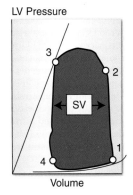

FIGURE 14-11 Pressure-volume loop representing the cardiac cycle. The end diastolic and the end systolic pressure-volume relationships represent the boundaries for the loops. The width of the pressure-volume loop represents the stroke volume (SV). Increases or decreases in myocardial contractility make the end systolic pressure-volume relationship steeper or shallower. The four segments of the loop (isovolumic contraction, ejection, isovolumic relaxation, ventricular filling) for the left ventricle are depicted in succession by mitral valve closure (1), aortic valve opening (2), aortic valve closure (3), and mitral valve opening (4).

venous return to the heart and, thus, maintaining cardiac output. Arterial constriction is responsible for initially maintaining systemic blood pressure despite decreases in cardiac output.

2. **Nonhemorrhagic Hypovolemic Shock**. Loss of plasma volume from the circulation can result in shock similar to that produced by hemorrhage (intestinal obstruction, burns, dehydration). Hypovolemic shock that results from a reduction in plasma volume has the same clinical characteristics as hemorrhagic shock except that selective reduction of the plasma volume greatly increases the viscosity of blood and exacerbates sluggish blood flow.

3. **Neurogenic shock** occurs in the absence of blood loss when vascular capacity increases so greatly that even a normal blood volume is not capable of maintaining venous return and cardiac output (traumatic transection of the spinal cord, acute blockade of the peripheral sympathetic nervous system by spinal or epidural anesthesia).

4. **Septic shock** is characterized by profound peripheral vasodilation, increased cardiac output secondary to decreased systemic vascular resistance, increased vascular permeability with fluid loss from the vascular compartment, and development of disseminated intravascular coagulation. Septic shock is most commonly caused by gram-positive bacteria. The end stages of septic shock are not greatly different from the end stages of hemorrhagic shock, even though the initiating factors are markedly different. Mortality approaches 50% in septic shock despite significant improvements in supportive care.

C. **Measurement of Cardiac Output**. The pulmonary artery thermodilution technique represents the clinical standard against which new techniques are compared.

1. **Echocardiographic techniques** can be used to estimate cardiac output by combining the Doppler principle to determine the velocity of blood in the aorta with two-dimensional views to determine aortic diameter. Transesophageal Doppler estimates of cardiac output require minimal operator training and allow rapid cardiac output estimation.

2. **Impedance cardiography** is based on the principle of thoracic electrical bioimpedance and involves the placement of electrodes to allow the transmission of current and measurement of voltage across the chest. The reliability of this technique is limited under several

circumstances including patient movement, poor electrocardiogram signal quality, cardiac tachydysrhythmias, excessive thoracic fluid, and open chest wounds with retractors.

IX. **Microcirculation** is the circulation of blood through the smallest vessels of the body—arterioles, capillaries, and venules. Capillaries, whose walls consist of a single layer of endothelial cells, serve as the site for the rapid transfer of oxygen and nutrients to tissues and receipt of metabolic byproducts (it is unlikely that any functional cell is $>50 \, \mu m$ away from a capillary). The muscular arterioles serve as the major resistance vessels and regulate regional blood flow to the capillary beds. Venules act primarily as collecting channels and storage vessels.

A. **Anatomy of the Microcirculation** (Table 14-6) (Fig. 14-12)

1. **Blood flow in capillaries** is approximately 1 mm per second and is intermittent rather than continuous. This intermittent blood flow reflects contraction and relaxation of metarterioles and precapillary sphincters in alternating cycles 6 to 12 times per minute (*vasomotion*).

a. Oxygen is the most important determinant of the degree of opening and closing of metarterioles and

---

Table 14-6

Anatomy of the Various Types of Blood Vessels

Vessel	Lumen Diameter	Approximate Cross-Sectional Area (cm^2)	Percentage of Blood Volume Contained
Aorta	2.5 cm	2.5	
Artery	0.4 cm	20	13
Arteriole	30 μm	40	1
Capillary	5 μm	2,500	6
Venule	20 μm	250	
Vein	0.5 cm	80	64[a]
Vena cava	3 cm	8	
Heart			7
Pulmonary circulation		18	9

[a]Blood volume contained in venules, veins, and vena cava.

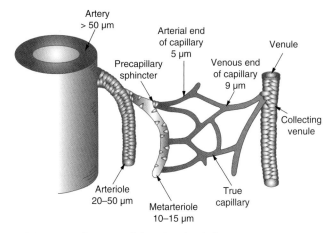

FIGURE 14-12 Anatomy of the microcirculation.

precapillary sphincters. A low PO_2 allows more blood to flow through capillaries to supply tissues.

b. In addition to nutritive blood flow through tissues that is regulated by oxygen, there is also nonnutritive (shunt) blood flow regulated by the autonomic nervous system (arteriovenous connections). In some parts of the skin, these arteriovenous anastomoses provide a mechanism to permit rapid inflow of arterial blood to warm the skin and dissipate the heat.

2. **Vasoactive Role of the Capillary Endothelium**

a. The notion that the endothelium of capillaries is an inert single layer of cells serving only as a passive filter to permit passage of water and small molecules across the blood vessel wall is no longer considered valid (now recognized as an important source of substances that cause contraction or relaxation of vascular smooth muscle).

b. One of these substances is prostacyclin that can relax vascular smooth muscle via an increase in cyclic adenosine monophosphate concentration. Prostacyclin is formed in the endothelium. The principal function of prostacyclin is to inhibit platelet adherence to the endothelium and platelet aggregation and thus prevent intravascular clot formation.

Table 14-7

Permeability of Capillary Membranes

	Molecular Weight (Daltons)	Relative Permeability
Water	18	1.0
Sodium chloride	58.5	0.96
Glucose	180	0.6
Hemoglobin	66,700	0.01
Albumin	69,000	0.0001

     c. The formation and release of nitric oxide is also
       important in the endothelium-mediated vascular
       dilation.

B. **Fluid Movement across Capillary Membranes**. Solvent
  and solute movement across capillary endothelial cells occurs by filtration, diffusion, and pinocytosis via endothelial
  vesicles (Table 14-7).

  1. **Filtration**. The four pressures that determine whether
     fluid will move outward across capillary membranes
     (filtration) or inward across capillary membranes
     (reabsorption) are capillary pressure, interstitial fluid
     pressure, plasma colloid osmotic pressure, and intersti-
     tial fluid colloid osmotic pressure (Tables 14-8 to 14-10).
     Any fluid that is not reabsorbed enters the lymph vessels.

Table 14-8

Filtration of Fluid at the Arterial Ends of Capillaries

Pressure favoring outward movement

Capillary pressure	25 mm Hg
Interstitial fluid pressure	−6.3 mm Hg
Interstitial fluid colloid osmotic pressure	5 mm Hg
Total	36.3 mm Hg

Pressure favoring inward movement

Plasma colloid osmotic pressure	28 mm Hg
Net filtration pressure	**8.3 mm Hg**

Table 14-9

Reabsorption of Fluid at the Venous Ends of Capillaries

Pressure favoring outward movement	
Capillary pressure	10 mm Hg
Interstitial fluid pressure	−6.3 mm Hg
Interstitial fluid colloid osmotic pressure	5 mm Hg
Total	21.3 mm Hg
Pressure favoring inward movement	
Plasma colloid osmotic pressure	28 mm Hg
Net reabsorption pressure	**6.7 mm Hg**

    a. **Capillary pressure** tends to move fluid outward across the arterial ends of capillary membranes. Changes in arterial pressure have little effect on capillary pressure and flow because of adjustments of precapillary resistance vessels.

    b. **Interstitial fluid pressure** tends to move fluid outward across capillary membranes. Loss of negative interstitial fluid pressure allows fluid to accumulate in tissue spaces as edema.

    c. **Plasma Colloid Osmotic Pressure**. Plasma proteins are principally responsible for the plasma colloid osmotic (oncotic) pressure that tends to cause movement of fluid inward through capillary

Table 14-10

Mean Values of Pressures Acting across Capillary Membranes

Pressure favoring outward movement	
Capillary pressure	17 mm Hg
Interstitial fluid pressure	−6.3 mm Hg
Interstitial fluid colloid osmotic pressure	5 mm Hg
Total	28.3 mm Hg
Pressure favoring inward movement	
Plasma colloid osmotic pressure	28 mm Hg
Net overall filtration pressure	**0.3 mm Hg**

membranes. Because there is about twice as much albumin as globulin in the plasma, about 70% of the total colloid osmotic pressure results from albumin and only about 30% from globulin and fibrinogen. A special phenomenon known as *Donnan equilibrium* causes the colloid osmotic pressure to be about 50% greater than that caused by proteins alone (reflects the negative charge characteristic of proteins that necessitates the presence of an equal number of positively charged ions, mainly sodium ions, on the same side of the capillary membrane as the proteins). These extra positive ions increase the number of osmotically active substances and thus increase the colloid osmotic pressure (about one-third of the normal plasma colloid osmotic pressure of 28 mm Hg is caused by positively charged ions held in the plasma by proteins). This is the reason that plasma proteins cannot be replaced by inert substances, such as dextran, without some decrease in plasma colloid osmotic pressure.

d. **Interstitial Fluid Colloid Osmotic Pressure**. Proteins present in the interstitial fluid are principally responsible for the interstitial fluid colloid osmotic pressure of about 5 mm Hg, which tends to cause movement of fluid outward across capillary membranes.

2. **Diffusion** is the most important mechanism for transfer of nutrients between the plasma and the interstitial fluid.

a. Oxygen, carbon dioxide, and anesthetic gases are examples of lipid-soluble molecules that can diffuse directly through capillary membranes independently of pores.

b. Sodium, potassium, and chloride ions and glucose are insoluble in lipid capillary membranes and therefore must pass through pores to gain access to interstitial fluids.

c. The diffusion rate of lipid-soluble molecules across capillary membranes in either direction is proportional to the concentration difference between the two sides of the membrane (large amounts of oxygen move from capillaries toward tissues, whereas carbon dioxide moves in the opposite direction).

X. **Lymphatics. Lymph vessels represent an alternate route by which fluids flow from interstitial spaces into the blood. The most important function of the lymphatic system is return**

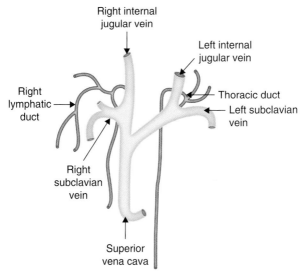

FIGURE 14-13 Depiction of the thoracic duct and right lymphatic duct as they enter the venous system.

of proteins into the circulation and maintenance of a low-protein concentration in the interstitial fluid.
A. **Anatomy** (Fig.14-13). The thoracic duct is the larger of the two (2 mm in diameter), entering the venous system in the angle of the junction of the left internal jugular and subclavian veins. Damage (surgical or traumatic) to a thoracic duct can cause intrathoracic fluid accumulation.
B. **Formation and flow of lymph**. Lymph is interstitial fluid that flows into lymphatic vessels. Flow of lymph through the thoracic duct is about 100 mL per hour. Skeletal muscle contraction and passive movements of the extremities facilitate flow of lymph. Elevations in CVP can impair the return of lymph to the central circulation.
C. **Edema** is the presence of excess interstitial fluid in peripheral tissues that results from the inability of lymph vessels to adequately transport fluid.
  1. Peripheral edema most common in dependent areas may be accompanied by accumulation of fluid in potential spaces (pleural cavity, pericardial space, peritoneal cavity, and synovial spaces).

2. The peritoneal cavity is susceptible to the development of edema fluid because any increased pressure in the liver (cirrhosis, cardiac failure) causes transudation of protein-containing fluids from the surface of the liver into the peritoneal cavity.

XI. **Pulmonary circulation is a low-pressure, low-resistance system in series with the systemic circulation. Blood passes through pulmonary capillaries in about 1 second, during which time it is oxygenated and carbon dioxide is removed.**

A. **Anatomy**

1. The right ventricle is semilunar in shape, wrapped around the medial aspect of the left ventricle. The thickness of the right ventricle is one-third that of the left ventricle, as it normally generates pressures approximately 25% that of the left side.

2. The pulmonary artery extends only about 4 cm beyond the apex of the right ventricle before division into the right and left main pulmonary arteries. Pulmonary blood vessels are innervated by the sympathetic nervous system (despite the presence of autonomic nervous system innervation, the resting vasomotor tone is minimal).

B. **Bronchial Circulation**

1. Bronchial arteries from the thoracic aorta supply oxygenated blood to supporting tissues of the lungs, including connective tissue and airways (majority of it empties into pulmonary veins and enters the left atrium rather than passing back to the right atrium).

2. The entrance of deoxygenated blood into the left atrium dilutes oxygenated blood and accounts for an anatomic shunt that is equivalent to an estimated 1% to 2% of the cardiac output. This anatomic shunt plus a part of coronary blood flow, which drains directly into the left side of the heart, are the reasons the cardiac output of the left ventricle slightly exceeds that of the right ventricle.

C. **Pulmonary Vascular Pressure** (Fig. 14-14)

1. Should the left ventricle fail, left atrial pressures can increase to greater than 15 mm Hg. Mean pulmonary artery pressures also increase, placing an increased workload on the right ventricle. If this occurs acutely, the right ventricle may also fail as it may not be able to generate an adequate stroke volume due to its structure.

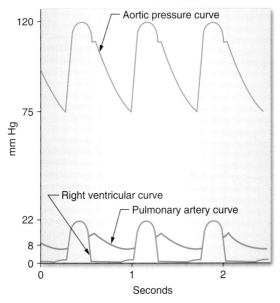

FIGURE 14-14 Comparison of intravascular pressures in the systemic and pulmonary circulations. (From Guyton AC, Hall JE. *Textbook of Medical Physiology*. 10th ed. Philadelphia, PA: Saunders; 2000, with permission.)

2. If pulmonary artery pressures rise gradually over time, the right ventricle may adapt with remodeling and dilatation but will eventually begin to fail.

D. **Measurement of Left Atrial Pressure**

1. The left atrial pressure can be estimated by inserting and inflating a balloon-tipped catheter into a small pulmonary artery (pressure measured immediately distal to the balloon is equivalent to that downstream in the pulmonary veins). This measurement is termed the *pulmonary artery occlusion pressure* ("wedge" pressure although the catheter is not truly wedged) and is usually 2 to 3 mm Hg higher than left atrial pressure.

2. When the balloon is deflated, flow will resume and the pulmonary artery end diastolic pressure can be measured (correlates with the pulmonary artery occlusion pressure in the absence of pulmonary hypertension).

E. **Interstitial Fluid Space**
1. The interstitial fluid space in the lung is minimal, and a continual negative pulmonary interstitial pressure of about −8 mm Hg dehydrates interstitial fluid spaces of the lungs and keeps the alveolar epithelial membrane in close approximation to the capillary membranes.
2. Negative pressure in pulmonary interstitial spaces draws fluid from alveoli through alveolar membranes and into the interstitium, keeping the alveoli dry (decreasing the likelihood of pulmonary edema).

F. **Pulmonary Blood Volume**
1. Blood volume in the lungs is about 450 mL. Cardiac failure or increased resistance to flow through the mitral valve causes pulmonary blood volume to increase.
2. Cardiac output can increase nearly four times before pulmonary artery pressure becomes increased (Fig. 14-15).
3. Pulmonary blood volume can increase up to 40% when an individual changes from the standing to the supine position (occurrence of orthopnea in the presence of left ventricular failure).

G. **Pulmonary Blood Flow and Distribution**. Optimal oxygenation depends on matching ventilation to pulmonary blood flow. Shunt occurs in lung areas that are perfused but inadequately ventilated, whereas dead space ventilation

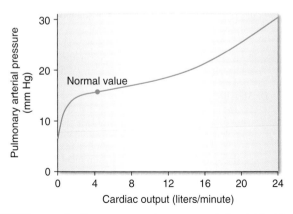

FIGURE 14-15 Cardiac output can increase nearly fourfold without greatly increasing the pulmonary arterial pressure. (From Guyton AC, Hall JE. *Textbook of Medical Physiology*. 10th ed. Philadelphia, PA: Saunders; 2000, with permission.)

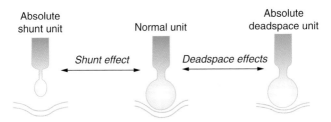

FIGURE 14-16 Gas exchange is maximally effective in normal lung units with optimal ventilation to perfusion (V/Q) relationships. The continuum of (V/Q) relationships is depicted by the ratios between normal and absolute shunt or dead space units.

occurs in lung areas that are ventilated but inadequately perfused (Fig. 14-16).

1. **Endothelial Regulation of Pulmonary Blood Flow**. The pulmonary vascular endothelium is responsible for the synthesis and secretion of various compounds that regulate smooth muscle activity in the pulmonary circulation. The primary vasodilatory compounds are nitric oxide and prostacyclin.

2. **Hypoxic Pulmonary Vasoconstriction**
   a. Alveolar hypoxia (Pao_2 <70 mm Hg) evokes vasoconstriction in the pulmonary arterioles supplying these alveoli. The net effect is to divert blood flow away from poorly ventilated alveoli (shunt effect is minimized, and the resulting Pao_2 is maximized).
   b. The mechanism for hypoxic pulmonary vasoconstriction is presumed to be locally mediated.
   c. Drug-induced inhibition of hypoxic pulmonary vasoconstriction could result in unexpected decreases in Pao_2 in the presence of lung disease (vasodilating drugs such as nitroprusside and nitroglycerin may be accompanied by decreases in Pao_2). Potent volatile anesthetics are acceptable choices for thoracic surgery requiring one-lung ventilation.

H. **Effect of Breathing**
   1. During spontaneous respiration, venous return to the heart is increased due to contraction of the diaphragm and abdominal muscles, which decreases intrathoracic pressure. The resulting augmented blood flow to the right atrium increases right ventricular stroke volume.

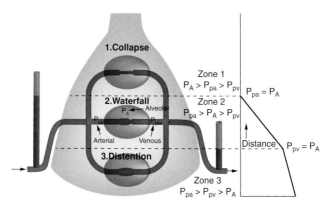

FIGURE 14-17 The lung is divided into three pulmonary blood flow zones reflecting the impact of alveolar pressure (P_A), pulmonary artery pressure (P_{pa}), and pulmonary venous pressure (P_{pv}) on the caliber of pulmonary blood vessels. (From West JB, Dollery CT, Naimark A. Distribution of blood flow in isolated lung: relation to vascular and alveolar pressures. *J Appl Physiol.* 1964;19:713–718, with permission.)

2. In contrast to spontaneous breathing, positive pressure ventilation increases intrathoracic pressure and thus impedes venous return to the heart and decreases right ventricular stroke volume.

I. **Regional Blood Flow in the Lungs.** The gravitational "zone" has a relatively minor role in blood flow distribution (Fig. 14-17). Approximately 75% of the distribution of pulmonary blood flow is determined by the branching structure of the pulmonary vascular tree.

J. **Pulmonary Circulatory Pathology**

1. **Pulmonary edema** is present when there are excessive quantities of fluid either in pulmonary interstitial spaces or in alveoli.

   a. The most common cause of acute pulmonary edema is greatly increased pulmonary capillary pressure resulting from left ventricular failure, and the lymphatic flow cannot adequately remove the increased fluid.

   b. Pulmonary edema can also result from local capillary damage that occurs with inhalation of acidic gastric fluid or irritant gases, such as smoke (called *permeability pulmonary edema* to distinguish it from "hydrostatic" pulmonary edema, which is due to increased pulmonary capillary pressure).

2. **Pulmonary Embolism**. Tachypnea and dyspnea are characteristic responses in awake patients experiencing pulmonary embolism; in the anesthetized patient, an acute decrease in end-tidal CO_2 may occur due to a sudden increase in dead space (loss of perfusion but not ventilation to major part of the lung).

3. **Pulmonary Hypertension** (Table 14-11). Many of the causes of pulmonary hypertension are associated with the development of hypoxemia. Lung transplant or in the case of right ventricular failure, heart–lung transplant may be required.

Table 14-11

Classification of Pulmonary Hypertension

I   Pulmonary arterial hypertension (PAH)
    Idiopathic PAH (majority) and heritable PAH
    Drug- and toxin-induced PAH
    Connective tissue disease–associated PAH
    HIV-associated PAH
    Portal hypertension–associated PAH
    Congenital heart diseases
    Schistosomiasis
II Pulmonary hypertension due to left heart disease
    LV systolic and diastolic dysfunction
    Valvular disease
    Congenital/acquired left heart inflow/outflow tract obstruction
    Developmental lung diseases
III Pulmonary hypertension due to lung diseases or hypoxia
    COPD, ILD, mixed restrictive/obstructive pattern disease
    Sleep disordered breathing and alveolar hypoventilation disorders
    Chronic exposure to high altitude
    Developmental lung diseases
IV Chronic thromboembolic pulmonary hypertension
V   Pulmonary hypertension due to multifactorial mechanisms
    Hematologic: chronic anemia, myoproliferative disorders, splenectomy
    Systemic: sarcoidosis, pulmonary histiocytosis, lymphangioleiomyomatosis
    Metabolic: glycogen storage disease, Gaucher's disease, thyroid disease
    Others: tumor obstruction, fibrosis mediastinitis

From Simonneau G, Gatzoulis MA, Adatia I, et al. Updated clinical classification of pulmonary hypertension. *J Am Coll Cardiol.* 2013;62(25)(suppl):D34–D41.

CHAPTER 15

Cardiac Physiology

I. **Introduction.** The heart has four chambers and can be characterized as two pumps connected in series, each composed of an atrium and a ventricle. The atria function primarily as conduits to the ventricles, but they also contract weakly to facilitate movement of blood into the ventricles during the filling phase, diastole. The ventricles serve as pumps during systole to supply the main force that propels blood through the systemic and pulmonary circulations. Specialized excitatory and conductive fibers in the heart maintain cardiac rhythm and transmit action potentials through cardiac muscle to initiate contraction.

II. **Cardiac Anatomy**

A. **Pericardium** is a fibrous sac that contains the heart and the proximal portions of great vessels.

1. The potential space between visceral and parietal pericardium normally contains 15 to 35 mL of pericardial fluid. Acutely, the pericardium can only accommodate a small amount of pericardial fluid without changes in intrapericardial pressure. Once the amount of pericardial fluid exceeds a limited reserve capacity, the intrapericardial pressure increases steeply with small amounts of pericardial fluid, leading to tamponade physiology.

2. Chronically, the pericardium can accommodate a large amount of fluid without causing tamponade because its size and compliance increase in compensation.

B. **Heart**

1. The heart consists of four chambers. The right atrium receives deoxygenated blood from the superior vena cava, the inferior vena cava, the coronary sinus, and Thebesian cardiac veins.

2. The chordae tendineae are fibrous collagenous structures that support the leaflets of tricuspid and mitral valves during systole.

3. The left atrium is normally smaller in size than the right but has thicker walls.

4. The left ventricle is a cone-shaped structure that is longer and narrower than the right ventricle. The aortic valve consists of three semilunar cusps that are supported within the three aortic sinuses of Valsalva.

C. **The Coronary Circulation**

1. A unique feature of the coronary circulation is that the heart requires a continuous delivery of oxygen by coronary blood flow to function. At rest, the myocardium extracts about 75% of the oxygen delivered by coronary blood flow (more than any other tissue in the body).

2. The right (RCA) and the left (LCA) coronary arteries arise respectively from the upper part of the right and the left coronary sinus of Valsalva and are the first branches of the aorta (Fig. 15-1).

   a. The RCA usually supplies the most of the right ventricle, a small part of the diaphragmatic aspect of left ventricle, the right atrium, part of left atrium, and posteroinferior one-third of interventricular septum.

   b. The RCA gives rise to the posterior descending artery (PDA). Coronary artery dominance is defined by the artery that supplies the PDA. In 70% of the population, the PDA is supplied by the RCA, coronary circulation referred to as *right dominant*. In 10% of the

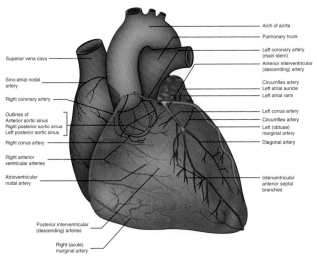

FIGURE 15-1 The coronary circulation.

population, the PDA is supplied by circumflex artery and is left dominant.

3. The left main coronary artery usually supplies the free wall of the left ventricle, a narrow strip of the right ventricle anteriorly, the anterior two-thirds of ventricular septum, and most of left atrium.

   a. After arising from the left coronary sinus, the left main coronary artery passes to the left atrioventricular groove, where it branches into left anterior descending artery (LAD) and the circumflex artery.

   b. The first septal branch of the LAD is usually targeted for ablation in interventional treatment for hypertrophic cardiomyopathy.

D. **The Cardiac Conduction System**

1. The cardiac conduction system consists of the sinoatrial (SA) node, the atrioventricular (AV) node, the AV bundle also known as the bundle of His, the bundle branches, and the Purkinje fibers (Fig. 15-2). The cardiac impulse is normally initiated by the SA node. This causes the atria to contract, first the right atrium followed by the left atrium.

2. From the SA node, the impulse is conducted to the AV node (supplied by the RCA in a large majority of population). The cardiac electrical impulse is delayed in the AV node about a fifth of a second before being conducted to the bundle of His and on to the ventricles, so that the atria contract just before the ventricles to augment end diastolic filling.

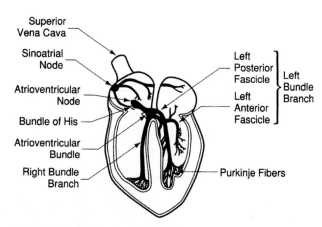

FIGURE 15-2 Cardiac conduction system.

3. The bundle of His branches into right and left bundle branches. The left bundle splits further into anterior and posterior fascicles. The bundle branches descend through the ventricular septum, where they continue on as the Purkinje fibers that end up directly stimulating the myocardium to contract.

III. **Clinical Electrophysiology and Electrocardiogram.** Body fluids are good electrical conductors, making it possible to record the sum of the action potentials of the cardiac cells on the surface of the body. Continuous monitoring of this electrocardiogram (ECG) during anesthesia is an essential tool for detecting myocardial ischemia, arrhythmias, and conduction system abnormalities.

A. **Electrocardiogram Leads**. The cardiac electrical activity is usually measured by electrodes placed on the skin (bipolar leads consist of two electrodes, one positive and one negative, and unipolar leads consist of one positive electrode [exploring] and a composite pole). Depolarization directed toward the positive electrode produces a positive deflection, whereas directed away from it produces a negative deflection. When the depolarization wave is perpendicular to the lead, a biphasic deflection is recorded (Fig. 15-3).

1. **Standard Limb Leads**. The standard limb leads (I, II, and III) record the potential difference between two

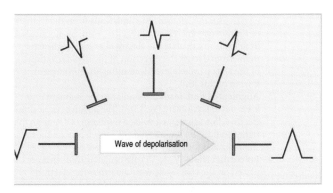

FIGURE 15-3 Wave of depolarization. Shape of QRS complex in any lead depends on orientation of that lead to vector of depolarization. (From Meek S, Morris F. Introduction. I—leads, rate, rhythm, and cardiac axis. *BMJ*. 2002;324[7334]:415–418.)

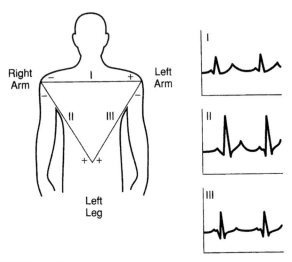

FIGURE 15-4 Standard limb leads of the electrocardiogram and typical recordings.

points of the body (Fig. 15-4). In lead I, the electrodes are placed on the left shoulder (positive) and right shoulder (negative). In lead II, the positive electrode is on the left leg and the negative is on the right shoulder. In lead III, the positive electrode is on the left leg and the negative on the left arm. The limb leads form the triangle of Einthoven which is used together with the augmented limb leads to calculate the electrical axis of the heart in the frontal axis. The direction of the depolarization of the atria parallels lead II, resulting in a prominent P wave in this lead.

2. **Augmented limb leads** are similar to the standard limb leads but are unipolar (Fig. 15-5). The positive (exploring) electrode for augmented voltage right arm (aVR) is on the right shoulder, for augmented voltage left arm on the left shoulder, and for augmented voltage foot on the left leg.

3. **Precordial leads** (V_1 to V_6) are unipolar leads that are placed on the chest wall, with the exploring electrode over one of six separate points (Table 15-1).

B. **Electrocardiographic axis of the heart** represents the overall direction of the electric impulse in the heart and is created by averaging all the action potentials. It is biased

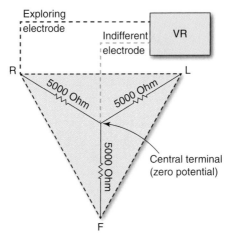

FIGURE 15-5 Unipolar limb lead circuit (VR).

toward the left because of the larger muscle mass of the left ventricle compared to the right (Fig. 15-6).

1. Left axis deviation (left ventricular hypertrophy) is defined as an axis less than −30 degrees and right axis deviation (right ventricular hypertrophy) as more than 90 degrees.
2. Abnormalities in the normal conduction pathway (blocks) in the heart also cause changes in the electrical axis.

C. **Electrocardiogram Lead Systems**

1. The three-lead system (most basic ECG system) consists of leads (I, II, and II) placed on the right arm, left arm, and left leg (provides adequate monitoring for arrhythmias; its use for detection myocardial ischemia

Table 15-1

Placement of Precordial Leads

V_1	Fourth intercostal space at the right sternal border
V_2	Fourth intercostal space at the left sternal border
V_3	Equidistant between V_2 and V_4
V_4	Fifth intercostal space in the left midclavicular line
V_5	Fifth intercostal space in the left anterior axillary line
V_6	Fifth intercostal space in the left midaxillary line

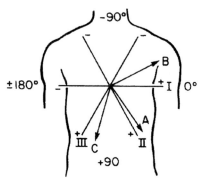

FIGURE 15-6 Electrical axis of the heart as determined from the standard limb leads of the electrocardiogram. In the normal heart, the electrical axis is approximately 59 degrees (A). Left axis deviation shifts the electrical axis to less than 0 degrees (B); right axis deviation is associated with an electrical axis of greater than 100 degrees.

is limited). For detecting intraoperative myocardial ischemia, V_5 has the greatest sensitivity. Lead II is superior in monitoring atrial arrhythmias.

2. It is important to differentiate artifacts from real ECG findings (modern ECG monitors have incorporated filters for signal processing to minimize the presence of electrical artifacts).

D. **Recording the Electrocardiogram**

1. The ECG is recorded on a graph paper consisting of 1-mm squares with every five squares separated by a darker line. Each 1-mm horizontal line represents 0.04 second and each 1-mm vertical line represents 0.1 mV, assuming proper calibration 1 cm/1 mV and standardized paper speed of 25 mm per second. Therefore, the distance between two darker lines represents 0.2 second and 0.5 mV on the horizontal and the vertical axes, respectively.

2. The heart rate in beats per minute can be calculated by dividing 60 by the number of seconds ($= 0.04$ second $\times$ number of small boxes) between two consecutive beats.

3. The electrical activity that activates the cardiac contraction is observed on a monitor display as a graph of voltage change through time.

E. **Normal Electrocardiographic Deflections.** The cardiac electrical impulse is initiated at the sinoatrial (SA) node, which is located at the junction of the superior vena cava to the right atrium. Any part of the conduction system can spontaneously depolarize and initiate an impulse, but the SA node normally has the highest rate of depolarization and is the pacemaker of the heart. The impulse is transmitted through right and left intraatrial pathways to the AV node and then to the bundle of His, through the Purkinje fibers to the ventricular subendocardium, which causes the myocardium to depolarize. The speed of conduction is different between the various areas of the system, with the slowest through the AV node producing atrioventricular synchrony for optimal end diastolic filling from atrial contraction. The normal ECG consists of a P wave (atrial systole), a QRS complex (ventricular systole), and a T wave (ventricular repolarization). The atrial repolarization wave is obscured by the larger QRS complex (Fig. 15-7).

1. **P wave** represents the atrial depolarization and has a normal duration and amplitude of 0.08 to 0.12 second and less than 2.5 mm in the limb leads. An enlarged P wave signifies atrial enlargement.

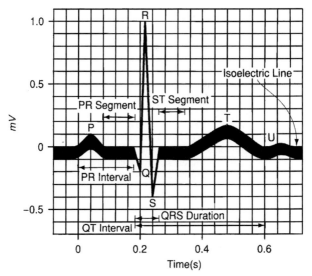

FIGURE 15-7 The normal waves and intervals on the electrocardiogram.

2. **P-R interval** corresponds to the time from the beginning of the atrial depolarization to the beginning of the ventricular depolarization. It is measured from the start of the P wave to the start of the QRS. The normal duration of the P-R interval is 0.12 to 0.2 second. Prolonged P-R interval is called *first-degree AV block*.

3. **Q wave** is defined as an initial negative deflection of the QRS and is usually absent in leads aVR, V_1, and V_2. A Q wave whose amplitude is more than one-third of the corresponding R wave, duration is longer than 0.04 second, and depth is greater than 1 mm, is indicative of myocardial infarction.

4. **QRS complex** is caused by the depolarization of the ventricles and normally has a duration of less than 0.10 second.

   a. A prolonged QRS duration may be due to left ventricular hypertrophy (LVH), impaired ventricular conduction (bundle branch block), beats initiated outside the conduction system (ectopic or paced beats), and beats passing through abnormal conduction pathways (Wolff-Parkinson-White syndrome).

   b. Normally, the QRS amplitude gradually increases in the precordial leads from V_1 to V_5 (called *R wave progression*).

5. **ST segment** starts when all myocardial cells are depolarized (end of QRS) and ends when ventricular repolarization begins (T wave). It is normally isoelectric and elevation or depression more than 1 mm from the baseline may indicate myocardial ischemia. Hyperkalemia and pericarditis may also cause ST elevation.

6. **T wave** is caused by the repolarization of the ventricles and is usually in the same direction as the QRS. Delay of conduction of cardiac impulses through the ventricles (prolonged depolarization), as occurs with myocardial ischemia, bundle branch blocks, or ectopic ventricular beats, may result in T-wave polarity opposite the QRS complex.

   a. Symmetrical or deeply inverted T waves may be indicative of myocardial ischemia.

   b. Peaked T waves may be present in hyperkalemia, LVH, and intracranial bleeding.

7. **QT interval** includes both ventricular depolarization and repolarization (measured from the beginning of the QRS to the end of the T wave and varies in duration according to heart rate).

IV. **Cardiac Physiology**
    A. **Myocardium** is the involuntary, striated muscle tissue in the heart between the epicardium and the endocardium. The primary structural proteins of the cardiac muscle are actin and myosin filaments, which interdigitate and slide along each other during contraction in a manner similar to skeletal muscle.
    B. **Cardiac Action Potential**. At the initiation of an action potential in a cardiomyocyte, the cell membrane rapidly depolarizes as the transmembrane potential rises from -85 mV to $+20$ mV. The membrane remains depolarized for about 0.2 second, the plateau phase, which is then followed by rapid repolarization. During the plateau phase, the cardiomyocyte cannot be restimulated for about 0.25 to 0.3 second, called the *refractory period*. This is followed for additional 0.05 second by the relative refractory period, when the myocardium can only be stimulated by a strong excitatory signal.

V. **Control of Cardiac Function**
    A. **Neural Control**
        1. Heart function is controlled by the autonomic nervous system by both adrenergic and muscarinic acetylcholine receptors, modulating the cardiac output by influencing heart rate and myocardial contraction. The atria are innervated by both the sympathetic and parasympathetic nervous system, but the ventricles are supplied principally by the sympathetic nervous system (Fig. 15-8).
        2. Maximal sympathetic nervous system stimulation can increase cardiac output by about 100% above normal. Conversely, maximal parasympathetic nervous system stimulation decreases ventricular contractile strength only by about 30%, as the vagal innervation is sparse in the ventricles.
    B. **Hormonal Control**. The hormones secreted by cardiomyocytes include natriuretic peptide, adrenomedullin, aldosterone, and angiotensin II. Atrial (ANP) and B-type natriuretic protein (BNP) are released from atria and ventricle in response to increased stretch of the chamber wall. The renin-angiotensin system is an important regulator of the cardiovascular system.

VI. **Cardiac Cycle**
    A. **Electrical and Mechanical Events**. The cardiac cycle is a series of coordinated electromechanical events that

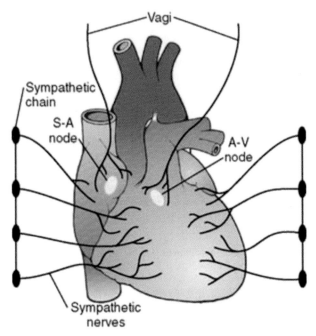

FIGURE 15-8 Cardiac sympathetic and parasympathetic nerves.

result in the ejection of blood from the heart into the great vessels (Fig. 15-9). The atrial pressure tracing, or central venous waveform, begins with an "a" wave that corresponds to atrial contraction at end diastole. The "c" wave represents ventricular systole during which time the right atrial pressure increases slightly as the right ventricle contracts against a closed tricuspid valve. The "y descent" represents a fall in right atrial pressures as the tricuspid valve opens and the right ventricle fills in diastole (Fig. 15-10).

B. **Myocardial Performance, Preload, and Afterload** (Fig. 15-11).

1. Afterload refers to the resistance or pressure against which the ventricle contracts. Mechanical obstruction such as aortic stenosis increases afterload and adversely affects myocardial performance. Pharmacologic

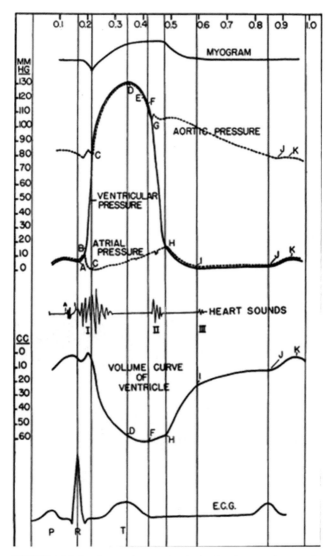

FIGURE 15-9 Cardiac cycle: mechanical, electrical, and acoustic events. (From Wiggers CJ. Dynamics of ventricular contraction under abnormal conditions. *Circulation*. 1952;5[3]:321–348.)

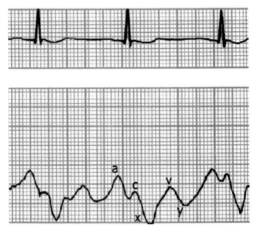

FIGURE 15-10 Central venous waveform. (From Pittman J, Ping JS, Mark JB. Arterial and central venous pressure monitoring. *Int Anesthesiol Clin.* 2004;42[1]:13–30.)

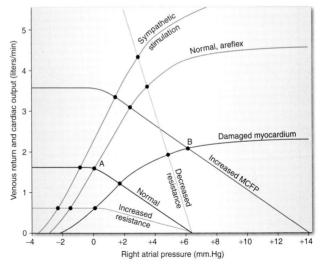

FIGURE 15-11 Determinants of cardiac output. (From Guyton AC. Determination of cardiac output by equating venous return curves with cardiac response curves. *Physiol Rev.* 1955;35[1]:123–129.)

interventions such as the administration of phenylephrine can increase afterload as well by increasing systemic vascular resistance. Afterload in its simplest interpretation often refers to the mean arterial pressure.
   2. Left ventricular (LV) pressure volume loops can be used to demonstrate how changes in preload and afterload affect stroke volume and end systolic and end diastolic pressure–volume relationships. The entire loop represents a single cardiac cycle with volume on the x-axis and pressure on the y-axis (Fig. 15-12A–C).
   C. **Hemodynamic Calculations** (Tables 15-2 and 15-3). Cardiac output is equal to heart rate multiplied by stroke volume (SV) and SV = end diastolic volume – end systolic volume. Mean arterial pressure (MAP) is two-third diastolic blood pressure plus one-third systolic blood pressure.

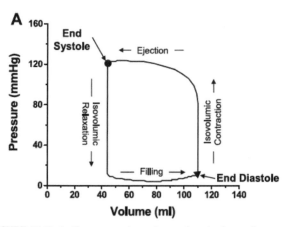

FIGURE 15-12 **A:** Pressure–volume loop of a single cardiac cycle. **B:** A reduction in ventricular filling pressure causes the loops to shift toward lower end systolic and end diastolic function. **C:** When afterload is increased, the loops get narrower and longer. EDPVR, end diastolic pressure–volume relationship; Ees, slope of linear ESPVR; ESPVR, end systolic pressure–volume relationship; Vo, volume axis intercept. (From Burkhoff D, Mirsky I, Suga H. Assessment of systolic and diastolic ventricular properties via pressure-volume analysis: a guide for clinical, translational, and basic researchers. *Am J Physiol Heart Circ Physiol.* 2005;289[2]:H501–512.)

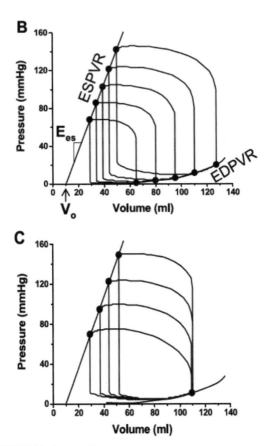

FIGURE 15-12 (Continued).

MAP is also cardiac output multiplied by systemic vascular resistance.

VII. Pathophysiology

A. **Ischemic heart disease** refers to atherosclerosis of the coronary arteries that obstructs blood flow to the myocardium resulting in either stable symptoms, which can be medically managed, or unstable acute coronary syndromes, which may call for more invasive intervention such as

Table 15-2

Hemodynamic Equations

$CO = HR \times SV$
$CI = CO / BSA$
$SV = EDV - ESV$
$MAP = CO \times SVR$
$MAP = 2/3 \text{ diastolic pressure} + 1/3 \text{ systolic pressure}$
$SVR = [(MAP - CVP) / CO] \times 80$
$PVR = [(\text{mean PAP} - \text{wedge}) / CO] \times 80$

CO, cardiac output; HR, heart rate; SV, stroke volume; CI, cardiac index; BSA, body surface area; EDV, end diastolic volume; ESV, end systolic volume; MAP, mean arterial pressure; SVR, systemic vascular resistance; CVP, central venous pressure; PVR, pulmonary vascular resistance; PAP, pulmonary artery pressure.

revascularization by percutaneous coronary intervention or coronary artery bypass graft surgery.
1. The development of atherosclerosis is an inflammatory process mediated by adherent leukocytes (phagocytes and T lymphocytes), cytokines, and smooth muscle cells that generate a lipid-rich necrotic plaque. Risk factors for ischemic heart disease include hypertension, cigarette smoking, hyperlipidemia, and abdominal obesity.

Table 15-3

Normal Hemodynamic Values

Cardiac index = 2.4 L/min
Cardiac output = 5–7 L/min
Stroke volume = 70–90 mL (1 mL/kg)
MAP = 60–90 mm Hg
CVP = 5–10 mm Hg
SVR = 800–1,200 dyne/s/cm^5
PVR = <250 dyne/s/cm^5
PAOP = 6–12 mm Hg
Mean PAP = 10–20 mm Hg

MAP, mean arterial pressure; CVP, central venous pressure; SVR, systemic vascular resistance; PVR, pulmonary vascular resistance; PAOP, pulmonary artery occlusion pressure; PAP, pulmonary artery pressure.

2. Acute coronary syndromes include the following three entities: unstable angina, non–ST elevation myocardial infarction (NSTEMI), and ST elevation myocardial infarction (STEMI).

3. Medical management of stable ischemic heart disease begins with risk factor reduction. β Blockade has been shown to confer a survival benefit in patients with prior myocardial infarction or a low ejection fraction and decreases myocardial oxygen consumption. Statins are indicated for their lipid-lowering effects and antiinflammatory properties.

B. **Heart failure** is a complex clinical syndrome that results from any structural or functional impairment of ventricular filling or ejection of blood (Table 15-4).

1. The most important risk factor for diastolic heart failure is hypertension. Diastolic heart failure is more common in the elderly, female, and obese populations and has now surpassed systolic heart failure as the leading class of heart failure.

2. Heart failure with reduced ejection fraction occurs in patients with an ejection fraction less than 40%. Patients often have concomitant diastolic dysfunction. One of the main risk factors for heart failure with reduced ejection fraction is coronary artery disease.

3. Treatment modalities range from oral medication to intravenous inotropes to mechanical assist devices. Diuretics, angiotensin-converting enzyme inhibitors, and β blockers have been the foundation of medical management.

4. Patients with decompensated systolic heart failure may require acute positive inotropic therapy with milrinone, dobutamine, or epinephrine. More invasive methods to support the failing ventricle include intraaortic balloon counterpulsation, ventricular assist devices, and cardiac transplantation.

C. **Valvular Heart Disease**

1. **Aortic stenosis** is the most common valvular heart disease in elderly patients. The typical presentation is either chest pain, syncope, or dyspnea (heart failure). Even with normal coronary arteries, patients are at risk for subendocardial ischemia due to the severity of LVH.

   a. Hemodynamic optimization of these patients, especially during induction of anesthesia, includes maintaining adequate preload, a higher MAP, and lower heart rate.

Table 15-4

ACCF/AHA Stages of Heart Failure and NYHA Functional Classification

ACC/AHA Stages of HF	NYHA Functional Classification	
A At high risk of HF but without structural heart disease or symptoms of HF	None	
B Structural heart disease but without signs or symptoms of HF	I	No limitation of physical activity. Ordinary physical activity does not cause symptoms of HF.
C Structural heart disease with prior or current symptoms of HF	I	No limitation of physical activity. Ordinary physical activity does not cause symptoms of HF.
	II	Slight limitation of physical activity. Comfortable at rest, but ordinary physical activity results in symptoms of HF.
	III	Marked limitation of physical activity. Comfortable at rest, but less than ordinary activity causes symptoms of HF.
	IV	Unable to carry on any physical activity without symptoms of HF or symptoms of HF at rest
D Refractory HF requiring specialized interventions	IV	Unable to carry on any physical activity without symptoms of HF or symptoms of HF at rest

ACCF, American College of Cardiology Foundation; AHA, American Heart Association; HF, heart failure; NYHA, New York Heart Association.
From Yancy CW, Jessup M, Bozkurt B, et al. 2013 ACCF/AHA guideline for the management of heart failure: a report of the American College of Cardiology Foundation/American Heart Association Task Force on Practice Guidelines. *J Am Coll Cardiol.* 2013;62(16):e147–e239.

  b. This allows more time for ventricular filling in the noncompliant heart while maintaining acceptable systemic perfusion to compensate for the increased transvalvular pressure gradient and relatively fixed cardiac output.
  2. **Aortic insufficiency** can be acute as a result of trauma, endocarditis, or dissection. With chronic regurgitation, the ventricle has time to compensate by dilating and

increasing diastolic compliance. This does not occur if the regurgitation occurs acutely. Chronic aortic insufficiency is characterized by volume and pressure overload of the left ventricle.

D. **Mitral stenosis** is most often due to rheumatic heart disease.
   1. Symptoms related to mitral stenosis are secondary to volume and pressure overload of the pulmonary circulation due to a fixed obstruction to LV filling.
   2. Hemodynamic goals include avoiding tachycardia, which further decreases diastolic filling time. Any factors that further increase pulmonary hypertension should be avoided.

E. **Mitral Regurgitation**
   1. Etiologies of mitral valve regurgitation include degenerative, rheumatic, congenital, and disorders related to coronary artery disease, endocarditis, or trauma.
   2. Patients with severe mitral regurgitation develop symptoms related to volume overload of the left atrium that may result in atrial fibrillation and secondary pulmonary hypertension.

VIII. **Cardiac Dysrhythmias. During the perioperative period, changes may take place that trigger cardiac dysrhythmias (important to monitor for arrhythmias throughout this time).**
   A. **Etiology.** Perioperative cardiac dysrhythmias are most likely to occur in patients with preexisting heart disease (coronary artery disease, valvular heart disease, or cardiomyopathies). Transient physiologic imbalances during the perioperative period make the heart more susceptible to abnormalities in the automaticity of pacemaker cells, the excitability of myocardial cells, and the conduction of the cardiac impulse (Table 15-5).

Table 15-5

Factors that Contribute to Imbalances that Predispose to Cardiac Dysrhythmias

Catecholamine release (laryngoscopy, tracheal intubation)
Electrolyte abnormalities, changes in Pao_2, $Paco_2$, pH
Drugs (inhaled anesthetics, succinylcholine, anticholinesterase–anticholinergic combinations, ketamine)
Blockade of the sympathetic nervous system (subarachnoid local anesthetics)
Direct stimulation of the heart during cardiothoracic procedures

B. **Mechanisms of Arrhythmia**
  1. **Automaticity**. Any cell of the cardiac conduction system can trigger its own action potential and act as a pacemaker. Normally, the highest rate of spontaneous depolarization occurs in the SA node making it the dominant pacemaker in the heart. Abnormal automaticity of any part of the conduction system can lead to arrhythmias.
  2. **Excitability** is the ability of the cardiac cell to respond to a stimulus by depolarizing. A measure of excitability is the difference between the resting transmembrane potential and the threshold potential of the cell. The smaller the difference between these potentials, the more excitable or irritable is the cell.
  3. **Ectopic Pacemaker**
     a. An ectopic pacemaker (abnormal focus) manifests as a premature contraction of the heart that occurs between normal beats.
     b. The AV node and the bundle of His are the most common areas for the presence of an ectopic pacemaker.
     c. Impulses generated outside the SA node follow a different pathway in the conductive system (usually slower) generating a change in the configuration of the QRS wave on the ECG.

IX. **Types of Dysrhythmias (Table 15-6)**
  A. **Heart Block**
    1. First-degree AV heart block is considered to be present when there is still one-to-one AV conduction but the

---

Table 15-6

Diagnosis of Cardiac Dysrhythmias from the Electrocardiogram

- Are P waves present and what is their relationship to the QRS complexes?
- Are the amplitudes, durations, and contours of the P waves, P-R intervals, QRS complexes, and Q-T intervals normal?
- During tachycardia, is the R-P long and P-R interval short (or vice versa)?
- What are the atrial and ventricular discharge rates (same or different)?
- Are the P-P and R-R intervals regular or irregular?

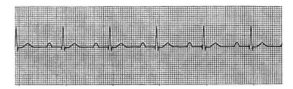

FIGURE 15-13 First-degree AV block.

P-R interval is longer than 0.2 second at a normal heart rate (Fig. 15-13).

2. Second-degree AV heart block is present when some AV conduction still is present but does not occur with every beat (classified as Mobitz type I [Wenckebach phenomenon] or Mobitz type II heart block) (Figs. 15-14 and 15-15).

   a. Wenckebach phenomenon is characterized by a progressive beat to beat prolongation of the P-R interval until conduction of the cardiac impulse is completely interrupted and a P wave is recorded without a subsequent QRS complex. After this dropped beat, the cycle is repeated.

   b. Mobitz type II heart block is the occurrence of a nonconducted atrial impulse without a prior change in the P-R interval and is considered a higher degree of AV block than Mobitz type I.

3. Third-degree AV heart block is present when there is no conduction of beats from the atria to the ventricles. The P waves are dissociated from the QRS complexes and the heart rate depends on the intrinsic discharge rate of the ectopic pacemaker beyond the site of conduction block.

   a. If the ectopic pacemaker is near the AV node, the QRS complexes appear normal and the heart rate is typically 40 to 60 beats per minute (Fig. 15-16). When the site of the block is infranodal, the escape ventricular

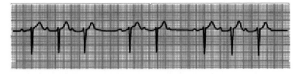

FIGURE 15-14 Mobitz type I (Wenckebach). (From Lange Instant Access EKG's and Cardiac Studies, Anil Patel.)

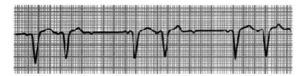

FIGURE 15-15 Mobitz type II. (From Lange Instant Access EKG's and Cardiac Studies, Anil Patel.)

pacemaker often has a discharge rate of less than 40 beats per minute and the QRS complexes are wide, resembling a bundle branch block (Fig. 15-17).

b. The treatment of patients with third-degree heart block usually requires insertion of a permanent artificial cardiac pacemaker. Temporary support may be provided with intravenous infusion of isoproterenol (chemical cardiac pacemaker) or a transvenous artificial cardiac pacemaker.

c. The safe perioperative management of patients with implanted rhythm control devices such as pacemakers and implantable cardioverter defibrillators (ICD) requires a basic understanding of the classification, function, and emergency management of these devices.

4. **Bundle Branch Block**

a. Blockage of the impulse conduction through the right or left bundle branches results in delay of activation of the corresponding ventricle, called *bundle branch block*, which may be complete or incomplete. Hemiblock or fascicular block refers to the blockade of either the anterior or posterior fascicle of the left bundle branch.

b. Left bundle branch block is clinically significant and cardiac disease must be ruled out.

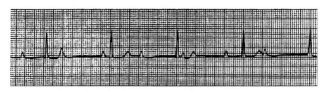

FIGURE 15-16 Third-degree atrioventricular heart block occurring at the level of the atrioventricular node (QRS complexes are narrow). There is no relation between the P waves and QRS complexes.

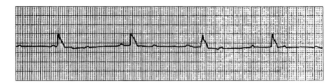

FIGURE 15-17 Third-degree atrioventricular heart block occurring at an infranodal level (QRS complexes are wide).

    c. Right bundle branch is commonly seen in healthy individuals but may be caused by right heart enlargement from conditions such as atrial septal defect, chronic lung disease, or pulmonary embolism.

B. **Reentry**
1. A reentry circuit is the most likely mechanism for supraventricular tachycardia, atrial flutter, atrial fibrillation, premature ventricular contractions, ventricular tachycardia, and ventricular fibrillation.
2. Reentry circuits can develop at any place in the heart where there is an imbalance between conduction and refractoriness creating a slow and fast pathway.
3. Reentry circuits can be eliminated by speeding conduction through normal tissues so cardiac impulses reach their initial site of origin when the fibers are still refractory or by prolonging the refractory period of normal cells so the returning impulses cannot reenter.

C. **Preexcitation Syndrome**
1. A preexcitation syndrome is present when atrial impulses bypass the AV node through an abnormal conduction pathway to produce premature excitation of the ventricle.
2. The most common accessory conduction pathway producing a direct connection (anatomic loop) of the atrium to the ventricle is known as Kent's bundle (usually left atrium to left ventricle) (Table 15-7).
3. Elimination of the pathologic conduction pathway can be achieved with radiofrequency catheter ablation.

D. **Sinus tachycardia** is usually defined as a sinus rhythm with a resting heart rate of greater than 100 beats per minute. A common cause of sinus tachycardia is sympathetic nervous system stimulation such as may occur during a noxious stimulus in the presence of low concentrations of anesthetic drugs.

Table 15-7

Accessory Pathways and Preexcitation Syndromes

	Connections
Kent's bundle	Atrium to ventricle
Mahaim bundle	Atrioventricular node to ventricle
Atriohisian fiber	Atrium to His bundle
James fiber	Atrium to atrioventricular node

Adapted from Atlee JL. Perioperative cardiac dysrhythmias: diagnosis and management. *Anesthesiology*. 1997;86:1397–1424.

E. **Sinus bradycardia** is usually defined as a sinus rhythm with heart rate of less than 60 beats per minute and may be caused by parasympathetic nervous system (vagal) stimulation of the heart, hypoxia, and medications.

F. **Sinus dysrhythmias** (normal variation in the SA node rate) is present during normal breathing with heart rate (R-R intervals) varying approximately 5% during various phases of the resting breathing cycle (during inspiration, the heart rate increases and during expiration, it decreases). In perioperative settings, sinus dysrhythmia is usually transient and often caused by autonomic nervous system imbalance as the result of an intervention (spinal or epidural anesthesia, laryngoscopy, surgical stimulation) or by the effects of drugs on the SA node.

G. **Premature atrial contractions** are recognized by an abnormal P wave and a shortened or prolonged P-R interval. Premature atrial contractions are usually benign and often occur in individuals without heart disease.

H. **Premature nodal (junctional) contractions** are characterized by the absence of normal P-waves and P-R intervals preceding the QRS complexes. Premature junctional contractions are less common than premature atrial and premature ventricular contractions and may be seen under normal conditions.

I. **Nodal (junctional) paroxysmal tachycardia** resembles atrial paroxysmal tachycardia except P waves may precede, follow, or be obscured by the QRS complex (common following heart surgery).

J. **Atrial paroxysmal tachycardia**, which often occurs in otherwise healthy young individuals, is caused by rapid rhythmic discharges of impulses from an ectopic atrial

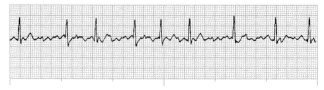

FIGURE 15-18 Atrial fibrillation.

pacemaker. The rhythm on the ECG is regular and the P waves are abnormal, often inverted, indicating a site of origin other than the SA node. Typically, the onset of atrial paroxysmal tachycardia is abrupt and may end just as suddenly with the pacemaker shifting back to the SA node. Atrial paroxysmal tachycardia may be terminated by parasympathetic nervous system stimulation of the heart with drugs or by carotid sinus massage.

K. **Atrial fibrillation** is characterized by normal QRS complexes occurring at a rapid and irregularly irregular rate in the absence of identifiable P waves (Fig. 15-18). SV is decreased during atrial fibrillation due to the loss of atrial contraction. A pulse deficit (heart rate by palpation is less than that of the ECG) reflects the inability of each ventricular contraction to eject a sufficient SV to produce a detectable peripheral pulse.

   1. There is an estimated 5% annual risk of thromboembolism in patients with atrial fibrillation who are not treated with anticoagulants.

   2. Treatment includes rate control therapy, direct current cardioversion, pharmacologic cardioversion (flecainide, dofetilide, propafenone, ibutilide, and amiodarone), catheter ablation, and surgical Maze procedure.

L. **Atrial flutter** is a regular contraction of the atria at a rate of 250 to 300 beats per minute and on the ECG is characterized by 2:1, 3:1, or 4:1 conduction of atrial impulses to the ventricle. Atrial flutter is seen commonly in patients with chronic pulmonary disease, dilated cardiomyopathy, myocarditis, ethanol intoxication, and thyrotoxicosis. Treatment is similar to that of atrial fibrillation.

M. **Premature ventricular contractions** result from reentry or an ectopic pacemaker in the ventricles and are not preceded by a P wave. They are classified unifocal or multifocal based on the morphology of the QRS depending on the number of sites of initiation. The QRS complex of the ECG is widened because the cardiac impulse is conducted through

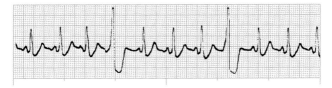

FIGURE 15-19 Multifocal premature ventricular contractions.

the slowly conducting muscle of the ventricle or an abnormal conduction pathway (Fig. 15-19).

1. A compensatory pause after a premature ventricular contraction occurs because the next impulse from the SA node reaches the ventricle during its refractory period.
2. Premature ventricular contractions often reflect significant cardiac disease (myocardial ischemia, valvular heart disease, high-catecholamine state, hypoxia, hypercapnia, cocaine, alcohol, caffeine, electrolyte abnormalities, and medications).
3. Treatment of premature ventricular contractions includes removal of trigger factors, β blockers, calcium channel blockers, lidocaine, amiodarone, and radiofrequency ablation depending on the symptoms.

N. **Ventricular tachycardia** on the ECG resembles a series of ventricular premature contractions that occur at a rapid (200 to 300 beats per minute) and regular rate (Fig. 15-20). It is classified as monomorphic or polymorphic and predisposes to ventricular fibrillation.

1. Common causes of ventricular tachycardia are myocardial ischemia, cardiomyopathies, electrolyte abnormalities (potassium, magnesium, calcium), and QT prolongation. Nonsustained ventricular tachycardia may be defined as three or more consecutive ventricular beats at a rate greater than 100 beats per minute lasting less than 30 seconds and is usually asymptomatic.

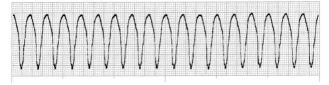

FIGURE 15-20 Ventricular tachycardia.

Coarse Ventricular Fibrillation

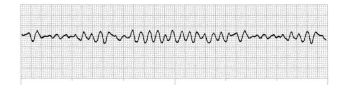

Fine Ventricular Fibrillation

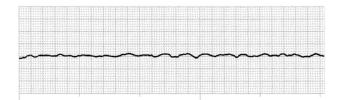

FIGURE 15-21 Ventricular fibrillation.

2. Sustained ventricular tachycardia usually leads to hemodynamic instability and necessitates termination with electrical cardioversion.

O. **Ventricular fibrillation** is characterized on the ECG by an irregular wavy line with voltages that range from 0.25 to 0.5 mV (Fig. 15-21). There is total absence of coordinated contractions with cessation of any effective pumping activity and disappearance of detectable pulse and systemic blood pressure.

1. The only effective treatment of ventricular fibrillation is the delivery of direct electric current through the ventricles (defibrillation), which simultaneously depolarizes all ventricular muscle. This depolarization allows the initiation of a cardiac pacemaker remote from the irritable focus responsible for the ventricular fibrillation.

2. Cardiopulmonary resuscitation must be initiated until a defibrillator becomes available. The survival rate of ventricular fibrillation may decrease by 7% to 10 % for every minute that defibrillation is delayed.

3. It is important to identify the patients at risk for ventricular fibrillation and place a prophylactic ICD.

CHAPTER 16

Renal Physiology

I. Introduction. The kidneys play a central role in the maintenance of homeostasis of the body (stabilize extracellular fluid electrolyte composition, maintain acid–base balance, regulate volume status and blood pressure, secrete of erythropoietin and renin, excrete toxins and metabolic waste). These functions involve complex interactions within the kidneys and with other organ systems and are frequently altered during anesthesia.

II. Kidney Structure and Function
   A. **Basic Anatomy of the Kidney**. Each kidney has an outer portion (cortex) and inner portion (medulla). The renal arteries arise from the abdominal aorta, and the renal veins direct blood flow into the inferior vena cava. The kidneys are prominently innervated by the sympathetic nervous system, from T4 through T12. The nephron is the functional unit of the kidney (Fig. 16-1).
      1. **The Glomerulus**
         a. Glomeruli are found in the renal cortex and consist of a tuft of capillaries surrounded by Bowman's capsule, the dilated blind end of the renal tubule. Glomerular capillaries are uniquely interposed between two sets of arterioles. Blood flows from the afferent arterioles through the glomerular capillaries and then on to the efferent arterioles. Glomerular capillary pressure causes water and low-molecular-weight substances to be filtered into Bowman's capsule and the renal tubule system.
         b. **Glomerular filtration rate (GFR)** is the volume of collective glomerular filtrate formed over time. Because 99% of this 180 L of glomerular filtrate is reabsorbed, daily urine output is 1 to 2 L. The kidneys have an autoregulatory mechanism to modulate the effect of mean arterial pressure on the GFR (a nearly constant filtration pressure leads to a consistent GFR

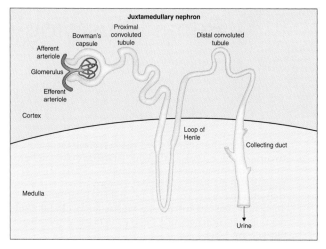

FIGURE 16-1 Schematic depiction of a juxtamedullary nephron.

across a range of mean arterial pressure, remaining relatively constant between mean arterial pressures of 60 and 160 mm Hg).

    2. **The renal tubule** (see Fig. 16-1)

B. **Glomerular filtrate** is converted into urine along the course of the renal tubule (Table 16-1).

    1. The process of reabsorption determines the volume of urine formed, whereas secretion is particularly important in determining the nature of the urine, such as concentration of potassium and hydrogen ions. The most important factors influencing the reabsorption of sodium and water are aldosterone, arginine vasopressin (AVP), renal prostaglandins, and atrial natriuretic factor (ANP).

    2. Reabsorption of sodium involves moving this ion against a concentration gradient from the lumen of the proximal tubule into peritubular capillaries (requires energy, supplied by the sodium-potassium adenosine triphosphatase [ATPase] system). The proximal convoluted renal tubules, driving the ATPase enzyme for sodium reabsorption, consume approximately 80% of renal oxygen consumption.

Table 16-1

Magnitude and Site of Solute Reabsorption or Secretion in the Renal Tubules

	Filtered (24 h)	Reabsorbed (24 h)	Secreted (24 h)	Excreted (24 h)	Percent Reabsorbed	Location
Water (L)	180	179		1	99.4	P,L,D,C
Sodium (mEq)	26,000	25,850		150	99.4	P,L,D,C
Potassium (mEq)	600	560	50	90	93.3	P,L,D,C
Chloride (mEq)	18,000	17,850		150	99.2	P,L,D,C
Bicarbonate (mEq)	4,900	4,900		0	10	P,D
Urea (mM)	870	460		410	53	P,L,D,C
Uric acid (mM)	50	49	4	5	98	P
Glucose (mM)	800	800		0	100	P

C, convoluted tubule; D, distal tubule; L, loop of Henle; P, proximal tubule.

3. More than 99% of the water in the glomerular filtrate is reabsorbed into peritubular capillaries as it passes through renal tubules. The distal tubules are almost completely impermeable to water, allowing for control of the specific gravity of the urine. The permeability of the collecting ducts is variable and determined by the action of AVP. Increased AVP leads to reabsorption of water from the collecting ducts, resulting in highly concentrated urine. Decreased AVP results in little water reabsorption and large amounts of dilute urine.

C. **Countercurrent System**
1. The ability of the kidneys to produce either dilute or concentrated urine depends on the gradient in osmolarity between the renal cortex and renal medulla that is created by the loop of Henle (Fig. 16-2).
2. The U-shaped arrangement of peritubular capillaries, known as the *vasa recta*, parallels the loops of Henle. This forms a countercurrent system, in which capillary inflow runs parallel and in an opposite direction to capillary outflow.

D. **Aquaporins** (tetramer protein structures and are found in the kidneys, brain, salivary and lacrimal glands, and respiratory tract) are channels that facilitate rapid passage of water across lipid cell membranes.

E. **Tubular transport maximum** (Tm or T_{max}) is the maximum amount of a substance that can be actively reabsorbed from the lumens of renal tubules each minute.
1. The Tm for glucose is approximately 220 mg per minute. When the amount of glucose that filters through the glomerular capillary exceeds this amount, the excess glucose cannot be reabsorbed and passes into urine (Fig. 16-3).
2. The presence of large amounts of unreabsorbed solutes in the urine such as glucose (or mannitol) produces osmotic diuresis by retaining water in the collecting system.

F. **Transport of Urine to the Bladder**
1. From the collecting ducts, urine travels into the renal pelvis. A ureter arises from the pelvis of each kidney. At its distal end, the ureter penetrates the bladder obliquely such that pressure in the bladder compresses the ureter, thereby preventing reflux of urine into the ureter when bladder pressure increases during micturition.
2. Each ureter is innervated by the sympathetic and parasympathetic nervous system (parasympathetic nervous

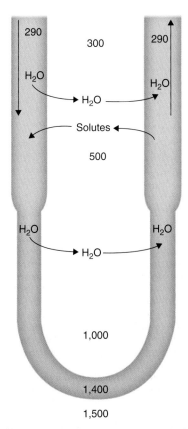

FIGURE 16-2 Countercurrent exchange of water and solutes in the vasa recta. (Adapted from Lote CJ, Harper L, Savage COS. Mechanisms of acute renal failure. *Br J Anaesth.* 1996;77:82–89, with permission.)

system stimulation increases the frequency of peristalsis, whereas sympathetic nervous system stimulation decreases peristalsis).
   a. Obstruction of a ureter by a stone causes intense reflex constriction and pain.
   b. Spinal cord damage above the sacral region leaves the micturition reflex intact but is no longer controlled by the brain.

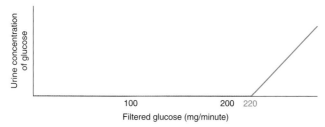

FIGURE 16-3 Transport maximum for glucose. Urinary concentration of glucose is negligible until the amount of filtered glucose exceeds the transport maximum.

III. **Renal Blood Flow.** Although the kidneys represent about 0.5% of total body weight, their blood flow is disproportionately large at 20% to 25% of the cardiac output. The ability to autoregulate keeps renal blood flow relatively constant across a range of systemic mean arterial pressures. Approximately 90% of the renal blood flow is distributed to the renal cortex, with less than 10% of renal blood flow going to the medulla. The generous delivery of blood to the cortex supports flow-dependent functions such as glomerular filtration and tubular reabsorption processes of the cortex. Low blood flow also makes the medulla more susceptible to ischemia than the cortex.

A. **Renal Cortex Blood Flow: Glomerular and Peritubular Capillaries** (Figs. 16-1 and 16-4)

B. **Autoregulation of Renal Blood Flow**

1. Renal blood flow and GFR are kept relatively constant within a range of mean arterial pressure between approximately 60 and 160 mm Hg (Fig. 16-5).

2. In the setting of decreased effective circulating volume, renal blood flow may be decreased despite adequate perfusion pressure (activation of the sympathetic nervous system shunts cardiac output away from the kidneys and adequate systemic blood pressure does not necessarily indicate adequate renal perfusion in the presence of hypovolemia).

C. **Juxtaglomerular Apparatus**

1. In response to decreased renal blood flow, juxtaglomerular cells release renin into the circulation (Fig. 16-6). Renin converts angiotensinogen to angiotensin I, which is then converted to angiotensin II by angiotensin-converting enzyme.

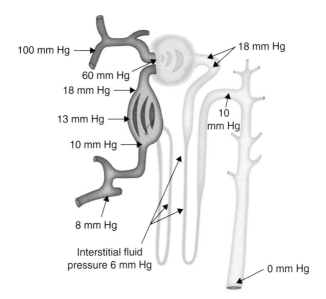

FIGURE 16-4 Intravascular pressures in the renal circulation. (From Guyton AC, Hall JE. *Textbook of Medical Physiology*. 10th ed. Philadelphia, PA: Saunders; 2000, with permission.)

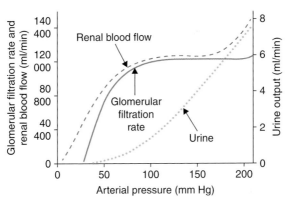

FIGURE 16-5 Autoregulation. Renal blood flow and glomerular filtration rate, but not urine output, are autoregulated between a mean arterial pressure of approximately 60 and 160 mm Hg. (From Guyton AC, Hall JE. *Textbook of Medical Physiology*. 10th ed. Philadelphia, PA: Saunders; 2000, with permission.)

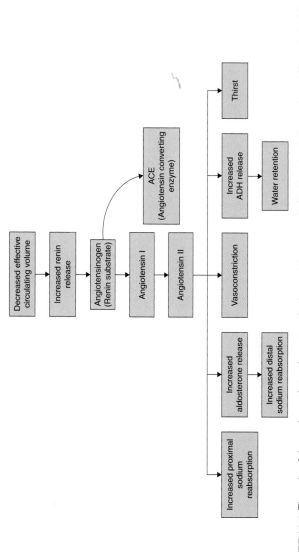

FIGURE 16-6 The role of the renin-angiotensin system in the maintenance of effective circulating volume. (From Lote CJ, Harper L, Savage COS. Mechanisms of acute renal failure. *Br J Anaesth.* 1996;77:82–89, with permission.)

2. Effects of angiotensin II include thirst, vasoconstriction, and salt and water reabsorption by the kidneys to maintain circulating volume and increase renal blood flow.

IV. **Regulation of Body Fluid.** The kidneys control blood and extracellular fluid volume, osmolarity of body fluids, and plasma concentration of ions and urea.

   A. **Blood and Extracellular Fluid Volume**
      1. Blood volume is maintained over a narrow range despite large daily variations in fluid and solute intake or loss.
         a. An increase in blood volume increases the cardiac output, which usually increases the systemic blood pressure. Increased cardiac output and systemic arterial pressure will increase renal blood flow and GFR, resulting in an increase in urine output. The negative feedback loop is completed by a consequent decrease in circulating blood volume.
         b. Regulation of normal circulating blood volume is impaired by factors directly affecting vascular capacitance (persistent vasoconstriction associated with essential hypertension or sympathetic nervous system stimulation results in a decrease in blood volume, whereas blood volume may be increased by chronic drug-induced vasodilation).
         c. The extracellular fluid space may be considered as a reservoir for excess intravenous fluid administered during the perioperative period.

   B. **Atrial and Renal Natriuretic Factors**
      1. Cardiac atrial muscle synthesizes and secretes a peptide hormone known as ANP, which is released in response to increased right and left atrial pressure and volume.
      2. The renal analogue of ANP is renal natriuretic peptide (urodilatin), which is synthesized in renal cortical nephrons.
         a. It is likely that ANP is primarily a cardiovascular regulator and relatively unimportant for sodium excretion, whereas renal natriuretic peptide participates in the intrarenal regulation of sodium excretion.
         b. In mechanical ventilation, positive end-expiratory pressure reduces atrial distension and atrial transmural pressure (reduces ANP release, which may contribute to sodium and water retention by the kidneys).

   C. **Osmolarity of Body Fluids**. The primary determinant of body fluid osmolarity is the concentration of sodium in the extracellular fluid. Sodium ion concentration is largely controlled by two mechanisms: the osmoreceptor–AVP response and the thirst reflex.

1. **Osmoreceptor–Arginine Vasopressin Hormone**
   a. In response to increased extracellular fluid osmolarity, osmoreceptors in the hypothalamus signal the posterior pituitary to increase the release of AVP (acts on renal collecting ducts to retain water and thus dilute serum sodium levels).
   b. A small change in osmolality (as little as 1%) can produce a large change in circulating AVP concentration, producing tight regulation of serum osmolality
2. **Thirst reflex** is primarily elicited by an increase in sodium concentration in the extracellular fluid.

V. **Plasma Concentration of Ions and Urea**
   A. **Sodium** (see Table 16-1)
      1. The kidneys control the concentration of sodium through the process of reabsorption.
      2. The renin-angiotensin-aldosterone system modulates the sodium reabsorption by the renal tubules. Angiotensin levels rise in the setting of hypotension or decreased circulating blood volume, is converted to angiotensin II in the lungs, and ultimately results in increased sodium reabsorption.
   B. **Potassium**, after being filtered in the glomerulus, is then reabsorbed by the proximal tubule and loop of Henle.
      1. Potassium is either reabsorbed or secreted in the distal tubule and collecting duct, depending on the level of aldosterone (Fig. 16-7).
      2. When aldosterone activity is blocked by certain diuretics, plasma potassium concentration depends more on dietary intake of potassium, making hypokalemia or hyperkalemia more likely (Fig. 16-8).
      3. The regulation of sodium and hydrogen ion concentrations also has an effect on urinary excretion of potassium.
         a. Hydrogen ions compete with potassium for secretion into the renal tubules. In the presence of alkalosis (vomiting and loss of gastric acid), potassium is excreted in the urine in order to maintain acid–base balance.
         b. Metabolic acidosis will lead to the secretion of hydrogen ions and retention of potassium, and plasma potassium concentration will increase.

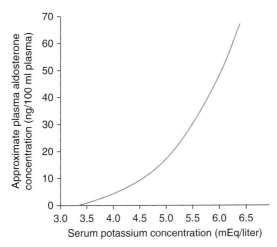

FIGURE 16-7 Small changes in the plasma concentrations of potassium evoke large changes in the plasma concentration of aldosterone. (From Guyton AC, Hall JE. *Textbook of Medical Physiology.* 10th ed. Philadelphia, PA: Saunders; 2000, with permission.)

C. **Acid–Base Balance**
   1. The kidneys secrete excess hydrogen ions by exchanging a hydrogen ion for a sodium ion, thus acidifying the urine, and by the synthesis of ammonia, which combines with hydrogen to form ammonium.
   2. In the presence of hypovolemia, bicarbonate reabsorption by the kidneys will lead to acidification of the urine and a metabolic alkalosis.

D. **Calcium and Magnesium**
   1. Calcium ion concentration is controlled principally by the effect of parathyroid hormone on bone reabsorption.
   2. Magnesium is reabsorbed by all portions of the renal tubules (urinary excretion of magnesium parallels the plasma concentration).

E. **Urea** elimination depends on the plasma concentration of urea (blood urea nitrogen or BUN) and the GFR.

VI. **Measuring Kidney Function**
   A. Formal measurement of kidney function requires labor-intensive studies such as collection of urine over time and

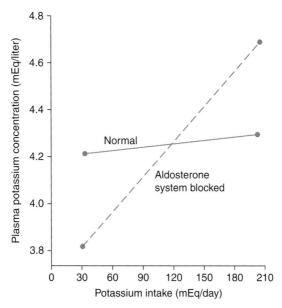

FIGURE 16-8 Plasma concentrations of potassium parallel intake when aldosterone activity is impaired. (From Guyton AC, Hall JE. *Textbook of Medical Physiology*. 10th ed. Philadelphia, PA: Saunders; 2000, with permission.)

measurement of blood and urine components. For clinical decision-making, estimates of GFR are accessible and inexpensive, requiring only basic laboratory work.

B. Serum creatinine (SCr), commonly used to measure changes in kidney function, is insensitive to small changes in GFR (needs to decrease by about 50% before a rise in SCr is seen).

VII. **Acute kidney injury results in an abrupt reduction in the kidney's ability to eliminate nitrogenous waste products and maintain fluid and electrolyte homeostasis. Despite the kidney's generous blood supply and large oxygen delivery, it remains at risk for ischemia in the perioperative period.**

A. **Classification** (Fig. 16-9)

1. **Prerenal azotemia** refers to decreases in renal function due to hypoperfusion in the setting of intact glomeruli and tubules. Correcting the underlying problems in circulation

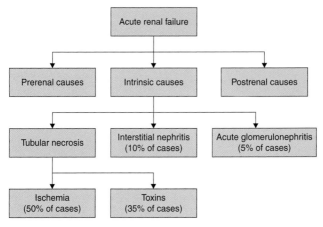

FIGURE 16-9 Classification of acute renal failure. (From Thadhani R, Pascual M, Bonventre JV. Acute renal failure. *N Engl J Med*. 1996;334: 1448–1460, with permission.)

will improve renal function. Common causes of prerenal azotemia in hospitalized patients include septic shock, heart failure, liver failure, and perioperative hemodynamic changes that lead to decreased renal perfusion.

2. **Intrinsic Causes of Acute Kidney Injury**

   a. The most common cause of intrinsic renal failure is acute tubular necrosis (ATN) caused by either ischemia or nephrotoxic agents.

   b. Renal tubule cells are particularly susceptible to ischemia because of their transport-related oxygen requirements and the low baseline blood flow to the renal medulla. ATN secondary to renal medullary ischemia is the most common cause of acute kidney injury (AKI) in the perioperative setting. In this setting, adequate urine output may be falsely reassuring (urine output does not correspond to the degree of cell damage or GFR in patients exposed to trauma, shock, or cardiovascular surgery).

B. **Postrenal Obstructive Nephropathy**. Perioperative patients with AKI should also be evaluated for postrenal etiologies, particularly those with acute oliguria (renal stones, prostatic hypertrophy, and mechanical obstruction of urinary catheters).

RIFLE criteria		
	GFR criteria	**Urine output criteria**
Risk	Increased SCr by 1.5× or GFR decrease by 25%	UO < 0.5 ml/kg/h for six hours
Injury	Increased SCr by 2× or GFR decrease by 50%	UO < 0.5 ml/kg/h for twelve hours
Failure	Increased SCr by 3× or GFR decrease by 75% or SCr > 4 mg/dL	UO < 0.3 ml/kg/h for 24 hours or Anuria for 12 hours
Loss	Persistent acute renal failure (four weeks duration)	
ESKD	End stage kidney disease (greater than three months)	

FIGURE 16-10 RIFLE criteria. GFR, glomerular filtration rate; ESKD, end-stage kidney disease; SCr, serum creatinine; UO, urine output. (Adapted from Bellomo R, Ronco C, Kellum JA, et al; Acute Dialysis Quality Initiative Workgroup. Acute renal failure—definition, outcome measures, animal models, fluid therapy and information technology needs: the Second International Consensus Conference of the Acute Dialysis Quality Initiative [ADQI] Group. *Crit Care*. 2004;8[4]:R204–R212.)

C. **Acute Kidney Injury Diagnosis**
1. **Diagnostic Criteria** (Fig. 16-10)
2. **Biomarkers**
   a. Serum creatinine and urine output are the most widely used diagnostic criteria to detect AKI. The rise in SCr lags an acute reduction in GFR.
   b. Neutrophil gelatinase–associated lipocalin (NGAL) has been identified as an early marker of AKI.

VIII. **Anesthesia and the Kidneys.** An understanding of kidney function is important as fundamental concepts of perioperative management include the maintenance of normal circulating volume, the regulation of electrolytes and acid–base status, and the clearance of metabolites and drugs. The perioperative time period is unique in that multiple potential insults, often concurrent or in rapid succession, challenge the kidney's functional ability.
   A. **Anesthesia and Renal Blood Flow**
   1. Regardless of the immediate cause, a fall in renal blood flow tends to decrease the GFR by diminishing blood

flow to the renal cortex and decreased renal blood flow puts the renal medulla at risk for ischemia because the blood supply to this region is already low at baseline. The sum effect of these changes is conservation of sodium and water and consequently a decrease in urine output.

2. Any factor that decreases the cardiac output will also lead to a release of AVP and an increase in the activity of both the sympathetic nervous system and the renin-angiotensin-aldosterone system.

3. Sustained changes in mean arterial pressure (greater than 10 minutes) are associated with a decreased ability to autoregulate renal blood flow. Autoregulation of GFR, by contrast, is sustained over longer periods of time.

4. Normal systemic arterial pressure does not ensure adequate renal blood flow and that renal ischemia may occur even in the absence of hypotension. Intraoperative urine output is a poor predictor of postoperative changes in renal function (Fig. 16-11).

B. **Perioperative Risk Assessment** (Table 16-2)

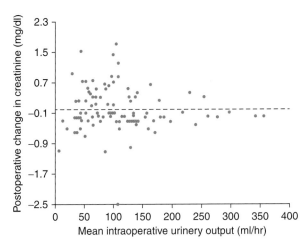

FIGURE 16-11 Intraoperative urine output. Mean intraoperative urine output does not correlate with postoperative changes in the plasma concentrations of creatinine. (From Alpert RA, Roizen MF, Hamilton WK, et al. Intraoperative urinary output does not predict postoperative renal function in patients undergoing abdominal aortic revascularization. *Surgery*. 1984;95:707–711, with permission.)

Table 16-2	

Risk Factors for Perioperative Acute Kidney Injury

Patient Risk Factors	Surgical Risk Factors
Age >56 years	Intraperitoneal surgery
Male gender	Emergent operation
Active congestive heart failure	
Ascites	
Diabetes	
Hypertension	

Adapted from Kheterpal S, Tremper KK, Heung M, et al. Development and validation of an acute kidney injury risk index for patients undergoing general surgery: results from a national data set. *Anesthesiology.* 2009;110(3):505–515.

C. **Intraoperative Management**
   1. The maintenance of renal blood flow can be accomplished by prompt correction of intravascular volume depletion and the maintenance of adequate systemic arterial pressure.
   2. The judicious use of positive end-expiratory pressure and the avoidance of unnecessary increases in mean airway pressure will help maintain cardiac output and adequate renal blood flow.
   3. Adequate analgesia will minimize sympathetic nervous system–mediated decreases in renal blood flow and is a potential benefit of regional anesthesia.
   4. Low-dose dopamine does not prevent AKI or improve morality.

CHAPTER 17

Intravenous Fluids and Electrolytes

I. **Introduction.** Total body water and electrolytes are divided between the intracellular and extracellular compartments. The major electrolytes in the intracellular compartment are potassium, magnesium, calcium, and phosphate. The extracellular compartment consists of the interstitial, plasma, and transcellular fluid components, where sodium and chloride are the major electrolytes.

II. **Total Body Fluid Composition (Fig. 17-1).** The adult body is composed of approximately 60% water, with some variation with age and gender, as well as significant variation. The cell membrane prevents sodium, the primary extracellular cation, from moving into the cell, except for a small amount by active pump transport, but isotonic fluids containing sodium added to the vascular space are distributed throughout the extracellular volume so that only 20% of the volume infused remains in the plasma.

III. **Intravenous Fluid Types**
   A. **Crystalloids** are fluid solutions containing ion salts and other low-molecular-weight substances (categorized based on their tonicity or osmotic pressure of the solution with respect to that of plasma) (Table 17-1). Administering large volumes of normal saline can result in hyperchloremic metabolic acidosis. "Balanced" or "physiologic" crystalloid solutions contain a composition approximating that of extracellular fluid but are usually slightly hypotonic because of lower sodium concentration.
   B. **Colloids (Table 17-2)**
      1. **Albumin (4% to 5%)** solution is produced from human blood and suspended in saline (heat-pasteurized at 60°C for 10 hours to reduce viral transmission). It is expensive to produce and distribute as compared to semisynthetic colloids and crystalloid solutions. The comparative effectiveness of fluid resuscitation with colloid versus

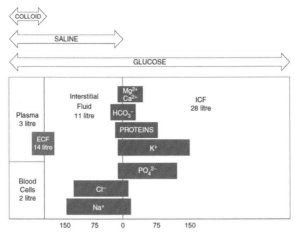

FIGURE 17-1 Body fluid compartments with main ion distribution. ECF, extracellular fluid; ICF, intracellular fluid.

crystalloid has been a long-standing controversy (studies show no difference in survival).

2. **Semisynthetic colloid solutions** (hydroxyethyl starch solutions [HES], succinylated gelatin, urea-linked gelatin–polygeline preparations, dextran solutions) (Table 17-3).

   a. HES is the most commonly used semisynthetic colloid solution.

   b. The maximum daily dose of HES is limited to 20 to 50 mL/kg of body weight/day but varies by solution.

   c. HES is removed from the circulation by redistribution and renal excretion.

   d. HES compounds have effects on coagulation with reductions in factor VIII, von Willebrand factor, and platelet function (noted even when used below recommended maximum doses). Solutions with more rapid degradation are associated with less effects on coagulation.

   e. The incidence of anaphylactoid reactions with HES use is 0.085%.

   f. When compared with saline, HES was associated with significantly more adverse events.

Table 17-1

Common Crystalloid Solutions

Solution	Osmolarity (mOsm/L)	Tonicity	pH	Calories (kcal/L)	Na$^+$ (mEq/L)	Cl$^-$ (mEq/L)	K$^+$ (mEq/L)	Glucose (g/L)	Lactate (mEq/L)	Acetate (mEq/L)	Gluconate (mEq/L)	Mg^{++} (mEq/L)	Ca^{++} (mEq/L)
NS	308	Iso	5		154	154							
D5NS	560	Hyper	4	170	154	154		50					
D51/2NS	406	Hyper	4	170	77	77		50					
LR	273	Iso	6.5	9	130	109	4		28				3
D5LR	525	Hyper	4.9	179	130	109	4	50	28				3
Plasmalyte	294	Iso		21	140	98	5			27	23	3	

D, dextrose; LR, lactated Ringer's; NS, normal saline.

Table 17-2

Common Colloid Solutions

Fluid	Trade Name	Source	Osmolarity (mOsm/L)	Na⁺ (mmol/L)	Cl⁻ (mmol/L)	K⁺ (mmol/L)
Albumin 4%	Albumex	Human donor	250	148	128	
Albumin 5%		Human donor	309	154	154	
HES 10% (200/0.5)	Hemohes	Potato starch	308	154	154	
HES 6% (450/0.7)	Hextend	Maize starch	304	143	124	3
HES 6% (130/0.4)	Voluven	Maize starch	308	154	154	
HES 6% (130/0.4)	Volulyte	Maize starch	286	137	110	4
HES 6% (130/0.42)	Venufundin	Potato starch	308	154	154	
HES 6% (130/0.42)	Tetraspan	Potato starch	296	140	118	4

Fluid	Ca⁺⁺ (mmol/L)	Mg⁺⁺ (mmol/L)	Lactate (mmol/L)	Acetate (mmol/L)	Octonate (mmol/L)	Malate (mmol/L)
Albumin 4%					6.4	
Albumin 5%						
HES 10% (200/0.5)						
HES 6% (450/0.7)	5	0.9	28			
HES 6% (130/0.4)						
HES 6% (130/0.4)		1.5		34		
HES 6% (130/0.42)		1		24		
HES 6% (130/0.42)	2.5					5

HES, hydroxyethyl starch.

Table 17-3

Black Box Warnings on Use of Hydroxyethyl Starch Solutions

Do not use in critically ill adult patients (sepsis, ICU patients, preexisting renal dysfunction)

Discontinue at first sign of renal injury

Avoid in patients undergoing cardiopulmonary bypass (excess bleeding)

Discontinue at first sign of coagulopathy

ICU, intensive care unit.

IV. **Assessing Fluid Responsiveness**
   A. Fluid responsiveness may be defined as a 15% increase in cardiac output following a 500-mL intravenous (IV) fluid bolus, indicating that the patient is still on the ascending limb of the cardiac output/end diastolic volume curve, also referred to as the *cardiac function curve*. Fluid administration to a patient on the plateau part of the curve may be of little benefit and result in adverse effects.
   B. Filling pressure measures, particularly central venous pressure, correlate poorly with blood volume, and changes in central venous pressure have been shown to poorly predict hemodynamic response to fluid challenge. Stroke volume changes due to increases or decreases in right ventricular preload may be used to assess fluid responsiveness.

V. **Important Fluid Constituents**
   A. **Magnesium.** Plasma magnesium level is normally 1.7 to 2.4 mg/dL and measurements may not be representative of total body magnesium stores (magnesium measurements can be falsely elevated with hemolysis of the blood sample, which releases the intracellular electrolytes). Excretion occurs via the kidney with more than 95% of the filtered magnesium being reabsorbed in the renal tubules, with this mechanism effectively regulating the plasma level.
      1. **Role of Magnesium**
         a. Magnesium plays a key role in many biologic processes including protein synthesis, neuromuscular function, and nucleic acid stability.
         b. Magnesium has antiarrhythmic properties related to calcium channel antagonism. IV magnesium administration can exert muscle-relaxing effects, enhance

nondepolarizing neuromuscular blockers, attenuate muscle fasciculations and potassium release with administration of succinylcholine, and precipitate skeletal muscle weakness in patients with Lambert-Eaton syndrome and myasthenia gravis. It has been used to reduce anesthetic requirements and attenuate cardiovascular effects of laryngoscopy and intubation. Magnesium decreases blood–brain barrier disruption and limits cerebral edema formation after brain injury.

   c. Side effects of IV administration include muscle weakness, hypotension, and bradycardia.

2. **Hypomagnesemia** may result from dietary deficiency (chronic alcoholism), gastrointestinal malabsorption or secretion (diarrhea, vomiting, laxative use), renal losses (medication effects, nephrotoxic agents, endocrine disease, diabetic nephropathy), and chelation (citrate binding in the case of massive transfusion).

   a. Hypomagnesemia is seen in as many as 11% of hospitalized patients and 65% of patients in the intensive care unit.

   b. Clinical manifestations of hypomagnesemia include cardiac and neuromuscular disorders, electrocardiogram (ECG) abnormalities (prolonged PR and QT intervals, diminished T-wave morphology, torsades de pointes), and accompanying hypokalemia and hypocalcemia.

3. **Hypermagnesemia** is rare and most commonly occurs with excessive administration of magnesium for therapeutic purposes.

   a. Clinical manifestations include QRS widening, hypotension, narcosis, diminution of deep tendon reflexes, respiratory depression from paralysis of muscles of ventilation, heart block, and cardiac arrest.

   b. Immediate treatment of life-threatening hypermagnesemia is with calcium gluconate, 10 to 15 mg/kg IV, followed by diuretics or dialysis, along with appropriate respiratory and circulatory support.

4. **Preeclampsia**

   a. Magnesium improves the clinical symptoms of preeclampsia by causing systemic, vertebral, and uterine vasodilation.

   b. Suggested dosing regimens of magnesium sulfate based on randomized trial data are 4 g IV loading dose over 10 to 15 minutes followed by infusion of 1 g per hour for 24 hours or 4 g IV loading dose with

10 g intramuscular (IM) followed by 5 g IM every 4 hours for 24 hours. Serum monitoring of magnesium levels should be performed for signs of toxicity or renal impairment.

c. Magnesium crosses the placenta and may result in neonatal lethargy, hypotension, and respiratory depression if administered for prolonged duration (more than 48 hours).

5. **Cardiac Dysrhythmias**

a. Excess magnesium blocks myocardial calcium influx resulting in decreased sinus node activity, prolonged atrioventricular (AV) conduction time, and increased AV node refractoriness. Arrhythmias associated with hypomagnesemia are often accompanied by hypokalemia (normalization of both electrolytes is recommended).

b. Prophylactic administration of magnesium during cardiopulmonary bypass has been shown to decrease the incidence of postoperative atrial fibrillation after coronary artery bypass graft surgery.

B. **Calcium**. The plasma concentration of calcium is maintained between 4.5 and 5.5 mEq/L (8.5 to 10.5 mg/dL) by an endocrine control system involving vitamin D, parathyroid hormone, and calcitonin. It is the ionized fraction of calcium that produces physiologic effects and is normally 2 to 2.5 mEq/L. The ionized concentration of calcium depends on arterial pH, with acidosis increasing and alkalosis decreasing the concentration. Plasma albumin binds nonionized calcium (in low-albumin states, less nonionized calcium is protein bound making more available to return to storage sites, such as bone and teeth). Nonionized plasma calcium levels must be interpreted with knowledge of the plasma albumin concentration.

1. **Role of Calcium**. Calcium is important for neuromuscular transmission, skeletal muscle contraction, cardiac muscle contractility, blood coagulation, and intracellular signaling in its function as a second messenger.

2. **Hypocalcemia** can result from decreased plasma concentration of albumin, hypoparathyroidism, acute pancreatitis, vitamin D deficiency, chronic renal failure associated with hyperphosphatemia, and citrate binding of calcium (in the case of transfused blood, particularly in hepatic failure and reduced citrate metabolism).

a. Symptoms of hypocalcemia include neuromuscular excitability, including muscle twitching, spasms,

tingling, numbness, carpopedal spasm, tetany, seizures, and cardiac dysrhythmias.
   b. Calcium can be administered by oral or IV route. IV preparations include calcium chloride which provides 27 mg of elemental calcium/mL and calcium gluconate which provides 9 mg.
3. **Hypercalcemia**
   a. Hyperparathyroidism is the most important cause of hypercalcemia and may be primary from parathyroid adenoma (85%), parathyroid hyperplasia (10%) which may be associated with multiple endocrine neoplasia syndromes, or, rarely (<1%), parathyroid carcinoma.
   b. Secondary hyperparathyroidism results from abnormal feedback loops present in failure and tertiary hyperparathyroidism from overactive responses to normal negative feedback mechanisms.
   c. Symptoms of hypercalcemia include decreased neuromuscular transmission (lethargy, hypotonia, confusion), renal effects (polyuria, dehydration, nephrolithiasis), cardiac rhythm abnormalities (QTc shortening, J waves following QRS complex), and pancreatitis.
   d. Treatment of hypercalcemia depends on the exact etiology but usually includes promoting renal excretion of calcium with IV fluids and loop diuretics while avoiding dehydration that would worsen any renal injury.
C. **Potassium** is the second most common cation in the body and the principal intracellular cation. With 98% of the body's potassium being intracellular, the concentration in the extracellular fluid is about 4 mEq/L, and the intracellular concentration is 150 mEq/L (estimation of total body potassium content from serum potassium values is inaccurate).
1. **Role of Potassium**. Disturbances of potassium homeostasis contribute to cardiac dysrhythmias, skeletal muscle weakness, and acid–base disturbances. The kidney is the principal organ involved in body potassium homeostasis, primarily through control of active potassium secretion in the urine.
2. **Drugs Causing Hypokalemia**. Diuretics that induce renal potassium loss are probably the most common cause of hypokalemia. Catecholamines shift potassium intracellularly and β agonists may be useful in the treatment of hyperkalemia. Insulin induces potassium to move into cells and is used to treat severe hyperkalemia.
3. **Drugs Causing Hyperkalemia**. Drugs that increase serum potassium concentrations do so by redistribution,

suppression of aldosterone secretion, inhibition of potassium secretion in the distal collecting duct, or by direct cell destruction.

a. Extracellular movement of potassium can result in plasma hyperkalemia without an increase in total body potassium (succinylcholine causes a release of potassium from skeletal muscle cells, resulting in an increase of the serum potassium concentration by as much as 0.5 mEq/L).

b. β-Adrenergic antagonists can cause a modest increase in the serum potassium concentration by virtue of an extracellular shift.

4. **Hypokalemia**. Skeletal muscle weakness and a predisposition to cardiac dysrhythmias are the most prominent symptoms of clinically significant hypokalemia. At the cellular level, hypokalemia causes hyperpolarity, increases resting potential, hastens depolarization, and increases automaticity and excitability of cardiac cells, predisposing to tachydysrhythmias.

a. **Treatment**. It is important to determine the cause of hypokalemia before aggressive potassium replacement is initiated (if serum potassium concentrations are acutely decreased due to intracellular redistribution and potassium therapy is initiated, potentially serious hyperkalemia could occur).

b. Life-threatening hypokalemia, presenting as malignant cardiac dysrhythmias or extreme neuromuscular collapse, requires supplemental IV potassium administration (rate of potassium infusion depends on the urgency of the indication, with a common recommendation being administration of IV potassium no greater than 10 mEq/hour peripherally).

5. **Hyperkalemia**. The earliest sign of hyperkalemia is peaked T waves on ECG, which typically occurs when the serum potassium concentration reaches 6 mEq/L. As the extracellular concentration increases further, the transmembrane gradient is decreased, with prolongation of the P-R interval and QRS widening on the ECG. At this point, the risk of asystole or ventricular fibrillation due to cardiac conduction blockade increases dramatically.

a. **Treatment**. The decision to treat hyperkalemia, in contrast to hypokalemia, is based on the degree of increase in the serum potassium concentration and the symptoms and signs that are present (if the serum potassium concentration is >6.5 mEq/L, the incidence of serious cardiac compromise is high and rapid intervention is indicated).

b. Calcium is administered to rapidly offset the adverse effects of potassium on cardiac conduction and contractility (IV administration of 10 to 20 mL of a 10% calcium chloride solution restores myocardial contractility in 1 to 2 minutes and lasts for 15 to 20 minutes).

c. Alkalization of the blood with sodium bicarbonate, 0.5 to 1.0 mEq/kg IV, rapidly moves potassium into cells decreasing the serum potassium level for as long as the arterial pH is increased.

d. Glucose-insulin infusion (50 mL of 50% glucose plus 10 units of regular insulin) produces a sustained transfer of extracellular potassium into cells, resulting in a 1.5 to 2.5 mEq/L decrease in the serum potassium concentration after approximately 30 minutes.

e. Potassium removal from the body also may be achieved by loop diuretics or, most rapidly and effectively, with hemodialysis.

D. **Phosphate** is the major intracellular anion and the normal plasma concentration of phosphate is 3.0 to 4.5 mg/dL, accounting for both organic and inorganic forms.

1. Phosphate is important in energy metabolism, intracellular signaling (cyclic adenosine monophosphate and cyclic guanosine monophosphate), cell structure (phospholipids), oxygen delivery (2,3-disphosphoglycerate), regulation of the glycolytic pathway, the immune system, the coagulation cascade, and buffering to maintain normal acid–base balance. Phosphorus regulation is a result of the interplay of phosphate and calcium levels, vitamin D, and parathyroid hormone on gastrointestinal absorption, renal reabsorption, and bone storage.

2. Hypophosphatemia (phosphorus concentration <1.5 mg/dL) causes a decrease in the concentration of adenosine triphosphate and 2,3-diphosphoglycerate in erythrocytes.

a. Profound skeletal muscle weakness sufficient to contribute to hypoventilation may be caused by hypophosphatemia, as well as central nervous system dysfunction and peripheral neuropathy.

b. Causes of hypophosphatemia include alcohol abuse, prolonged parenteral nutrition, hemodialysis, salicylate poisoning, and gram-negative bacteremia.

E. **Iron.** Iron present in food is absorbed from the proximal small intestine into the circulation, where it is bound to transferrin. Approximately 80% of the iron in plasma enters the bone marrow to be incorporated into new erythrocytes. Hemoglobin synthesis is the principal determinant of the plasma iron turnover rate.

1. **Iron deficiency** is estimated to be present in 20% to 40% of menstruating females but only about 5% of adult males and postmenopausal females.

2. **Causes** of iron-deficiency anemia include inadequate dietary intake of iron, increased iron requirements due to pregnancy or blood loss, or interference with absorption from the gastrointestinal tract. Partial gastrectomy, malabsorptive bariatric surgery, and sprue are causes of inadequate iron absorption.

3. **Diagnosis**. Iron deficiency initially results in a decrease in iron stores and a parallel decrease in the erythrocyte content of iron. Depleted iron stores are indicated by decreased plasma concentrations of ferritin and the absence of reticuloendothelial hemosiderin in a bone marrow aspirate. Plasma ferritin concentrations of less than 12 μg/dL are diagnostic of iron deficiency.

4. **Treatment**. Prophylactic use of iron preparations should be reserved for individuals at high risk for developing iron deficiency (pregnant and lactating females, low-birth-weight infants, females with heavy menses). In iron-deficiency anemia, administration of medicinal iron increases the rate of erythrocyte production resulting in a rise in hemoglobin concentration within 72 hours. There is no justification for continuing iron therapy beyond 3 weeks if a favorable response has not occurred.

   a. **Oral Iron**. Ferrous sulfate administered orally is the most frequent choice for the treatment of iron-deficiency anemia and is available as syrup, pills, or tablets.

   b. **Parenteral iron** acts similarly to oral iron but should be used only if patients cannot tolerate or do not respond to oral therapy.

F. **Copper** is present is a constituent of enzymes and is an essential component of several proteins. Copper deficiency is rare in the presence of an adequate diet. Supplements of copper should be given during prolonged hyperalimentation.

G. **Zinc** is an enzymatic cofactor essential for cell growth and the synthesis of nucleic acid, carbohydrates, and proteins. Adequate zinc is provided by a diet containing sufficient animal protein. Diets in which protein is obtained primarily from vegetable sources may not supply adequate zinc.

CHAPTER 18

Sympathomimetic Drugs

I. **Naturally Occurring Catecholamines (Table 18-1) (Fig. 18-1)**

   A. **Epinephrine** is a circulating hormone synthesized, stored, and released from the adrenal medulla. Its natural functions upon release into the circulation include regulation of myocardial contractility, heart rate, vascular and bronchial smooth muscle tone, glandular secretions, and metabolic processes such as glycogenolysis and lipolysis. It is a potent activator of α-adrenergic receptors and also activates β_1 and β_2 receptors. Oral administration is not effective as epinephrine is rapidly metabolized in the gastrointestinal mucosa and liver (administered subcutaneously, intravenously [IV], or intramuscularly). Epinephrine is poorly lipid soluble, preventing its ready entrance into the central nervous system and accounting for the lack of cerebral effects.

     1. **Clinical uses** of epinephrine include treatment of life-threatening allergic reactions/anaphylaxis, treatment of severe asthma and bronchospasm, administration during cardiopulmonary resuscitation as a vital therapeutic drug, administration during periods of hemodynamic instability to promote myocardial contractility and increase vascular resistance, and continuous infusion for continuous support of myocardial contractility and vascular resistance. Epinephrine is added to local anesthetic solutions to decrease systemic absorption prolonging the duration of action of the anesthetic for regional and local anesthesia.

     2. **Cardiovascular Effects**. The cardiovascular effects of epinephrine result from stimulation of α- and β-adrenergic receptors (see Table 18-1).

     3. **Airway Smooth Muscle**. Smooth muscles of the bronchi are relaxed by epinephrine-induced activation of β_2 receptors. The bronchodilating effects of epinephrine are not seen in the presence of β-adrenergic blockade.

Table 18-1

Classification and Comparative Pharmacology of Sympathomimetics

	Receptors Stimulated				Cardiac Effects			Peripheral Vascular Resistance
	α	β₁	β₂	Mechanism of Action	Cardiac Output	Heart Rate	Dysrhythmias	
Nature catecholamines								
Epinephrine	+	++	++	Direct	++	++	+++	±
Norepinephrine	+++	++	0	Direct	−	−	+	+++
Dopamine	++	++	+	Direct	+++	+	+	+
Synthetic catecholamines								
Isoproterenol	0	+++	+++	Direct	+++	+++	+++	−−
Dobutamine	0	+++	+	Direct	+++	+	±	NC
Synthetic noncatecholamines								
Ephedrine	++	+	+	Direct and Indirect	++	++	++	+
Phenylephrine	+++	0	0	Direct	−	−	NC	+++

(continued)

Table 18-1

Classification and Comparative Pharmacology of Sympathomimetics *(continued)*

	Renal Blood Flow	Mean Arterial Pressure	Airway Resistance	Central Nervous System Stimulation	Single Intravenous Dose (70-kg Adult)	Continuous Infusion Dose (70-kg Adult)
Nature catecholamines						
Epinephrine	– –	+	– –	Yes	2–8 µg	1–20 µg/min
Norepinephrine	– – –	+++	NC	No	Not used	4–16 µg/min
Dopamine	+++	+	NC	No	Not used	2–20 µg/kg/min
Synthetic catecholamines						
Isoproterenol	–	±	– – –	Yes	1–4 µg	1–5 µg/min
Dobutamine	++	+	NC		Not used	2–10 µg/kg/min
Synthetic noncatecholamines						
Ephedrine	– –	++	– –	Yes	10–25 µg	Not used
Phenylephrine	– – –	+++	NC	No	50–100 µg	20–50 µg/min

0, none; +, minimal increase; ++, moderate increase; +++, marked increase; –, minimal decrease; – –, moderate decrease; – – –, marked decrease; NC, no change.

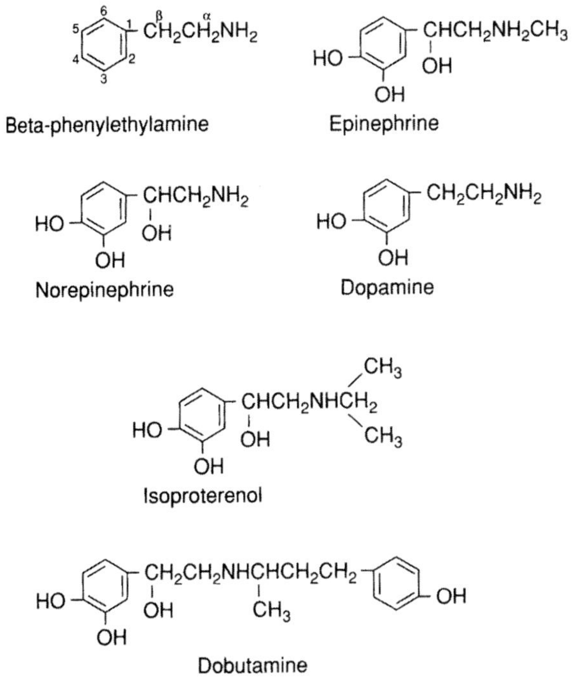

FIGURE 18-1 Sympathomimetics are derived from β-phenyleth-ylamine, with a catecholamine being any compound that has hy-droxyl groups on the 3 and 4 carbon positions of the benzene ring. The naturally occurring catecholamines are epinephrine, norepi-nephrine, and dopamine. Isoproterenol and dobutamine are syn-thetic catecholamines.

4. **Metabolic Effects**. Epinephrine has the most significant effect on metabolism of all the catecholamines.
   a. β_1 Receptor stimulation due to epinephrine increases liver glycogenolysis and adipose tissue lipolysis, whereas α_1 receptor stimulation inhibits release of insulin.
   b. Release of endogenous epinephrine and the resulting glycogenolysis and inhibition of insulin secretion is the most likely explanation for perioperative hyperglycemia.

5. **Electrolytes**
   a. Selective β_2-adrenergic agonist effects of epinephrine are speculated to reflect activation of the sodium-potassium pump in skeletal muscles, leading to a transfer of potassium ions into cells (Fig. 18-2).
   b. The observation that serum potassium measurements in blood samples obtained immediately before induction of anesthesia are lower than measurements 1 to 3 days preoperatively is presumed to reflect stress-induced release of epinephrine (Fig. 18-3). In making therapeutic decisions based on a preinduction serum potassium measurement, especially in patients without a reason to experience hypokalemia, one should consider the possible role of preoperative anxiety and the release of epinephrine.

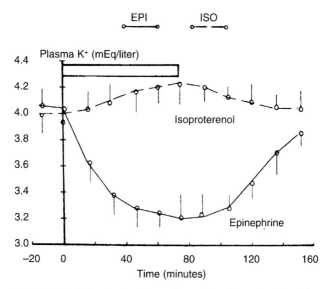

FIGURE 18-2 Selective β_2-adrenergic agonist effects of epinephrine are responsible for stimulating the movement of potassium ions (K^+) into cells, with a resulting decrease in the serum potassium concentration. (From Brown MJ, Brown DC, Murphy MB. Hypokalemia from beta2-receptor stimulation by circulating epinephrine. *N Engl J Med.* 1983;309[23]:1414–1419, with permission.)

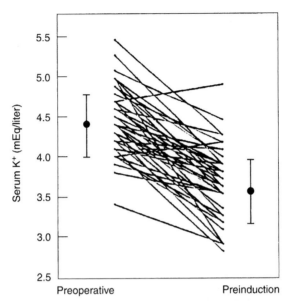

FIGURE 18-3 Individual and mean (± SD) plasma potassium (K^-) concentrations determined 1 to 3 days preoperatively and immediately before the induction (preinduction) of anesthesia. (From Kharasch ED, Bowdle TA. Hypokalemia before induction of anesthesia and prevention by beta 2 adrenoceptor antagonism. *Anesth Analg*. 1991;72[2]:216–220, with permission.)

6. **Ocular Effects**. Epinephrine causes contraction of the radial muscles of the iris, producing mydriasis.
7. **Gastrointestinal and Genitourinary Effects**
   a. Epinephrine, norepinephrine, and isoproterenol produce relaxation of gastrointestinal smooth muscle.
   b. Activation of β-adrenergic receptors relaxes the detrusor muscle of the bladder, whereas activation of α-adrenergic receptors contracts the trigone and sphincter muscles.
   c. Hepatosplanchnic vasoconstriction occurs as well as impaired renal blood flow as cardiac output is diverted to the dilated skeletal muscle vasculature.
8. **Coagulation** is accelerated by epinephrine. A hypercoagulable state present during the intraoperative and

postoperative period may reflect stress-associated release of epinephrine.

B. **Norepinephrine** is the endogenous neurotransmitter
synthesized and stored in postganglionic sympathetic nerve
endings and released with sympathetic nerve stimulation.
Norepinephrine stimulates β_1- and α_1-adrenergic receptors
(see Table 18-1). A continuous infusion of norepineph-
rine, 2 to 16 μg per minute, may be used to treat refractory
hypotension.

1. **Clinical Uses**. The primary utility of norepinephrine is
as a potent vasoconstrictor to increase total peripheral
vascular resistance and mean arterial pressure. It is a
first-line agent in the treatment of refractory hypotension during severe sepsis. Norepinephrine-induced
vasoconstriction and redistribution of flow may increase
splanchnic blood flow and urine output in severely
hypotensive septic patients.

2. **Side Effects**. The use of norepinephrine as an inotropic
agent is limited by its action as a potent vasoconstrictor.
Excessive vasoconstriction and decreased perfusion of
renal, splanchnic, and peripheral vascular beds may lead
to end-organ hypoperfusion and ischemia.

C. **Dopamine** is an endogenous catecholamine that regulates
cardiac, vascular, and endocrine function and is an important neurotransmitter in the central and peripheral nervous
systems. Dopamine receptors may also be associated with
the neural mechanism for "reward" that is associated
with cocaine and alcohol dependence. Traditionally, the
pharmacokinetics of dopamine has been attributed to
dose-dependent effects on varying receptors (too simplistic as even in healthy individuals there are a wide range
of clinical responses depending on individual variability
in pharmacokinetics). Despite identical IV infusion rates,
there may be a 10- to 75-fold variability in plasma dopamine concentrations produced even in healthy individuals
with normal drug metabolism. The effects of dopamine
cannot be predicted based on the dose, and the drug must
be titrated to effect. Dopamine increases cardiac output by
stimulation of β_1 receptors, increasing stroke volume (less
dysrhythmogenic than epinephrine). Rapid metabolism of
dopamine with an elimination half-life of 1 to 2 minutes
mandates its use as a continuous infusion (1 to 20 μg/kg/
minute) to maintain therapeutic plasma concentrations.

1. **Clinical Uses**

a. Dopamine is used clinically to increase cardiac
output in patients with decreased contractility, low

systemic blood pressure, and low urine output as may be present after cardiopulmonary bypass or with chronic heart failure (unique among the catecholamines in being able to simultaneously increase myocardial contractility, renal blood flow, glomerular filtration rate, excretion of sodium, and urine output).

b. The divergent pharmacologic effects of dopamine and dobutamine make their use in combination potentially useful (infusions of dopamine and dobutamine produce a greater improvement in cardiac output, at lower doses, than can be achieved by either drug alone). The objective of combination therapy is to increase coronary perfusion and cardiac output while decreasing afterload, similar to an intraaortic balloon pump.

2. **Renal-Dose Dopamine**

a. The term *renal-dose dopamine* or *low-dose dopamine* refers to the continuous infusion of small doses (1 to 3 μg/kg/minute) of dopamine to patients to promote renal blood flow. In healthy individuals, low-dose dopamine increases renal blood flow and induces natriuresis and diuresis.

b. The term *renal-dose* or *low-dose dopamine* is misleading as dopamine has many effects at sites other than the kidneys, even at low doses.

c. In the absence of data confirming the efficacy of dopamine in preventing acute renal failure, renal-dose dopamine cannot be recommended.

3. **Cardiovascular Effects**. Dopamine is associated more than dobutamine or epinephrine with dose-related sinus tachycardia and the potential to cause ventricular arrhythmias and may predispose to myocardial ischemia by precipitating tachycardia, increasing contractility, increasing afterload, and precipitating coronary artery vasospasm.

4. **Gastrointestinal Effects**. There is no evidence that low-dose dopamine has beneficial effects on splanchnic function or reduces the progression to multiorgan failure in sepsis.

5. **Endocrine and Immunologic Effects**

a. Dopamine disrupts metabolic and immunologic functions through its effects on hormones and lymphocyte function.

b. In the acute phase of an illness, dopamine induces the pattern of hypopituitarism seen in prolonged critical illness and chronic stress. When dopamine is used in the chronic phase of illness, it further suppresses the circulating concentrations of pituitary hormones.

c. Dopamine's overall effect is to suppress the secretion and function of anterior pituitary hormones, aggravating catabolism and cellular immune function and inducing central hypothyroidism.

6. **Respiratory Effects**. The infusion of low-dose dopamine interferes with the ventilatory response to arterial hypoxemia and hypercapnia, reflecting the role of dopamine as an inhibitory neurotransmitter at the carotid bodies (result is depression of ventilation in patients who are being treated with dopamine to increase myocardial contractility).

II. **Synthetic Catecholamines** (see Table 18-1) (see Fig. 18-1)

A. **Isoproterenol** is the most potent activator of all the sympathomimetics with β_1 and β_2 receptor activity (two to three times more potent than epinephrine and at least 100 times more active than norepinephrine, devoid of α agonist effects). The cardiovascular effects of isoproterenol reflect activation of β_1 receptors in the heart and β_2 receptors in skeletal muscle. Although cardiac output may increase thereby increasing systolic blood pressure, the mean arterial pressure may decrease due to decreases in systemic vascular resistance and associated decreases in diastolic blood pressure. Compensatory baroreceptor-mediated reflex slowing of the heart rate does not occur during infusion of isoproterenol because mean arterial pressure is not increased. Metabolism of isoproterenol in the liver by catechol-O-methyltransferase is rapid, necessitating a continuous infusion to maintain therapeutic plasma concentrations.

1. **Clinical Uses**. A continuous infusion of isoproterenol, 1 to 5 μg per minute, is effective in increasing the heart rate in adults in the presence of heart block. Isoproterenol is used to provide sustained increases in heart rate before insertion of a temporary or permanent cardiac pacemaker.

2. **Adverse Effects**. Vasodilation and decreased blood pressure may limit the use of isoproterenol. The combination of decreased diastolic blood pressure and increased heart rate and dysrhythmias may lead to myocardial ischemia.

B. **Dobutamine** is a synthetic catecholamine derived from isoproterenol consisting of a 50:50 racemic mixture of two stereoisomers. Dobutamine has potent β_1-adrenergic effects with weaker β_2-adrenergic activity. Its effect on α receptors increases at higher doses. Because dobutamine does not possess clinically important vasoconstrictor activity, it may be ineffective in patients who require increased systemic vascular resistance rather than augmentation of cardiac output to increase systemic blood pressure. Dobutamine affects heart rate through its action on β_1-adrenergic receptors. Dobutamine stimulates sinoatrial node automaticity as well as atrioventricular nodal and ventricular conduction. At low doses, increases in heart rate may be minimal. However, high doses of dobutamine (>10 μg/kg/minute IV) may predispose the patient to tachycardia and cardiac dysrhythmias. Unlike dopamine, dobutamine does not act indirectly by stimulating the release of endogenous norepinephrine. Dobutamine does not activate dopaminergic receptors to increase renal blood flow. Renal blood flow, however, may improve as a result of drug-induced increases in cardiac output. Rapid metabolism of dobutamine (half-life of 2 minutes) necessitates its administration as a continuous infusion of 2 to 10 μg/kg/minute to maintain therapeutic plasma concentrations.

1. **Clinical Uses**
   a. Dobutamine produces potent β-adrenergic agonist effects at doses less than 5 μg/kg/minute IV increasing myocardial contractility (β_1 and α_1 receptors) and causing a modest degree of peripheral vasodilation (β_2 receptors).
   b. Dobutamine is used to improve cardiac output in patients with congestive heart failure and is also useful for weaning from cardiopulmonary bypass. Vasodilators may be combined with dobutamine or dopamine to decrease afterload, optimizing cardiac output in the presence of increased systemic vascular resistance.
2. **Adverse Effects**. The use of dobutamine may be limited by the occurrence of tachyarrhythmias (occur more frequently at higher dosages or in patients with underlying arrhythmias or heart failure).

III. **Synthetic Noncatecholamines (Fig. 18-4)**
   A. **Ephedrine** is an indirect (stimulation of release of endogenous norepinephrine) and direct (stimulates α- and β-adrenergic receptors) acting synthetic sympathomimetic. The slow inactivation and excretion of ephedrine

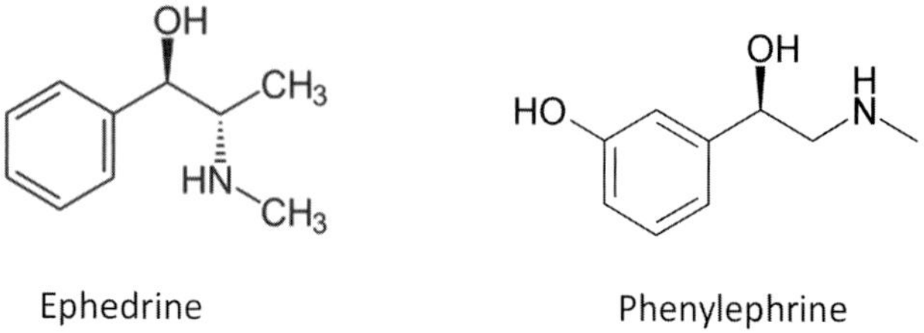

Ephedrine   Phenylephrine

FIGURE 18-4 Synthetic noncatecholamine sympathomimetics.

are responsible for the prolonged duration of action of this sympathomimetic.

1. **Clinical Uses**
   a. Ephedrine, 5 to 10 mg IV administered to adults, is a commonly selected sympathomimetic to increase systemic blood pressure in the presence of sympathetic nervous system blockade produced by regional anesthesia or hypotension due to inhaled or injected anesthetics.
   b. Until recently, ephedrine was considered the preferred sympathomimetic for administration to parturients experiencing decreased systemic blood pressure owing to spinal or epidural anesthesia. Recent reviews of trials of ephedrine versus phenylephrine have concluded that systemic blood pressure control is similar with both drugs but phenylephrine is associated with a higher umbilical artery pH at delivery than ephedrine (seems that α agonists such as phenylephrine may be preferable to ephedrine for treatment of maternal hypotension).

2. **Cardiovascular effects** of ephedrine resemble those of epinephrine, but its systemic blood pressure–elevating response is less intense and lasts approximately 10 times longer.
   a. IV ephedrine results in increases in systolic and diastolic blood pressure, heart rate, and cardiac output.
   b. The principal mechanism for cardiovascular effects produced by ephedrine is increased myocardial contractility due to activation of β_1 receptors. In the presence of preexisting β-adrenergic blockade, the cardiovascular effects of ephedrine may resemble

responses more typical of α-adrenergic receptor stimulation.

   c. A second dose of ephedrine produces a less intense systemic blood pressure response than the first dose (tachyphylaxis, occurs with many sympathomimetics).

B. **Phenylephrine** mimics the effects of norepinephrine but is less potent and longer lasting (principally stimulates α_1-adrenergic receptors by a direct effect, with only a small part of the pharmacologic response being indirect-acting due to its ability to evoke the release of norepinephrine). Phenylephrine exerts minimal effects on β-adrenergic receptors. The dose of phenylephrine necessary to stimulate α_1 receptors is far less than the dose that stimulates α_2 receptors. Phenylephrine primarily causes venoconstriction rather than arterial constriction.

   1. **Clinical Uses**

     a. Phenylephrine, 50 to 200 μg IV bolus, is often administered to adults to treat systemic blood pressure decreases that accompany sympathetic nervous system blockade produced by a regional anesthetic and peripheral vasodilation following administration of injected or inhaled anesthetics.

     b. Phenylephrine is believed to be particularly useful in patients with coronary artery disease and in patients with aortic stenosis because it increases coronary perfusion pressure without chronotropic side effects, unlike most other sympathomimetics.

     c. Phenylephrine has been used as a continuous infusion (20 to 100 μg per minute) in adults to maintain normal blood pressure during surgery.

     d. The reflex vagal effects produced by phenylephrine can be used to slow heart rate in the presence of hemodynamically significant supraventricular tachydysrhythmias.

     e. Topically applied, phenylephrine is a widely available nasal decongestant (brand name Neo-Synephrine).

   2. **Cardiovascular Effects**

     a. Rapid IV injection of phenylephrine to patients with coronary artery disease produces dose-dependent peripheral vasoconstriction and increases in systemic blood pressure that are accompanied by decreases in cardiac output (Fig. 18-5).

     b. Decreases in cardiac output may reflect increased afterload but more likely are due to

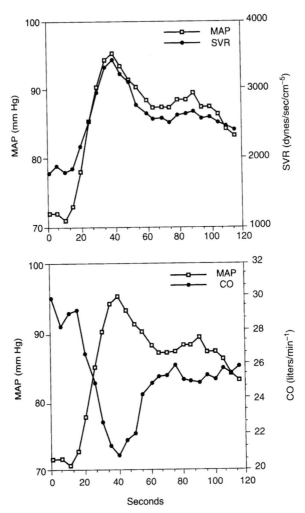

FIGURE 18-5 Hemodynamic response to rapid intravenous injection of phenylephrine in a single patient. Mean arterial pressure (MAP) and systemic vascular resistance (SVR) increase and cardiac output (CO) decreases in response to phenylephrine, with peak effects occurring 42 seconds after drug administration. (From Schwinn DA, Reves JG. Time course and hemodynamic effects of alpha-1-adrenergic bolus administration in anesthetized patients with myocardial disease. *Anesth Analg.* 1989;68[5]:571–578, with permission.)

baroreceptor-mediated reflex bradycardia in response
to drug-induced increases in diastolic blood pressure.
c. Pulmonary artery pressure is increased by
phenylephrine.

3. **Metabolic Effects**. Stimulation of α receptors by a continuous infusion of phenylephrine during acute potassium
loading interferes with the movement of potassium ions
across cell membranes into cells (Fig. 18-6). Administration of phenylephrine in the absence of an acute
potassium load does not change the plasma potassium
concentration.

4. **Treatment of Overdose**
   a. Systemic manifestations of sympathetic nervous system activation (systemic hypertension, tachycardia,
   baroreceptor-mediated bradycardia) may accompany
   vascular absorption of α agonists (phenylephrine,
   epinephrine) when used as topical or injected vasoconstrictors in the surgical field.
   b. Because β1 receptor blockades reduces cardiac
   output, treatment of phenylephrine-induced

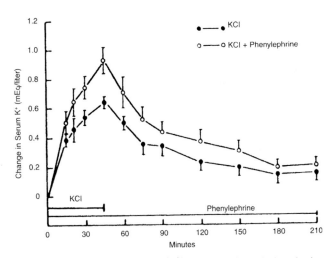

FIGURE 18-6 Plasma potassium (K^+) concentrations during the infusion of potassium chloride (KCl) increase more in patients also receiving phenylephrine. (From Williams ME, Rosa RM, Silva P, et al.
Impairment of extrarenal potassium disposal by alpha-adrenergic
stimulation. *N Engl J Med*. 1984;311[3]:145–149, with permission.)

hypertensive crisis with β-adrenergic blocking drugs is *contraindicated*.

c. Systemic hypertension induced by intravenously administered α agonists may not require treatment. The duration of action of IV phenylephrine and epinephrine is brief and hypertension may resolve spontaneously without pharmacologic interventions. Severe hypertension may require pharmacologic interventions but treatment must not decrease the ability of the stressed myocardium to increase contractility and heart rate (vasodilating drugs such as nitroprusside or nitroglycerin are indicated).

IV. **Selective β$_2$-adrenergic agonists relax bronchiole and uterine smooth muscle but, in contrast to isoproterenol, generally lack stimulating (β$_1$) effects on the heart (Table 18-2) (Fig. 18-7).**

A. **Clinical Uses**

1. β$_2$-Adrenergic agonists are the preferred treatment for acute episodes of asthma and the prevention of exercise-induced asthma (divided into those with an intermediate duration of action [3 to 6 hours] and those that are long-acting [>12 hours]).

2. β$_2$-Adrenergic agonists may be administered as continuous infusions to stop premature uterine contractions (tocolytics).

B. **Route of Administration**

1. β$_2$-Adrenergic bronchodilators can be administered orally, by inhalation, subcutaneously, or via IV injection. The inhaled route is preferred because the side effects are fewer for any given degree of bronchodilation.

2. With optimal inhalation technique (discharge the inhaler while taking a slow deep breath over 5 to 6 seconds, and then hold the breath at full inspiration for 10 seconds), approximately 12% of the drug is delivered from the metered-dose inhaler to the lungs; the remainder is deposited in the mouth, pharynx, and larynx.

3. The presence of an endotracheal tube decreases by approximately 50% to 70% the amount of drug delivered by a metered-dose inhaler that reaches the trachea. Actuation of the metered-dose inhaler during a mechanically delivered inspiration increases the amount of drug that passes beyond the distal end of the tracheal tube.

Table 18-2

Comparative Pharmacology of Selective β₂-Adrenergic Agonist Bronchodilators

	β₂ Selectivity	Peak Effect (min)	Duration of Action (h)	Concentration (μg per puff)	Method of Administration
Albuterol	High	30–60	4	90	MDI, oral
Metaproterenol	Moderate	30–60	3–4	200	Oral, subcutaneous
Terbutaline	High	60	4	200	MDI, oral, subcutaneous

MDI, metered-dose inhaler.

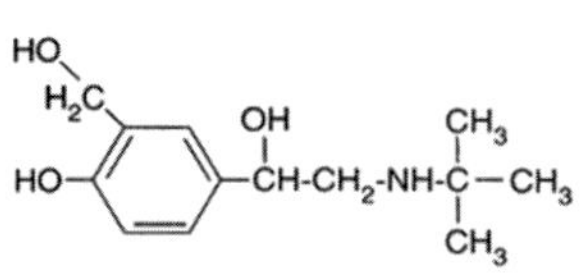

Albuterol

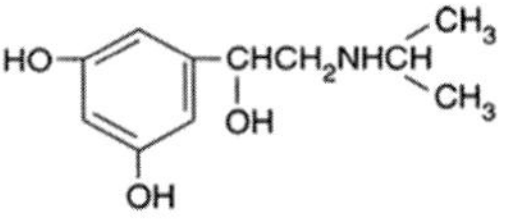

Metaproterenol

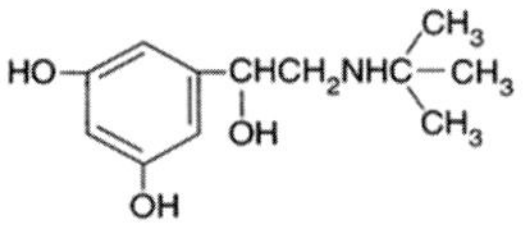

Terbutaline

FIGURE 18-7 Selective β_2-adrenergic agonists.

C. **Side Effects.** The widespread distribution of β_2-adrenergic receptors makes it likely that undesired responses may result when β_2-adrenergic agonists undergo systemic absorption.
   1. The principal side effect in awake subjects of β_2-adrenergic agonists treatment is tremor (caused by direct stimulation of β_2 receptors in skeletal muscles). Increased heart rate is less common with the selective β_2-adrenergic agonists.
   2. In patients with acute, severe asthma, β_2-adrenergic agonists may cause a transient decrease in arterial oxygenation presumed to reflect relaxation of compensatory vasoconstriction in areas of decreased ventilation (supplemental oxygen indicated).
   3. Increased mortality in patients with severe asthma treated with β_2-adrenergic agonists is most likely a reflection of the severity of the asthma rather than a toxic effect of the drug therapy.
   4. Acute metabolic responses to β_2-adrenergic agonists include hyperglycemia, hypokalemia, and hypomagnesemia.

D. **Albuterol** (known as salbutamol outside the United States), is the preferred selective β_2-adrenergic agonist for the treatment of acute bronchospasm due to asthma.
   1. Administration is most often by metered-dose inhaler, producing about 100 μg per puff; the usual dose is two

puffs delivered during deep inhalations 1 to 5 minutes apart. This dose may be repeated every 4 to 6 hours, not to exceed 16 to 20 puffs daily.

2. Alternatively, 2.5 to 5 mg of albuterol (0.5 to 1 ml of 0.5% solution in 5 ml of normal saline) may be administered by nebulization every 15 minutes for three to four doses, followed by treatments hourly during the initial hours of therapy. The duration of action of an inhaled dose is about 4 hours, but significant relief of symptoms may persist up to 8 hours.

3. The effects of albuterol and volatile anesthetics on bronchomotor tone are additive.

E. **Metaproterenol** is a selective β_2-adrenergic agonist used to treat asthma.

F. **Terbutaline** is a predominantly β_2-adrenergic agonist that may be administered orally, subcutaneously, or by inhalation to treat asthma. The subcutaneous administration of terbutaline (0.25 mg) produces responses that resemble those of epinephrine, but the duration of action is longer.

V. **Cardiac glycosides (Fig. 18-8)**

A. **Digoxin** is used most often during the perioperative period for the management of supraventricular tachydysrhythmias. The use of digoxin to treat acute decreases in left ventricular

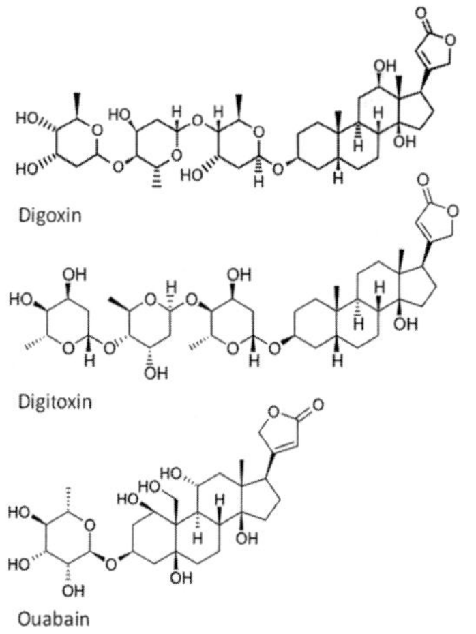

FIGURE 18-8 Cardiac glycosides.

contractility is uncommon because of the availability of more potent and less toxic drugs. Digoxin may be selected only for treatment of symptoms that persist after administration of angiotensin-converting enzyme inhibitors or β-adrenergic antagonists.

1. IV administration of propranolol or esmolol combined with digoxin may provide more rapid control of supraventricular tachydysrhythmias and minimize the likelihood of toxicity by permitting decreases in the dose of both classes of drugs.

2. Direct current cardioversion in the presence of digoxin may be hazardous because of increased risk for developing cardiac dysrhythmias, including ventricular fibrillation.

3. In approximately 30% of patients with Wolff-Parkinson-White syndrome, digitalis decreases refractoriness in the accessory conduction pathway to the point that rapid atrial impulses can cause ventricular fibrillation.

4. Digoxin may be harmful in patients with hypertrophic subaortic stenosis because increased myocardial contractility intensifies the resistance to ventricular ejection.

B. **Pharmacokinetics**. Digoxin is eliminated almost entirely by renal excretion, with a half-life of 1 to 2 days. The half-life is inversely proportional to glomerular filtration rate and thus increases with age or renal disease.

C. **Mechanism of Action**

1. Cardiac glycosides selectively and reversibly inhibit the sodium-potassium adenosine triphosphatase (ATPase) ion transport system (sodium pump) located in the sarcolemma (cell wall) of cardiac cells.

2. In addition to positive inotropic effects, cardiac glycosides enhance parasympathetic nervous system activity, leading to delayed conduction of cardiac impulses through the atrioventricular node and decreases in heart rate.

3. The electrophysiologic effects of therapeutic plasma concentrations of cardiac glycosides manifest on the electrocardiogram (ECG) as (a) prolonged P-R intervals due to delayed conduction of cardiac impulses through the atrioventricular node, (b) shortened QTc intervals because of more rapid ventricular repolarization, (c) ST segment depression (scaphoid or scooped-out) due to a decreased slope of phase 3 depolarization of cardiac action potentials, and (d) diminished amplitude or inversion of T waves. The P-R interval is rarely prolonged to longer than 0.25 second.

4. When digitalis is discontinued, the changes on the ECG disappear in several weeks.

D. **Toxicity**. Cardiac glycosides have a narrow therapeutic range (estimated that approximately 20% of patients who are being treated with cardiac glycosides experience some form of digitalis toxicity). The most frequent cause of digitalis toxicity in the absence of renal dysfunction is the concurrent administration of diuretics that cause potassium depletion. During anesthesia, hyperventilation of the patient's lungs can decrease the serum potassium concentration an average of 0.5 mEq/L for every 10 mm Hg decrease in $Paco_2$. Hypokalemia probably increases myocardial binding of cardiac glycosides, resulting in an excess drug effect.

1. **Diagnosis**. Digoxin is often administered in situations where digitalis toxicity is difficult to distinguish from the effects of the cardiac disease.

   a. Determination of the plasma digoxin concentration may be used to indicate the likely presence of digitalis toxicity. A plasma digoxin concentration of less than 0.5 ng/mL eliminates the possibility of digitalis toxicity. Anorexia, nausea, and vomiting are early manifestations of digitalis toxicity. These symptoms, when present preoperatively in patients receiving cardiac glycosides, should arouse suspicion of digitalis toxicity.

   b. There are no unequivocal features on the ECG that confirm the presence of digitalis toxicity. Nevertheless, toxic plasma concentrations of digitalis typically cause atrial or ventricular cardiac dysrhythmias (increased automaticity) and delayed conduction of cardiac impulses through the atrioventricular node (prolonged P-R interval on the ECG), culminating in incomplete to complete heart block.

2. **Treatment** of digitalis toxicity includes (a) correction of predisposing causes (hypokalemia, hypomagnesemia, arterial hypoxemia), (b) administration of drugs (phenytoin, lidocaine, atropine) to treat cardiac dysrhythmias, and (c) insertion of a temporary artificial transvenous cardiac pacemaker if complete heart block is present.

   a. Supplemental potassium decreases the binding of digitalis to cardiac muscle and directly antagonizes the cardiotoxic effects of cardiac glycosides. Serum potassium concentrations should be determined before treatment because supplemental potassium in the presence of a high preexisting plasma level of potassium will intensify atrioventricular block and depress the automaticity of ectopic pacemakers in the ventricles, leading to complete heart block.

   b. If renal function is normal and atrioventricular conduction block is not present, it is acceptable to administer potassium, 0.025 to 0.050 mEq/kg IV, to treat life-threatening cardiac dysrhythmias associated with digitalis toxicity, obviously with continuous ECG monitoring.

   c. Phenytoin (0.5 to 1.5 mg/kg IV over 5 minutes) or lidocaine (1 to 2 mg/kg IV) is effective in suppressing ventricular cardiac dysrhythmias caused by digitalis.

   d. Atropine, 35 to 70 μg/kg IV, can be administered to increase heart rate by offsetting excessive parasympathetic nervous system activity produced by toxic plasma concentrations of digitalis.

   e. Propranolol is effective in suppressing increased automaticity produced by digitalis toxicity, but its tendency to increase atrioventricular node refractoriness limits its usefulness when conduction blockade is present.

   f. Life-threatening digitalis toxicity can be treated by administering digoxin antibodies thus decreasing the plasma concentration of digoxin.

E. **Drug Interactions**

   1. Quinidine produces a dose-dependent increase in the plasma concentration of digoxin that becomes apparent within 24 hours after the first dose. This effect of quinidine may be due to displacement of digoxin from binding sites in tissues.

   2. Clinical experience does not support the occurrence of an increased incidence of cardiac dysrhythmias in patients being treated with cardiac glycosides and receiving succinylcholine.

   3. Sympathomimetics with β-adrenergic agonist effects may increase the likelihood of cardiac dysrhythmias in the presence of cardiac glycosides.

   4. IV administration of calcium may precipitate cardiac dysrhythmias in patients receiving cardiac glycosides.

VI. **Selective Phosphodiesterase Inhibitors. Phosphodiesterase inhibitors are a heterogeneous group of noncatecholamine nonglycoside compounds that exert a competitive inhibitory** action on phosphodiesterase enzymes (Fig. 18-9). Selective inhibitors of phosphodiesterase fraction III (PDE III) decrease the hydrolysis of cyclic adenosine monophosphate (cAMP), leading to increased intracellular concentrations of cAMP in the myocardium and vascular smooth muscle. Selective PDE III inhibitors act independently of β-adrenergic receptors and will increase myocardial contractility in patients with myocardial depression from β receptor blockade and in patients who have downregulation of β-adrenergic receptors and are refractory to catecholamine therapy. The PDE III inhibitors have their greatest clinical usefulness in patients who would benefit from combined inotropic and vasodilator therapy.

A. **Amrinone (inamrinone)** acts as a selective PDE III inhibitor and produces dose-dependent positive inotropic and vasodilator effects manifesting as increased cardiac output and decreased left ventricular end diastolic pressure. The name amrinone was changed to inamrinone in the United States in 2000 to avoid confusion with amiodarone. IV administration of a loading dose, 0.5 to 1.5 mg/kg, increases cardiac output within 5 minutes, with detectable positive inotropic effects persisting for approximately 2 hours. After the initial dose, a maintenance infusion of 2 to 10 μg/kg/minute produces positive inotropic effects that are maintained during the infusion (tachyphylaxis does not occur).

B. **Milrinone** is a derivative of amrinone with almost 30 times the inotropic potency of amrinone but less adverse side effects. Because of its reduced incidence of side effects, milrinone has replaced amrinone in clinical use. Cardiac output improves both as a result of increased inotropy as well as vascular smooth muscle relaxation of peripheral

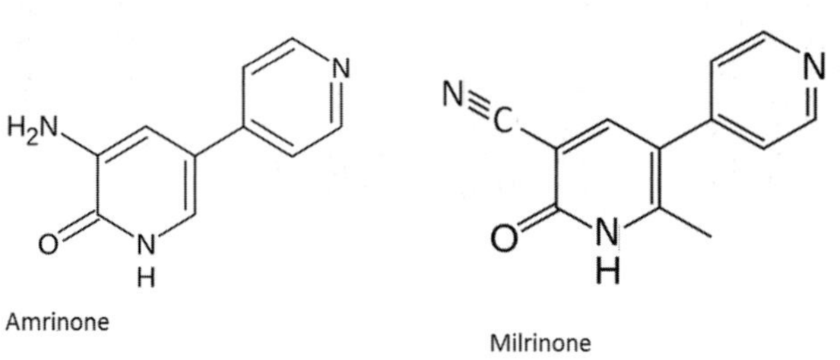

Amrinone

Milrinone

FIGURE 18-9 Selective inhibitors of phosphodiesterase subtype III, amrinone and milrinone.

and pulmonary vessel. Milrinone is administered as an IV bolus of 50 μg/kg over 10 minutes followed by a continuous infusion of 0.375 to 0.75 μg/kg/minute to maintain plasma milrinone concentrations at or above therapeutic levels.

1. **Clinical Uses**
   a. Milrinone may be useful in the management of acute left ventricular dysfunction (successful weaning of high-risk patients from cardiopulmonary bypass may be enhanced by administration of milrinone).
   b. Milrinone may potentiate the effects of adrenergic agents as well as help increase inotropy in chronic heart failure patients who have downregulation of β_1-adrenergic receptors.
   c. Milrinone is particularly useful in the setting of pulmonary hypertension (decreases pulmonary artery pressures more effectively than other positive inotropic agents).
   d. Milrinone is associated with more vasodilation and greater decreases in systemic vascular resistance and blood pressure than dobutamine. Unlike dobutamine, milrinone rarely causes tachycardia.
   e. The choice between dobutamine and milrinone may be based on hemodynamic differences. Milrinone may be preferred in situations with high filling pressures, elevated pulmonary artery pressure, need for continued β blockade, decreased responsiveness to catecholamine therapy, and increased risk for tachyarrhythmias. Dobutamine may be preferred in situations with significant vasodilation or renal dysfunction.

2. **Side Effects**
   a. Rapid administration of milrinone may decrease systemic vascular resistance, decrease venous return, and result in hypotension.
   b. Rapid administration of large IV loading doses may also be associated with arrhythmias (enhanced atrioventricular nodal conduction).

VII. **Calcium is present in the body in greater amounts than any other mineral. Calcium is important for (a) neuromuscular transmission, (b) skeletal muscle contraction, (c) cardiac muscle contractility, (d) blood coagulation, and (e) exocytosis necessary for release of neurotransmitters. In addition, calcium is the principal component of bone. Calcium is a potent inotrope. Increasing the plasma concentrations of** ionized calcium with exogenous administration of calcium chloride or calcium gluconate is commonly used to treat cardiac depression as may accompany delivery of volatile anesthetics, transfusion of citrated blood, and following termination of cardiopulmonary bypass.

A. **Calcium Measurement**

1. The plasma concentration of calcium is maintained between 4.3 and 5.3 mEq/L (8.5 to 10.5 mg/dL) by endocrine control of ion transport in the kidney, intestine, and bone, mediated by vitamin D, parathyroid hormone, and calcitonin.

2. Total plasma calcium consists of (a) calcium bound to albumin, (b) calcium complexed with citrate and phosphorus ions, and (c) freely diffusible ionized calcium.

3. It is the ionized calcium, and not the total plasma calcium, that produces the physiologic effects of calcium (hypoalbuminemia and hypophosphatemia typically are not associated with signs of hypocalcemia but large transfusions may be associated with acute hypocalcemia because of the binding of ionized calcium to the citrate anticoagulant).

4. Ionized calcium typically represents approximately 45% of the total plasma concentration. The ionized fraction of calcium changes with pH because calcium and hydrogen ions compete for the binding site on albumin. Acidosis increases ionized calcium, whereas alkalosis reduces ionized calcium. Most laboratories directly measure ionized calcium, the moiety of clinical interest. A normal plasma ionized calcium concentration is 1 to 1.26 mmol/L (2 to 2.5 mEq/L or 4 to 5 mg/dL).

CHAPTER 19

Sympatholytics

I. **α- and β-Adrenergic receptor antagonists** prevent the interaction of the endogenous neurotransmitter norepinephrine or sympathomimetics with the corresponding adrenergic receptors and attenuate sympathetic nervous system homeostatic mechanisms and evoke predictable pharmacologic responses.

II. **α-Adrenergic receptor antagonists** bind selectively to α-adrenergic receptors and interfere with the ability of catecholamines or other sympathomimetics to provoke α responses at the heart and peripheral vasculature. Orthostatic hypotension, baroreceptor-mediated reflex tachycardia, and impotence are invariable side effects of α-adrenergic blockade.

  A. **Mechanism of Action**. Phentolamine, prazosin, and yohimbine are competitive (reversible binding with receptors) α-adrenergic antagonists, whereas phenoxybenzamine binds covalently to α-adrenergic receptors to produce an irreversible and insurmountable type of α receptor blockade (even massive doses of sympathomimetics are ineffective until the effect of phenoxybenzamine is terminated by metabolism).

  B. **Phentolamine** produces transient nonselective α-adrenergic blockade (administered intravenously [IV] produces peripheral vasodilation and a decrease in systemic blood pressure that reflects α_1 receptor blockade and a direct action of phentolamine on vascular smooth muscle). Decreases in blood pressure elicit baroreceptor-mediated increases in sympathetic nervous system activity manifesting as cardiac stimulation.

    1. **Clinical Uses**

      a. The principal use of phentolamine is the treatment of acute hypertensive emergencies, as may accompany intraoperative manipulation of a pheochromocytoma or autonomic nervous system hyperreflexia (30 to 70 µg/kg IV [to 5 mg], produces a prompt but transient decrease in systemic blood pressure).

A continuous infusion of phentolamine (0.1 to 2 mg per minute) may be used to maintain normal blood pressure during the intraoperative resection of a pheochromocytoma.

b. Local infiltration with a phentolamine-containing solution (5 to 15 mg in 10 mL of normal saline) is appropriate when a sympathomimetic is accidentally administered extravascularly.

C. **Phenoxybenzamine** acts as a nonselective α-adrenergic antagonist by combining covalently with α-adrenergic receptors (blockade at postsynaptic α_1 receptors is more intense than at α_2 receptors).

1. **Pharmacokinetics.** Onset of α-adrenergic blockade is slow, taking up to 60 minutes to reach peak effect even after IV administration. This delay in onset is due to the time required for structural modification of the phenoxybenzamine molecule, which is necessary to render the drug pharmacologically active.

2. **Cardiovascular Effects**

   a. Phenoxybenzamine administered to a supine, normovolemic patient in the absence of increased sympathetic nervous system activity produces little change in systemic blood pressure. Orthostatic hypotension, however, is prominent, especially in the presence of preexisting hypertension or hypovolemia.

   b. Despite decreases in blood pressure, cardiac output is often increased and renal blood flow is not greatly altered unless preexisting renal vasoconstriction is present.

3. **Noncardiac Effects**

   a. Phenoxybenzamine prevents the inhibitory action of epinephrine on the secretion of insulin.

   b. Stimulation of the radial fibers of the iris is prevented, and miosis is a prominent component of the response to phenoxybenzamine.

4. **Clinical Uses**

   a. Phenoxybenzamine, 0.5 to 1.0 mg/kg orally (prazosin is an alternative), is administered preoperatively to control blood pressure in patients with pheochromocytoma. Chronic α-adrenergic blockade, by relieving intense peripheral vasoconstriction, permits expansion of intravascular fluid volume as reflected by a decrease in the hematocrit.

   b. Treatment of peripheral vascular disease characterized by intermittent claudication is not favorably influenced by α-adrenergic blockade because cutaneous rather than skeletal muscle blood flow is increased. The most beneficial clinical responses to α-adrenergic blockade are in diseases with a large component of cutaneous vasoconstriction, such as Raynaud's disease.

D. **Yohimbine** is a selective antagonist at presynaptic α_2 receptors, leading to enhanced release of norepinephrine from nerve endings. As a result, this drug may be useful in the treatment of the rare patient suffering from idiopathic orthostatic hypotension. In the past, impotence had been successfully treated with yohimbine in male patients with vascular, diabetic, and psychogenic origins.

E. **Prazosin** is a selective postsynaptic α_1 receptor antagonist that leaves intact the inhibiting effect of α_2 receptor activity on norepinephrine release from nerve endings. As a result, prazosin is less likely than nonselective α-adrenergic antagonists to evoke reflex tachycardia.

F. **Terazosin** is a long-acting orally effective α_1-adrenergic antagonist that may be useful in the treatment of benign prostatic hyperplasia by virtue of its ability to relax prostatic smooth muscle.

G. **Tamsulosin** is an orally effective α_{1a}-adrenergic antagonist that is indicated for the treatment of the signs and symptoms of benign prostatic hyperplasia.

H. **Tolazoline** is a competitive nonselective α-adrenergic receptor antagonist (has been used to treat persistent pulmonary hypertension of the newborn but its use for this purpose has been largely replaced by nitric oxide).

III. **β-Adrenergic receptor antagonists bind selectively to β-adrenergic receptors and interfere with the ability of catecholamines or other sympathomimetics to provoke β responses. Drug-induced β-adrenergic blockade prevents the effects of catecholamines and sympathomimetics on the heart and smooth muscles of the airways and blood vessels. β Antagonist therapy should be continued throughout the perioperative period to maintain desirable drug effects and to avoid the risk of sympathetic nervous system hyperactivity associated with abrupt discontinuation of these drugs.**

A. **Mechanism of Action**

1. β-Adrenergic receptor antagonists exhibit selective affinity for β-adrenergic receptors, where they act by competitive inhibition (binding is reversible such that the drug can be displaced from the occupied receptors if sufficiently large amounts of agonist become available).

2. Chronic administration of β-adrenergic antagonists is associated with an increase in the number of β-adrenergic receptors.
B. **Structure–Activity Relationships** (Fig. 19-1)
C. **Classification** (Tables 19-1 and 19-2)
D. **Pharmacokinetics** (see Table 19-1)
  1. The principal difference in pharmacokinetics between all the β-adrenergic receptor antagonists is the

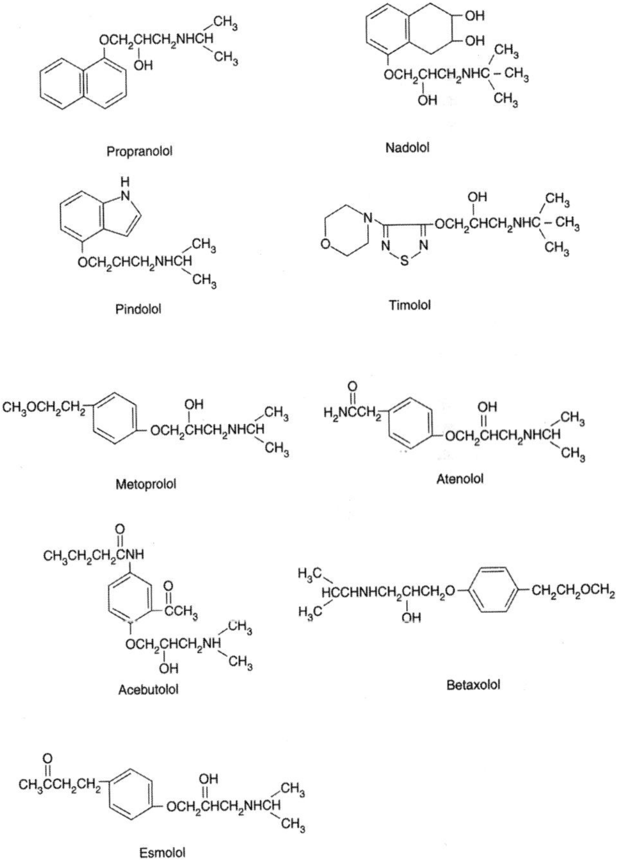

FIGURE 19-1 β-Adrenergic antagonists.

Table 19-1

Comparative Characteristics of β-Adrenergic Receptor Antagonists

	Propranolol	Nadolol	Pindolol	Timolol	Metoprolol
Cardiac selectivity	No	No	No	No	Yes
Partial agonist activity	No	No	Yes	No	No
Protein binding (%)	90–95	30	40–60	10	10
Clearance	Hepatic	Renal	Hepatic/Renal	Hepatic	Hepatic
Active metabolites	Yes	No	No	No	No
Elimination half-time (h)	2–3	20–24	3–4	3–4	3–4
First-pass hepatic metabolism (estimate) (%)	75	Minimal	10–15	50	60
Blood level variability	+ + + +	+	+ +	+ + +	+ + + +
Adult oral dose (mg)	40–360	40–320	5–20	10–30	50–400
Adult intravenous dose (mg)	1–10		0.4–2	0.4–1	1–15

Table 19-1

Comparative Characteristics of β-Adrenergic Receptor Antagonists *(continued)*

	Atenolol	Acebutolol	Betaxolol	Esmolol
Cardiac selectivity	Yes	Yes	Yes	Yes
Partial agonist activity	No	Yes	No	No
Protein binding (%)	5	25		55
Clearance	Renal	Hepatic/Renal	Hepatic/Renal	Plasma hydrolysis
Active metabolites	No	Yes		No
Elimination half-time (h)	6–7	3–4	11–22	0.15
First-pass hepatic metabolism (estimate) (%)	10	60		
Blood level variability	+	+ +		
Adult oral dose (mg)	50–200	200–800	10–20	
Adult intravenous dose (mg)	5–10	12.5–50		10–80 IV 50–300 μg/ kg/min

+, minimal; + +, modest; + + +, moderate; + + + +, marked.

| Table 19-2 |

Comparative Characteristics of β-Adrenergic Receptor Antagonists Effective in the Treatment of Congestive Heart Failure

	Metoprolol (Extended Release)	Carvedilol	Bisoprolol
Cardiac selectivity	Yes	No	Yes
Partial agonist activity	No	No	No
Initial oral dose[a]	6.25 mg twice daily	3.125 mg twice daily	1.25 mg daily
Desired dosage range[a]	50–150 mg daily	25–50 mg twice daily	5 mg daily

[a]Recommended doses for treatment of patients with mild to moderate congestive heart failure.

elimination half-time ranging from brief for esmolol (about 10 minutes) to hours for the other drugs.

2. β-Adrenergic receptor antagonists are eliminated by several different pathways and this must be considered in the presence of renal and/or hepatic dysfunction.

3. The therapeutic plasma concentration varies greatly among these drugs and between patients (interpatient variability). Explanations for interpatient variability include differences in basal sympathetic nervous system tone, flat dose-response curves for the drug so changes in plasma concentrations evoke minimal changes in pharmacologic effects, impact of active metabolites, and genetic differences in β-adrenergic receptors that influence how an individual patient responds to a given drug and plasma concentration.

E. Propranolol is a nonselective β-adrenergic receptor antagonist that lacks intrinsic sympathomimetic activity and thus is a pure antagonist (antagonism of β_1 and β_2 receptors is about equal) (see Table 19-1). As the first β-adrenergic antagonist introduced clinically, propranolol is the standard drug to which all β-adrenergic antagonists are compared. Typically, propranolol is administered in stepwise increments until physiologic plasma concentrations have been attained, as indicated by a resting heart rate of 55 to 60 beats per minute.

1. **Cardiac Effects**
   a. Propranolol decreases heart rate and myocardial contractility by β_1 receptor blockade, resulting in decreased cardiac output.
   b. Heart rate slowing induced by propranolol lasts longer than the negative inotropic effects, suggesting a possible subdivision of β_1 receptors.
   c. Concomitant blockade of β_2 receptors by propranolol increases peripheral vascular resistance, including coronary vascular resistance but drug-induced decreases in myocardial oxygen requirements predominate.

2. **Pharmacokinetics**. Propranolol is rapidly and almost completely absorbed from the gastrointestinal tract, but systemic availability of the drug is limited by extensive hepatic first-pass metabolism (may account for 90% to 95% of the absorbed dose). There is considerable individual variation in the magnitude of hepatic first-pass metabolism, accounting for up to 20-fold differences in plasma concentrations of propranolol in patients after oral administration of comparable doses. Hepatic first-pass metabolism is the reason the oral dose of propranolol (40 to 800 mg per day) must be substantially greater than the IV dose (0.05 mg/kg given in increments of 0.5 to 1.0 mg every 5 minutes).
   a. **Protein Binding**. Propranolol is extensively bound (90% to 95%) to plasma proteins. Heparin-induced increases in plasma concentrations of free fatty acids due to increased lipoprotein lipase activity result in decreased plasma protein binding of propranolol (Fig. 19-2).
   b. **Metabolism**. Clearance of propranolol from the plasma is by hepatic metabolism. An active metabolite, 4-hydroxypropranolol, is equivalent in activity to the parent compound. Elimination of propranolol is greatly decreased when hepatic blood flow decreases. Renal failure does not alter the elimination half-time of propranolol, but accumulation of metabolites may occur.
   c. **Clearance of Local Anesthetics**. Propranolol decreases clearance of amide local anesthetics by decreasing hepatic blood flow and inhibiting metabolism in the liver.

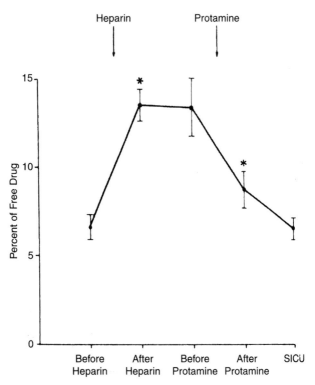

FIGURE 19-2 Heparin administration is associated with decreased plasma protein binding of propranolol manifesting as an increased plasma concentration of free (unbound) drug. (Mean ± SE; *$P < .05$.) SICU, surgical intensive care unit. (From Wood M, Shand DG, Wood AJ. Propranolol binding in plasma during cardiopulmonary bypass. *Anesthesiology.* 1979;51:512–516, with permission.)

      d. **Clearance of Opioids**. Pulmonary first-pass uptake of fentanyl is substantially decreased in patients being treated chronically with propranolol.

  F. **Nadolol and pindolol** are nonselective β-adrenergic receptor antagonists; nadolol is unique in that its long duration of action permits once daily administration.

    1. **Pharmacokinetics**. Nadolol is slowly and incompletely absorbed (an estimated 30%) from the gastrointestinal

tract. Metabolism does not occur, with about 75% of the drug being excreted unchanged in urine and the remainder in bile.

G. **Timolol** is a nonselective γ-adrenergic receptor antagonist that is as effective as propranolol for various therapeutic indications. In addition, timolol is effective in the treatment of glaucoma because of its ability to decrease intraocular pressure, presumably by decreasing the production of aqueous humor. Timolol is administered as eye drops in the treatment of glaucoma, but systemic absorption may be sufficient to cause resting bradycardia and increased airway resistance.

   1. **Pharmacokinetics**. Timolol is rapidly and almost completely absorbed after oral administration but extensive first-pass hepatic metabolism limits the amount of drug reaching the systemic circulation to about 50% of that absorbed from the gastrointestinal tract.

H. **Metoprolol** is a selective β_1-adrenergic receptor antagonist that prevents inotropic and chronotropic responses to β-adrenergic stimulation, whereas bronchodilator, vasodilator, and metabolic effects of β_2 receptors remain intact (metoprolol is less likely to cause adverse effects in patients with chronic obstructive airway disease or peripheral vascular disease). Selectivity is dose related, and large doses of metoprolol are likely to become nonselective, exerting antagonist effects at β_2 receptors as well as β_1 receptors (airway resistance may increase in asthmatic patients).

   1. **Pharmacokinetics**. Metoprolol is readily absorbed from the gastrointestinal tract, but this is offset by substantial hepatic first-pass metabolism such that only about 40% of the drug reaches the systemic circulation.

I. **Atenolol** is the most selective β_1-adrenergic antagonist that may have specific value in patients in whom the continued presence of β_2 receptor activity is desirable. In patients at risk for coronary artery disease, treatment with IV atenolol before and immediately after surgery, followed by oral therapy during the remainder of the hospitalization, decreases mortality and the incidence of cardiovascular complications for as long as 2 years. Perioperative administration of atenolol to patients at high risk for coronary artery disease significantly decreases the incidence of postoperative myocardial ischemia.

   1. **Pharmacokinetics**. Atenolol undergoes little or no hepatic metabolism and is eliminated principally by renal excretion.

J. **Betaxolol** is a cardioselective β_1-adrenergic antagonist with no intrinsic sympathomimetic activity and weak membrane-stabilizing activity.

K. **Bisoprolol** is a β_1 selective antagonist drug without significant intrinsic agonist activity. The most prominent pharmacologic effect of bisoprolol is a negative chronotropic effect. Bisoprolol is useful in the treatment of essential hypertension and has been shown to improve survival in patients with mild to moderate congestive heart failure (see Table 19-2).

L. Esmolol is a rapid-onset and short-acting selective β_1-adrenergic receptor antagonist that is administered only IV. After a typical initial dose of 0.5 mg/kg IV over about 60 seconds, the full therapeutic effect is evident within 5 minutes, and its action ceases within 10 to 30 minutes after administration is discontinued (useful for preventing or treating adverse systemic blood pressure and heart rate increases that occur intraoperatively in response to noxious stimulation, as during tracheal intubation). Esmolol, 150 mg IV, administered about 2 minutes before direct laryngoscopy and tracheal intubation provides reliable protection against increases in both heart rate and systolic blood pressure, which predictably accompanies tracheal intubation (Fig. 19-3).

1. **Pharmacokinetics**
   a. Esmolol is available for IV administration only (only other β-adrenergic antagonists that may be administered IV are propranolol and metoprolol).
   b. Plasma esterases responsible for the hydrolysis of esmolol are distinct from plasma cholinesterase, and the duration of action of succinylcholine is not predictably prolonged in patients treated with esmolol.
   c. Evidence of the short duration of action of esmolol is return of the heart rate to predrug levels within 15 minutes after discontinuing the drug.

M. **Side Effects**. The side effects of β-adrenergic antagonists are similar for all available drugs, although the magnitude may differ depending on their selectivity and the presence or absence of intrinsic sympathomimetic activity. The principal contraindication to administration of β-adrenergic antagonists is preexisting atrioventricular heart block or cardiac failure not caused by tachycardia.

1. **Cardiovascular System**. β-Adrenergic antagonists produce negative inotropic and chronotropic effects. Patients with peripheral vascular disease do not

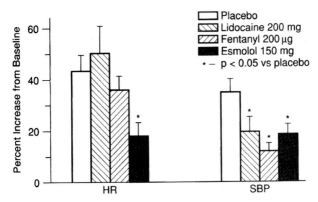

FIGURE 19-3 Maximum percent increases in heart rate (HR) and systolic blood pressure (SBP) after induction of anesthesia and direct laryngoscopy with tracheal intubation in patients pretreated with saline, lidocaine, fentanyl, or esmolol. All three drugs blunt the increase in SBP, but only esmolol is also effective in attenuating the increase in HR. (From Helfman SM, Gold MI, DeLisser EA, et al. Which drug prevents tachycardia and hypertension associated with tracheal intubation: lidocaine, fentanyl, or esmolol? *Anesth Analg.* 1991;72:482–486, with permission.)

tolerate well the peripheral vasoconstriction associated with β$_2$ receptor blockade produced by nonselective β-adrenergic antagonists. The principal antidysrhythmic effect of β-adrenergic blockade is to prevent the dysrhythmogenic effect of endogenous or exogenous catecholamines or sympathomimetics.

a. **Treatment of Excess Myocardial Depression.** The usual clinical manifestations of excessive myocardial depression produced by β-adrenergic blockade include bradycardia, low cardiac output, hypotension, and cardiogenic shock. Excessive bradycardia and/or decreases in cardiac output due to drug-induced β blockade should be treated initially with atropine in incremental doses of 7 μg/kg IV. Atropine is likely to be effective by blocking vagal effects on the heart and thus unmasking any residual sympathetic nervous system innervation. If atropine is ineffective, continuous infusion of isoproterenol in doses sufficient to overcome competitive β blockade is appropriate.

Glucagon administered to adults, 1 to 10 mg IV followed by 5 mg per hour IV, effectively reverses myocardial depression produced by β-adrenergic antagonists at normal doses because these drugs do not exert their effects by means of β-adrenergic receptors. In the presence of bradycardia that is unresponsive to pharmacologic therapy, it may be necessary to place a transvenous artificial cardiac pacemaker.

2. **Airway Resistance**. Nonselective β-adrenergic antagonists such as propranolol consistently increase airway resistance as a manifestation of bronchoconstriction due to blockade of β_2 receptors (exaggerated in patients with preexisting obstructive airway disease).

3. **Metabolism**. Nonselective β-adrenergic antagonists such as propranolol interfere with glycogenolysis that ordinarily occurs in response to release of epinephrine during hypoglycemia. Tachycardia, which is an important warning sign of hypoglycemia in insulin-treated diabetics, is blunted by β-adrenergic antagonists (nonselective β-adrenergic antagonists are not recommended for administration to patients with diabetes mellitus who may be at risk for developing hypoglycemia).

4. **Distribution of extracellular potassium** across cell membranes is influenced by sympathetic nervous system activity as well as insulin (stimulation of β_2-adrenergic receptors seems to facilitate movement of potassium intracellularly).

5. **Interaction with anesthetics**. Additive myocardial depression with β-adrenergic antagonists and anesthetics is not excessive, and treatment with β-adrenergic antagonists may therefore be safely maintained throughout the perioperative period (an exception may be patients treated with timolol in whom profound bradycardia has been observed in the presence of inhaled anesthetics).

6. **Nervous System**. β-Adrenergic antagonists may cross the blood–brain barrier to produce side effects (fatigue and lethargy). Atenolol and nadolol are less lipid soluble than other β-adrenergic antagonists and thus may be associated with a lower incidence of central nervous system effects.

7. **Fetus**. β-Adrenergic antagonists can cross the placenta and cause bradycardia, hypotension, and hypoglycemia in newborn infants of mothers who are receiving the drug.

N. **Withdrawal Hypersensitivity**. Acute discontinuation of β-adrenergic antagonist therapy can result in excess sympathetic nervous system activity that manifests in 24 to 48 hours.

Table 19-3

Clinical Uses of β-Adrenergic Blockers

Treatment of essential hypertension
Management of angina pectoris
Treatment of acute coronary syndrome
Perioperative β-adrenergic receptor blockade
Treatment of intraoperative myocardial ischemia
Suppression of cardiac dysrhythmias
Management of congestive heart failure
Prevention of excessive sympathetic nervous system activity
Preoperative preparation of hyperthyroid patients
Treatment of migraine headache

Presumably, this enhanced activity reflects an increase in the number of β-adrenergic receptors (upregulation) during chronic therapy with β-adrenergic antagonists.

O. **Clinical Uses** (Table 19-3). It is accepted that patients being treated with β-adrenergic receptor antagonists should have their medication continued uninterrupted through the perioperative period. It is also recommended that patients at high risk for myocardial ischemia and presenting for major surgery should be treated with β-adrenergic receptor antagonists beginning preoperatively and continuing into the postoperative period.

1. **Treatment of Essential Hypertension**

a. The antihypertensive effect of β-adrenergic blockade is largely dependent on decreases in cardiac output due to decreased heart rate. An important advantage in the use of β-adrenergic antagonists for the treatment of essential hypertension is the absence of orthostatic hypotension.

b. Often a β-adrenergic antagonist is used in combination with a vasodilator to minimize reflex baroreceptor–mediated increases in heart rate and cardiac output produced by the vasodilator.

2. **Management of Angina Pectoris**. Orally administered β-adrenergic antagonists are equally effective in decreasing the likelihood of myocardial ischemia manifesting as angina pectoris (reflects drug-induced decreases in myocardial oxygen requirements secondary to decreased heart rate and myocardial contractility).

3. **Treatment of Acute Coronary Syndrome**. It is recommended that all patients who experience an acute myocardial infarction receive IV β-adrenergic antagonists (contraindicated in the presence of severe bradycardia, unstable left ventricular failure, atrioventricular heart block). β-Adrenergic antagonist prophylaxis after acute myocardial infarction is considered to be one of the most scientifically substantiated, cost-effective preventive medical treatments.

4. **Perioperative β-adrenergic receptor blockade** is recommended for patients considered at risk for myocardial ischemia (known coronary artery disease, positive preoperative stress tests, diabetes mellitus treated with insulin, left ventricular hypertrophy) during high-risk surgery (vascular surgery, thoracic surgery, intraperitoneal surgery, anticipated large blood loss).

   a. The goal of preoperative therapy is a resting heart rate between 65 and 80 beats per minute.

   b. The mechanism for the beneficial effects of perioperative β-adrenergic receptor blockade is not known but is most likely multifactorial (Table 19-4). It is not known if patients with cardiac risk factors but no signs of underlying coronary artery disease will benefit from perioperative administration of a β-adrenergic antagonist.

   c. Preoperatively, oral therapy can be initiated with atenolol 50 mg or bisoprolol 5 to 10 mg daily or

---

Table 19-4

Possible Explanations for Cardioprotective Effects Produced by Perioperative β-Adrenergic Receptor Blockade

Decreased myocardial oxygen consumption and demand
Less stress on potentially ischemic myocardium owing to decreased heart rate and myocardial contractility
Attenuation of effects of endogenous catecholamines
Redistribution of coronary blood flow to ischemic areas
Increased coronary blood flow owing to increased diastolic time
Plaque stabilization owing to decrease in shear forces
Cardiac antidysrhythmic effects
Antiinflammatory effects (?)

metoprolol 25 to 50 mg twice daily. If the patient is seen the morning of surgery, atenolol 5 to 10 mg IV or metoprolol 5 to10 mg IV can be titrated. Esmolol is an acceptable drug to achieve β-adrenergic receptor blockade during surgery and postoperatively in the intensive care unit where continuous IV infusions can be monitored.

5. **Treatment of Intraoperative Myocardial Ischemia**
   a. Appearance of evidence of myocardial ischemia on the electrocardiogram or as wall motion abnormalities on the transesophageal echocardiogram may benefit from treatment with a β-adrenergic receptor blocking drug, assuming the absence of contraindications (severe reactive airway disease, shock, left ventricular failure) and the presence of an adequate concentration of inhaled anesthetic drugs.
   b. The drug selected should be titrated IV to the desired heart rate (about 60 beats per minute) to attenuate myocardial ischemia.
   c. Treatment options include esmolol (1 to 1.5 mg/kg IV followed by a continuous infusion of 50 to 300 μg/kg/minute), metoprolol (5 mg IV), atenolol (5 to 10 mg IV), or propranolol (1 to 10 mg IV). The advantage of esmolol is the ability to titrate its effects to the desired heart rate. Nitroglycerin is often added to this treatment regimen.

6. **Suppression of Cardiac Dysrhythmias**
   a. β-Adrenergic receptor blocking drugs are effective in the treatment of cardiac dysrhythmias as a result of enhanced sympathetic nervous system stimulation.
   b. Esmolol and propranolol are effective for controlling the ventricular response rate to atrial fibrillation and atrial flutter (also effective for controlling atrial dysrhythmias following cardiac surgery).

7. **Management of Congestive Heart Failure**. Metoprolol, carvedilol, and bisoprolol improve ejection fraction and increase survival in patients in chronic heart failure (see Table 19-2). When β blocking drugs are used to treat congestive heart failure, the initial doses of β blockers should be minimal and gradually increased.

8. **Prevention of Excessive Sympathetic Nervous System Activity**. β-Adrenergic blockade is associated with attenuated heart rate and blood pressure changes in response to direct laryngoscopy and tracheal intubation.

9. **Preoperative Preparation of Hyperthyroid Patients**. Thyrotoxic patients can be prepared for surgery in

an emergency by IV administration of propranolol or esmolol or electively by oral administration of propranolol (40 to 320 mg daily).

IV. **Combined α- and β-Adrenergic Receptor Antagonists**

A. **Labetalol** is a unique parenteral and oral antihypertensive drug that exhibits selective α_1- and nonselective β_1- and β_2-adrenergic antagonist effects, whereas presynaptic α_2 receptors are spared such that released norepinephrine can continue to inhibit further release of catecholamines via the negative feedback mechanism resulting from stimulation of α_2 receptors. The β to α blocking potency ratio is 3:1 for oral labetalol and 7:1 for IV labetalol.

1. **Pharmacokinetics**. Metabolism of labetalol is by conjugation of glucuronic acid and the elimination half-time is prolonged in the presence of liver disease and unchanged by renal dysfunction.

2. **Cardiovascular Effects**. Labetalol lowers systemic blood pressure by decreasing systemic vascular resistance (α_1 blockade), whereas reflex tachycardia triggered by vasodilation is attenuated by simultaneous β blockade. Cardiac output remains unchanged. The maximum systemic blood pressure–lowering effect of an IV dose of labetalol (0.1 to 0.5 mg/kg) is present in 5 to 10 minutes.

3. **Clinical Uses**

a. Labetalol is a safe and effective treatment for hypertensive emergencies (epinephrine overdose as may occur during submucosal injection to produce surgical hemostasis). Caution has been urged in using β-adrenergic blockers to treat phenylephrine and epinephrine overdose resulting from systemic absorption following topical application. Labetalol, 20 to 80 mg IV, may be administered about every 10 minutes until the desired therapeutic response is achieved.

b. Rebound hypertension after withdrawal of clonidine therapy and hypertensive responses in patients with pheochromocytoma can be effectively treated with labetalol.

c. Labetalol, 0.1 to 0.5 mg/kg IV, can be administered to anesthetized patients to attenuate increases in heart rate and blood pressure that are presumed to result from abrupt increases in the level of surgical stimulation.

d. Controlled hypotension produced with intermittent injections of labetalol, 10 mg IV, is not associated with increases in heart rate, intrapulmonary shunt, or cardiac output (in contrast to nitroprusside).

4. **Side Effects**. Orthostatic hypotension is the most common side effect of labetalol therapy. Bronchospasm is possible in susceptible patients, reflecting the β-adrenergic antagonist effects of labetalol. Fluid retention in patients treated chronically with labetalol is the reason for combining this drug with a diuretic during prolonged therapy.

B. **Carvedilol** is a nonselective β-adrenergic receptor antagonist with α_1 blocking activity. This drug has no intrinsic β-adrenergic agonist effect. Carvedilol is indicated for the treatment of mild to moderate congestive heart failure owing to ischemia or cardiomyopathy (see Table 19-2).

V. **Calcium channel blockers** (also known as *calcium entry blockers* and *calcium antagonists*) are a diverse group of structurally unrelated compounds that selectively interfere with inward calcium ion movement across myocardial and vascular smooth muscle cells (Tables 19-5, 19-6, and 19-7). The phenylalkylamines and benzothiazepines are selective for the atrioventricular node, whereas the dihydropyridines are selective for the arteriolar beds.

A. **Mechanism of Action**
   1. Calcium channel blockers bind to receptors on voltage-gated calcium ion channels (L, long-lasting; N, neural;

Table 19-5

Classification of Calcium Channel Blockers

Phenylalkylamines
Verapamil

Dihydropyridines
Nifedipine
Nicardipine
Nimodipine
Isradipine
Felodipine
Amlodipine

Benzothiazepines
Diltiazem

Table 19-6

Comparative Pharmacologic Effects of Calcium Channel Blockers

	Verapamil	Nifedipine	Nicardipine	Diltiazem
Systemic blood pressure	Decrease	Decrease	Decrease	Decrease
Heart rates	Decrease	Increase to no change	Increase to no change	Decrease
Myocardial depression	Moderate	Moderate	Slight	Moderate
Sinoatrial node depression	Moderate	None	None	Slight
Atrioventricular node conduction	Marked	None	None	Moderate depression
Coronary artery dilation	Moderate	Marked	Greatest	Moderate
Peripheral artery dilation	Moderate	Marked	Marked	Moderate

Table 19-7

Pharmacokinetics of Calcium Channel Blockers

	Verapamil	Nifedipine	Nicardipine	Nimodipine	Diltiazem
Dosage					
Oral	80–160 mg every 8 h	10–30 mg every 8 h	20 mg every 8 h	30–60 mg every 4–6 h	60–90 mg every 8 h
Intravenous	75–150 µg/kg	5–15 µg/kg		10 µg/kg	75–150 µg/kg
Absorption (%)					
Oral	>90	>90		>90	
Bioavailability (%)	10–20	65–70	30	5–10	40
Onset of effect (min)					
Oral	<30	<20	20–60	30–90	30
Sublingual		3			
Intravenous	1–3	1–3	1–3	1–3	
First-pass hepatic extraction after oral administration (%)	75–90	40–60	20–40	90	70–80

(continued)

Table 19-7

Pharmacokinetics of Calcium Channel Blockers *(continued)*

	Verapamil	Nifedipine	Nicardipine	Nimodipine	Diltiazem
Protein binding (%)	83–93	92–98	95	99	98
Clearance					
Renal (%)	70	80	55	20	35
Hepatic (%)	15	<15	45	80	60
Active metabolites	Yes	No		Yes	
Therapeutic plasma concentration (ng/mL)	50–250	10–100	5–100	10–30	100–250
Elimination half-time (h)	3–7	3–7	3–5	2	4–6

From Reves JG, Kissin I, Lell WA, et al. Calcium entry blockers: uses and implications for anesthesiologists. *Anesthesiology.* 1982;57:504–518; Durand PG, Lehot JJ, Foex P. Calcium-channel blockers and anaesthesia. *Can J Anaesth.* 1991;38:75–89.

and T, transient opening subtypes) resulting in maintenance of these channels in an inactive (closed) state (Fig. 19-4). As a result, calcium influx is decreased and there is a reduction in intracellular calcium.

2. Blockade of slow calcium channels by calcium channel blockers predictably results in slowing of the heart rate, reduction in myocardial contractility, decreased speed of conduction of cardiac impulses through the atrioventricular node, and vascular smooth muscle relaxation.

B. **Pharmacologic Effects** (see Table 19-6)

C. **Phenylalkylamines** (Fig. 19-5)

1. **Verapamil** is a synthetic derivative of papaverine that is supplied as a racemic mixture.

   a. **Side Effects**. Verapamil has a major depressant effect on the atrioventricular node, a negative chronotropic effect on the sinoatrial node, a negative inotropic effect on cardiac muscle, and a moderate vasodilating effect on coronary and systemic arteries.

   b. **Clinical Uses**. Verapamil is effective in the treatment of supraventricular tachydysrhythmias, reflecting its primary site of action on the atrioventricular node. The mild vasodilating effects produced by verapamil make this drug useful in the treatment of vasospastic angina pectoris and essential hypertension. Verapamil may be useful in the treatment of maternal and fetal tachydysrhythmias as well as premature labor.

   c. **Pharmacokinetics**. Oral verapamil is almost completely absorbed, but extensive hepatic first-pass metabolism limits bioavailability to 10% to 20% (see Table 19-7). As a result, the oral dose (80 to 160 mg three times daily) is about 10 times the IV dose.

D. **Dihydropyridines** prevent calcium entry into the vascular smooth cells by extracellular allosteric modulation of the L-type voltage-gated calcium ion channels (see Fig. 19-5).

1. **Nifedipine** is a dihydropyridine derivative with greater coronary and peripheral arterial vasodilator properties than verapamil. Unlike verapamil, nifedipine has little or no direct depressant effect on sinoatrial or atrioventricular node activity. Peripheral vasodilation and the resulting decrease in systemic blood pressure produced by nifedipine activates baroreceptors, leading to increased peripheral sympathetic nervous system activity most often manifesting as an increased heart rate.

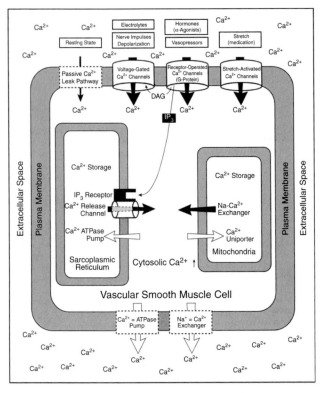

FIGURE 19-4 Calcium ion entry and exit from a vascular smooth muscle cell. Calcium enters the cytosol *(black arrows)* of the vascular smooth muscle cell either from the extracellular space through the plasma membrane *(top of diagram)* or from the intracellular storage areas. The primary entry sites for calcium ions are the voltage-gated channels. (From Kanneganti M, Halpern NA. Acute hypertension and calcium-channel blockers. *New Horiz*. 1996;4:19–25, with permission.)

The presence of aortic stenosis may also exaggerate the cardiac depressant effects of nifedipine.

a. **Clinical Uses.** Nifedipine is administered orally to treat patients with angina pectoris, especially that due to coronary artery vasospasm.

b. **Pharmacokinetics** (see Table 19-7)

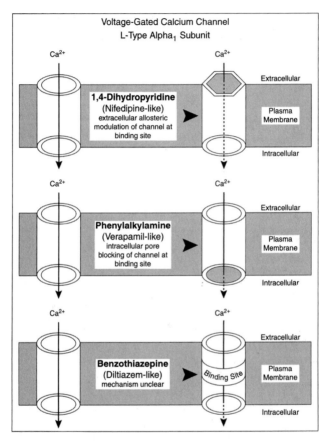

FIGURE 19-5 Mechanism of action of the three classes of calcium channel blockers. (From Kanneganti M, Halpern NA. Acute hypertension and calcium-channel blockers. *New Horiz.* 1996;4:19–25, with permission.)

    c. **Side effects** of nifedipine include flushing, vertigo, and headache. Nifedipine may induce renal dysfunction. Abrupt discontinuation of nifedipine has been associated with coronary artery vasospasm.

  2. **Nicardipine** lacks effects on the sinoatrial node and atrioventricular node and has minimal myocardial

depressant effects. This drug has the greatest vasodilating effects of all the calcium entry blockers, with vasodilation being particularly prominent in the coronary arteries.

  a. **Clinical Uses**. Nicardipine is used as a tocolytic drug having a similar tocolytic effect as salbutamol but with fewer side effects.

3. **Nimodipine** is a highly lipid-soluble analogue of nifedipine (lipid solubility facilitates its entrance into the central nervous system).

  a. **Clinical Uses**. The lipid solubility of nimodipine and its ability to cross the blood–brain barrier is responsible for the potential value of this drug in treating patients with subarachnoid hemorrhage.

  b. **Cerebral Vasospasm**. The vasodilating effect of nimodipine on cerebral arteries is uniquely valuable in preventing or attenuating cerebral vasospasm that often accompanies subarachnoid hemorrhage.

4. **Amlodipine** has minimal detrimental effects on myocardial contractility and provides antiischemic effects comparable to β blockers in patients with acute coronary syndrome.

E. **Benzothiazepines**

1. **Diltiazem** like verapamil, blocks predominantly the calcium channels of the atrioventricular node and is therefore a first-line medication for the treatment of supraventricular tachydysrhythmias. It may also be used for the chronic control of essential hypertension. Diltiazem exerts minimal cardiodepressant effects and is unlikely to interact with β-adrenergic blocking drugs to decrease myocardial contractility.

F. **Drug Interactions**. Verapamil and diltiazem have depressant effects on the generation of cardiac action potentials at the sinoatrial node and slow the movement of cardiac impulses through the atrioventricular node (patients with preexisting cardiac conduction abnormalities may experience greater degrees of atrioventricular heart block with concurrent administration of β blockers or digoxin). Treatment with calcium channel blockers can be continued until the time of surgery without risk of significant drug interactions, especially with respect to conduction of cardiac impulses. Toxicity reflecting an overdose of calcium channel blockers may be partially reversed with IV administration of calcium or dopamine.

1. **Anesthetic Drugs**

  a. Calcium channel blockers must be administered with caution to patients with impaired left ventricular function or hypovolemia.

      b. Treatment of cardiac dysrhythmias with calcium channel blockers in anesthetized patients produces only transient decreases in systemic blood pressure and infrequent prolongation of the P-R interval on the electrocardiogram.

      c. Because of the tendency to produce atrioventricular heart block, verapamil should be used cautiously in patients being treated with digitalis or β-adrenergic blocking drugs (Table 19-8).

      d. There is no evidence that patients being treated chronically with calcium channel blockers are at increased risk for anesthesia.

  2. **Neuromuscular blocking drugs** potentiate the effects of depolarizing and nondepolarizing neuromuscular blocking drugs. This potentiation resembles that produced by mycin antibiotics in the presence of neuromuscular blocking drugs.

      a. The neuromuscular effects of verapamil may be more likely to manifest in patients with a compromised margin of safety of neuromuscular transmission.

      b. Antagonism of neuromuscular blockade may be impaired because of diminished presynaptic release of acetylcholine in the presence of a calcium channel blocker.

  3. **Local Anesthetics**. Verapamil and diltiazem have potent local anesthetic activity, which may increase the risk of local anesthetic toxicity when regional anesthesia is administered to patients being treated with this drug.

  4. **Potassium-Containing Solutions.** Calcium channel blockers slow the inward movement of potassium ions such that hyperkalemia may occur after much smaller amounts of exogenous potassium infusion (potassium chloride to treat hypokalemia, administration of stored whole blood).

  5. **Dantrolene**. Whenever calcium channel blockers, especially verapamil or diltiazem, and dantrolene must be administered concurrently, invasive hemodynamic monitoring and frequent measurement of the plasma potassium concentration are recommended.

G. **Risks of Chronic Treatment**. Despite the popularity of calcium channel blockers in the treatment of cardiovascular diseases (essential hypertension, angina pectoris), there is increasing concern about the long-term safety of these drugs, especially the short-acting dihydropyridine derivatives (risk of developing cardiovascular complications). Treatment with calcium channel blockers, especially

Table 19-8

Effect of Chronic Antianginal Therapy on Perioperative Heart Rate (beats per minute) and P-R Interval (ms)

	Before Induction	After Induction	10 min after Cardiopulmonary Bypass
Control			
Heart rate	72	71	87
P-R interval	160	156	164
Calcium channel blockers			
Heart rate	69	70	86
P-R interval	168	169	175
β-Adrenergic antagonists			
Heart rate	59	65	78
P-R interval	168	171	183
Nifedipine plus β-adrenergic antagonists			
Heart rate	67	69	86
P-R interval	175	177	186

From Henling CE, Slogoff S, Kodali SV, et al. Heart block after coronary artery bypass effect of chronic administration of calcium-entry blockers and β-blockers. *Anesth Analg.* 1984;63:515–520.

short-acting dihydropyridine derivatives, should generally be reserved for second-step rather than initial therapy.

H. **Cytoprotection**
1. Drug-induced calcium channel blockade may provide cytoprotection against ischemic reperfusion injury by limiting the accumulation of oxygen free radicals.
2. Calcium channel blockers may attenuate renal injury from nephrotoxic drugs such as cisplatinum and iodinated radiographic contrast media.

CHAPTER 20

Vasodilators

I. **Introduction.** Control of vascular tone in the peripheral and pulmonary circulations is a complex interplay of local metabolism, endothelial function, and regulation by the sympathetic nervous and endocrine systems.

II. **Systemic hypertension** is estimated to affect 30% of adults in the United States and is defined as 150 to 159/90 to 99 mm Hg (stage 1) or greater than or equal to 160/100 mm Hg (stage 2). By far, the most common type of hypertension is "essential" or "primary" for which there is no clear unifying pathophysiology. Hypertension is a major risk factor for cardiovascular disease including atherosclerosis, heart failure, stroke, renal disease, and overall decreased survival.

III. **Specific Antihypertensive Drugs and Anesthesia** (Table 20-1). Hypertensive patients are likely to be receiving one or more of thiazide diuretics, calcium channel blockers, angiotensin-converting enzyme (ACE) inhibitors/angiotensin II receptor blocker medications, and β-adrenergic blockers. Severe or poorly controlled hypertension is a relatively common cause for postponement of surgery although evidence supporting this practice comes from small studies mostly more than 20 years old.

  A. **Sympatholytics**

    1. **β-Adrenergic blockers** are less commonly used as first-line agents in hypertension as other agents may have a better safety profile for this indication in those older than the age of 60 years. β Blockers are indicated for long-term treatment of patients with coronary artery disease and heart failure and for their antihypertensive action in these patients.

      a. **Mechanism of Action.** β Blockers can be classified according to whether they exhibit β_1 selective versus nonselective properties and whether they possess intrinsic sympathomimetic activity.

Table 20-1

Intravenous Antihypertensive Drugs Commonly Used in the Perioperative Setting

DRUG Mechanism	DOSE Bolus	Infusion	Onset	DURATION Plasma Half-Life Clinical Effect[a]
Metoprolol β₁ Blocker	1–5 mg		1–5 min	Half-life: 3–7 h Clinical: 1–4 h
Labetalol α₁, β₁, β₂ Blocker	5–20 mg	0.5–2 mg/min	1–5 min	Half-life: 6 h Clinical: 1–4 h
Esmolol β₁ Blocker		50–300 µg/kg/min	1–2 min	Half-life: 9 min
Nicardipine Dihydropyridine Ca blocker	100 µg	5–15 mg/h	2–10 min	Half-life: 2–4 h Clinical: 30–60 min
Hydralazine Arteriolar dilator	5–20 mg		5–20 min	Half-life: 2–8 h Clinical: 1–8 h
Fenoldopam Dopamine type 1 agonist		0.05–1.6 µg/kg/min	5–10 min	Half-life: 5 min Clinical: 30–60 min
Nitroprusside NO donor		0.25–4 µg/kg/min	1–2 min	Half-life: <10 min Clinical: 1–10 min
Nitroglycerin NO donor		5–300 µg/kg/min	1–2 min	Half-life: 1–3 min Clinical: 5–10 min

[a]Clinical effect commonly seen after bolus dose or stopping infusion.
Ca, calcium; NO, nitric oxide.

b. **Side Effects**. Treatment of hypertension with β blockers involves certain risks, including bradycardia and heart block, congestive heart failure, bronchospasm, claudication, masking of hypoglycemia, sedation, impotence, and when abruptly discontinued may precipitate angina pectoris or even myocardial infarction. Patients with any degree of congestive heart failure cannot generally tolerate more than modest doses of β blockers, yet it is clear that when dosage is slowly increased and the drugs are given chronically, the antiadrenergic effect provides a significant benefit in chronic systolic heart failure. In patients with symptomatic asthma, β blockers should be avoided. β Blockers potentially increase the risk of serious hypoglycemia in diabetic patients because they blunt autonomic nervous system responses that would warn of hypoglycemia. Nevertheless, the incidence of hypoglycemia has not been shown to be increased in diabetic patients being treated with β-adrenergic antagonists to control hypertension.

c. **Intravenous β Blockers**. Perioperative β blockade can be used to continue preoperative therapy, but due to extensive first-pass activity for oral agents, the conversion to intravenous dosing is somewhat unpredictable.

2. **α_1 Receptor Blockers**. Prazosin, terazosin, and doxazocin are oral, selective postsynaptic α_1-adrenergic receptor antagonists resulting in vasodilating effects on both arterial and venous vasculature. Absence of presynaptic α_2 receptor antagonism leaves intact the normal inhibitory effect on norepinephrine release from nerve endings. In addition to treating essential hypertension, prazosin may be of value for decreasing afterload in patients with congestive heart failure. Prazosin may also be a useful drug for the preoperative preparation of patients with pheochromocytoma.

a. **Pharmacokinetics**. Prazosin is nearly completely metabolized, and less than 60% bioavailability after oral administration suggests the occurrence of substantial first-pass hepatic metabolism (the fact that this drug is metabolized in the liver permits its use in patients with renal failure without altering the dose).

b. **Cardiovascular Effects**. Prazosin decreases systemic vascular resistance without causing reflex-induced tachycardia or increases in renin activity as occurs during treatment with hydralazine or minoxidil.

    c. **Side Effects**. The side effects of prazosin include vertigo, fluid retention, and orthostatic hypotension.

3. **α_2 Agonists**. Clonidine is a centrally acting selective partial α_2-adrenergic agonist (220:1 α_2 to α_1 activity) that acts as an antihypertensive drug by virtue of its ability to decrease sympathetic output from the central nervous system. This drug has proved to be particularly effective in the treatment of patients with severe hypertension or renin-dependent disease. The usual daily adult dose is 0.2 to 0.3 mg orally. Another drug of the same class is intravenous dexmedetomidine, a much more α_2 selective drug which is approved for sedation rather than hypertension, although it does have a blood pressure–lowering action.

    a. **Mechanism of Action**. α_2-Adrenergic agonists produce clinical effects by binding to α_2 receptors (Fig. 20-1). Decreased sympathetic nervous system activity is manifested as peripheral vasodilation and decreases in systemic blood pressure, heart rate, and cardiac output.

    b. **Pharmacokinetics**. Clonidine is rapidly absorbed after oral administration and reaches peak plasma concentrations within 60 to 90 minutes. The transdermal route requires about 48 hours to produce steady-state therapeutic plasma concentrations.

    c. **Cardiovascular Effects**. The ability of clonidine to decrease systemic blood pressure without paralysis of compensatory homeostatic reflexes is highly desirable. Renal blood flow and glomerular filtration rate are maintained in the presence of clonidine therapy.

    d. **Side Effects**. The most common side effects produced by clonidine are sedation and xerostomia. Consistent with sedation is a 50% decrease in anesthetic requirements for inhaled anesthetics (minimum alveolar concentration) and injected drugs in patients pretreated with clonidine administered in the preanesthetic medication.

    e. **Rebound Hypertension**. Abrupt discontinuation of clonidine therapy can result in rebound hypertension as soon as 8 hours and as late as 36 hours after the last dose. Rebound hypertension can usually be controlled by reinstituting clonidine therapy or by administering a vasodilating drug such as hydralazine or nitroprusside.

    f. **Other Clinical Uses**. α-Adrenergic agonists (clonidine and dexmedetomidine) induce sedation,

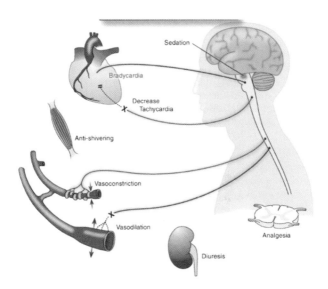

FIGURE 20-1 Schematic depiction of effects that are mediated by α_2-adrenergic receptors. The site for sedation is the locus ceruleus of the brainstem, whereas the principal site of analgesia is most likely the spinal cord. In the heart, the dominant effect of α_2 stimulation is attenuation of tachycardia through block of the cardioaccelerator nerves and bradycardia through vagal stimulation. In the peripheral vasculature, there are vasodilatory effects reflecting sympatholysis and vasoconstriction mediated by α_2 receptors in smooth muscle cells. (From Kamibayashi T, Maze M. Clinical uses of alpha$_2$-adrenergic agonists. *Anesthesiology*. 2000;93:1345–1349, with permission.)

decrease anesthetic requirements, and improve perioperative hemodynamic (attenuate blood pressure and heart rate responses to surgical stimulation) and sympathoadrenal stability.

B. **ACE inhibitors** are most effective in treating systemic hypertension secondary to increased renin production. These drugs have been established as first-line therapy in patients with systemic hypertension, congestive heart failure, and mitral regurgitation.

1. **Mechanism of Action**. Angiotensin II normally binds to a specific cell membrane receptor (AT_1) that ultimately leads to increased release of calcium from sarcoplasmic reticulum to produce vasoconstriction. Administration

of ACE inhibitors as prodrugs increases oral bioavailability prior to their hepatic metabolism to the active drug.

2. **Side Effects**
   a. Cough, upper respiratory congestion, rhinorrhea, and allergic-like symptoms seem to be the most common side effects of ACE inhibitors.
   b. Decreases in glomerular filtration rate may occur in patients treated with ACE inhibitors.
   c. Hyperkalemia is possible due to decreased production of aldosterone. The risk of hyperkalemia is greatest in patients with recognized risk factors (congestive heart failure with renal insufficiency).

3. **Preoperative Management**
   a. Adverse circulatory effects during anesthesia are recognized in patients chronically treated with ACE inhibitors, but continuation of these drugs until the time of surgery is not associated with adverse consequences.
   b. Exaggerated hypotension attributed to continued ACE inhibitor therapy has been responsive to crystalloid fluid infusion and/or administration of a catecholamine or vasopressin infusion.

C. **Angiotensin II receptor inhibitors** produce antihypertensive effects by blocking the vasoconstrictive actions of angiotensin II without affecting ACE activity. As with ACE inhibitors, hypotension following induction of anesthesia has been observed in patients being treated with angiotensin II receptor blockers causing some to recommend these drugs be discontinued on the day before surgery.

D. **Calcium Channel Blocking Drugs**. Calcium channel blocking drugs used as antihypertensives inhibit calcium influx through the voltage-sensitive L-type calcium channels in vascular smooth muscle. They are arterial specific, with little effect on venous circulation.

E. **Phosphodiesterase (PDE) Inhibitors**
   1. The PDEs variably inhibit the breakdown of intracellular cyclic adenosine monophosphate and cyclic guanosine monophosphate (GMP). The intravenous PDE-3 inhibitor milrinone has replaced amrinone due to its reduced side effect profile. Its combined inotropic and vasodilator actions make it an ideal drug in the short-term treatment of heart failure, both in the intensive care and operative settings.
   2. Concurrent administration of nitroglycerin and erectile dysfunction drugs within 24 hours is not recommended

as life-threatening hypotension from exaggerated systemic vasodilation may occur.

IV. **Nitric Oxide and Nitrovasodilators**

   A. **Nitric Oxide (NO)**. NO is recognized as a chemical messenger in a multitude of biologic systems, with homeostatic activity in the modulation of cardiovascular tone (synthesized in endothelial cells from the amino acid L-arginine by NO synthetase). NO production has a large role in regulation of vascular tone throughout the body. As a therapeutic agent, inhaled NO (iNO) affects the pulmonary circulation but not the systemic circulation due its extremely rapid uptake by hemoglobin.

      1. **NO as a Pulmonary Vasodilator**. iNO causes pulmonary arterial vasodilation that is proportional to the degree of pulmonary vasoconstriction (Fig. 20-2). By dilating vessels in alveoli where it is locally delivered, iNO usually improves oxygenation by improving ventilation: perfusion matching. iNO, 10 to 20 ppm, has been used for therapy of persistent pulmonary hypertension of the newborn.

         a. **Toxicity**. iNO increases methemoglobin levels as NO combines with hemoglobin (increases in methemoglobin concentrations are usually modest). Life-threatening rebound arterial hypoxemia and pulmonary hypertension may accompany discontinuation of iNO therapy. NO is oxidized to nitrogen dioxide (NO_2) especially in the presence of high concentrations of oxygen. NO_2 is a known pulmonary toxin ("silo-filler's disease"). In the presence of left heart dysfunction or failure, the increased pulmonary blood flow caused by iNO can precipitate acute left heart failure and pulmonary edema.

   B. **Nitrodilators** (sodium nitroprusside and nitroglycerin) work through the generation of NO, which then augments cGMP in vascular smooth muscle, both arteries and veins, leading to vasodilation. The more recent availability of intravenous nicardipine and other arterial-specific dilators such as clevidipine and fenoldopam has to some degree replaced the use of the nitrodilators, especially nitroprusside.

   C. **Sodium nitroprusside (SNP)** is a direct-acting, nonselective peripheral vasodilator that causes relaxation of arterial and venous vascular smooth muscle. The extreme potency of SNP necessitates careful titration of dosage as provided by continuous infusion devices and frequent monitoring of systemic blood pressure, often by intraarterial monitoring.

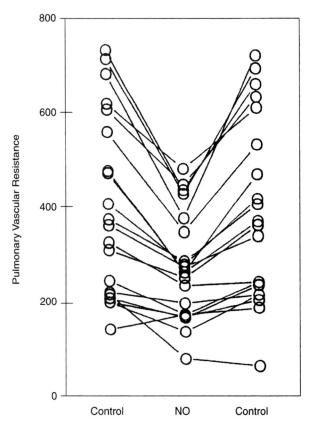

FIGURE 20-2 Inhalation of nitric oxide. Pulmonary vascular resistance (dyne/cm/s^{-5}) before, during, and after inhalation of nitric oxide (NO) for each patient before cardiopulmonary bypass. (From Rich GF, Murphy GD, Roos CM, et al. Inhaled nitric oxide: selective pulmonary vasodilation in cardiac surgical patients. *Anesthesiology.* 1993;78:1028–1035, with permission.)

1. **Mechanism of Action**. SNP interacts with oxyhemoglobin, dissociating immediately and forming methemoglobin while releasing cyanide and NO that is responsible for the direct vasodilating effect of SNP.
2. **Metabolism** of SNP begins with the transfer of an electron from the iron of oxyhemoglobin to SNP, yield-

ing methemoglobin and an unstable SNP radical that promptly breaks down, releasing all five cyanide ions, one of which reacts with methemoglobin to form cyanomethemoglobin. The remaining free cyanide ions are available to rhodanese enzyme in the liver and kidneys for conversion to thiocyanate. Rhodanese uses thiosulfate ions as sulfur donors, and most adults can detoxify approximately 50 mg of SNP using existing sulfur stores. Normal adult methemoglobin concentrations (about 0.5% of all hemoglobin) are capable of binding the cyanide released from 18 mg of SNP. Cyanomethemoglobin remains in dynamic equilibrium with free cyanide and is nontoxic.

3. **Dose and Administration**. Patients receiving SNP should have blood pressure monitored continuously via an arterial catheter. The recommended initial dose of SNP is 0.3 μg/kg/minute IV titrated to a maximum rate of 10 μg/kg/minute IV, with the maximum rate not to be infused longer than 10 minutes. SNP infusion rates of greater than 2 μg/kg/minute IV result in dose-dependent accumulation of cyanide and the risk of cyanide toxicity must be considered. Delivery of the SNP infusion as protected from light by aluminum foil is most often via an infusion pump.

4. **Organ-Specific Effects of SNP**

   a. **Cardiovascular**. Baroreceptor-mediated reflex responses to SNP-induced decreases in systemic blood pressure manifest as tachycardia and increased myocardial contractility. These reflex-mediated responses may oppose the blood pressure–lowering effects of SNP. SNP may increase the area of damage associated with a myocardial infarction through a phenomenon called *coronary steal.*

   b. **Renal**. SNP-induced decreases in systemic blood pressure may result in decreases in renal function. Release of renin may accompany blood pressure decreases produced by SNP and contribute to blood pressure overshoots when the drug is discontinued.

   c. **Hepatic**. Hepatic blood flow does not change when cardiac output is maintained in anesthetized patients, despite 20% to 60% decreases in systemic blood pressure produced by SNP.

   d. **Cerebral**. SNP increases cerebral blood flow and cerebral blood volume, and in patients with decreased intracranial compliance, this may increase intracranial pressure (greater than the increase produced by nitroglycerin). Decreasing blood pressure slowly over

5 minutes with SNP in the presence of hypocarbia and hyperoxia negates the increase in intracranial pressure that accompanies the rapid infusion of SNP. Patients with known inadequate cerebral blood flow as associated with dangerously increased intracranial pressure or carotid artery stenosis should probably not be treated with SNP.

e. **Pulmonary**. Decreases in the Pao_2 may accompany the infusion of SNP and other peripheral vasodilators used to produce controlled hypotension (attenuation of hypoxic pulmonary vasoconstriction by peripheral vasodilators is the presumed mechanism). The addition of positive end-expiratory pressure may reverse vasodilator-induced decreases in the Pao_2.

f. **Hematologic**. Increased intracellular concentrations of cGMP, as produced by SNP and nitroglycerin, have been shown to inhibit platelet aggregation.

5. **Cyanide Toxicity**. Clinical evidence of cyanide toxicity may occur when the rate of IV SNP infusion is greater than 2 μg/kg/minute or when sulfur donors and methemoglobin are exhausted, thus allowing cyanide radicals to accumulate. Mixed venous Po_2 is increased in the presence of cyanide toxicity, indicating paralysis of cytochrome oxidase and inability of tissues to use oxygen. Metabolic acidosis develops as a reflection of anaerobic metabolism in the tissues.

a. **Treatment of Cyanide Toxicity**. Appearance of tachyphylaxis in a previously sensitive patient in association with metabolic acidosis and increased mixed venous Po_2 mandates immediate discontinuation of SNP and administration of 100% oxygen despite normal oxygen saturation. Sodium bicarbonate is administered to correct metabolic acidosis. Sodium thiosulfate, 150 mg/kg IV administered over 15 minutes, is a recommended treatment for cyanide toxicity. Another treatment is methylene blue, 1 to 2 mg/kg IV, administered over 5 minutes, to facilitate the conversion of methemoglobin to hemoglobin.

6. **Thiocyanate toxicity** is rare, as thiocyanate is 100-fold less toxic than cyanide. In patients with normal renal function, 7 to 14 days of SNP infusion in the 2 to 5 μg/kg/minute range may be required to produce potentially toxic thiocyanate blood concentrations. Clinical evidence of neurotoxicity produced by thiocyanate

includes hyperreflexia, confusion, psychosis, and miosis. Toxicity may progress to seizures and coma. Increased thiocyanate concentrations competitively inhibit uptake and binding of iodine in the thyroid gland, sometimes producing clinical hypothyroidism.

7. **Methemoglobinemia**. Adverse effects from methemoglobinemia produced by SNP breakdown are unlikely even in patients with a congenital inability to convert methemoglobin to hemoglobin (methemoglobin reductase deficiency).

8. **Clinical Use**. The use of SNP has significantly declined with the introduction of more selective arterial agents which have a greater margin of safety and much less or absent toxicity. Before the availability of these drugs, SNP was used widely in the settings of controlled hypotension, hypertensive emergencies, aortic and cardiac surgery, and heart failure.

D. **Nitrates**. Nitroglycerin is an organic nitrate that acts principally on venous capacitance vessels and large coronary arteries to produce peripheral pooling of blood and decreased cardiac ventricular wall tension. As the dose of nitroglycerin is increased, there is also relaxation of arterial vascular smooth muscle. The most common clinical use of nitroglycerin is sublingual or IV administration for the treatment of angina pectoris.

1. **Mechanism of Action**. Nitroglycerin, like SNP, generates NO, which stimulates production of cGMP to cause peripheral vasodilation. In contrast to SNP, which spontaneously produces NO, nitroglycerin requires the presence of thio-containing compounds. Nitroglycerin is not recommended in patients with hypertrophic obstructive cardiomyopathy or in the presence of severe aortic stenosis.

2. **Route of Administration**. Nitroglycerin is most frequently administered by the sublingual route, but it is also available as an oral tablet, a buccal or transmucosal tablet, a sublingual spray, and a transdermal ointment or patch. Continuous infusion of nitroglycerin, via special delivery tubing to decrease absorption of the drug into plastic, is a useful approach to maintain a constant delivered concentration of nitroglycerin.

3. **Methemoglobinemia**. The nitrite metabolite of nitroglycerin is capable of oxidizing the ferrous ion in hemoglobin to the ferric state with the production

of methemoglobin. High doses of nitroglycerin may produce methemoglobinemia especially in patients with hepatic dysfunction.

4. **Tolerance.** A limitation to the use of all nitrates is the development of tolerance to their vasodilating effects. Tolerance is dose-dependent and duration-dependent, usually manifesting within 24 hours of sustained treatment. A drug-free interval of 12 to 14 hours is recommended to reverse tolerance to nitroglycerin and other nitrates.

5. **Clinical Use**

a. Perioperatively, nitroglycerin in all its forms is used to treat suspected myocardial ischemia as well as volume overload in the setting of heart failure (preload reduction).

b. As a systemic antihypertensive, both for treatment and achieving controlled hypotension, nitroglycerin infusion can be effective but its preferential effect on veins rather than arteries can make it less effective in severe hypertension than drugs which preferentially act on the arteries (use for hypertension has declined with the availability of intravenous nicardipine and fenoldopam).

E. **Isosorbide dinitrate** is a commonly administered oral nitrate for the prophylaxis of angina pectoris and for preload reduction in patients with heart failure. Its effects are very similar to that of nitroglycerin but as an oral agent, isosorbide dinitrate is well absorbed from the gastrointestinal tract and it is not subject to the extensive first-pass metabolism that limits oral use of nitroglycerin.

F. **Hydralazine** is a direct systemic arterial vasodilator that produces reflex sympathetic nervous system stimulation with resulting increases in heart rate and myocardial contractility (not recommended for patients with myocardial ischemia or coronary disease). It is an effective afterload-reducing agent and is still used in combination with nitrates for outpatient treatment of congestive heart failure and for intermittent intravenous dosing in the perioperative period or critical care setting.

G. **Fenoldopam** is a dopamine type 1 receptor agonist, causing systemic arterial dilation (increases renal blood flow and urine output). Fenoldopam is only available in an intravenous preparation. There is a baroreflex-mediated increase in heart rate. Adverse effects are limited to an increase in intraocular pressure making this drug unsuitable for patients with glaucoma.

H. **Diuretics** continue to be first-line oral agents used for essential hypertension. Both thiazide and loop diuretics cause potassium loss and their use generally mandates supplementation with potassium and often magnesium.

CHAPTER 21

Antiarrhythmic Drugs

I. **Introduction**

A. Cardiac arrhythmias occur commonly in the perioperative period, most of which are relatively benign and are due to transient changes in physiology, surgical stimuli, or the effect of anesthetic agents.

B. Improved survival for patients receiving implantable cardiac defibrillator devices compared with antiarrhythmic drugs has altered the treatment paradigms for patients with ventricular arrhythmias.

C. Catheter ablation techniques are preferred treatments for many supraventricular arrhythmias including atrial and certain types of atrial fibrillation.

D. Pharmacologic treatment of cardiac arrhythmias is principally used to suppress atrial fibrillation and atrial flutter that is not responsive to catheter ablation treatment and for patients with implantable cardioverter-defibrillator devices who are receiving frequent indicated electrical shocks.

E. The two major physiologic mechanisms that cause ectopic cardiac arrhythmias are reentry and enhanced automaticity.

1. Factors encountered in the perioperative period that facilitate cardiac arrhythmias due to both mechanisms include hypoxemia, electrolyte and acid–base abnormalities, myocardial ischemia, altered sympathetic nervous system activity, bradycardia, and the administration of certain drugs.

2. Alkalosis is even more likely than acidosis to trigger cardiac arrhythmias.

3. Hypokalemia and hypomagnesemia predispose to ventricular arrhythmias and must be suspected in patients who are being treated with diuretics.

4. Increased sympathetic nervous system activity lowers the threshold for ventricular fibrillation, a phenomenon that is attenuated by β blockade and vagal stimulation.

F. Drugs administered for the chronic suppression of cardiac arrhythmias pose little threat to the uneventful course

of anesthesia and should be continued up to the time of
induction of anesthesia.

1. Cardiac arrhythmias, however, do require treatment
   when hemodynamic function is compromised, or
   the disturbance predisposes to more serious cardiac
   arrhythmias.
2. General anesthetic–related cardiac arrhythmias have
   been ascribed to abnormal pacemaker activity characterized by suppression of the sinoatrial node, with the
   emergence of latent pacemakers within or below the
   atrioventricular tissues.

II. **Mechanism of Action**
   A. Antiarrhythmic drugs produce pharmacologic effects by
      blocking passage of ions across sodium, potassium, and cal-
      cium ion channels present in the heart (Fig. 21-1).

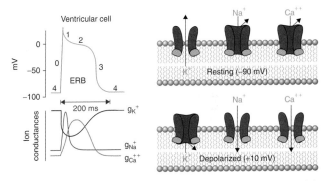

FIGURE 21-1 The physiologic basis of the cardiac action potential.
Phase 0 represents rapid depolarization as a result of opening of
Na^+ channels and closing of K^+ channels. Phase 1 is the period of
initial repolarization that results from closure of Na^+ and opening
of K^+ channels. Phase 2 is the plateau phase that results from the
sustained Ca^{++} current that began with the initial depolarization.
Phase 3 is repolarization due to opening of K^+ and closure of Ca^{++}
channels. Phase 4 is the resting potential during which time K^+ channels are open and Na^+ and Ca^{++} channels are closed. The effective
refractory period (ERP) is the time during which the cell cannot be
depolarized again. (Adapted from Klabunde RE, ed. *Cardiovascular
Physiology Concepts*. 2nd ed. Philadelphia, PA: Lippincott Williams
& Wilkins; 2011.)

B. The effects of cardiac antiarrhythmic drugs on the action potential and effective refractory period of the cardiac action potential determine the clinical effect of these drugs.

III. **Classification**

A. Cardiac arrhythmic drugs are most commonly classified into four groups based primarily on the ability of the drug to control arrhythmias by blocking specific ion channels and currents during the cardiac action potential (Tables 21-1 and 21-2).

Table 21-1

Classification of Cardiac Antiarrhythmic Drugs

Class I (inhibit fast sodium ion channels)

Class IA
Quinidine
Procainamide
Disopyramide
Moricizine

Class IB
Lidocaine
Tocainide
Mexiletine

Class IC
Flecainide
Propafenone

Class II (decrease rate of depolarization)
Esmolol
Propranolol
Acebutolol

Class III (inhibit potassium ion channels)
Amiodarone
Sotalol
Ibutilide
Dofetilide
Bretylium

Class IV (inhibit slow calcium channels)
Verapamil
Diltiazem

Table 21-2

Electrophysiologic and Electrocardiographic Effects of Cardiac Antiarrhythmic Drugs

	Class IA	Class IB	Class IC	Class II	Class III	Class IV
Depolarization rate (phase 0)	Decreased	No effect	Greatly decreased	No effect	No effect	No effect
Conduction velocity	Decreased	No effect	Greatly decreased	Decreased	Decreased	No effect
Effective refractory period	Greatly increased	Decreased	Increased	Decreased	Greatly increased	No effect
Action potential duration	Increased	Decreased	Increased	Increased	Greatly increased	Decreased
Automaticity	Decreased	Decreased	Decreased	Decreased	Decreased	No effect
P-R duration	No effect	No effect	Increased	No effect or increased	Increased	No effect or increased
QRS duration	Increased	No effect	Greatly increased	No effect	Increased	No effect
QTc duration	Greatly increased	No effect or decreased	Increased	Decreased	Greatly increased	No effect

B. Antiarrhythmic drugs also differ in their pharmacokinetics and efficacy in treating specific types of arrhythmias (Tables 21-3 and 21-4).

IV. **Proarrhythmic effects describe bradyarrhythmias or tachyarrhythmias that represent new cardiac arrhythmias associated with antiarrhythmic drug treatment.**
   A. **Torsades de pointes** manifests as prolongation of the QTc interval on the electrocardiogram (ECG).
      1. Class IA drugs (quinidine and disopyramide) and class III drugs (amiodarone) prolong the QTc interval by potassium channel blockade providing the setting for torsades de pointes.
      2. Drug-induced torsades de pointes is often associated with bradycardia because the QTc interval is longer at slower heart rates.
   B. **Incessant ventricular tachycardia** may be precipitated by drugs that slow conduction of cardiac impulses (class IA and class IC drugs) sufficiently to create a continuous ventricular tachycardia circuit (reentry). Incessant ventricular tachycardia is more likely to occur with high doses of class IC drugs and in patients with a prior history of sustained ventricular tachycardia and poor left ventricular function.
   C. **Wide complex ventricular rhythm** is usually associated with class IC drugs in the setting of structural heart disease.

V. **Efficacy and Results of Treatment with Cardiac Antiarrhythmic Drugs**
   A. Chronic suppression of ventricular ectopy with an antiarrhythmic drug other than amiodarone does not prevent future life-threatening arrhythmias and may increase mortality.
      1. Patients treated with class IC drugs experienced a higher incidence of sudden cardiac arrest reflecting the proarrhythmia effects of these drugs.
      2. β-Adrenergic antagonists that do not typically suppress ventricular arrhythmias appear to decrease mortality and the risk of life-threatening ventricular arrhythmias.
   B. Survivors of cardiac arrest have a high risk of subsequent ventricular fibrillation and treatment of these patients with amiodarone results in fewer life-threatening cardiac events.
   C. The proarrhythmic and negative inotropic effects of class IA and class IC drugs precludes their administration to patients with congestive heart failure. In these patients, administration of amiodarone appears to be safe and effective.

Table 21-3

Pharmacokinetics of Cardiac Antiarrhythmic Drugs

	Principal Clearance Mechanism	Protein Binding (%)	Elimination Half-Time (h)	Therapeutic Plasma Concentration
Quinidine	Hepatic	80–90	5–12	1.2–4.0 µg/mL
Procainamide	Renal/hepatic	15	2.5–5.0	4–8 µg/mL
Disopyramide	Renal/hepatic	15	8–12	2–4 µg/mL
Lidocaine	Hepatic	55	1.4–8.0	1–5 µg/mL
Tocainide	Hepatic/renal	10–30	12–15	4–10 µg/mL
Mexiletine	Hepatic	60–75	6–12	0.75–2.00 µg/mL
Flecainide	Hepatic	30–45	13–30	0.3–1.5 µg/mL
Propafenone	Hepatic	>95	5–8	
Propranolol	Hepatic	90–95	2–4	10–30 ng/mL
Amiodarone	Hepatic	96	8–107 d	1.5–2.0 µg/mL
Sotalol	Renal			
Verapamil	Hepatic	90	4.5–12.0	100–300 ng/mL

Table 21-4

Efficacy of Cardiac Antiarrhythmic Drugs

	Conversion of Atrial Fibrillation	Paroxysmal Supraventricular Tachycardia	Premature Ventricular Contractions	Ventricular Tachycardia
Quinidine	+	++	++	+
Procainamide	+	++	++	++
Disopyramide	+	++	++	++
Lidocaine	0	0	++	++
Tocainide	0	0	++	++
Mexiletine	0	0	++	++
Moricizine	0	0	++	++
Flecainide	0	+	++	++
Propafenone	0	++	++	+
Propranolol	+	++	+	++
Amiodarone	+	++	++	++
Sotalol	++	+	0	0
Verapamil	++	++	0	0
Diltiazem	++	++	0	0
Digitalis	++	++	0	0
Adenosine	0	++		0

0, no effect; +, effective; ++, highly effective.

VI. **Prophylactic Antiarrhythmic Drug Therapy**
   A. Although commonly used in the past, lidocaine is no longer recommended as prophylactic treatment for patients in the early stages of acute myocardial infarction and without malignant ventricular ectopy.
   B. Calcium channel antagonists are not recommended as routine treatment of patients with acute myocardial infarction because mortality is not decreased by these drugs.
   C. Data on the ability of magnesium to decrease mortality following myocardial infarction are conflicting. Treatment with magnesium is indicated in patients following an acute myocardial infarction who develop torsades de pointes ventricular tachycardia.
   D. In patients with heart failure, amiodarone reduces the risk of sudden cardiac death and therefore represents a viable alternative in patients who are not eligible for or who do not have access to implanted cardiac defibrillator (ICD) therapy for the prevention of sudden cardiac death from arrhythmias.
   E. Atrial fibrillation after heart surgery is a common complication that has been associated with prolonged hospitalization and cardiovascular morbidity. Prophylactic therapy with amiodarone, β blockers, sotalol, and magnesium has been effective in reducing the occurrence of atrial fibrillation, length of hospital stay, and cost of hospital treatment and may be effective in reducing the risk of stroke.

VII. **Decision to Treat Cardiac Arrhythmias**
   A. Drug treatment of cardiac arrhythmias is not uniformly effective and frequently causes side effects. The benefit of antiarrhythmic drugs is clearest when it results in the immediate termination of a sustained tachycardia (termination of ventricular tachycardia by lidocaine or supraventricular tachycardia by adenosine or verapamil). The mechanism by which β-adrenergic antagonists decrease mortality after an acute myocardial infarction is not known.
   B. The value of monitoring plasma drug concentrations in minimizing the risks associated with therapy is not established.

VIII. **Antiarrhythmic Drug Pharmacology**
   A. **Quinidine** is a class IA drug that is effective in the treatment of acute and chronic supraventricular arrhythmia (rarely used because of its side effects). Supraventricular

tachyarrhythmias associated with Wolff-Parkinson-White syndrome are effectively suppressed by quinidine.

1. **Mechanism of Action**. Quinidine decreases the slope of phase 4 depolarization, which explains its effectiveness in suppressing cardiac arrhythmias caused by enhanced automaticity.

2. **Metabolism and Excretion**
   a. Quinidine is hydroxylated in the liver to inactive metabolites, which are excreted in the urine.
   b. The concurrent administration of phenytoin or rifampin may lower blood levels of quinidine by enhancing liver clearance.

3. **Side Effects**. Quinidine has a low therapeutic ratio, with heart block, hypotension, and proarrhythmia being potential adverse side effects.

B. **Procainamide** is as effective as quinidine for the treatment of ventricular tachyarrhythmias but less effective in abolishing atrial tachyarrhythmias. Premature ventricular contractions and paroxysmal ventricular tachycardia are suppressed in most patients within a few minutes after intravenous (IV) administration, which is better tolerated than IV quinidine but may still cause hypotension.

1. **Mechanism of Action**
   a. Procainamide is an analogue of the local anesthetic procaine.
   b. Procainamide possesses an electrophysiologic action similar to that of quinidine but produces less prolongation of the QTc interval on the ECG (paradoxical ventricular tachycardia is a rare feature of procainamide therapy).
   c. Procainamide has no vagolytic effect and can be used in patients with atrial fibrillation to suppress ventricular irritability without increasing the ventricular rate.

2. **Metabolism and Excretion**
   a. Procainamide is eliminated by renal excretion and hepatic metabolism (dose of procainamide must be decreased when renal function is abnormal).
   b. The activity of the *N*-acetyltransferase enzyme response for the acetylation of procainamide is genetically determined (in patients who are rapid acetylators, the elimination half-time of procainamide is 2.5 hours compared with 5 hours in slow acetylators).

3. **Side Effects**
   a. Similar to quinidine, use of procainamide has dramatically decreased due to its side effect profile and availability of newer agents.
   b. Hypotension that results from procainamide is more likely to be caused by direct myocardial depression than peripheral vasodilation.
   c. Chronic administration of procainamide may be associated with a syndrome that resembles systemic lupus erythematosus.

C. **Disopyramide** is comparable to quinidine in effectively suppressing atrial and ventricular tachyarrhythmias. About 50% of the drug is excreted unchanged by the kidneys.
   1. **Side Effects**
      a. The most common side effects of disopyramide are dry mouth and urinary hesitancy, both of which are caused by the drug's anticholinergic activity.
      b. Prolongation of the QTc interval on the ECG and paradoxical ventricular tachycardia (similar to quinidine) may occur.
      c. Disopyramide has significant myocardial depressant effects and can precipitate congestive heart failure and hypotension.

D. **Moricizine** is a phenothiazine derivative that is reserved for the treatment of life-threatening ventricular arrhythmias when other drugs such as amiodarone are not available or contraindicated (e.g., allergy).
   1. **Side Effects**. Proarrhythmic effects occur in 3% to 15% of patients treated chronically with moricizine.

E. **Lidocaine** is used principally for suppression of ventricular arrhythmias, having minimal if any effect on supraventricular tachyarrhythmias. The efficacy of prophylactic lidocaine therapy for preventing early ventricular fibrillation after acute myocardial infarction has not been documented and is no longer recommended. Advantages of lidocaine over quinidine or procainamide are the more rapid onset and prompt disappearance of effects when the continuous infusion is terminated, greater therapeutic index, and a much reduced side effect profile. Lidocaine for IV administration differs from that used for local anesthesia because it does not contain a preservative.
   1. **Mechanism of Action**
      a. The effectiveness of lidocaine in suppressing premature ventricular contractions reflects its ability to decrease the rate of spontaneous phase 4 depolarization.

b. The ineffectiveness of lidocaine against supraventricular tachyarrhythmias presumably reflects its inability to alter the rate of spontaneous phase 4 depolarization in atrial cardiac cells.

2. **Metabolism and Excretion**. Lidocaine is metabolized in the liver, and resulting metabolites may possess cardiac antiarrhythmic activity.

3. **Side Effects**
   a. Lidocaine is essentially devoid of effects on the ECG or cardiovascular system when the plasma concentration remains less than 5 μg/mL (does not alter the duration of the QRS complex on the ECG, and activity of the sympathetic nervous system is not changed).
   b. Toxic plasma concentrations of lidocaine (>5 to 10 μg/mL) produce peripheral vasodilation and direct myocardial depression, resulting in hypotension.
   c. Stimulation of the central nervous system (CNS) occurs in a dose-related manner, with symptoms appearing when plasma concentrations of lidocaine are greater than 5 μg/mL. Seizures are possible at plasma concentrations of 5 to 10 μg/mL.
   d. CNS depression, apnea, and cardiac arrest are possible when plasma lidocaine concentrations are greater than 10 μg/mL.
   e. The convulsive threshold for lidocaine is decreased during arterial hypoxemia, hyperkalemia, or acidosis (importance of monitoring these parameters during continuous infusion of lidocaine to patients for suppression of ventricular arrhythmias).

F. **Mexiletine** is an orally effective amine analogue of lidocaine that is used for the chronic suppression of ventricular cardiac tachyarrhythmias. As it is a lidocaine analog, mexiletine may be effective in decreasing neuropathic pain for patients in whom alternative pain medications have been unsatisfactory.

1. **Side Effects**
   a. Neurologic side effects include tremulousness, diplopia, vertigo, and occasionally slurred speech.
   b. Increases in liver enzymes may occur especially in patients manifesting congestive heart failure.

G. **Tocainide** is an orally effective amine analogue of lidocaine that is used for the chronic suppression of ventricular cardiac tachyarrhythmias.

H. **Phenytoin** is particularly effective in suppression of ventricular arrhythmias associated with digitalis toxicity and may be useful in the treatment of paradoxical ventricular tachycardia or torsades de pointes. The IV dose is 100 mg (1.5 mg/kg) every 5 minutes until the cardiac arrhythmia is controlled or 10 to 15 mg/kg (maximum 1,000 mg) has been administered. Because phenytoin can precipitate in 5% dextrose in water, it is preferable to give the drug via a delivery tubing containing normal saline.

1. **Mechanism of Action**
   a. Phenytoin exerts a greater effect on the electrocardiographic QTc interval than does lidocaine and shortens the QTc interval more than any of the other antiarrhythmic drugs.
   b. The ability of some volatile anesthetics to depress the sinoatrial node is a consideration if administration of phenytoin during general anesthesia is planned.

2. **Metabolism and Excretion**
   a. Phenytoin is hydroxylated and then conjugated with glucuronic acid for excretion in the urine (impaired hepatic function may result in higher than normal blood levels of the drug).
   b. Warfarin, phenylbutazone, and isoniazid may inhibit metabolism and increase phenytoin blood levels.

3. **Side Effects**
   a. Phenytoin toxicity most commonly manifests as CNS disturbances, especially cerebellar disturbances (ataxia, nystagmus, vertigo, slurred speech, sedation, mental confusion).
   b. Phenytoin partially inhibits insulin secretion and may lead to increased blood glucose levels in patients who are hyperglycemic.
   c. Leukopenia, granulocytopenia, and thrombocytopenia may occur as a manifestation of drug-induced bone marrow depression.

I. Flecainide is a fluorinated local anesthetic analogue of procainamide that is more effective in suppressing ventricular premature beats and ventricular tachycardia than quinidine and disopyramide. Flecainide is also effective for the treatment of atrial tachyarrhythmias (effective for the treatment of tachyarrhythmias).

1. **Metabolism and Excretion**
   a. Oral absorption of flecainide is excellent, and a prolonged elimination half-time (about 20 hours) makes

a twice daily dose of 100 to 200 mg acceptable (not available in an IV formulation).

b. Elimination of flecainide is decreased in patients with congestive heart failure or renal failure and decreased left ventricular function.

2. **Side Effects**

a. Proarrhythmic effects occur in a significant number of treated patients especially in the presence of left ventricular dysfunction.

b. Flecainide prolongs the QRS complex and may depress sinoatrial node function as do β-adrenergic antagonists and calcium channel blockers (not administered to patients with second- and third-degree atrioventricular heart block).

c. The most common noncardiac adverse effect of flecainide is dose-related blurred vision.

d. Flecainide increases the capture thresholds of pacemakers.

J. **Propafenone**, like flecainide, is an effective oral antiarrhythmic drug for suppression of ventricular and atrial tachyarrhythmias. The rate of metabolism is genetically determined with about 90% of patients able to metabolize propafenone efficiently in the liver (availability of propafenone increases significantly in the presence of liver disease).

1. **Side Effects**

a. Propafenone depresses the myocardium and may cause conduction abnormalities such as sinoatrial node slowing, atrioventricular block, and bundle branch block.

b. Propafenone interferes with the metabolism of propranolol and metoprolol resulting in increased plasma concentrations of these β blockers. This drug also increases the plasma concentration of warfarin and may prolong the prothrombin time.

K. **β-Adrenergic antagonists** are effective for treatment of cardiac arrhythmias related to enhanced activity of the sympathetic nervous system (perioperative stress). Multifocal atrial tachycardia may respond to esmolol or metoprolol but is best treated with amiodarone. Acebutolol is effective in the treatment of frequent premature ventricular contractions. β-Adrenergic antagonists, especially propranolol, may be effective in controlling torsades de pointes for patients with prolonged QTc intervals. Acebutolol, propranolol, and metoprolol are approved for prevention of sudden death following myocardial infarction.

1. **Mechanism of Action**
   a. The antiarrhythmic effects of β-adrenergic antagonists most likely reflect blockade of the responses of β receptors in the heart to sympathetic nervous system stimulation, as well as the effects of circulating catecholamines (rate of spontaneous phase 4 depolarization is decreased and the rate of sinoatrial node discharge is decreased).
   b. β-Adrenergic antagonists can depress the myocardium not only by β blockade but also by direct depressant effects on cardiac muscle.
   c. The usual oral dose of propranolol for chronic suppression of ventricular arrhythmias is 10 to 80 mg every 6 to 8 hours. Effective β blockade is usually achieved in an otherwise normal person when the resting heart rate is 55 to 60 beats per minute. For emergency suppression of cardiac arrhythmias in an adult, propranolol may be administered IV in a dose of 1 mg per minute (3 to 6 mg).

2. **Metabolism and Excretion**
   a. Orally administered propranolol is extensively metabolized in the liver, and a hepatic first-pass effect is responsible for the variation in plasma concentration.
   b. Propranolol readily crosses the blood–brain barrier.
   c. The principal metabolite of propranolol is 4-hydroxypropranolol, which possesses weak β-adrenergic antagonist activity.

3. **Side Effects**
   a. Bradycardia, hypotension, myocardial depression, and bronchospasm are side effects of β-adrenergic antagonists that reflect the ability of these drugs to inhibit sympathetic nervous system activity. The use of propranolol in patients with preexisting atrioventricular heart block is not recommended.
   b. Interference with glucose metabolism may manifest as hypoglycemia in patients being treated for diabetes mellitus.
   c. Upregulation of β-adrenergic receptors occurs with chronic administration of β-adrenergic antagonists such that abrupt discontinuation of treatment may lead to supraventricular tachycardia.

L. **Amiodarone** is a potent antiarrhythmic drug with a wide spectrum of activity against refractory supraventricular and ventricular tachyarrhythmias. In the presence of ventricular tachycardia or fibrillation that is resistant to electrical defibrillation, amiodarone 300 mg IV is recommended.

Preoperative oral administration of amiodarone decreases the incidence of atrial fibrillation after cardiac surgery. It is also effective for suppression of tachyarrhythmias associated with Wolff-Parkinson-White syndrome. Similar to β blockers and unlike class I drugs, amiodarone decreases mortality after myocardial infarction. After initiation of oral therapy, a decrease in ventricular tachyarrhythmias occurs within 72 hours. After discontinuation of chronic oral therapy, the pharmacologic effect of amiodarone lasts for a prolonged period (up to 60 days), reflecting the prolonged elimination half-time of this drug (Fig. 21-2).

1. **Mechanism of Action**. Amiodarone prolongs the effective refractory period in all cardiac tissues and also has an antiadrenergic effect (noncompetitive blockade of α and β receptors). Amiodarone acts as an antianginal drug by dilating coronary arteries and increasing coronary blood flow.

2. **Metabolism and Excretion**
   a. Amiodarone has a prolonged elimination half-time (29 days) and is minimally dependent on renal excretion.

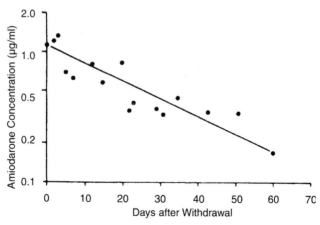

FIGURE 21-2 After discontinuation of amiodarone, the plasma concentration decreases slowly, resulting in a prolonged elimination half-time. (From Kannan R, Nademannee K, Hendrickson JA, et al. Amiodarone kinetics after oral doses. *Clin Pharmacol Ther.* 1982;31:438–444, with permission.)

    b. The principal metabolite, desethylamiodarone, is pharmacologically active and has a longer elimination half-time than the parent drug, resulting in accumulation of this metabolite with chronic therapy.

3. **Side effects** in patients treated chronically with amiodarone are common, especially when the daily maintenance dose exceeds 400 mg. Screening tests, such as chest radiographs and tests for pulmonary function, thyroid-stimulating hormone, and liver function, are recommended.

    a. **Pulmonary toxicity** (pulmonary alveolitis) is the most serious side effect of amiodarone (estimated at 5% to 15% of treated patients, with a reported mortality of 5% to 10%). The cause of this drug-induced pulmonary toxicity is not known but may reflect the ability of amiodarone to enhance production of free oxygen radicals in the lungs. For this reason, it may be prudent to restrict the inspired concentration of oxygen in patients receiving amiodarone and undergoing general anesthesia to the lowest level capable of maintaining adequate systemic oxygenation.

    b. **Cardiovascular**. Like quinidine and disopyramide, amiodarone may prolong the QTc interval on the ECG, which may lead to an increased incidence of ventricular tachyarrhythmias, including torsades de pointes (proarrhythmic effect). Heart rate often slows and is resistant to treatment with atropine. The potential need for a temporary artificial cardiac (ventricular) pacemaker and administration of a sympathomimetic such as isoproterenol may be a consideration in patients being treated with this drug and scheduled to undergo surgery.

    c. **Ocular, Dermatologic, Neurologic, and Hepatic**. Corneal microdeposits occur in most patients during amiodarone therapy, but visual impairment is unlikely. Optic neuropathy has been found in 1.8% of patients treated with amiodarone compared to 0.3% of the general population. Neurologic toxicity may manifest as peripheral neuropathy, tremors, sleep disturbance, headache, or proximal skeletal muscle weakness. Transient, mild increases in plasma transaminase concentrations may occur, and fatty liver infiltration has been observed.

4. **Pharmacokinetic**
   a. Amiodarone inhibits hepatic P450 enzymes resulting in increased plasma concentrations of digoxin, procainamide, quinidine, warfarin, and cyclosporine.
   b. Amiodarone also displaces digoxin from protein-binding sites. The digoxin dose may be decreased as much as 50% when administered in the presence of amiodarone.
   c. The anticoagulant effects of warfarin are potentiated because amiodarone may directly depress vitamin K–dependent clotting factors.
5. **Endocrine**. Amiodarone contains iodine and has effects on thyroid metabolism, causing either hypothyroidism or hyperthyroidism in 2% to 4% of patients. Amiodarone-induced hyperthyroidism reflecting the release of iodine from the parent drug is often refractory to conventional therapy. When medical management fails, the performance of surgical thyroidectomy provides prompt metabolic control. Bilateral superficial cervical plexus blocks have been described for anesthetic management of subtotal thyroidectomy in these patients.

M. **Dronedarone** is a noniodinated benzofuran derivative of amiodarone that has been developed as an alternative for the treatment of atrial fibrillation and atrial flutter. The clinical use of dronedarone is limited by its contraindication in patients with permanent atrial fibrillation or patients with advanced or recent congestive heart failure exacerbations.

1. **Mechanism of Action**. Dronedarone has the pharmacologic ability to block multiple ion channels. It also has sympatholytic effects.
2. **Metabolism and Excretion**
   a. Dronedarone is well absorbed after oral administration undergoes significant first-pass metabolism that reduces its net bioavailability to 15%.
   b. Dronedarone is a substrate for and a moderate inhibitor of CYP3A4 (should not be coadministered with other CYP3A4 inhibitors such as antifungals, macrolide antibiotics, or protease inhibitors). When coadministered with moderate CYP3A4 inhibitors (verapamil, diltiazem), lower doses of concomitant drugs should be used to avoid severe bradycardia and conduction block.
3. **Side Effects**. The most frequently reported adverse effect of dronedarone is nausea and diarrhea. Treated patients do not have an increased rate of interstitial lung disease, hyperthyroid, or hypothyroidism.

N. **Sotalol** is a nonselective β-adrenergic antagonist drug that is usually restricted for use in patients with life-threatening ventricular tachycardia or fibrillation.

1. **Side Effects.** The most dangerous side effect of sotalol is torsades de pointes. The β blocking effects of sotalol result in decreased myocardial contractility, bradycardia, and delayed conduction of cardiac impulses through the atrioventricular node.

O. **Ibutilide** is effective for the conversion of recent onset atrial fibrillation or atrial flutter to normal sinus rhythm. Polymorphic ventricular tachycardia may occur during ibutilide treatment, especially in patients with predisposing factors (impaired left ventricular function, preexisting prolonged QTc intervals, hypokalemia, hypomagnesemia).

P. **Bretylium** is no longer recommended for treatment of ventricular fibrillation during cardiopulmonary resuscitation as it is less effective than amiodarone.

Q. **Verapamil and Diltiazem**. Verapamil is highly effective in terminating paroxysmal supraventricular tachycardia, controls reentrant tachycardia, and effectively controls the ventricular rate in most patients who develop atrial fibrillation or flutter. Verapamil does not have a depressant effect on accessory tracts and thus will not slow the ventricular response rate in patients with Wolff-Parkinson-White syndrome. Verapamil has little efficacy in the therapy for ventricular ectopic beats. The usual dose of verapamil for suppression of paroxysmal supraventricular tachycardia is 5 to 10 mg IV (75 to 150 μg/kg) over 1 to 3 minutes followed by a continuous infusion of about 5 μg/kg/minute to maintain a sustained effect. The administration of calcium gluconate, 1 g IV, approximately 5 minutes before administration of verapamil may decrease verapamil-induced hypotension without altering the drug's antiarrhythmic effects. Diltiazem, 20 mg IV, produces antiarrhythmic effects similar to those of diazepam, and the potential side effects are similar.

1. **Mechanism of Action**

a. Verapamil and the other calcium channel blockers inhibit the flux of calcium ions across the slow channels of vascular smooth muscle and cardiac cells (manifests as a decreased rate of spontaneous phase 4 depolarization).

b. Verapamil has a substantial depressant effect on the atrioventricular node and a negative chronotropic effect on the sinoatrial node. This drug exerts a negative inotropic effect on cardiac muscle and produces a moderate degree of vasodilation of the coronary arteries and systemic arteries.

2. **Metabolism and Excretion**

   a. An estimated 70% of an injected dose of verapamil is eliminated by the kidneys, whereas up to 15% may be present in the bile.

   b. The need for a large oral dose is related to the extensive hepatic first-pass effect that occurs with the oral route of administration.

3. **Side Effects**

   a. Atrioventricular heart block is more likely in patients with preexisting defects in the conduction of cardiac impulses.

   b. Direct myocardial depression and decreased cardiac output are likely to be exaggerated in patients with poor left ventricular function.

   c. Peripheral vasodilation may contribute to hypotension.

   d. There may be potentiation of anesthetic-produced myocardial depression, and the effects of neuromuscular blocking drugs may be exaggerated.

IX. **Other Cardiac Antiarrhythmic Drugs**

A. **Digitalis**

   1. Digitalis preparations such as digoxin are effective cardiac antiarrhythmics for stabilization of atrial electrical activity and the treatment and prevention of atrial tachyarrhythmias.

   2. Because of their vagolytic effects, these drugs can also slow conduction of cardiac impulses through the atrioventricular node and thus slow the ventricular response rate in patients with atrial fibrillation. Conversely, digitalis preparations enhance conduction of cardiac impulses through accessory bypass tracts and can dangerously increase the ventricular response rate in patients with Wolff-Parkinson-White syndrome.

   3. The usual oral dose of digoxin is 0.5 to 1.0 mg in divided doses over 12 to 24 hours.

   4. Digitalis toxicity is a risk and may manifest as virtually any cardiac arrhythmia (most commonly atrial tachycardia with block).

B. **Adenosine** is an endogenous nucleoside that slows conduction of cardiac impulses through the atrioventricular node, making it an effective alternative to calcium channel blockers (verapamil) for the acute treatment of paroxysmal supraventricular tachycardia, including that due to conduction through accessory pathways in patients with Wolff-Parkinson-White syndrome. This drug is not effective in the treatment of atrial fibrillation, atrial flutter, or ventricular tachycardia. The usual dose of adenosine is 6 mg IV followed, if necessary, by a repeat injection of 6 to 12 mg IV about 3 minutes later. Adenosine receptors represent a logical target for treatment of pain.

1. **Mechanism of Action**
   a. Adenosine stimulates cardiac adenosine$_1$ receptors to increase potassium ion currents, shorten the action potential duration, and hyperpolarize cardiac cell membranes.
   b. Its short-lived cardiac effects (elimination half-time 10 seconds) are due to carrier-mediated cellular uptake and metabolism to inosine by adenosine deaminase.
   c. Methylxanthines inhibit the actions of adenosine by binding to adenosine$_1$ receptors. Conversely, dipyridamole (adenosine uptake inhibitor) and cardiac transplantation (denervation hypersensitivity) potentiate the effects of adenosine.

2. **Side Effects**
   a. Adenosine may produce transient atrioventricular heart block.
   b. Bronchospasm, although an uncommon complication, has been observed after the IV administration of adenosine, even in the absence of preexisting symptoms (use with caution, if at all, in patients known to have active wheezing).
   c. The pharmacologic effects of adenosine are antagonized by methylxanthines (theophylline, caffeine) and potentiated by dipyridamole.

C. **Ranolazine** has been noted to have efficacy in treatment of atrial arrhythmias and suppression of nonsustained ventricular tachycardia and for the adjunctive treatment of chronic stable angina.

CHAPTER 22

Diuretics

I. **Introduction.** Most diuretics produce their clinical effect by blocking sodium (Na^+) reabsorption in different locations of the nephron, resulting in increased sodium ion delivery to the distal tubules (Fig. 22-1).

II. **Carbonic Anhydrase Inhibitors**

A. Acetazolamide is the prototype of a class of sulfonamide drugs that bind avidly to the enzyme carbonic anhydrase, producing noncompetitive inhibition of enzyme activity, principally in the proximal renal tubules as well as the collecting ducts (Table 22-1) (see Fig. 22-1).

1. **Pharmacokinetics and Pharmacodynamics.** After oral administration, acetazolamide is excreted unchanged by the kidneys (dose should be adjusted in patients with renal failure and the elderly). Acetazolamide completely blocks membrane-bound and cytoplasmic carbonic anhydrase in the proximal tubule and to a lesser extent in the collecting ducts, preventing Na^+ and HCO_3^- absorption. This increased excretion of HCO_3^- results in an alkaline urine and metabolic acidosis.

2. **Clinical Uses**

a. In addition to its diuretic properties, acetazolamide is administered to decrease intraocular pressure in the treatment of glaucoma.

b. Formation of cerebrospinal fluid is inhibited by acetazolamide and it has been used in the treatment of idiopathic intracranial hypertension.

c. Acetazolamide may be beneficial in the management of familial periodic paralysis because the drug-induced metabolic acidosis increases the local concentration of potassium in skeletal muscles.

d. Acetazolamide, by producing metabolic acidosis, may stimulate the respiratory drive in patients who are hypoventilating in a compensatory response to respiratory alkalosis, as occurs with altitude sickness.

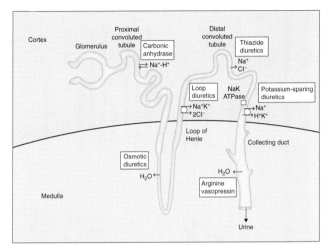

FIGURE 22-1 The sites of action of the different diuretics.

3. **Side Effects**
   a. There is a high incidence of systemic side effects associated with the use of acetazolamide (fatigue, decreased appetite, depression, paresthesias), which could be secondary to the development of acidosis.
   b. Acetazolamide dose should be reduced in patients with chronic renal insufficiency and avoided in patients with severe chronic renal insufficiency because of the increased risk of metabolic acidosis.

III. **Loop diuretics are first-line therapy in patients with fluid retention resulting from heart failure.**
   A. **Pharmacokinetics and Pharmacodynamics**
   1. **Furosemide** is effective when administered orally (absorption varies between patients from 10% to 100%, with an average bioavailability of 50%) or intravenously. Furosemide has a rapid onset, producing diuresis within 5 to 10 minutes of administration, with a peak effect at 30 minutes and duration of action of 2 to 6 hours. In patients with normal renal function, 40 mg of intravenous (IV) furosemide will produce maximal natriuresis.

Table 22-1

Diuretics and Their Sites of Action

	Receptors	Main Site of Action	Clinical Uses	Notable Side Effects
Carbonic anhydrase	Carbonic anhydrase	Proximal convoluted tubule	Altitude sickness Glaucoma	Metabolic acidosis
Loop diuretics	Na-K-2Cl cotransport	Medullary thick ascending loop of Henle	First-line diuretics in renal impairment	Ototoxicity Alkalosis Hypokalemia
Thiazides	Na-Cl cotransport	Cortical ascending loop of Henle	First line therapy of hypertension	Alkalosis Hypokalemia Diabetes and dyslipidemia Hyperuricemia
Osmotic diuretics		Proximal convoluted tubule and loop of Henle	Increased intracranial pressure Oxygen free radical scavenging	Volume overload in CHF patients Hypokalemia, hyponatremia, hypomagnesemia
Potassium-sparing diuretics	Epithelial Na channel	Collecting duct	Adjuncts to loop diuretics or thiazides	Hyperkalemia
Aldosterone blockers	Na-K-ATPase	Collecting duct	Heart failure with low ejection fraction	Hyperkalemia

Table 22-1

Diuretics and Their Sites of Action *(continued)*

	Receptors	Main Site of Action	Clinical Uses	Notable Side Effects
Dopamine and fenoldopam	D1	Proximal tubule and loop of Henle	Renal protection and hypertension treatment in critically ill patients	Effectiveness not substantiated
Brain natriuretic peptide	Na-K-ATPase	Collecting duct	Management of decompensated heart failure	
Vasopressin	V_2	Collecting duct	SIADH, CHF, cirrhosis	
Aquaporins	AQP	Collecting duct		

CHF, congestive heart failure; SIADH, syndrome of inappropriate antidiuretic hormone.

2. **Bumetanide and Torasemide**
   a. Bumetanide is 40 times more potent than furosemide except in its effect on potassium excretion.
   b. Torasemide is twice as potent as furosemide and has a longer duration of action allowing for a once a day dosing regimen.

B. **Clinical Uses**
   1. Loop diuretics are the first line of treatment of hypertension in patients with renal insufficiency. The antihypertensive effect of loop diuretics is due to their ability to decrease intravascular fluid volume and eliminate salt. Compared to furosemide, the long-acting drug azosemide produces better blood pressure control while preserving the normal 10% decline in blood pressure in many individuals that occurs at night (nocturnal dipping).
   2. Loop diuretics are commonly used in patients admitted with acute exacerbation of heart failure. Diuresis leads to loss of water and salt with resulting decrease in intravascular volume thus lowering ventricular filling pressure and reducing pulmonary edema.
   3. Furosemide decreases intracranial pressure by inducing systemic diuresis and decreasing cerebrospinal fluid production. Furosemide can be administered as single-drug therapy (0.5 to 1.0 mg/kg IV) or as a lower dose (0.1 to 0.3 mg/kg IV) in combination with mannitol (combination of furosemide and mannitol is more effective in decreasing intracranial pressure than either drug alone but severe dehydration and electrolyte imbalance are also more likely).

C. **Side effects** of loop diuretics most often manifest as abnormalities of fluid and electrolyte balance (can lead to hypokalemia and increase the likelihood of digitalis toxicity).
   1. Acute or chronic treatment of patients with diuretics, including loop diuretics, may result in tolerance to the diuretic effect ("braking phenomenon").
      a. Acute tolerance is presumed to reflect activation of the renin-angiotensin system to retain sodium and water in the presence of a contracted extracellular fluid volume.
      b. With chronic use of diuretics, there is evidence of a compensatory hypertrophy of those portions of the renal tubule (especially distal convoluted tubules) responsible for sodium retention, leading to decreased diuretic effectiveness. When tolerance develops in a

patient treated chronically with furosemide, it may be possible to reestablish a diuretic effect with the administration of a thiazide diuretic, which blocks the hypertrophied Na^+ reabsorption sites.

2. Loop diuretics should only be administered to patients with a normal or increased intravascular fluid volume. Hypotension may result from administration of loop diuretics to hypovolemic patients exacerbating renal ischemic injury and concentrating nephrotoxins in the renal tubules.

3. Furosemide increases renal tissue concentrations of aminoglycosides and enhances the possible nephrotoxic effects of these antibiotics. Cephalosporin nephrotoxicity may also be increased by furosemide.

4. Loop diuretics potentiate nondepolarizing neuromuscular blockade.

5. The renal clearance of lithium is decreased in the presence of diuretic-induced decreases in sodium reabsorption, and plasma concentrations of lithium may be acutely increased by the IV administration of furosemide in the perioperative period.

6. Ototoxicity, either transient or permanent, is a rare, dose-dependent complication associated with the use of loop diuretics.

IV. **Thiazide diuretics are most often administered for long-term treatment of essential hypertension in which the combination of diuresis, natriuresis, and vasodilation are synergistic (thiazides are usually administered in combination with other antihypertensives).**

    A. **Pharmacokinetics and Pharmacodynamics** (see Fig. 22-1)

        1. Thiazide diuretics are readily absorbed when administered orally (hydrochlorothiazide has a 60% to 70% bioavailability).

        2. Thiazides' effectiveness markedly decreases in patients with renal insufficiency.

        3. Thiazide diuretics have a long half-life of 8 to 12 hours, allowing for a convenient once-a-day dosing.

    B. **Clinical Uses**

        1. Thiazide diuretics are recommended as first-line therapy for essential hypertension and the use of chlorthalidone specifically has been shown to decrease the risk of major cardiovascular events. The antihypertensive effect of thiazide diuretics is due initially to a decrease in extracellular fluid volume, often with a decrease in cardiac

Table 22-2

Side Effects of Thiazide Diuretics

Hypokalemic, hypochloremic, metabolic alkalosis
Cardiac dysrhythmias (hypokalemia or hypomagnesemia)
Hypercalcemia (patients receiving calcium supplements)
Potentiate nondepolarizing muscle relaxants (hypokalemia)
Decreased efficacy in presence of nonsteroidal anti-inflammatory drugs
Promote lithium reabsorption (risk of lithium toxicity)
Glucose intolerance (aggravate glucose control especially in combination with β blockers)
Orthostatic hypotension (hypovolemia)

output, which normalizes after several weeks. The sustained antihypertensive effect of thiazide diuretics is due to peripheral vasodilation, which requires several weeks to develop.

2. Because they stimulate calcium reabsorption, thiazide diuretics are used in the treatment of calcium-containing renal calculi.

C. **Side Effects** (Table 22-2)

V. **Osmotic diuretics (mannitol, urea, isosorbide, glycerin) are inert substances that do not undergo metabolism and are filtered freely at the glomerulus. Their administration causes increased plasma and renal tubular fluid osmolality, with resulting osmotic diuresis.**

A. **Mannitol** is the only osmotic diuretic in current use. Structurally, mannitol is a six-carbon sugar alcohol that does not undergo metabolism.

1. **Pharmacokinetics and Pharmacodynamics.** After administration, mannitol is completely filtered at the glomeruli, and none of the filtered drug is subsequently reabsorbed from the renal tubules. By increasing tubular fluid osmolality, it decreases water reabsorption and promotes water diuresis.

2. **Clinical Uses**

a. Mannitol is used primarily in the acute management of elevated intracranial pressure and in the treatment of glaucoma. Mannitol decreases intracranial pressure by increasing plasma osmolarity, which draws water from tissues, including the brain, along an osmotic gradient. Mannitol begins to exert an effect within 10 to 15 minutes, with a peak effect at 30 to 45 minutes and a duration of 6 hours. An intact blood–brain barrier is necessary for the cerebral effects of mannitol. If the blood–brain barrier is not intact, mannitol may enter the brain, drawing fluid with it and causing worsening of the cerebral edema. In addition, a rebound increase in intracranial pressure may occur following mannitol use.

b. Mannitol has been used to prevent perioperative kidney failure in the setting of acute tubular necrosis.

c. Mannitol also has free radical scavenging properties, which may protect transplanted kidneys following reperfusion.

d. Despite its common use during cardiac and major vascular surgery for renal protection, it has not been shown to prevent perioperative acute renal failure.

3. **Side Effects**

a. The initial increase in intravascular volume associated with the administration of mannitol may be poorly tolerated in patients with left ventricular dysfunction, leading to pulmonary edema (furosemide may be a preferred drug for treatment of increased intracranial pressure in patients with left ventricular dysfunction).

b. Prolonged use of mannitol may cause hypovolemia, electrolyte disturbances with hypokalemic hypochloremic alkalosis, and plasma hyperosmolarity due to excessive excretion of water and sodium.

VI. **Potassium-Sparing Diuretics.** Potassium-sparing diuretics act on the collecting ducts and are grouped in two categories: pteridine analogs (triamterene, amiloride) and aldosterone receptor blockers (spironolactone, eplerenone).

A. **Pharmacokinetics and Pharmacodynamics.** Oral absorption of amiloride and triamterene is limited (25% and 50%, respectively). Amiloride is more potent than triamterene and is not metabolized but excreted unchanged in the kidneys. Triamterene is a pteridine with a structural resemblance to folic acid.

B. **Clinical Uses.** Potassium-sparing diuretics are most often used in combination with loop diuretics or thiazide diuretics to augment diuresis and limit renal loss of potassium.

C. **Side Effects.** Hyperkalemia is the principal side effect of therapy with potassium-sparing diuretics, especially when combined with angiotensin-converting enzyme inhibitors or angiotensin II receptor blockers or in presence of non-steroidal anti-inflammatory drugs.

VII. **Aldosterone Antagonists. Spironolactone bears a close structural resemblance to aldosterone and results in potassium-sparing diuresis. Eplerone is a selective aldosterone receptor blocker and has less affinity for other mineralocorticoid receptors and is less potent than spironolactone.**

A. **Pharmacokinetics and Pharmacodynamics**. Spironolactone and eplerenone are the only diuretics that do not need to reach the renal tubule to exert their effect (they provide competitive blockade of epithelial aldosterone receptors in the distal tubule and the collecting duct).

B. **Clinical Uses**

1. Spironolactone and eplerenone are often prescribed for the treatment of essential hypertension, in combination with thiazides, particularly in patients with a low renin state (African Americans, the elderly, and diabetics) or patients with metabolic syndrome (group of risk factors that raises risk for heart disease).

2. The combination of spironolactone with a thiazide diuretic results in improved diuresis and blood pressure control, in addition to prevention of the thiazide-induced hypokalemia and hypomagnesemia.

3. Spironolactone and eplerenone are used in the treatment of patients demonstrating "aldosterone escape," which results from incomplete aldosterone blockade during antihypertensive therapy with blockers of the renin-angiotensin-aldosterone system.

C. **Side Effects**

1. Hyperkalemia, especially in the presence of impaired renal function, is the most serious side effect of treatment with spironolactone (combination of spironolactone with angiotensin-converting enzyme inhibitors can exacerbate hyperkalemia in these patients).

2. Spironolactone can block androgen and progesterone receptors, leading to gynecomastia and breast tenderness.

VIII. **Dopamine receptor agonists (dopamine, fenoldopam) result in natriuresis and increased renal blood flow via their actions on renal tubular dopamine-1 (D_1) receptors.**

A. **Pharmacokinetics and Pharmacodynamics**

1. Endogenous dopamine is synthesized locally in the epithelial cells of the renal tubules and exerts its effect

directly. Activation of D_1 receptors in the proximal renal tubule and in the loop of Henle increases cyclic adenosine monophosphate formation, resulting in inhibition of the Na^+-H^+ exchange and Na^+-K^+-ATPase pump. In addition, D_1 receptors mediate an increase in renal blood flow leading to a small increase in glomerular filtration rate.

2. With increasing doses of dopamine, sympathetic activation begins to predominate (β activation results in increased inotropy, increased cardiac output, and elevation in systemic blood pressure and at even higher doses, α activation prevails, leading to vasoconstriction).

3. Fenoldopam is a fast-acting IV antihypertensive used in the short-term treatment of patients with severe hypertension. Fenoldopam is a relatively selective D_1 receptor agonist with moderate affinity to α_2 receptors. It has no effect on D_2, β, or α_1 receptors.

B. **Clinical Uses**

1. Dopamine is used to maintain renal blood flow in patients in cardiogenic shock with low or normal systemic vascular resistance. Similarly, fenoldopam is used for its renal vasodilation properties and, even at higher doses, it lacks sympathetic activity, thus it is used to treat resistant hypertension.

2. Both drugs have been used at very low doses to provide renal protection in high-risk patients, such as after cardiac or major vascular surgery, or following radioiodine contrast injection (randomized trials have not found a reduction in the incidence of perioperative acute renal failure).

IX. **Natriuretic Peptides.** Atrial natriuretic peptide and brain natriuretic peptide are normally produced in the atria and ventricles of the heart, respectively, in response to myocardial wall stretch. They exert their diuretic effect on the collecting duct of the kidneys.

X. **Vasopressin receptor antagonists,** or vaptans, competitively inhibit V_2 receptor in the renal collecting duct, thereby leading to decreased water reabsorption.

XI. **Neprilysin Antagonists.** Neprilysin (NEP) is a ubiquitous, membrane-bound metalloproteinase with greatest concentration in cardiovascular tissues and the kidneys. Specific NEP inhibition has been shown to increase circulating levels of natriuretic peptides, thus promoting natriuresis and also reducing the cardiovascular remodeling that is inherent to end-stage heart failure.

XII. Aquaporin Modulators. Aquaporins are recently described membrane channels facilitating water movement across cells in response to osmotic gradient.

CHAPTER 23

Lipid-Lowering Drugs

I. **Lipoprotein Metabolism. Lipoproteins are macromolecular lipid protein complexes responsible for the transport of lipids to and from the peripheral tissues (Table 23-1). Lipoprotein metabolism can be divided into the exogenous and endogenous pathways (Fig. 23-1).**

II. **Lipid Disorders**

   A. Familial hypercholesterolemia arises from a defect in the gene for low-density lipoprotein receptors (LDL-R). Heterozygotes for this defect experience accelerated atherosclerosis and represent about 1 in 500 persons.

   B. Hyperlipidemia may also arise from secondary causes including obesity, diabetes, alcohol abuse, hypothyroidism, glucocorticoid excess, and hepatic or renal dysfunction.

   C. Most cases of hyperlipidemia in adults arise from a combination of secondary causes, genetic predisposition, and environmental factors, including poor diet and a lack of exercise.

   D. It has been recognized for several decades that increased plasma concentrations of total and LDL cholesterol are associated with an increased risk of cardiovascular disease. Conversely, higher high-density lipoprotein (HDL) cholesterol levels appear to reduce the risk of atherosclerosis and cardiovascular events because of the critical role of HDL in reverse cholesterol transport. The safety and efficacy of 3-hydroxy-3-methylglutaryl coenzyme A reductase (HMG-CoA reductase) inhibitors, or statins, have been particularly well established (Table 23-2).

III. **Drugs for Treatment of Hyperlipidemia (Table 23-3)**

   A. **Statins** are drugs that act as inhibitors of HMG-CoA reductase, the enzyme that catalyzes the rate-limiting step of cholesterol biosynthesis in which HMG-CoA is converted to mevalonate (see Fig. 23-1). The drugs in this class (atorvastatin, fluvastatin, lovastatin, pravastatin, simvastatin, and

Table 23-1

Classification of Lipoproteins

Lipoprotein	Density (g/mL)	Diameter (nm)
Chylomicrons	<0.95	75–1,200
Very-low-density lipoproteins (VLDL)	0.95–1.006	30–90
Intermediate-density lipoproteins (IDL)	1.006–1.019	~30
Low-density lipoproteins (LDL)	1.019–1.063	~20
High-density lipoproteins (HDL)	1.063–1.21	8–12

rosuvastatin) are considered equivalent and relatively free of side effects. Randomized clinical trials have shown that statins lower cardiac events in patients with or without atherosclerosis. The reduction in cardiac events observed with statin use may not be only secondary to the LDL lowering effects. Statins are thought to stabilize existing atherosclerotic plaques and there is evidence that statins have many

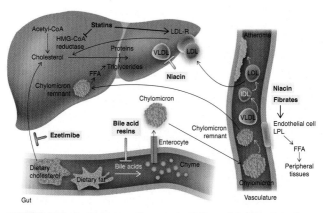

FIGURE 23-1 A diagrammatic representation of lipid metabolism. T-shaped markers indicate inhibition, arrow-shaped markers indicate enhancement.

Table 23-2

Statin Benefit Groups

1. Clinical evidence of ASCVD
2. LDL-C >190 mg/dL
3. Age 40–75 years with diabetes and an LDL-C 70–189 mg/dL
4. Age 40–75 years without diabetes, an LDL-C 70–189 mg/dL, and an estimated 10-year risk of ASCVD >7.5% (10-year risk of ASCVD based on Pooled Cohort Equations available at my.americanheart.org/cvriskcalculator)

ASCVD, atherosclerotic cardiovascular disease; LDL-C, low-density lipoprotein cholesterol.
Adapted from Stone NJ, Robinson JG, Lichtenstein AH, et al. 2013 ACC/AHA guideline on the treatment of blood cholesterol to reduce atherosclerotic cardiovascular risk in adults: a report of the American College of Cardiology/American Heart Association Task Force on Practice Guidelines. *Circulation.* 2014;63(25, pt B):2889–2934.

pleiotropic effects, including antiinflammatory, antioxidant, and vasodilatory properties.

1. **Pharmacokinetics**
   a. Statins are variably absorbed from the gastrointestinal tract following oral ingestion.
   b. Lovastatin and simvastatin are prodrugs that require metabolism to the open β-hydroxy acid form to be pharmacologically active.

Table 23-3

Drugs for Treatment of Hyperlipidemia

	LDL	HDL	Triglycerides
Diet change	↓10%–15%	Variable increase	↓10%–20%
Statins	↓20%–60%	↑10%–15%	↓10%–20%
Bile acids resins	↓15%–30%	↑3%–5%	No change or mild increase
Fibrates	↓5%–20% or increase	↑10%–35%	↓40%–50%
Ezetimibe	↓18%–22%	↑1%–3%	↓8%–12%
Niacin	↓15%–30%	↑20%–30%	↓20%–50%

      c. All of the statins are highly protein bound with the exception of pravastatin.

      d. Except for pravastatin, all of the statins undergo extensive metabolism by hepatic P450 enzymes.

  2. **Side Effects**. Statins are usually well tolerated with the most common complaints being gastrointestinal upset, fatigue, and headache.

      a. **Muscle-Related Adverse Effects**. The most common adverse side effects from statins are skeletal muscle related (can range in severity from simple myalgias to myositis with mild creatine kinase elevation to life-threatening rhabdomyolysis) (Table 23-4). Myopathy appears to be most frequent in patients treated with simvastatin and lovastatin. Drugs likely to be administered during anesthesia, including succinylcholine, have not been shown to increase the incidence of statin-induced myopathy.

      b. **Hepatic Dysfunction**. Persistent increases in plasma aminotransferase concentrations occur in 0.5% to 2% of treated patients and are dose-dependent.

B. **Bile acid resins** are effective for the treatment of lipid disorders in which the primary abnormality is an increased plasma LDL cholesterol concentration with a normal or near normal triglyceride level. These drugs in this class have a low potential for toxicity and are well tolerated.

  1. **Side Effects**

      a. Palatability and constipation are common complaints in patients being treated with cholestyramine.

      b. Because cholestyramine is a chloride form of an ion exchange resin, hyperchloremic acidosis can occur, especially in younger and smaller patients in whom the relative dose is larger.

Table 23-4

Statin Myotoxicity Risk Factors

1. Age >80 years
2. Female sex
3. Asian ancestry
4. Renal/hepatic failure
5. Excessive alcohol use
6. History of prior muscle disease
7. Poorly controlled hypothyroidism

        c. Absorption of fat-soluble vitamins as well as other pharmacologic agents may be impaired.

C. **Niacin** (nicotinic acid) is a water-soluble B complex vitamin that inhibits synthesis of very-low-density lipoproteins in the liver by an unknown mechanism. In addition, niacin inhibits release of free fatty acids from adipose tissue and increases the activity of lipoprotein lipase. The result of these effects is a dose-related 15% to 30% decrease in plasma LDL cholesterol concentrations, a 20% to 50% decrease in triglycerides, and a 20% to 30% increase in HDL.

    1. **Pharmacokinetics**. Niacin is readily absorbed from the gastrointestinal tract and undergoes extensive hepatic first-pass metabolism.

    2. **Side Effects**. Niacin, unlike the resins and statins, has many side effects, which may limit its usefulness.

        a. The most common side effect is intense prostaglandin-induced cutaneous flushing that occurs in about 10% of patients.

        b. Hepatic dysfunction manifesting as increased plasma transaminase activity and cholestatic jaundice may be associated with large doses of niacin (not recommended for administration to patients with liver disease).

        c. Hyperglycemia and abnormal glucose tolerance may occur in nondiabetic patients treated with niacin.

        d. Niacin may exaggerate the orthostatic hypotension associated with antihypertensive drugs and the myopathy associated with statins.

D. **Fibrates** are derivatives of fibric acid and are the most effective drugs for decreasing plasma concentrations of triglycerides. In the postoperative period, treatment with fibrates is restarted when the patient is well hydrated and able to ingest oral medications. Fibrates produce a dose-dependent 40% to 50% decrease in plasma triglycerides and 10% to 35% increase in HDL concentrations, whereas the effect on LDL concentrations is variable. Drug-induced increases in the activity of lipoprotein lipase is the likely mechanism for the triglyceride lowering effects of these drugs.

    1. **Pharmacokinetics**

        a. Gemfibrozil is well absorbed from the gastrointestinal tract following oral administration.

        b. Fenofibrate is a prodrug that is hydrolyzed by esterases to the active metabolite, fenofibric acid. Increased plasma concentrations of liver transaminase enzymes are more likely to occur with fenofibrate than with the other fibrates.

2. **Side Effects**
   a. The most common side effects of the fibrates are gastrointestinal (abdominal pain, nausea) and headache.
   b. Gemfibrozil increases the cholesterol content of bile (lithogenicity) and may increase the formation of gallstones.
   c. The incidence of skeletal muscle myopathy and risk of rhabdomyolysis is increased when this drug is administered in combination with statins, especially lovastatin.
   d. The anticoagulant effect of warfarin is potentiated by gemfibrozil, presumably reflecting its displacement from binding sites on albumin.
   e. A mild increase in plasma transaminase enzymes may occur in treated patients. Considering the dependence on renal excretion for elimination and occasional increases in liver function tests, it may be prudent to avoid administration of this drug to patients with preexisting renal or hepatic disease.

E. **Ezetimibe** acts as a selective inhibitor of cholesterol absorption, which leads to a secondary upregulation of LDL-R.

F. **Omega-3 Fatty Acids (Fish Oil).** The primary effect of this fatty acid is to decrease plasma concentrations of triglycerides. Fish oil supplements are not regarded as drugs and thus are not regulated by the U.S. Food and Drug Administration. The long-term safety of taking fish oil capsules is not known, and there is no evidence that fish oil supplementation prevents heart disease.

CHAPTER 24

Gas Exchange

I. **Introduction.** During surgery, an applied respiratory physiologist and an understanding of the physiology and pharmacology pertaining to the respiratory system is fundamental to anesthetic management.

II. Functional Anatomy
   A. **Upper Airway Anatomy and Gas Flow**
      1. **Oropharynx and Nasopharynx**
         a. The air passages extending from the nares and lips through the nasopharynx and oropharynx, through the larynx to the cricoid cartilage make up the functional upper airway. The upper airway serves a host of functions: warming and humidifying passing air, filtering particulate matter, and preventing aspiration.
         b. The upper airway mucosa is highly vascular and well innervated (must be appreciated when performing nasopharyngeal intubation with endotracheal tubes, nasogastric sumps or feeding tubes, or fiberoptic bronchoscopes).
         c. The pharynx is 12- to 15-cm long and is divided into the nasopharynx, the oropharynx, and the laryngopharynx (lying posterior to the larynx). The supine position, sleep, and general anesthesia may promote obstruction of the oropharynx by the tongue, soft palate, and pharyngeal musculature as their tone decreases.
      2. **Larynx**
         a. The larynx is a complex structure that lies anterior to the 4th to the 6th cervical vertebrae and consists of several muscles, their ligaments, and associated cartilaginous structures (Fig. 24-1).
         b. The larynx serves as the organ of phonation, plays an important role in coughing, and in airway protection from aspiration.

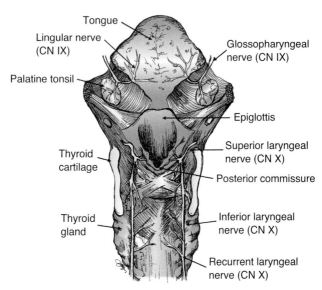

FIGURE 24-1 Diagram of the larynx from the base of the tongue to below the thyroid cartilage as viewed from its posterior aspect. Note the relationship of the superior laryngeal, inferior laryngeal, and recurrent laryngeal nerves and the posterior aspect of the larynx, thyroid, and trachea. Tracheal and thyroid surgery places these nerves at risk. (From Jaeger JM. Blank RS. Essential anatomy and physiology of the respiratory system and pulmonary circulation. In: Slinger P, ed. *Principles and Practice of Anesthesia for Thoracic Surgery.* New York, NY: Springer; 2011:51–69, with permission.)

    c. The paired vocal cords attach posteriorly to the vocal process of each arytenoid and anteriorly meet at the junction of the thyroepiglottic ligament of the anterior portion of the thyroid cartilage. The triangular opening formed by the vocal ligaments is the glottis with its apex anteriorly (Fig. 24-2).

  B. **Pharyngeal Innervation.** Innervation of the pharynx is supplied via sensory and motor branches of the glossopharyngeal nerve (CN IX) and vagus nerve (CN X) (external and internal branches of the superior laryngeal nerves, recurrent laryngeal nerves).

  C. **Tracheal and Bronchial Structure**

    1. The trachea originates at the cricoid cartilage (at the level of vertebra C6) and extends approximately 10 to

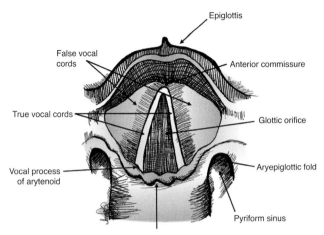

FIGURE 24-2 Diagram of the glottis as seen from above using a laryngoscope or fiberoptic bronchoscope. Note the triangular-shaped glottic introitus with its narrowest aspect at the anterior commissure. Passage of bronchoscopes, endotracheal tubes, and especially, double-lumen tubes should be directed posteriorly where the vocal cords will spread the widest. Note that the vocal process of the arytenoid cartilage pivots on a small point and can be traumatized and displaced with rough handling. (From Jaeger JM, Blank RS. Essential anatomy and physiology of the respiratory system and pulmonary circulation. In: Slinger P, ed. *Principles and Practice of Anesthesia for Thoracic Surgery*. New York, NY: Springer; 2011:51–69, with permission.)

12 cm (females) and 12 to 14 cm (males) to terminate in a bifurcation (carina) at the T4/5 vertebral level (2nd intercostal space, the angle of Louis) (Fig. 24-3).

2. The right main bronchus is wider (16 vs. 13 mm), shorter (1.5 to 2.5 vs. 4.5 to 5 cm) and more vertical than the left (Fig. 24-4).

D. **Respiratory Airways and Alveoli**. The airways continue to divide into smaller diameter conduits until one arrives at the bronchioles with diameters less than 0.8 mm. The immune defenses of the lung are extremely important because of the direct exposure of this organ to the external environment via the airways. Exaggerated inflammatory response and the activity of these cells and others may be harmful to the lung; acute respiratory distress syndrome (ARDS) and emphysema are examples.

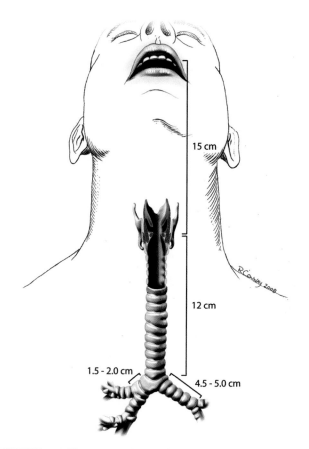

FIGURE 24-3 The average length from the incisors to the vocal cords is approximately 15 cm, and the distance from the vocal cords to the tracheal carina is 12 cm. The average distance from the tracheal carina to the take-off of the right upper bronchus is 2.0 cm in men and 1.5 cm in women. The distance from the tracheal carina to the take-off of the left upper and left lower lobe is approximately 5.0 cm in men and 4.5 cm in women. These anatomic distances apply to individuals with a height of 170 cm. (From Campos J. Lung isolation in patients with difficult airways. In: Slinger P, ed. *Principles and Practice of Anesthesia for Thoracic Surgery*. New York, NY: Springer; 2011:247–258, with permission.)

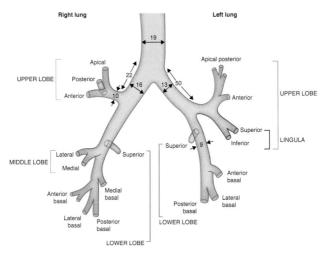

FIGURE 24-4 Diagram of the trachea, lobar, and segmental bronchi showing median lengths and diameters for a 170 cm height patient. The lengths and diameters of the bronchi vary considerably between individuals.

III. **Pulmonary Circulation**
  A. Blood flow through the pulmonary circulation is normally equal to the blood flow through the systemic circulation (a major exception being intracardiac shunting when it exceeds systemic circulation).
  B. Pressures in the pulmonary circulation are normally lower than the systemic circulation because the pulmonary vascular resistance (PVR) is lower than the systemic resistance (approximately one-sixth of systemic resistance).
  C. Only one-third of the bronchial circulation returns to the systemic venous system; the remainder drains into the pulmonary veins and this constitutes the largest portion of the normal extrapulmonary venoarterial shunt. This bronchial shunt is less than 1% of the cardiac output in healthy individuals but may increase to 10% in bronchiectasis, emphysema, and some congenital cardiac conditions.

IV. **Thorax and Muscles of Respiration.** The bony thorax is composed of the 12 ribs, the sternum anteriorly, and the thoracic vertebral column posteriorly. The caudal end of the thorax is formed by the diaphragm, and the cranial end of the thorax is the thoracic inlet, within the ring formed by the first ribs, containing the trachea, esophagus, and the neurovascular supply to the head and arms. Bulk movement of air into and out of the lungs occurs as a result of changes in intrathoracic pressure created by rhythmic changes in the volume of the thorax. Expansion of the chest cavity occurs when three respiratory muscle groups (diaphragm, intercostal, and accessory) work in concert.

A. **Inspiration**

1. The diaphragm is unique in that its muscle fibers radiate from a central tendinous structure to insert peripherally on the ventrolateral aspect of the first three lumbar vertebrae, the aponeurotic arcuate ligaments, the xiphoid process, and the upper margins of the lower six ribs.

2. Contraction of the diaphragm causes a large caudal displacement of the central tendon resulting in a longitudinal expansion of the chest cavity.

3. The fall in pleural pressure and accompanying lung expansion produce an increase in abdominal pressure and outward movement of the abdominal wall. The supine and Trendelenburg positions or surgical retractors can significantly interfere with this abdominal motion especially in the morbidly obese, necessitating controlled ventilation under anesthesia.

B. **Expiration** is a passive process in quiet breathing and is largely the response to relaxation of the inspiratory muscles and the balance of forces generated by the elastic recoil of the lungs and chest wall.

1. When high levels of ventilation are required as in exercise or if airway resistance increases (as in exacerbations of asthma or COPD), the expiratory phase becomes an active process with forceful contraction of the rectus abdominis, the transverse abdominis, and the internal and external oblique muscles.

2. Innervation of the abdominal musculature is from thoracic nerves 7 through 12 and the first lumbar nerve.

V. **Respiratory Mechanical Function.** The basics of mechanical function of the respiratory system are the interaction of two opposing springs: the chest wall, which at rest is trying to expand, and the lungs, which at rest are trying to contract. The lungs and chest wall move together as a unit (made possible by the enclosed, air-tight thoracic cavity where the outer surface of the lungs and its visceral pleura are in close proximity to the parietal pleura, covering the inner surface of the chest wall and the mediastinal structures). The volume of gas contained in the lungs at this resting point is termed *functional residual capacity* (FRC). For a healthy young adult male, total lung capacity (TLC) will be approximately 6 to 6.5 L and FRC will be 2.5 to 3 L. The oxygen contained in the FRC (500 to 600 mL) is the only reservoir of oxygen in the body. Pathologic conditions such as the introduction of air or blood into the intrapleural space (pneumothorax, empyema, pleural effusion, bronchopleural fistula) can rapidly disrupt this lung–chest wall interaction, leading to a compromise in respiratory function but also interfere with cardiovascular function.

A. **Lung Volumes and Spirometry**

1. By convention, the static and dynamic subdivisions of gas contained within the lung are given a common nomenclature of volumes and capacities (Table 24-1) (Fig. 24-5).

Table 24-1

Lung Volumes and Capacities

Lung Volumes	Definition
Tidal volume (V_T)	Air volume inspired and expired during a relaxed breathing cycle
Residual volume (RV)	Volume remaining in the lung after a maximal expiratory effort
Expiratory reserve volume (ERV)	The volume of air that can be forcibly exhaled between the resting end-expiratory volume and RV
Inspiratory reserve volume (IRV)	The volume of air that can be inspired with maximal effort above the normal resting end-expiratory position of a V_T
Forced expiratory volume in 1 second (FEV_1)	The volume of air that can be exhaled in 1 second with maximal effort from the point of maximal inspiration
Lung Capacities	
Vital capacity (VC)	The amount of air that can be exhaled from the point of maximal inspiration to the point of maximal expiration (IRV + ERV)
Forced vital capacity (FVC)	The volume of air that can be exhaled with maximal effort from TLC
Total lung capacity (TLC)	Total volume of air in the lungs after a maximal inspiration (IRV + ERV + RV)
Functional residual capacity (FRC)	Amount of air in the lung at the end of a quiet exhalation (ERV + RV)

Lung volumes and capacities

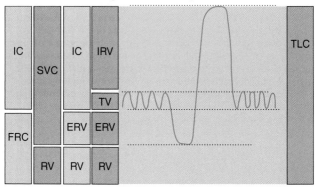

FIGURE 24-5 Complete pulmonary function testing will provide data on lung volumes and capacities to differentiate obstructive from restrictive lung diseases. IC, inspiratory capacity; RV, residual volume; SVC, slow vital capacity; ERV, expiratory reserve volume; TV, tidal volume; IRV, inspiratory reserve volume; TLC, total lung capacity. Functional residual capacity (FRC) = ERV + RV. Measuring closing volume and closing capacity requires insoluble gas washout techniques and is not included in routine pulmonary function testing. However, an appreciation of the variable relationship between closing capacity and FRC and the effects of anesthesia on FRC are essential for the anesthesiologist to understand the changes in gas exchange that occur during anesthesia. (From Slinger P, Darling G. Preanesthetic assessment for thoracic surgery. In: Slinger P, ed. *Principles and Practice of Anesthesia for Thoracic Surgery*. New York, NY: Springer; 2011:11–34, with permission.)

2. Volumes are most commonly measured by spirometry (Figs. 24-6 and 24-7) and capacities are then calculated as the sum of specific volumes.
3. Complete pulmonary function testing in the laboratory will commonly report measurements of volume ratios, flows, lung resistance, and lung diffusion capacity for carbon monoxide (DLCO).

B. **Closing Capacity and Closing Volume**
1. The key to understanding the complex changes that develop in the respiratory system during anesthesia is to appreciate the relationship between FRC and closing capacity (CC). CC is the sum of closing volume (CV) and RV.

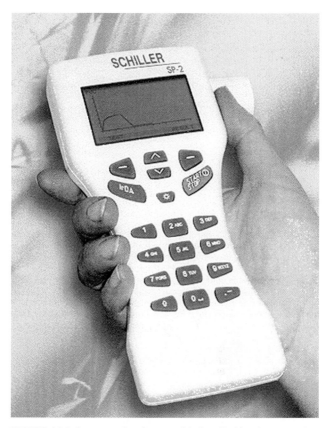

FIGURE 24-6 An example of a portable handheld spirometer that can be easily used in the preoperative assessment clinic or at the bedside to measure the majority of the clinically important lung volumes and capacities. (From Slinger P, Darling G. Preanesthetic assessment for thoracic surgery. In: Slinger P, ed. *Principles and Practice of Anesthesia for Thoracic Surgery.* New York, NY: Springer; 2011:11–34, with permission.)

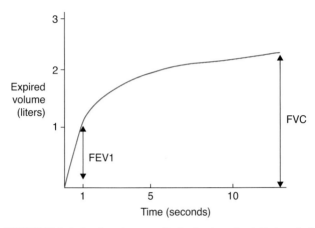

FIGURE 24-7 A simple spirogram. Expired volume is plotted against time. The total volume exhaled during a forced expiration from total lung capacity is the forced vital capacity (FVC). The fraction of the FVC that is exhaled in the first second is the forced expiratory volume in 1 second (FEV_1). These values are compared to normal data for age, sex, and height and given a percentage of predicted value (e.g., FEV_1%). (From Slinger P, Darling G. Preanesthetic assessment for thoracic surgery. In: Slinger P, ed. *Principles and Practice of Anesthesia for Thoracic Surgery.* New York, NY: Springer; 2011:11–34, with permission.)

2. CV is the lung volume below which small airways begin to close (or at least cease to contribute expiratory gas) during expiration.
3. When an alveolar unit falls below its CC, even for a brief period during one respiratory cycle, the concentration of oxygen (PAO_2) in that unit falls slightly. This results in the increase of venoarterial admixture ("shunt") and decrease in arterial oxygen tension (PaO_2) seen in the elderly and during general anesthesia.
   a. When a region of the lung is kept below its CC, the loss in volume will eventually lead to atelectasis as the gas trapped in the alveoli is absorbed.
   b. An important goal in the perioperative period is restoring the balance between FRC and CC. Because CC cannot be changed, this involves improving FRC by a variety of techniques to improve the mechanical advantage of the chest wall (adequate reversal of neuromuscular blockers, upright positioning,

regional analgesia, and possibly the use of positive end-expiratory pressure [PEEP] or continuous positive airway pressure [CPAP]).

    c. When positive pressure is applied during expiration to the airway of a patient who is having positive pressure ventilation, this applied airway pressure is referred to as **PEEP**. When a patient is breathing spontaneously, an applied airway pressure is referred to as **CPAP**.

C. **Compliance** is the change in lung volume for a given change in airway pressure. It is the reciprocal of "elastance." Monitoring changes in respiratory compliance is extremely important in ventilated patients as an early warning of changes in the lung or chest–abdominal wall complex that may negatively affect gas exchange.

D. **Resistance** in the respiratory system is important because, in the perioperative period, complications such as bronchospasm or secretions in an endotracheal tube or partial circuit obstruction will present primarily as increased resistance.

E. **Work of breathing** is commonly used to denote the ongoing energy expenditure required by the respiratory system. During normal quiet breathing, expiration is passive and does not require work.

    1. The oxygen requirement for the work of breathing is less than 2% of the normal basal oxygen consumption (3 to 4 mL/kg/minute).

    2. In patients with COPD due to the mechanical inefficiency of the respiratory system, increasing the minute ventilation to 20 L per minute may increase the oxygen consumption of the muscles of respiration to levels of 200 mL per minute.

F. **Respiratory fatigue** may occur at any point from the central nervous system (CNS) to the muscles of respiration (diaphragm is possibly the most fatigue-resistant skeletal muscle and can sustain resistive loads of up to 40% of maximal indefinitely).

    1. Because the oxygen supply requirement for the diaphragm is high in proportion to its mass, it is susceptible to hypoxia either due to decreased oxygen content of the arterial blood or due to decreased cardiac output.

    2. The diaphragm can be rested for a short period by mechanical ventilation but histologic evidence of muscle fiber atrophy can be seen after as little as 18 hours of mechanical ventilation and clinical evidence of weakness is seen within days.

VI. **Distribution of Ventilation**
   A. **Pulmonary circulation** is composed of the pulmonary circulation from the main pulmonary artery and the smaller bronchial circulation arising from the aorta. The pulmonary circulation dominates, by volume, and serves to deliver the mixed venous blood to the alveolar capillaries to facilitate gas exchange and to act as a large, low-resistance reservoir for the entire cardiac output from the right ventricle. The bronchial circulation serves to provide nutritional support to the airways and their associated pulmonary blood vessels.
   B. **Pulmonary Hemodynamics**
      1. Despite receiving all of the cardiac output from the right ventricle, the pulmonary vasculature maintains a relatively low pulmonary blood pressure. The normal adult mean pulmonary artery pressure (P_{PA}) is 9 to 16 mm Hg with systolic P_{PA} of 18 to 25 mm Hg.
      2. PVR can change as a result of numerous factors (hypoxia, acidosis, mitral valve stenosis or regurgitation, left ventricular failure, primary pulmonary hypertension, or pulmonary emboli).
   C. **Distribution of Perfusion**. There is a gradient of distribution of perfusion of the lung that is similar but not identical to the gradient of distribution of ventilation, with increased perfusion of regions in the central and lower regions compared to the upper regions (Fig. 24-8). Gravity, posture, and alveolar pressure will also have effects on the distribution of pulmonary blood flow.
   D. **Matching of Ventilation and Perfusion**
      1. Within certain limits, the lung attempts to match ventilation to perfusion (never ideal because the ventilation and perfusion gradients are not identical) (Fig. 24-9).
      2. This matching is closer during spontaneous ventilation than during positive pressure ventilation. With positive pressure ventilation, the effects of alveolar pressure are increased and pulmonary blood flow distribution becomes less homogeneous (concept of perfusion zones of the lung) (Fig. 24-10A,B).
   E. **Dead Space**
      1. Any portion of an inspired breath that does not enter gas exchanging lung units is dead space (V_D). Minute ventilation (V_E) is the sum of alveolar ventilation (V_A) and dead space ventilation (V_D).
      2. Dead space can be subdivided into physiologic dead space and apparatus dead space (breathing circuit).

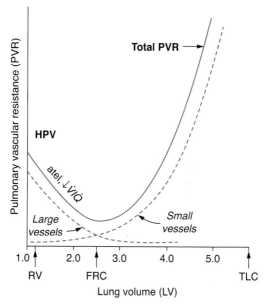

FIGURE 24-8 The relationship between pulmonary vascular resistance (PVR) and lung volume. PVR is lowest at functional residual capacity (FRC) and increases as the lung volume decreases toward residual volume (RV), owing primarily to the increase in resistance of large pulmonary vessels. PVR also increases as lung volume increases above FRC toward total lung capacity (TLC) because of an increase in resistance of small interalveolar lung vessels.

Physiologic dead space is further subdivided into airway dead space and alveolar dead space (Fig. 24-11).

3. Airway dead space is relatively constant but does vary directly with lung volume and bronchodilation increases airway dead space. Airway dead space is decreased by endotracheal intubation. For most correctly functioning modern anesthetic apparatus, equipment dead space is not clinically important.

4. A healthy person, breathing spontaneously, will have practically no alveolar dead space.

   a. Tidal volume breathing will usually result in a V_D/V_T ratio of approximately 0.3, entirely due to airway dead space.

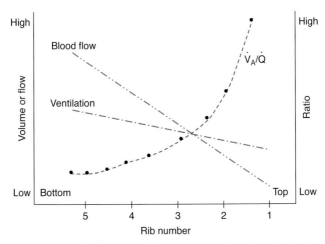

FIGURE 24-9 Distribution of blood flow (perfusion) and alveolar ventilation and the ventilation-to-perfusion ratio (V_A/Q) as a function of the distance from the base of the lung (to the left in the figure) to the apex (to the right). In the upright position, both ventilation and blood flow are greater at the base of the lung than at the apex. However, the gradient is steeper for blood flow than ventilation. Thus, the V_A/Q ratio is higher at the apex than in the mid- or dependent lung regions. (Reproduced with permission from Slinger P. *Principles and Practice of Anesthesia for Thoracic Surgery*. New York, NY: Springer; 2011.)

     b. Alveolar dead space, however, becomes clinically important during positive pressure ventilation and in any condition of altered hemodynamics. Decreased cardiac output, pulmonary embolism, and changes in posture will all have clinically important effects on alveolar dead space.

F. **Shunt** or venous admixture is the portion of the venous blood returned to the heart that passes to the arterial circulation without being exposed to normally ventilated lung units.

    1. Shunt may be extrapulmonary (blood does not pass through the lungs, thebesian veins, and bronchial circulation; <1% total pulmonary circulation) or pulmonary (venous blood passing through lung regions with decreased or no alveolar ventilation) (see Fig. 24-11).

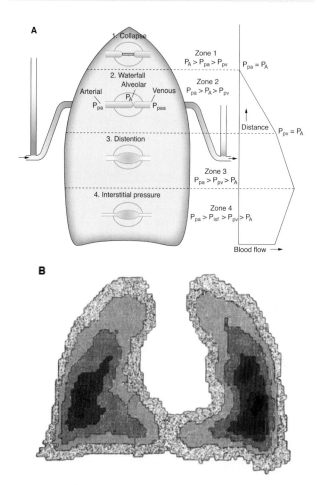

FIGURE 24-10 The distribution of pulmonary blood flow in the up-right position. **A.** Pulmonary blood flow as affected by gravity and alveolar pressure. This classic description based on the work of West divides pulmonary blood flow into four zones. P_A, alveolar pressure; P_{pa}, pulmonary arteriolar pressure; P_{pv}, pulmonary venous pressure; P_{isf}, pulmonary interstitial pressure. **B.** Subsequent investigations with lung scanning have shown that blood flow is actually distributed more in a central to peripheral pattern. (Reproduced with permission from Slinger P. *Principles and Practice of Anesthesia for Thoracic Surgery.* New York, NY: Springer; 2011.)

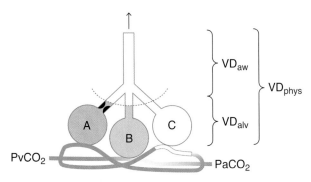

FIGURE 24-11 A simplified three-compartment model of the lung with *A* representing shunt; *B* an ideal gas unit; and *C* alveolar dead space (VD_{alv}). Physiologic dead space (VD_{phys}) is filled with air containing no CO_2, shown as the *white area*. VD_{phys} is the sum of airway dead space (VD_{aw}) and VD_{alv}. The airway–alveolar interface is demonstrated by the *dotted line*. (Reproduced with permission from Tusman G, Sipmann S, Bohm SH. Rationale of dead space measurement by volumetric capnography. *Anesth Analg.* 2012;114:866–874.)

2. Shunt and dead space are the extremes of the continuum of ventilation and perfusion matching (Fig. 24-12). Shunt has a large effect on Pao_2 but a limited effect on $Paco_2$. Shunt is the commonest cause of hypoxemia during anesthesia (Fig. 24-13).

G. **Alveolar–arterial oxygen difference (A-aD_{O_2})** can be used as a crude monitor of shunt (proportional to shunt but the absolute gradient increases as F_{IO_2} increases). If F_{IO_2} and PvO_2 (cardiac output and temperature) remain relatively constant, the trend of the A-aD_{O_2} is a reasonably reliable monitor of changes in shunt.

H. **Matching of Ventilation and Perfusion**

1. Due to the combined effects of the architecture of the lung parenchyma and vasculature and gravity, there is a matching of ventilation and perfusion (V_A/Q) in the lung.

2. Typical resting values in an adult are 4 and 5 L per minute for alveolar ventilation and cardiac output for a V_A/Q ratio of 0.8 (see Fig. 24-11).

3. Positive pressure ventilation, decreased cardiac output, and atelectasis interfere with normal V_A/Q matching.

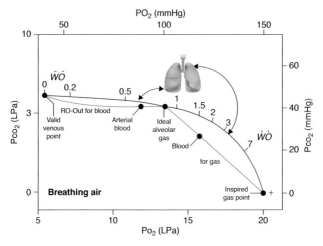

FIGURE 24-12 The *heavy line* indicated all possible values of alveolar O_2 (P_{AO_2}) and CO_2 (P_{ACO_2}) with ventilation perfusion (V/Q) ratios ranging from zero (to the left, lung base) to infinity (to the right, lung apex) for a person breathing air. Mixed expired gas is a mixture of ideal alveolar gas and dead space. Arterial blood is a mixture of blood with the same gas tensions as ideal alveolar gas and shunt (mixed venous blood).

   I. **Hypoxic pulmonary vasoconstriction (HPV)** is a unique reflex to try and minimize these perturbations in V_A/Q matching (pulmonary arterioles respond to regional hypoxemia by constricting). The arterioles in essentially all other tissues in the body vasodilate in response to hypoxemia.

     1. This reflex will tend to redirect blood flow from poorly or nonventilated lung regions to better ventilated regions.

     2. The primary stimulus for HPV is alveolar hypoxia (Fig. 24-14).

 VII. **Oxygen Transport.** Oxygen diffuses into the plasma of the pulmonary capillary blood, driven by its concentration gradient from the alveolus. This oxygen is then taken up by partially desaturated hemoglobin (Hb) molecules in the red blood cells of mixed venous blood to form oxyhemoglobin. Due to the high affinity of Hb for oxygen, a large proportion (normally

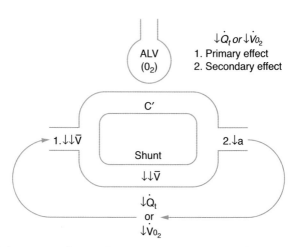

FIGURE 24-13 A simplified diagram of the effects of a decrease in mixed venous oxygen saturation *(v)* on arterial oxygenation *(a)*. Mixed venous blood passes either though ventilated lung regions (ALV), where it is oxygenated in the pulmonary capillaries *(c′)* or through nonventilated (shunt) lung regions. A decrease in mixed venous oxygen due to either a decrease in cardiac output (Q_t) or an increase in oxygen consumption (Vo_2) will pass through the pulmonary shunt and result in a fall in arterial oxygenation. (From *Nunn's Applied Respiratory Physiology*. 7th ed. Edinburgh, United Kingdom: Churchill Livingstone Elsevier; 2010, with permission.)

>98%) of the total oxygen in arterial blood is carried within the red blood cells as oxyhemoglobin.

A. Less than 2% is circulated as dissolved oxygen (the tension of the oxygen dissolved in plasma [Pao_2] that is measured in an arterial [or venous (PvO_2)] blood gas sample).

  1. The quantity of oxygen dissolved in blood is directly proportional to its partial pressure.

    a. For each mm Hg of PO_2, there is 0.003 mL of dissolved oxygen per 100 mL of blood (for a Pao_2 of 100 mm Hg, there will be 0.3 mL of dissolved O_2 in 100 mL of blood vs. approximately 20 mL of O_2 bound to Hb).

    b. Dissolved oxygen can approach 1.5 mL with an FIO_2 of 1.0 and can be clinically even more important in hyperbaric environments.

B. The release of oxygen by Hb as the PO_2 in the surrounding plasma falls (and conversely the uptake of O_2 by Hb as the

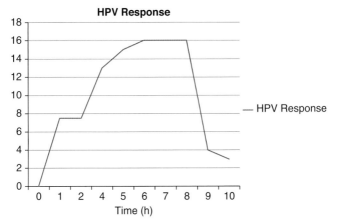

FIGURE 24-14 The relationship between hypoxic pulmonary vaso-constriction (HPV) (vertical axis) and time in hours (h) (horizontal axis) in humans exposed to isocapnic hypoxia (approximate inspired PO_2 60 mmHg), beginning at 0h with a return to normoxia at 8h. HPV response was measured as the increase in echocardiographic right ventricular systolic pressure. Note the two-phase, rapid and slow, onset of HPV. Also note that after prolonged HPV, the pulmonary pressures do not return to baseline for several hours. (Based on data from Talbot NP, Balanos GM, Dorrington KL, et al. Two temporal components within the human pulmonary vascular response to 2 h of isocapnic hypoxia. *J Appl Physiol.* 2005;98:1125–1139.)

PO_2 rises) is not in a linear correlation with PO_2 but curvilinear producing the oxyhemoglobin saturation curve (or dissociation curve) (Fig. 24-15). PO_2 values of 40, 50, and 60 will correspond (approximately) to saturations of 70%, 80%, and 90%.

   C. **Shifts of the Oxyhemoglobin Desaturation Curve**

      1. By convention, to compare these curves, the PO_2 at the point of 50% saturation (P_{50}) is used as a reference. For HbA, the P_{50} is 26 mm Hg.

      2. The normal HbA oxygen saturation curve shifts to the left or right secondary to a variety of physiologic changes (pH, temperature, 2,3-diphosphoglycerate).

VIII. **Carbon Dioxide Transport**

   A. Carbon dioxide (CO_2) is the main product of aerobic metabolism of proteins, fats, and carbohydrates.

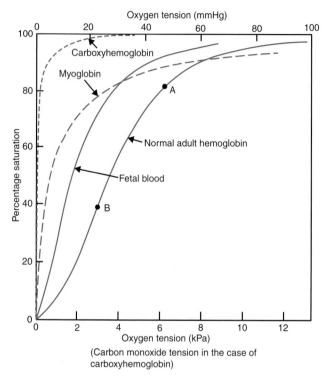

(Carbon monoxide tension in the case of carboxyhemoglobin)

FIGURE 24-15 Dissociation curves of normal adult (HbA) and fetal (HbF) hemoglobin. Curves for myoglobin and carboxyhemoglobin are shown for comparison.

Carbon dioxide is moderately soluble in all body fluids (approximately 20 times more soluble than oxygen) and diffuses down its concentration gradient from its site of intracellular production into the capillary and venous blood.

B. Similar to oxygen, the tension of dissolved CO_2 in blood is the portion measured in blood gas analysis.

1. The majority of CO_2 in the blood is transported in the blood as bicarbonate (HCO_3^-) after diffusion into red cells and enzymatic conversion (Fig. 24-16).

2. The difference in PCO_2 between venous and arterial blood is normally only 5 mm Hg, whereas the difference between arterial and venous PO_2 is typically 60 mm Hg.

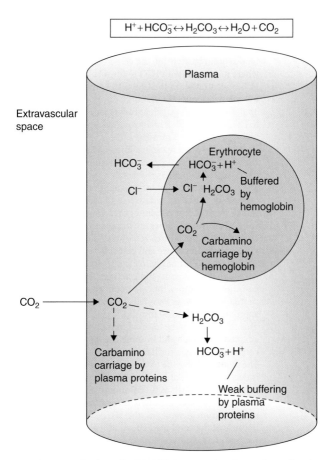

$$H^+ + HCO_3^- \leftrightarrow H_2CO_3 \leftrightarrow H_2O + CO_2$$

FIGURE 24-16 Carbon dioxide (CO_2) enters the plasma in molecular form from the tissues. The majority of CO_2 is transformed into bicarbonate (HCO_3^-) in the red blood cells; this reaction is catalyzed by carbonic anhydrase. A small proportion of plasma CO_2 is attached to plasma proteins as carbamino compounds or directly converted to HCO_3^- in the plasma. Some CO_2 in the red cell is also attached to hemoglobin as carbamino compounds. The excess hydrogen (H^+) ions generated in the red blood cell are transferred to the plasma in exchange for chloride ion (Cl^-). This is called the "chloride shift." (From *Nunn's Applied Respiratory Physiology.* 7th ed. Edinburgh, United Kingdom: Churchill Livingstone Elsevier; 2010, with permission.)

IX. **Respiratory Control**
  A. **Central Nervous System** (Fig. 24-17)
    1. Dissolved CO_2 in plasma diffuses easily across the blood–brain barrier into the cerebrospinal fluid (CSF) where it interacts with H_2O to form H^+ and HCO_3^-. The H^+ concentration in the CSF is the primary controller for normal minute ventilation.
    2. The brainstem central chemoreceptor is acutely sensitive to changes in pH. Normally, an awake individual's $Paco_2$ will vary less than 3 mm Hg.
    3. Ventilation will increase in a linear fashion as $Paco_2$ rises until a maximal stimulation somewhere over a $Paco_2$ of 100 mm Hg is reached.
    4. The central chemoreceptor is acutely sensitive to CNS depressants. Opioids, sedatives, and most general anesthetics decrease the respiratory response to hypercapnia.
  B. **Peripheral chemoreceptors** are located primarily in the carotid bodies at the bifurcation of the carotid arteries and also in aortic bodies above and below the aortic arch. These receptors respond primarily to changes in Pao_2.
    1. Although there is some tonic activity from these peripheral chemoreceptors, they do not normally stimulate ventilation until the Pao_2 falls to below a threshold of approximately 70 to 80 mm Hg.
    2. This threshold will be lowered in individuals who are adapted to altitude and in some chronic respiratory or congenital hypoxic cardiac diseases.
    3. The hypoxic drive due to the peripheral chemoreceptors is decreased by volatile anesthetics (even in very low concentrations such as 0.1 minimum alveolar concentration [MAC], which are often present immediately after recovery from general anesthesia).
    4. Because of the combined effects of residual opioids on the central chemoreceptors and the blunting of hypoxic drive by trace amounts of volatile anesthetics, it is a common practice to initially administer supplemental oxygen to patients in the recovery room after general anesthesia then to follow the oxygen saturation using pulse oximetry as the supplemental oxygen is decreased prior to discharge.

X. **Abnormal Breathing Patterns.** Several recognized abnormal patterns involve dysfunction of the central chemoreceptors.
  A. Primary alveolar hypoventilation syndrome (Ondine's curse) is a congenital insensitivity of the central

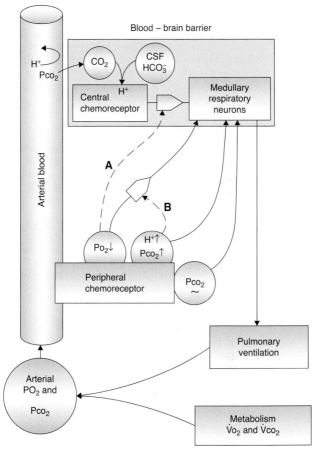

FIGURE 24-17 A diagram of the connections between individual components of the chemical and neural portions of the physiologic control of respiration (see text for details). (From *Nunn's Applied Respiratory Physiology*. 7th ed. Edinburgh, United Kingdom: Churchill Livingstone Elsevier; 2010, with permission.)

chemoreceptor to changes in CSF pH. It results in apnea and hypoventilation, particularly during sleep.

B. Cheyne-Stokes respiration is a pattern of 10- to 20-second periods of apnea followed by periods of hyperventilation. It is caused by a delayed response interval in the central chemoreceptor. Cheyne-Stokes is the most severe form of periodic breathing, which is seen to some degree in neonates and the elderly and during sleep at all ages.

XI. **Altered Physiologic Conditions**

A. **Anesthesia**

1. The near universal finding of rapid lung collapse upon induction of anesthesia and the rapid reappearance after discontinuation of PEEP has led to the conclusion that atelectasis is due to compression of lung tissue rather than alveolar gas absorption behind occluded airways.

2. The geometry of the chest and diaphragm is altered under general anesthesia with relaxation of the chest wall and a marked cephalad displacement of the most dorsal portion of the diaphragm at end-expiration.

3. Absorption atelectasis can occur when the rate of gas uptake into the blood exceeds the rate of ventilation of the alveolus (rate of gas absorption from unventilated areas is dependent on the initial F_{IO_2}).

B. **Position**

1. In the spontaneously breathing patient, awake or during anesthesia, the majority of gas exchange is due to caudal displacement of the diaphragm, which occurs primarily in the dorsal portions of the thoraces.

2. During deep anesthesia and paralysis, the diaphragm becomes relatively flaccid. The weight of the abdominal contents pushes cranially on the dorsal diaphragm and during inspiration, with positive pressure ventilation, gas preferentially distributes to the now more compliant ventral portions of the lungs.

   a. Matching of ventilation/perfusion is decreased with induction of anesthesia and further decreased with paralysis and positive pressure ventilation. The addition of low levels of PEEP (<10 cm H_2O, after recruitment) will usually ameliorate this mismatch.

   b. Matching of ventilation to perfusion will usually be superior in the prone position when compared with the supine position (unlike the supine position, the

addition of PEEP in the prone position may lead to
deterioration in ventilation/perfusion matching).

C. **Obesity**

1. The increased weight of the abdominal contents and
chest wall impose a restrictive ventilatory pattern on the
respiratory system with a decrease of all lung volumes
but a preservation of the FEV_1/FVC ratio (a fall in FRC
leads to increased venoarterial shunt and a tendency to
desaturate during induction and maintenance of anesthesia and in the postoperative period).

2. The challenge in respiratory management of the obese
patient perioperatively is to minimize the fall in FRC
(regional anesthesia/analgesia, avoiding long-acting
muscle relaxants, positioning, and use of postoperative
CPAP).

D. **Sleep-Disordered Breathing**

1. Approximately 20% of the population has disorders of
respiration during sleep, ranging from simple snoring to
obstructive sleep apnea.

   a. Obstructive sleep apnea (OSA) is defined by more
   than 5 episodes per hour of apnea, each >10 seconds.

   b. The disturbance of normal sleep leads to daytime
   somnolence and the periods of hypoxia may contribute to cardiovascular morbidity.

2. The obesity hypoventilation syndrome is a combination
of obesity, hypoventilation, and severe OSA, which has
been called the *Pickwickian* syndrome.

E. **Altered Barometric Pressures**

1. **Altitude**. The ambient PO_2 decreases proportionally as
the barometric pressure falls with increases in altitude
(PO_2 is 149 mm Hg at sea level, 122 at 5,000 ft of elevation, and may be as low as 108 mm Hg in a commercial
airliner pressurized to 8,000 ft [maximum permitted
altitude-equivalent]).

   a. There are acute and chronic adaptations to the
   hypoxia associated with altitude. Rapid adaptation
   involves hyperventilation, driven by the peripheral
   chemoreceptors to decrease the alveolar PCO_2 and
   thus increase the alveolar PAO_2. Secondary alkalinization of blood and CSF returns to normal after several
   days at altitude as bicarbonate is excreted.

   b. Increased pulmonary pressures due to HPV triggered by hypoxia can lead to high altitude pulmonary edema (treated with oxygen, diuretics, and
   pulmonary vasodilators).

    c. Anesthesia at mild elevations is generally uncomplicated as long as oxygen saturation is monitored and adequate supplemental oxygen is provided.

    d. Most modern commercial vaporizers deliver reasonably accurate dosages of volatile anesthetics at modest elevations (<6,000 ft).

    e. Pressure in the air-filled cuff of an endotracheal tube or laryngeal mask airway will increase and decrease significantly with changes in ambient pressure, which may be associated with medical air transport.

2. **Hyperbaric oxygen** is delivered in a chamber pressurized to two to three times atmospheric pressure (ATM) (1,400 to 2,100 mm Hg).

    a. Indications include gas embolism, decompression sickness, necrotizing soft tissue infections, and carbon monoxide poisoning.

    b. At high FIO_2 levels, above 2 ATM, hyperoxia may cause convulsions. Prolonged exposure to a high PaO_2 causes pulmonary oxygen toxicity and a restrictive lung disease.

F. **Age**

1. **Infants and Children**. The overall compliance of the respiratory system is low in newborns and increases until late adolescence (predisposes infants to a significant fall in FRC during anesthesia).

    a. All airways are proportionally smaller in infants than adults and airway resistance is higher, resulting in increased work of breathing at rest and particularly during upper or lower airway infections (croup).

    b. The narrowest portion of the upper airway is at the cricoid cartilage until age 5 years.

    c. Control of breathing in the newborn is unique. Hypoxia initially causes increased ventilation, as in the adult, but then leads to a decrease in ventilation.

    d. Oxygen consumption is higher in newborns than adults (6 to 8 mL/kg/minute). The increased oxygen requirements are met by both increased minute ventilation and increased cardiac output.

    e. Fetal hemoglobin has a low P_{50} (18 to 19 mm Hg), which increases oxygen loading in the placenta but decreases oxygen unloading in the tissues. Fetal hemoglobin predominates at birth until 3 to 6 months of age.

2. **The Elderly**. Changes in the respiratory system with age include decrease of muscle tone in the dilators of

the pharynx, predisposing to upper airway obstruction during anesthesia.

a. With the loss of structural support of peripheral airways, the CC increases significantly, which has major anesthetic implications (fall of FRC below CC leads to increased venoarterial shunt and is responsible for the decrease in Pao_2 with age). The mean Pao_2 of healthy patients will decline to approximately 80 mm Hg at age 70 years, after which it remains stable.

b. The responsiveness of both central and peripheral chemoreceptors to hypercarbia and hypoxemia decreases with age.

XII. **Chronic respiratory disease is divided into obstructive and restrictive. In obstructive disease, the FEV_1/FVC ratio is typically less than normal ($<80\%$) with a decreased FEV_1. Restrictive disease typically has a normal FEV_1/FVC ratio and a decreased FEV_1.**

A. **Chronic obstructive pulmonary disease (COPD)** includes emphysema, peripheral airways disease, and chronic bronchitis. Any individual patient may have one or all of these conditions, but the dominant clinical feature is impairment of expiratory airflow.

1. Some moderate and severe COPD patients have an elevated $Paco_2$ at rest ($Paco_2$ rises in these patients when supplemental Fio_2 is administered). Supplemental oxygen must be administered postoperatively to prevent the hypoxemia associated with the unavoidable fall in functional residual capacity. The attendant rise in $Paco_2$ should be anticipated and monitored.

2. To identify these patients preoperatively, all moderate or severe COPD patients need an arterial blood gas analysis (important to know the patient's baseline preoperative $Paco_2$ to guide weaning if mechanical ventilation becomes necessary in the postoperative period).

3. COPD patients desaturate more frequently and severely than normal patients during sleep (due to the rapid/shallow breathing pattern that occurs in all patients during REM sleep).

4. Right ventricular dysfunction occurs in up to 50% of moderate to severe COPD patients.

a. The dysfunctional right ventricle is poorly tolerant to sudden increases in afterload such as the change from spontaneous to controlled ventilation.

   b. Chronic recurrent hypoxemia is the cause of the right ventricle dysfunction and the subsequent progression to cor pulmonale. COPD patients who have resting Pao_2 less than 55 mm Hg should receive supplemental home oxygen.

5. Many patients with moderate or severe COPD will develop cystic air spaces in the lung parenchyma known as *bullae*.

   a. Positive pressure ventilation can be used safely in patients with bullae, provided the airway pressures are kept low.

   b. Due to the lower solubility of nitrogen in plasma compared to nitrous oxide, when a patient is converted from breathing air to breathing a mixture containing nitrous oxide during anesthesia, the nitrous oxide will diffuse into a bulla faster than the nitrogen can be absorbed, and the bulla will increase in size with the attendant risk of rupture.

6. Patients with severe COPD often breathe in a pattern that interrupts expiration before the alveolar pressure has fallen to atmospheric pressure (leads to an elevation of the end-expiratory lung volume above the FRC and has been termed *auto-PEEP* or *intrinsic-PEEP*).

B. **Restrictive lung diseases** are often part of a multisystemic disease process such as connective tissue disorders.

1. Patients with mild to moderate restrictive lung disease are, in general, less of a problem to manage intraoperatively (compared to COPD) and more of a problem postoperatively.

2. Due to the decrease in FRC in restrictive disease, these patients tend to develop an increased shunt during anesthesia and postoperatively (restoration of the FRC postoperatively is important).

XIII. **One-lung ventilation (OLV) is performed during thoracic surgery to facilitate the surgical exposure in the chest. OLV is commonly obtained by placement of a double-lumen endobronchial tube or a bronchial blocker with a standard endotracheal tube.**

A. It is important to thoroughly denitrogenate the operative lung, by ventilating with oxygen, immediately before it is allowed to collapse.

B. Although nitrous oxide is even more effective than oxygen in speeding lung collapse (because of its solubility), it is not commonly used in thoracic anesthesia because many patients may have blebs or bullae.

C. A major concern that influences anesthetic management for thoracic surgery is the occurrence of hypoxemia during OLV (Fig. 24-18).

   1. The goal during OLV is to maximize PVR in the non-ventilated lung while minimizing PVR in the ventilated lung. PVR is lowest at FRC and increases as lung volume rises or falls above or below FRC.

   2. Patients having OLV in the lateral position have significantly better Pao_2 levels than patients during OLV in the supine position due to a preferential distribution of blood flow to the dependent lung caused by gravitational forces.

Factors affecting the distribution of blood flow during OLV:

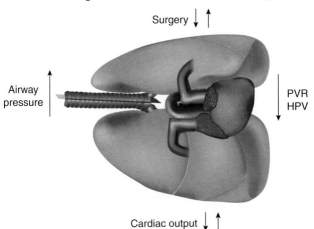

FIGURE 24-18 Factors affecting the distribution of pulmonary blood flow during one-lung ventilation (OLV). Hypoxic pulmonary vaso-constriction (HPV) and the collapse of the nonventilated lung, which increase pulmonary vascular resistance (PVR), tend to distribute blood flow toward the ventilated lung. The airway pressure gradient between the ventilated and nonventilated thoraces tends to encourage blood flow to the nonventilated lung. Surgery and cardiac output can have variable effects either increasing or decreasing the proportional flow to the ventilated lung. Gravity will also increase the blood flow to the dependent lung.

CHAPTER 25

Respiratory Pharmacology

I. **Pharmacology of the Airways.** The delivery of medications to the lungs can have systemic effects and/or direct effects on the airway (inhaled anesthetics have bronchodilatory effects, whereas β-adrenergic agonists delivered via aerosol exert direct effects on bronchial smooth muscle with few systemic effects).

A. **Influence of the Autonomic Nervous System on the Airways**

1. The parasympathetic nervous system regulates airway caliber, airway glandular activity, and airway microvasculature.

   a. Acetylcholine activates the muscarinic (M3) receptor of postganglionic fibers of the parasympathetic nervous system to produce bronchoconstriction.

   b. Anticholinergics can provide bronchodilation even in the resting state because the parasympathetic nervous system produces a basal level of resting bronchomotor tone.

2. Although the sympathetic nervous system plays no direct role in control of airway muscle tone, β_2-adrenergic receptors are present on airway smooth muscle cells and cause bronchodilation via stimulatory G mechanisms (allows for pharmacologic manipulation of airway tone).

B. **Inhaled Adrenergic Agonists** (Table 25-1)

1. The mainstay of therapy for bronchospasm, wheezing, and airflow obstruction is β-adrenergic agonists (typically delivered via inhalers or nebulizers).

2. Short-acting β_2 agonists such as albuterol, levalbuterol, metaproterenol, and pirbuterol are prescribed for the rapid relief (rescue therapy) of wheezing, bronchospasm, and airflow obstruction. Clinical effect is seen in a matter of minutes and lasts up to 4 to 6 hours.

3. Long-acting β_2 agonists are prescribed for control of symptoms when rescue therapies are used more than two times per week.

Table 25-1

Pharmacologic Influence on the Autonomic Nervous System

Systemic Adrenergic Agonists	Inhaled Adrenergic Agonists	Inhaled Cholinergic Antagonists	Systemic Cholinergic Antagonists
	Short Acting	**Short Acting**	
Terbutaline	Albuterol	Ipratropium	Atropine
Epinephrine	Levalbuterol		Scopolamine
Albuterol	Metaproterenol		Glycopyrrolate
	Pirbuterol		
	Long Acting	**Long Acting**	
	Salmeterol	Tiotropium	
	Formoterol		
	Arformoterol		

From Wojciechowski P, Hurford W. Pharmacology of the airways. In: Slinger P, ed. *Principles and Practice of Anesthesia for Thoracic Surgery*. New York, NY: Springer; 2011:121–132, with permission.

4. Systemic absorption of inhaled β_2 agonists is responsible for a myriad of side effects (tremors, tachycardia), most of which are not serious. Hyperglycemia, hypokalemia, and hypomagnesemia also can occur with β_2-agonist therapy but the severity of these side effects tends to diminish with regular use.

5. Tolerance to β_2 agonists can occur with regular use over a period of weeks and, while not affecting peak bronchodilation, can be evidenced by a decrease in the duration of bronchodilation and the magnitude of side effects.

C. **Systemic Adrenergic Agonists.** Oral, intravenous (IV), or subcutaneous administration of β-specific or nonspecific adrenergic agonists is now reserved for rescue therapy.

1. Terbutaline can be given orally, subcutaneously, or intravenously; albuterol (salbutamol) can be given intravenously; and epinephrine is usually given subcutaneously or intravenously. Regardless of the route of administration, all three will produce bronchodilation.

2. The side effect profile of systemic adrenergic agonists is similar to the side effect profile for inhalational adrenergic agonists (tremor, tachycardia).

D. **Inhaled Cholinergic Antagonists** (see Table 25-1)

1. The use of inhaled anticholinergics in chronic obstructive pulmonary disease (COPD) as maintenance and rescue therapy is considered standard treatment.

2. Anticholinergics are not used for maintenance therapy in asthma and are only recommended for use in acute exacerbations.

3. Ipratropium is classified as a short-acting anticholinergic and is commonly used as maintenance therapy for COPD and as rescue therapy for both COPD and asthmatic exacerbations. It is not indicated for the routine management of asthma.

4. Tiotropium is the only long-acting anticholinergic available for COPD maintenance therapy.

5. Inhaled anticholinergics are poorly absorbed and therefore serious side effects are uncommon (dry mouth, urinary retention, pupillary dilation, blurred vision).

E. **Systemic Cholinergic Antagonists**

1. The systemically administered anticholinergics atropine and glycopyrrolate act via the same mechanisms as inhaled anticholinergics, but their use is generally limited by side effects.

2. Atropine, because of its tertiary ammonium structure, has a tendency to cause tachycardia, gastrointestinal upset, blurred vision, dry mouth, and central nervous system effects secondary to its ability to cross the blood–brain barrier.

3. Glycopyrrolate has a quaternary ammonium structure and is insoluble in lipids, similar to ipratropium and tiotropium, and has fewer systemic side effects than atropine.

II. **Influence of Inflammation on the Airway.** Asthma and COPD, the most common obstructive airway diseases, have a component of inflammation as part of their pathogenesis. Patients presenting to the operating room with obstructive airway diseases have a high likelihood of taking antiinflammatory therapies for control of their disease (Table 25-2).

A. **Inhaled Corticosteroids**

1. Inhaled corticosteroids (ICS) reduce the inflammatory changes associated with asthma, thereby improving lung function and reducing exacerbations, whereas the use of ICS as monotherapy in COPD is discouraged.

Table 25-2			
Pharmacologic Influence on Inflammation			
Inhaled Corticosteroids	Leukotriene Modifiers	Mast Cell Stabilizers	Methylxanthines
Monotherapy Beclomethasone	**Antagonists** Montelukast	Cromolyn Sodium	Theophylline
Budesonide Ciclesonide	Zafirlukast Pranlukast (not in U.S.)	Nedocromil	Aminophylline
Flunisolide Fluticasone Mometasone Triamcinolone	**Inhibitors** Zileuton		
Combination Therapy Budesonide/ Formoterol Fluticasone/ Salmeterol			

From Wojciechowski P, Hurford W. Pharmacology of the airways. In: Slinger P, ed. *Principles and Practice of Anesthesia for Thoracic Surgery*. New York, NY: Springer; 2011:121–132, with permission.

    2. In COPD, ICS are used as a part of combination therapy along with long-acting β-adrenergic agonists (LABA).

    3. Side effects with the use of ICS in asthma and COPD include an increase in pneumonia but not deaths, oropharyngeal candidiasis, pharyngitis, osteoporosis, dysphonia, and cough.

B. **Systemic Corticosteroids**

    1. Systemic corticosteroids given in IV or oral form are used for treatment of asthma and COPD exacerbations.

    2. Patients who are hospitalized with a COPD exacerbation will typically receive IV corticosteroids to suppress any inflammatory component that may be contributing.

    3. In asthma, corticosteroids are recommended for exacerbations that are either severe, with a peak expiratory flow of less than 40% of baseline, or a mild to moderate

exacerbation with no immediate response to short-acting β-adrenergic agonists.

4. The recommended duration of therapy is 3 to 10 days without tapering (some patients with difficult to manage asthma and COPD will be receiving long-term oral corticosteroid therapy).

C. **Leukotriene modifiers** for the treatment of asthma are usually prescribed for long-term control in addition to short-acting β-adrenergic agonists or in conjunction with ICS and short-acting β agonists.

D. **Mast Cell Stabilizers**. Cromolyn sodium and nedocromil are used in the treatment of asthma (delivered by powder inhaler and are not first-line therapy).

E. **Methylxanthines**. Currently, theophylline is recommended only as an alternative therapy and is not a first-line choice for asthma or COPD (significant side effect profile and the need for monitoring of blood level).

III. **Influence of Anesthetics on the Airways**

A. **Volatile Anesthetics** (Table 25-3). Volatile anesthetics reduce bronchomotor tone and all commonly used volatile anesthetics, except desflurane, produce a degree of bronchodilatation (may be helpful in patients with obstructive lung disease or in patients that experience any degree of bronchoconstriction).

B. **Intravenous Anesthetics** (see Table 25-3). IV anesthetics can decrease bronchomotor tone when used for induction or IV anesthesia. Ketamine is thought to have a direct relaxant effect on smooth muscle, whereas propofol is thought to reduce vagal tone and have a direct effect on muscarinic

Table 25-3	
Anesthetics with a Favorable Influence on Bronchomotor Tone	
Volatile Anesthetics	**Intravenous Anesthetics**
Isoflurane	Propofol
Sevoflurane	Ketamine
Halothane	Midazolam

From Wojciechowski P, Hurford W. Pharmacology of the airways. In: Slinger P, ed. *Principles and Practice of Anesthesia for Thoracic Surgery*. New York, NY: Springer; 2011:121–132, with permission.

receptors (propofol or ketamine can be beneficial in patients with bronchospasm or obstructive airway disease).
C. **Local anesthetics** are primarily used to suppress coughing and blunt the hemodynamic response to tracheal intubation.

IV. **Pharmacology of the Pulmonary Circulation. Patients with pulmonary hypertension (PHTN) are high-risk candidates for both cardiac and noncardiac surgery (have poor cardiorespiratory reserve and are at risk of having perioperative complications including pulmonary hypertensive crises with resultant heart failure, respiratory failure, and dysrhythmias). Drugs affecting the pulmonary vascular bed are routinely administered during anesthesia and reducing the consequences of an elevated pulmonary vascular resistance and the resulting right ventricular dysfunction should be considered as the primary goal of therapy with pulmonary vasodilators.**
A. **Anesthetic Drugs**
1. **Ketamine** causes pulmonary vasoconstriction and should be used with extreme caution in this group.
2. **Propofol** is commonly used in anesthesia, including for patients with PHTN (frequently used to maintain anesthesia during and after lung transplantation).
3. **Opioids** seem to have little to no deleterious effects on the pulmonary vascular system.
4. **Volatile Anesthetics**. At clinically relevant concentrations, modern volatile anesthetics likely have little to no direct vasodilating effect on the pulmonary vasculature. Nitrous oxide is typically avoided in patients with PHTN as it is believed to cause pulmonary vasoconstriction.
5. **Magnesium** is a vasodilator in both the systemic and pulmonary circulations.
6. **Regional Analgesia**. Pain can increase PVR and perioperative thoracic epidural analgesia (TEA) is commonly used in abdominal and thoracic surgery. As with most anesthetic interventions in patients with PHTN, careful titration and monitoring is paramount.
B. **Pulmonary vasodilators** are typically employed to improve right ventricular function in the setting of PHTN or in an effort to enhance regional pulmonary blood flow and improve intrapulmonary shunt. Vasodilators are hampered by their relatively nonselective actions in the pulmonary vascular bed (hypotensive systemic hemodynamic effects,

perfusion of underventilated alveoli, worsen intrapulmonary shunt, and, in turn, worsen oxygenation).

1. **Nitric oxide (NO)** is preferentially delivered to ventilated lung units leading to improved perfusion to alveoli that are able to participate in gas exchange.

    a. At present, NO is only approved for infants with respiratory distress syndrome.

    b. Methemoglobin levels need to be monitored when NO is administered for more than 24 hours.

    c. Heart and lung transplantation represent two distinct areas where acute pulmonary vasodilation has strong theoretic benefit as it relates to improving acute right ventricular failure and attenuating reperfusion injury.

2. **Prostaglandins.** Prostanoids induce relaxation of vascular smooth muscle, inhibit growth of smooth muscle cells, and are powerful inhibitors of platelet aggregation.

3. **Phosphodiesterase Inhibitors.** Owing to the relatively higher expression of phosphodiesterase 5 (PDE5) in the pulmonary circulation relative to the systemic circulation, PDE5 inhibitors have a relatively selective effect on PVR as opposed to SVR. In the acute setting, sildenafil has been demonstrated to enhance the effects of inhaled NO and may also be useful in blunting the rebound in pulmonary pressures that occur during weaning of inhaled NO.

V. **Hypoxic Pulmonary Vasoconstriction. IV anesthetic agents have no effect on hypoxic pulmonary vasoconstriction (HPV), whereas all of the volatile anesthetics inhibit HPV in a dose-dependent fashion. HPV is decreased by systemic vasodilators such as nitroglycerin and nitroprusside (cause some deterioration in Pao_2 during anesthesia).**

VI. **Intrinsic Pharmacologic Effects of the Lungs. The lungs receive essentially the entire cardiac output and there is ample blood-endothelial interface for surface enzyme activity as well as uptake and secretion. "First-pass" uptake is used to describe the amount of substance removed from the blood on the first cycle through the lungs. The lungs have a pronounced impact on the blood concentration of substances even when it does not ultimately break them down or secrete them (reflects uptake and retention of substances, often followed by release back into the blood ["capacitor effect"]). The** lungs have been found to have substantial concentrations of P-450 isoenzymes.

A. **Opioids**. Fentanyl has been shown to have a markedly variable first-pass uptake up to 90% in humans. Sufentanil demonstrates uptake that is a little more than half that of fentanyl. Morphine has a much lower uptake of about 10%.

B. **Local anesthetics**
    1. For lidocaine, there is a first-pass uptake of approximately 50% with significant retention at 10 minutes.
    2. The issue of pulmonary uptake and delayed release of local anesthetics must be considered in the treatment of suspected local anesthetic toxicity with emulsified lipid.

C. **Hypnotics**
    1. Thiopental has been found to have nearly 15% first-pass uptake in humans with little or no metabolism.
    2. The pulmonary uptake of ketamine was found to be slightly less than 10% without subsequent metabolism.
    3. Propofol shows about 30% first-pass uptake and negligible metabolism by the lungs.

CHAPTER 26

Acid–Base Disorders

I. **Introduction**
   A. The management of acid–base disorders requires establishing the cause(s) of the disorder and then treating the underlying physiologic derangement (Table 26-1). The acid–base disturbance is often evolving rapidly (ischemia, shock) and there is a delay getting laboratory results.
   B. With just blood gas and common serum biochemistry data, we can manage the majority of clinical acid–base disorders.
   C. The central focus of treating acid–base disturbances is the understanding of the biochemistry of the hydrogen ion.
      1. Deviations in hydrogen ion concentrations from the normal range can cause marked alterations in protein structure and function, enzyme activity, and cellular function.
      2. The largest contribution of metabolic acids arises from the oxidation of carbohydrates, principally glucose, to produce carbon dioxide (volatile acid, approximately 24,000 mEq/day).
      3. The hydrogen ion concentration is regulated to maintain the arterial blood pH between 7.35 and 7.45.
         a. The expression of the hydrogen ion concentration as pH masks large variations in hydrogen ion concentration despite small changes in pH.
         b. For example, a pH range of 7.0 to 7.7 is associated with a fivefold change (100 nmol/L to 20 nmol/L) in hydrogen ion concentration. The pH of venous blood and interstitial fluid is lower than that of arterial blood (approximately 7.35).

II. **Mechanisms for Regulation of Hydrogen Ion Concentration.** Regulation of pH over a narrow range depends on (a) buffer systems, (b) ventilatory responses, and (c) renal responses. The buffer system mechanism is local and immediate but incomplete. Ventilatory responses are slower (minutes) and

Table 26-1

Basic Definitions

p: a mathematical notation for a concentration expressed as the $-\log$ to the base 10, useful to describe substances present in the plasma in very low concentrations

pH: the concentration of free hydrogen ions (H^+) in a solution. The pH of water is 7.0 at 25°C and 6.8 at 37°C. The normal pH of most body fluids is 7.4 (range 7.35–7.45). This means that there are 40 nmol/L of H^+ in plasma (for comparison, there are 140 million nmol/L of Na^+ [140 mmol/L] in plasma).

pH_i: intracellular pH

Acid: a substance that increases the hydrogen ion concentration of a fluid (proton donor)

Alkali (or base): a substance that decreases the hydrogen ion concentration of a fluid (proton acceptor)

Buffer: a substance which reduces the change of pH in a solution when amounts of acid or base are added

K_a: the dissociation constant for a dissolved acid (HA), that is, the equilibrium ratio: $[H^+]\,[A^-]/[HA]$

pK_a: the $-\log$ of K_a for a given acid, for example, for carbonic acid (H_2CO_3), $pK_a = 6.2$. By convention, "strong" acids (e.g., HCl) have a $pK_a < -2$ (more free H^+ at equilibrium) and "weak" acids (e.g., H_2CO_3) have a pK_a -2 to $+12$ (this is confusing, but due to the negative logarithmic notation, a smaller number indicates a higher concentration of free H^+)

Anions: a negative ionized particle (e.g., HCO_3^-, Cl^-), that is, an excess of electrons vs. protons

Cations: a positively charged particle (e.g., Na^+, K^+), that is, an excess of protons vs. electrons

Strong ions: the ions of substances, which are completely dissociated in body fluids (e.g., Na^+, Cl^-, K^+, SO_4^{2-}, Mg^{2+}, Ca^{2+})

Mole (mol): a fixed number [6.022×10^{23} (Avogadro's number)] of elementary entities (atoms, molecules, ions, electrons, etc.)

Molecular weight (MW) (actually, the "molecular mass"): the mass of 1 mole of a specific entity

Equivalent (Eq): The amount of a substance that will supply or react with 1 mole of H^+ ions (in acid–base reactions) or supply 1 mole of electrons (in oxidation–reduction reactions) mmol = mol/1,000, mEq = Eq/1,000. For singly charged particles (e.g., Na^+), 1 mmol/L = 1 mEq/L; for doubly changed particles (e.g., Mg^{2+}), 1 mmol/L = 2 mEq/L

Mole day: an informal annual holiday based on Avogadro's number on October 23 (10/23) from 6:02 AM to 6:02 PM

$$HHb \rightleftharpoons H^+ + Hb^-$$

$$HProt \rightleftharpoons H^+ + Prot^-$$

$$H_2PO_4^- \rightleftharpoons H^+ + HPO_4^{2-}$$

$$H_2CO_3 \rightleftharpoons H^+ + HCO_3^-$$

FIGURE 26-1 Buffering systems present in the body. Hb, hemoglobin; Prot, protein.

usually incomplete. Renal responses develop very slowly (hours) but can produce nearly complete pH correction.

A. **Buffer Systems** (Fig. 26-1). Body fluids contain acid–base buffer systems that immediately combine with acid or alkali to prevent excessive changes in the hydrogen ion concentration.

1. **Bicarbonate buffering system** consists of carbonic acid (H_2CO_3) and sodium bicarbonate ($NaHCO_3$). Bicarbonate buffer is primarily a product of the approximately 200 mL of carbon dioxide produced per minute (Figs. 26-2 and 26-3). The bicarbonate buffer system accounts for >50% of the total buffering capacity of blood and approximately one-third of the bicarbonate buffering capacity of blood occurs within erythrocytes.

2. **Hemoglobin Buffering System**. Dissociation of oxyhemoglobin to deoxyhemoglobin facilitates the binding of hydrogen ions produced by the dissociation of carbonic acid. This situation is reversed in the pulmonary circulation where the conversion of deoxyhemoglobin to oxyhemoglobin facilitates the release of hydrogen ions.

B. **Protein Buffering System**. Like hemoglobin, other histidine-containing proteins are important intracellular buffers. Although the relatively low concentration of plasma proteins limits their role as extracellular buffers, hypoproteinemia will further reduce buffering capacity, especially in the critically ill patient.

$$CO_2 + H_2O \rightleftharpoons H_2CO_3 \rightleftharpoons HCO_3^- + H^+$$

FIGURE 26-2 Hydration of carbon dioxide results in carbonic acid (H_2CO_3), which can subsequently dissociate into bicarbonate and hydrogen ions.

$$pH = 6.10 + \log \frac{HCO_3^-}{Paco_2 \, (0.03)}$$

FIGURE 26-3 The Henderson-Hasselbalch equation can be used to calculate the pH of a solution from the concentration of bicarbonate and the Pco_2.

    C. **Phosphate buffering system** is important in most fluid compartments but is especially important in renal tubules, where phosphate is concentrated. Phosphate is a very important intracellular buffer because it is the most abundant intracellular anion.

  III. **Intracellular pH regulation. Although blood pH is commonly measured clinically, it is the intracellular pH (pH_i) that is of functional importance (Table 26-2).**
    A. **Ventilatory Responses**
       1. Ventilation is quantitatively the most important mechanism of acid removal, given the enormous daily production of volatile acid compared to nonvolatile acid.
       2. Ventilatory responses cannot return pH to 7.4 when a metabolic abnormality is responsible for the acid–base disturbance (intensity of the stimulus responsible for increases or decreases in alveolar ventilation will begin to diminish as pH returns toward 7.4).
       3. Most patients cannot hyperventilate to below 20 mm Hg.
       4. It is likely that the insult causing severe metabolic acidosis will also adversely affect respiratory muscle function, thus compromising the respiratory response.

Table 26-2

Intracellular Functions Affected by Local pH

Cellular metabolism
Cytoskeletal structure
Muscle contractility
Cell–cell coupling
Membrane conductance
Intracellular messengers
Cell activation, growth, and proliferation
Cell volume regulation
Intracellular membrane flow

B. **Renal Responses**
   1. The day-to-day renal contribution to acid–base regulation is directed toward the conservation of bicarbonate and the excretion of hydrogen ions.
   2. Almost all filtered bicarbonate must be reabsorbed from the glomerular filtrate to maintain the normal plasma bicarbonate concentration (25 mEq/L) and plasma pH.
      a. Carbonic anhydrase facilitates the dissociation of carbonic acid into water and carbon dioxide that both enter the renal tubular cell. Inhibition of carbonic anhydrase by acetazolamide interferes with the reabsorption of bicarbonate ions from renal tubular fluid. As a result, excess bicarbonate ions are lost in the urine and the plasma bicarbonate concentration is decreased (Fig. 26-4).

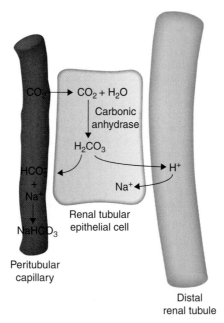

FIGURE 26-4 Schematic depiction of the renal tubular secretion of hydrogen ions, which are formed from the dissociation of carbonic acid in renal tubular epithelial cells.

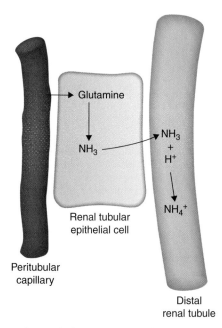

FIGURE 26-5 Ammonia formed in renal tubular epithelial cells combines with hydrogen ions in the renal tubules to form ammonium.

      b. Hydrogen ions are secreted into renal tubules by epithelial cells lining proximal renal tubules, distal renal tubules, and collecting ducts (facilitated by aldosterone).

      c. Active hydrogen ion transport is inhibited when the urinary pH drops below 4.0. Thus, hydrogen ions must combine with ammonia and phosphate buffers in the renal tubular lumen to prevent the pH from decreasing below this critical level (Fig. 26-5).

   3. The value of renal regulation of hydrogen ion concentration is not its rapidity but instead its ability to nearly completely neutralize any excess acid or alkali that enters the body fluids.

IV. **Classification of Acid–Base Disturbances (Table 26-3).** Acid–base disturbances are categorized as respiratory or metabolic acidosis (pH <7.35) or alkalosis (pH >7.45). An acid–base disturbance that results primarily from changes

---

Table 26-3

Distinguishing Respiratory and Metabolic Acidosis versus Alkalosis

	pH	Paco$_2$	Bicarbonate
Respiratory acidosis			
Acute	↓↓	↑↑↑	↑
Chronic	NC	↑↑↑	↑↑
Respiratory alkalosis			
Acute	↑↑	↓↓↓	↓
Chronic	NC	↓↓↓	↓↓
Metabolic acidosis			
Acute	↓↓↓	↓	↓↓↓
Chronic	↓	↓↓↓	↓↓↓
Metabolic alkalosis			
Acute	↑↑↑	↑	↑↑↑
Chronic	↑↑	↑↑	↑↑↑

↑, increase; ↓, decrease; NC, no change from normal.

in alveolar ventilation is described as respiratory acidosis or alkalosis. An acid–base disturbance unrelated to changes in alveolar ventilation is designated as metabolic acidosis or alkalosis. Compensation describes the secondary renal or ventilatory responses that occur as a result of the primary acid–base disturbance. The principal manifestation of severe respiratory or metabolic acidosis is depression of the central nervous system. The principal manifestation of respiratory or metabolic alkalosis is increased excitability of the peripheral nervous system (tetany) and central nervous system (seizures).

A. **Respiratory Acidosis**. Any event (drug or disease) that decreases alveolar ventilation results in an increased concentration of dissolved carbon dioxide in the blood (increased Paco$_2$), which in turn leads to formation of carbonic acid and hydrogen ions. By convention, carbonic acid resulting from dissolved carbon dioxide is considered a respiratory acid, and respiratory acidosis is present when the pH is <7.35 and Paco$_2$ is >45 mm Hg.

1. Acidosis, respiratory or metabolic, often has profound effects on many drug and enzyme interactions in the body, which function optimally only within normal pH ranges.

    2. Of particular importance is the clinical scenario of increasing respiratory acidosis due to inadequate reversal of muscle relaxants.

B. **Respiratory Alkalosis**. Respiratory alkalosis is present when increased alveolar ventilation removes sufficient carbon dioxide from the body to decrease the hydrogen ion concentration to the extent that pH becomes >7.45.

    1. A physiologic cause of respiratory alkalosis is hyperventilation due to stimulation of chemoreceptors by a low Po_2 associated with ascent to altitude.

    2. Kidneys compensate with time for this loss of carbon dioxide by excreting bicarbonate ions in association with sodium and potassium ions. This renal compensation is evident in individuals residing at altitude who have a nearly normal pH despite a low $Paco_2$.

    3. A frequent cause of acute respiratory alkalosis is iatrogenic hyperventilation of the lungs as during anesthesia.

C. **Metabolic Acidosis**

    1. The most common and most confusing acid–base disorder that clinicians are required to manage is metabolic acidosis. Any acid formed in the body other than carbonic acid from carbon dioxide is considered a metabolic acid, and its accumulation results in metabolic acidosis.

    2. Acidosis impairs myocardial contractility and the responses to endogenous or exogenous catecholamines.

        a. Hemodynamic deterioration is usually minimal (in the awake state) when the pH remains >7.2 due to compensatory increases in sympathetic nervous system activity (accentuated detrimental effects of metabolic acidosis in individuals with underlying left ventricular dysfunction or myocardial ischemia or in those in whom sympathetic nervous system activity may be impaired, as by drug-induced β-adrenergic blockade or general anesthesia).

        b. Respiratory acidosis may produce more rapid and profound myocardial dysfunction than does metabolic acidosis, reflecting the ability of carbon dioxide to freely diffuse across cell membranes and exacerbate intracellular acidosis.

    3. Acute metabolic acidosis has been treated with intravenous administration of an exogenous buffer, usually sodium bicarbonate, in the hope that normalizing pH will attenuate the detrimental effects of acidosis

(effectiveness of the use of sodium bicarbonate to treat metabolic acidosis is debatable).

    a. Sodium bicarbonate administration increases the carbon dioxide load to the lungs, leading to further increases in arterial and intracellular Pco_2 if alveolar ventilation is not concomitantly increased (estimated that 1 mEq/kg sodium bicarbonate, given intravenously, produces approximately 180 mL of carbon dioxide and necessitates a transient doubling of alveolar ventilation to prevent hypercarbia).

    b. If alveolar ventilation can be increased to deal with the increased carbon dioxide load from administration of sodium bicarbonate (initial bolus dose 0.5 to 1 mEq/kg), then it can be useful as a temporizing measure to help restore hemodynamic stability in shock combined with severe metabolic acidosis.

4. **Lactic Acidosis**

    a. Normal clearance of lactate maintains its serum concentration between 0.5 and 1.0. Most lactate is cleared by the liver, where it undergoes oxidation, gluconeogenesis, and eventual conversion to bicarbonate (severe reductions in hepatic blood flow, which occur during shock, will decrease hepatic lactate clearance).

    b. Lactic acid is a strong acid and therefore dissociates almost completely under physiologic conditions into the lactate anion and a hydrogen ion (traditionally thought to occur mainly during anaerobic glycolysis but is not recognized, can form under normoxic conditions).

    c. In the critically ill patient, lactate production may increase while lactate clearance is impaired and lactic acidosis may occur (point-of-care testing allows almost instantaneous lactate determinations to be performed in the operating room and intensive care unit). A serum lactate >1.5 mmol/L upon admission is an independent predictor of mortality in critically ill patients.

5. **Dilutional acidosis** occurs when the plasma pH is decreased by extracellular volume expansion with chloride-containing solutions such as normal saline (Table 26-4). Clinically, a hyperchloremic metabolic acidosis may accompany large-volume infusion of isotonic saline.

6. **Differential Diagnosis of Metabolic Acidosis**

    a. Base excess (BE) is defined as the amount of strong acid or base to return the plasma pH to 7.4, assuming $Paco_2$ is 40 mm Hg and normothermia. The BE is

Table 26-4

Electrolytes in Plasma and Commonly Available Crystalloid Solutions

Solution	Na	Cl	K	Ca	Mg	Lactate	Acetate	Gluconate	pH	mOsm
				(mEq/L)						
Plasma	144	107	5	2	1.5				7.4	290
NS	154	154							5.5	308
RL	130	109	4	3		28			6.5	273
Plasmalyte	140	98	5		3		27	23 (mmol)	7.4	294
Ionolyte	137	110	4		1.5		34		7.4	287

mOsm, osmolarity; NS, normal saline; RL, Ringer's lactate.

calculated (not measured) by modern blood gas analyzers from an algorithm based on measured HCO_3^- and pH.

b. In isolated acute respiratory acidosis or alkalosis, the BE should not change (normal value = 0).

7. **Anion Gap**

   a. Calculation of the anion gap may assist in the evaluation of acid–base disorders. The anion gap is a derived value based on the principle of electrochemical neutrality such that the sum of the positive (cationic) charges in a solution must equal the sum of the negative (anionic) charges.

   b. Under normal circumstances, the concentration of the predominant cation (sodium) exceeds that of the combined predominant anions (chloride and bicarbonate) [anion gap = $Na^+ - (HCO_3^- + Cl^-)$] by 9 to 13 mEq/L.

   c. The term *anion gap* refers solely to the difference in concentration between the traditionally measured anions and cations.

   d. Metabolic acidosis is most often associated with an increase in the anion gap (Table 26-5).

8. **Simplified Approach to Metabolic Acidosis of Uncertain Etiology.** When the cause of a metabolic acidosis is unclear, measure the serum lactate, blood urea nitrogen (BUN), creatinine, and glucose (if this does not identify the etiology

Table 26-5

Causes of Metabolic Acidosis

Increased Anion Gap	Normal Anion Gap
• Lactic acidosis	• Hyperchloremic acidosis (excess saline administration)
• Ketoacidosis	
• Chronic renal failure (accumulation of sulfates, phosphates, urea)	• Diarrhea (long-standing bicarbonate loss)
• Intoxication: organic acids (salicylates, ethanol, methanol, formaldehyde, ethylene glycol, paraldehyde), INH, sulfates, metformin	• Pancreatic fistula
	• Renal tubular acidosis
	• Intoxication: ammonium chloride, acetazolamide, toluene
• Massive rhabdomyolysis	

of the acidosis, then send serum for toxicology to measure salicylates, methanol, ethylene glycol).

D. **Metabolic alkalosis** is commonly iatrogenic. Causes include vomiting with excess loss of hydrochloric acid, nasogastric suction, chronic administration of diuretics, hypoalbuminemia, and excess secretion of aldosterone.

V. **Compensation for Acid–Base Disturbances**

A. Respiratory acidosis is compensated for within 6 to 12 hours by increased renal secretion of hydrogen ions, with a resulting increase in the plasma bicarbonate concentration.

1. After a few days, the pH will be normal despite persistence of an increased $Paco_2$.

2. Sudden correction of chronic respiratory acidosis, by iatrogenic hyperventilation, may result in acute metabolic alkalosis because increased plasma bicarbonate is not promptly eliminated by the kidneys.

B. Respiratory alkalosis is compensated for by decreased reabsorption of bicarbonate ions from renal tubules. As a result, more bicarbonate ions are excreted in the urine, which decreases the plasma concentration of bicarbonate and returns the pH toward normal despite persistence of a decreased $Paco_2$.

C. Metabolic acidosis stimulates alveolar ventilation, which causes rapid removal of carbon dioxide from the body and decreases the hydrogen ion concentration toward normal (compensation only partial because pH remains somewhat below normal).

D. Metabolic alkalosis diminishes alveolar ventilation, which in turn causes accumulation of carbon dioxide and a subsequent increase in hydrogen ion concentration. As with metabolic acidosis, the respiratory compensation for metabolic alkalosis is only partial.

1. During prolonged vomiting, there may be excessive loss of chloride ions along with sodium and potassium (kidneys preferentially conserve sodium and potassium ions and the urine becomes paradoxically acidic).

2. The presence of paradoxical aciduria indicates electrolyte depletion.

VI. **Effects of Temperature on Acid–Base Status (Table 26-6)**

A. As blood is cooled, carbon dioxide becomes more soluble (carbon dioxide partial pressure will decrease as the temperature falls).

1. The magnitude of this change is approximately 4.5% per degree Celsius and will tend to increase the pH.

Table 26-6		
α-Stat versus pH-Stat Management during Hypothermia		
	α Stat	**pH Stat**
Carbon dioxide added to oxygenator	No	Yes
Enzyme function	Near normal	Decreased
Cerebral blood flow	Normal	Increased
Blood gas temperature correction required	No	Yes
Hb-O_2 dissociation curve	Marked left shift	Less marked left shift

    2. These changes are probably insignificant within the physiologic temperature range but are important when interpreting blood gas and acid–base data during induced cooling during cardiopulmonary bypass.

B. **pH-Stat Management**

    1. During hypothermic conditions, blood pH is increased and P_{CO_2} is decreased. The pH-stat strategy seeks to return the pH and P_{CO_2} of hypothermic blood to normal.

    2. Temperature correction of blood gas samples is required to interpret the values obtained from a hypothermic patient but measured at 37°C.

C. **α-Stat Management**. The α-stat strategy seeks to replicate the alkalinization of blood that occurs during cooling in poikilothermic mammals.

CHAPTER 27

Physiology of Blood and Hemostasis

I. **Introduction.** Understanding the physiology of coagulation and blood interactions is important in determining the preoperative bleeding risk of patients and in managing hemostatic therapy perioperatively. At the center of hemostasis is the ability to generate thrombin, a serine protease, and the subsequent role for thrombin in the activation of additional coagulation factors (Figs. 27-1 and 27-2). Managing perioperative hemostasis also requires consideration of the postoperative hypercoagulability that may follow.

II. Hemostasis and History (see Figs. 27-1 and 27-2) (Table 27-1)

A. **Initiation of Coagulation.** Initiation of coagulation by procoagulant activities has been traditionally separated into extrinsic, intrinsic, and common pathways (a better understanding of the complex interactions has created a better conceptual integration of these pathways). Following tissue injury and vascular endothelial disruption, activation of hemostasis occurs by tissue factor (TF) expression on the subendothelial vascular basement of the blood vessel. As part of the activation, there are also checks and balances in the system to prevent an over exuberant prothrombotic effect from occurring.

B. **Propagation of Coagulation.** Platelets further amplify or potentially initiate clot formation at the site of vascular injury. Inflammatory cells all contain adhesion molecules to facilitate binding in the rapid flow of blood vessels. Thrombin activation of platelets further amplifies clot formation by multiple mechanisms. In the absence of factor VIIIa or factor IXa, as is clinically observed in hemophilia A or B, the initiation of coagulation is normal, but amplification/propagation is altered. Patients with hemophilia clot, but they develop bleeding in muscle and joints due to low TF expression.

503

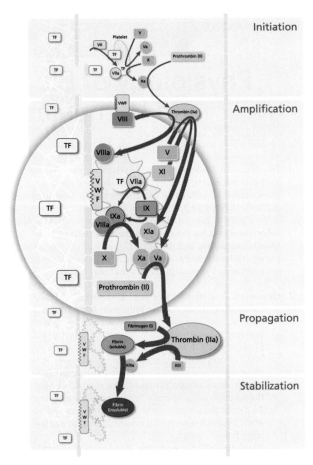

FIGURE 27-1 Initiation, amplification, propagation, and stabilization of hemostasis and clot formation. This describes the complexity of the clotting process and illustrates the interaction between coagulation factors and the cell surfaces of platelets in what has been described as the cellular model of hemostasis. Four sequential and interrelated stages include initiation, amplification, propagation, and stabilization as shown. This model also combines multiple aspects of the classic waterfall/cascade model, and further explains additional aspects of hemostasis that the classic acellular model does not. (Modified from Monroe DM, Hoffman M. What does it take to make the perfect clot? *Arterioscler Thromb Vasc Biol.* 2006;26:41–48.)

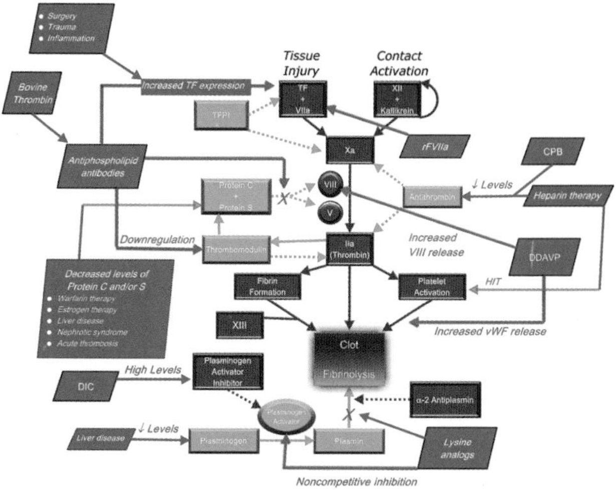

FIGURE 27-2 Procoagulant forces *(red)* and natural anticoagulant/ fibrinolytic forces *(green)* and diagrammed. Dashed lines indicated an inhibitory effect. Acquired risk factors are presented in blue boxes with white lettering and arrows indicating the mechanism for the hypercoagulable effect. "X's" denote a specific block in a pathway. Note that some acquired risk factors have multiple effects; see text for full details. CPB, cardiopulmonary bypass; DDAVP, desmopressin; DIC, disseminated intravascular coagulation; TF, tissue factor; TFPI, tissue factor pathway inhibitor. (From Sniecinski RM, Hursting MJ, Paidas MJ, et al. Etiology and assessment of hypercoagulability with lessons from heparin-induced thrombocytopenia. *Anesth Analg.* 2010;112:46–58.)

1. **Tissue Factor, Thrombin, and Fibrin(ogen) in Clot Formation and Stability**. When generated, thrombin facilitates the proteolytic conversion of circulating, soluble fibrinogen to an insoluble fibrin meshwork (provides structural support to the clot).
2. **Role of Fibrinogen** (Fig. 27-3). Fibrinogen is a critical protein for clot formation and has a critical role in hemostasis.
   a. Of all the coagulation factors, fibrinogen circulates at the highest concentration (7.6 μM, ~200 to 400 mg/dL). In pregnancy and during acute inflammatory responses that often occur postoperatively, fibrinogen is an acute-phase reactant.
   b. In patients with hemophilia and other bleeding abnormalities, lower levels of thrombin generation

	Table 27-1	

Plasma Levels, Half-lives of Coagulation Factors

Factor	Level (μM)	Half-life (h)
Fibrinogen	7.6	72–120
Prothrombin	1.4	72
Factor V	0.03	36
Factor VII	0.01	3–6
Factor VIII	0.00003	12
Factor IX	0.09	24
Factor X	0.17	40
Factor XI	0.03	80
Factor XIII	0.03	120–200
vWF	0.03	10–24
Protein C	0.08	10
Protein S	0.14	42
Antithrombin	2.6	48–72

vWF, von Willebrand factor.
Modified from Tanaka KA, Key NS, Levy JH. Blood coagulation: hemostasis and thrombin regulation. *Anesth Analg.* 2009;108:1433–1446.

occur and as a result clot formation is altered, thus hemophiliacs commonly bleed into joints.

3. **Critical factor levels for hemostasis.** A critical question is what levels of fibrinogen, platelets, and other coagulation proteins are necessary to optimize hemostasis in the surgical patients (many recommend treating fibrinogen levels if they have decreased below <1.0 g/L [100 mg/dL]).

4. **Role of Factor XIII.** Factor XIII plays a major role in the terminal phase of the clotting cascade that promotes formation of cross-linked fibrin polymers and generation of a stable hemostatic plug.

5. **Role of Platelets and von Willebrand Factor.** Platelets adhere to sites of vascular injury and to each other by direct and indirect effects that are part of a complex cellular mechanism required for hemostasis.

a. Following vascular injury, the subendothelial surface is exposed which then binds to vWF that is synthesized in the endothelium and critical for platelet adhesion in arteries and arterioles that have high shear rates.

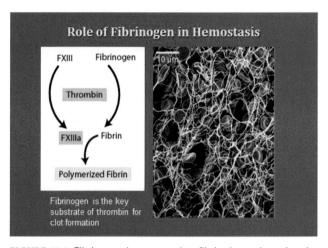

FIGURE 27-3 Fibrinogen is converted to fibrin that polymerizes by the action of thrombin. The electron micrograph shows a fibrin clot with red blood cells trapped. Platelets also are critical to fibrin formation, but they are 8 to 10 microns and not visible in the photo. Fibrinogen receptors on the platelet surface (called **IIb/IIIa receptors**) facilitate the lattice network of fibrin formation. Factor XIII, a trans-glutamase, is also important for cross-linking the fibrin clot to create a stronger clot that is resistant to fibrinolysis. (Modified from Tanaka KA, Key NS, Levy JH. Blood coagulation: hemostasis and thrombin regulation. *Anesth Analg.* 2009;108:1433–1446.)

      b. Platelets provide a catalytic membrane surface for further thrombin generation and clot formation.

      c. When activated, platelets may also form occlusive thrombi in cardiovascular diseases that result in myocardial infarction, stroke, or other acute ischemic syndromes of other organs.

   C. **Endothelial Regulation of Coagulation** (see Fig. 27-2). The vascular endothelium provides an extensive interface that is critical for both anticoagulant and procoagulant functions as shown.

      1. Increased shear forces and flow across the endothelium release important anticoagulation agents (Table 27-2).

      2. Endothelial activation also provides anticoagulation by releasing tissue-type plasminogen activator (t-PA) from the endothelial stores.

Table 27-2

Endothelial Proteins and Mediators of Hemostasis

ADAMTS-13
Endothelial protein C receptor
Glycocalyx
Heparan sulfate
Nitric oxide
Plasminogen activator inhibitor-1
Prostacyclin
Protein C
Protein S
Thrombomodulin
Tissue factor
Tissue factor pathway inhibitor
Tissue-type plasminogen activator
von Willebrand factor

ADAMTS-13, *a* *d*isintegrin *a*nd *m*etalloprotease with a *t*hrombo*s*pondin
type 1 motif, member *13*.

---

3. Endothelial damage following vascular injury or inflammatory responses initiates an array of procoagulant responses that include release of TF, vWF, plasminogen activator inhibitor (PAI)-1, and protease activated receptors (PARs).

4. This complex equilibrium of hemostasis continues and is constantly scavenged by many of these important mechanisms to localize hemostasis to the site of vascular injury through this multitude of regulatory mechanisms.

D. **Antithrombin, protein C, and protein S** are important serine proteases that exert anticoagulant and antiinflammatory activities (activated protein C binds protein S, and together they function as a critical anticoagulant by inhibiting factor Va and factor VIIIa).

III. **Inflammation and Coagulation: An Important Link.** Coagulation is closely linked to inflammatory responses (hemostatic initiation, contact activation, and other pathways amplify inflammatory responses and can collectively produce end-organ damage in the process of their normal function as host defense mechanisms).

A. Surgical injury and additional activation that can occur following cardiopulmonary bypass produce inflammatory responses initiated by contact of blood with the damaged vasculature and other nonendothelial extracorporeal circuits.

B. In vascular surgical and trauma patients, ischemia-reperfusion injury of organs can also occur.

IV. **Coagulation Testing**

A. The two tests most frequently used in the perioperative setting, other than blood counts, include the prothrombin time, used to evaluate the extrinsic coagulation cascade, and the activated partial thromboplastin time, used to evaluate the intrinsic pathway of the classic coagulation system.

1. The prothrombin time is affected by reductions of factors VII, X, V, and prothrombin and is used to measure the effect of warfarin and other agents with vitamin K antagonist activity or the consequences of decreased synthetic activity resulting from hepatic dysfunction.

a. Although prothrombin time is used commonly for perioperative coagulation screening, its use and target values are still controversial and often based on consensus rather than supportive data.

b. Clinical hemostasis may not be adequately evaluated with prothrombin times alone as is apparent in patients with hemophilia who have isolated factor VIII or IX deficiency despite normal prothrombin times.

2. The partial thromboplastin time is another widely used coagulation test that assesses the intrinsic coagulation cascade. The partial thromboplastin time is used to monitor lower doses of unfractionated heparin (up to ~1.0 units/mL). At higher heparin concentrations used during cardiac surgery, the activated clotting time (ACT) is used.

B. Although these coagulation tests are used to evaluate bleeding, they only examine specific components of the overall coagulation cascade and may not be useful to determine the exact cause of the coagulopathy.

C. Whole blood viscoelastic tests including thromboelastography and thromboelastometry provide multiple insights in to coagulation factor interaction and allow assessment of individual characteristics of either individual limbs of hemostasis or global monitoring of coagulation (widely used in the perioperative and trauma setting). The commonly used thromboelastometric variables include coagulation time (onset in seconds), clot formation time (initial rate of fibrin polymerization in seconds), angle (a; in degrees), maximum clot firmness (in millimeters), and lysis time (in seconds, used for the diagnosis of premature lysis or hyperfibrinolysis).

V. **Perioperative Changes in Coagulation.** In surgical patients, there are multiple perioperative events that influence hemostatic function and produce coagulopathy. Vascular and tissue injury are important contributors to bleeding, but with significant hemorrhage and resuscitation with crystalloids/colloids, a dilutional coagulopathy can occur resulting from significant reductions in platelet counts/dilutional thrombocytopenia and factor deficiencies.

VI. **Hemostatic Therapy.** Red blood cells and hemostatic factors that include plasma/fresh frozen plasma, platelet concentrates, and cryoprecipitate are used when bleeding occurs. Postoperatively, an important anabolic state occurs that increases hemostatic factors for several days (create a hypercoagulable, procoagulant response). This is integral to the current practice of use of anticoagulation for postoperative venous thromboembolic prophylaxis because of the increased thrombotic potential postoperatively.

   A. **Postoperative Hypercoagulability.** The complex balance in hemostatic function can be readily altered in the postoperative setting. Embolic and other thrombotic events occurring locally at the site of an atherosclerotic plaque can result in myocardial infarction and ischemic stroke. Abnormalities present in cancer patients can also initiate coagulation and other prothrombotic events that increase the risk of venous thromboembolic events.

      1. Congenital coagulation factor deficiencies or polymorphisms of critical proteins including hemophilia A or B, vWF, antithrombin, protein C, protein S, factor V Leiden, and prothrombin (polymorphisms) can present with either bleeding or thrombosis.

      2. Acquired or congenital absence of the anticoagulant proteins reduces normal clot formation and regulation, and untreated patients are at an increased risk for venous thromboembolic problems, including pulmonary embolism.

      3. A more common occurrence is the antiphospholipid syndrome that is caused by the lupus anticoagulant, which is a phospholipid binding antibody (patients may present with prolonged prothrombin times and

partial thromboplastin times, but they are actually hypercoagulable).

B. **Disseminated intravascular coagulation (DIC)** is a coagulation disorder that occurs when pathologic activation of the hemostatic systems occurs following major tissue injury (trauma, sepsis).

1. Activation of the coagulation system occurs; however, the multiple endothelial and circulating anticoagulation mechanisms that are part of hemostatic mechanisms are unable to inhibit systemic thrombin formation (microvascular deposition of clot/fibrin and thrombotic microangiopathy).

2. Platelets are also activated, resulting in either a hemorrhagic coagulopathy or procoagulant state. Thrombocytopenia occurs in DIC, but the most common cause of perioperative thrombocytopenia is the dilutional effect following volume resuscitation.

3. The current strategy for treating massive transfusion coagulopathy in the setting of trauma and surgery includes the administration of platelets and other clotting factors (platelets, fresh frozen plasma, and/or cryoprecipitate).

CHAPTER 28

Blood Products and Blood Components

I. **Introduction**
   A. Millions of blood components are transfused annually, especially in surgical and trauma patients (benefit/risk of transfusions has become part of informed consent).
   B. Transfusion-related acute lung injury (TRALI) followed by hemolytic transfusion reactions are the most common causes of mortality and morbidity associated with transfusions.
      1. Decisions to transfuse require multiple clinical considerations including risk factors, comorbidities, hemodynamic stability, and the rate of bleeding.
      2. Guidelines and transfusion algorithms for the management of bleeding in surgical patients are available. Multiple risk factors are important when considering patients at risk for bleeding (Tables 28-1 and 28-2).

II. **Transfusion Therapy for Bleeding.** Critical bleeding in the perioperative setting requires volume replacement (crystalloid, colloid, red blood cells [RBCs]) (none provide coagulation factors or platelets and thus their use can exacerbate coagulopathy). Severe bleeding requires use of fresh frozen plasma (FFP), platelets, cryoprecipitate, and factor concentrates (e.g., fibrinogen and prothrombin complex concentrates) to restore circulating levels of hemostatic factors. Following massive transfusion therapy, hypothermia and acidosis (temperature and pH) must be monitored and corrected during any ongoing transfusion.
   A. **Red Blood Cells**
      1. There is no single minimum acceptable hemoglobin level that can be applied to all patients when deciding when to transfuse RBCs. With acute anemia, compensatory mechanisms that increase cardiac output and improve oxygen transport depend on the patient's cardiovascular reserve. In surgical patients with heart failure and/or flow-restricting lesions, compensation during acute anemia may be limited.

Table 28-1

Predictors of Postoperative Bleeding: Cardiothoracic Surgery

Advanced age
Small body size or preoperative anemia (low RBC volume)
Antiplatelet and antithrombotic drugs
Prolonged operation (CPB time)—high correlation with OR type
Emergency operation
Other comorbidities (CHF, COPD, HTN, PVD, renal failure)

RBC, red blood cell; CPB, cardiopulmonary bypass; CHF, congestive heart failure; COPD, chronic obstructive pulmonary disease; HTN, hypertension; OR, operating room; PVD, peripheral vascular disease.
From Ferraris VA, Ferraris SP, Saha SP, et al. Perioperative blood transfusion and blood conservation in cardiac surgery: the STS and the SCA Clinical Practice Guideline. *Ann Thorac Surg.* 2007;83:S27–S86.

2. The decision to transfuse must include multiple factors (intravascular volume, whether the patient is actively bleeding, and the need for improvement in oxygen transport).
    a. The American Society of Anesthesiologists Task Force on Perioperative Blood Transfusion noted in its recommendations that transfusion of RBCs should usually be administered when the hemoglobin concentration is low (e.g., <6 g/dL in a young, healthy patient), especially when the anemia is acute.
    b. RBCs are usually unnecessary when the hemoglobin concentration is more than 10 g/dL.
    c. Hemoglobin triggers for transfusion are not to be taken as absolute; patients with significant cardiac disease should be transfused if signs or symptoms of inadequate myocardial oxygenation appear.
B. **RBC Storage Lesions**
    1. RBCs develop a complex series of biochemical and metabolic changes during storage in the blood bank. As the blood ages, RBCs undergo shape changes with increased fragility.
    2. Because of increased red cell–endothelial cell interaction, bioreactive lipids and other substances are released that may initiate inflammatory responses leading to TRALI.
C. **RBC Storage and Tissue Oxygenation Parameters**
    1. Transfusion of RBCs is used therapeutically to increase the oxygen-carrying capacity of blood and thereby improve oxygen delivery to tissues.

Table 28-2

Evidence-Based Indications for Transfusing Red Blood Cells, Platelets, Fresh Frozen Plasma, and Cryoprecipitate in Perioperative Settings Guidelines

1. The risks of bleeding in surgical patients are determined by the extent and type of surgery, the capacity to control bleeding, the expected rate of bleeding, and the outcomes of uncontrolled bleeding.

2. RBC transfusions should not be dictated by a single hemoglobin "trigger" but instead should be based on each individual patient's risk of developing complications of inadequate oxygenation. RBC transfusions are rarely indicated when the hemoglobin concentration is >10 g/dL and are nearly always indicated when it is <6 g/dL. The indications for autologous transfusion may be more liberal than for allogeneic transfusion.

3. Prophylactic platelet transfusion is ineffective when thrombocytopenia is due to increased platelet destruction. Surgical patients with microvascular bleeding usually need platelet transfusion if the platelet count is <50,000 platelets/μL and rarely platelet transfusion if is the platelet count is >100,000 platelets/μL.

4. Fresh frozen plasma (FFP) is indicated for urgent reversal of warfarin therapy, correction of known coagulation factor deficiencies for which specific concentrates are unavailable, and correction of microvascular bleeding when prothrombin and partial thromboplastin times are >1.5 times normal. FFP is not indicated for increasing plasma volume or albumin concentration.

5. Cryoprecipitate should be considered for patients with von Willebrand's disease unresponsive to desmopressin, bleeding patients with von Willebrand's disease, and bleeding patients with fibrinogen levels <80–100 mg/dL.

RBC, red blood cell.

Practice guidelines for perioperative blood transfusion and adjuvant therapies: an updated report by the American Society of Anesthesiologists Task Force on Perioperative Blood Transfusion and Adjuvant Therapies. *Anesthesiology*. 2006;105:198–208.

2. The true impact of the age of stored RBC on patient outcomes remains in question, but an answer should emerge from these ongoing clinical trials.

D. **Plasma/fresh frozen plasma (FFP)** are used to replace volume and coagulation factors during massive transfusion (Table 28-3).

1. FFP is used for treating bleeding because of coagulopathies that are associated with a prolongation of either the activated partial thromboplastin time or prothrombin time/international normalized ratio greater than 1.5 times normal.

Table 28-3

Plasma Transfusion Indications

1. Management of bleeding or to prevent bleeding prior to an urgent invasive procedure in patients requiring replacement of multiple coagulation factors
2. Massively transfused patients who have clinically significant coagulation deficiencies and hypovolemia
3. Patients on warfarin therapy with bleeding or that need to undergo an invasive procedure before vitamin K could reverse the effects of warfarin or who need only transient reversal of warfarin effects
4. For transfusion or plasma exchange in patients with thrombotic thrombocytopenic purpura (TTP) and some cases of hemolytic uremic syndrome (HUS)
5. Management of patients with selected coagulation factor deficiencies, congenital or acquired, for which no specific coagulation concentrates are available
6. Management of patients with rare specific plasma protein deficiencies, when recombinant products or purified products are unavailable
7. Fresh frozen plasma (FFP) is the product of choice for patients specifically requiring replacement of the labile clotting factors or other proteins with poor storage stability because the other plasma products may be deficient in these factors during liquid storage; deficiencies due to consumption/hemodilution rarely fall to levels that are inadequately treated with non-FFP components; consultation with a hematologist or transfusion medicine physician is recommended for assistance with indications

2. When FFP is indicated, it should be administered in a dose calculated to achieve a minimum of 30% of plasma factor concentration (10 to 15 mL/kg of FFP will generally result in a rise of most coagulation proteins by 25% to 30%).

3. Plasma is overused in surgery, most often because of the empirical nature of transfusion therapy.
   a. The most common cause of bleeding after surgery is platelet dysfunction.
   b. The prothrombin time and partial thromboplastin times, which are widely used to evaluate bleeding, have never been demonstrated to accurately reflect the cause of bleeding in surgical patients.

4. Plasma transfusions, like all blood products, have the potential for adverse effects (transfusion-associated circulatory overload, TRALI).

E. **Solvent treated plasma** is human pooled plasma that has been solvent/detergent (S/D) treated (kills certain viruses and minimizes the risk of serious virus transmission) and is thought to reduce the risk of TRALI. This product is indicated for replacement of multiple coagulation (administration is based on ABO blood group compatibility).

F. **Cryoprecipitate** contains therapeutic amounts of factor VIII:C, factor XIII, von Willebrand factor, and fibrinogen.

1. Cryoprecipitate is used not only to increase fibrinogen levels depleted because of massive hemorrhage or coagulopathy but also for the treatment of congenital or acquired factor XIII deficiency.

2. One unit of cryoprecipitate per 10 kg body weight increases plasma fibrinogen by roughly 50 to 70 mg/dL in the absence of continuing consumption or massive bleeding. The minimum hemostatic level of fibrinogen is traditionally suggested to be around 100 mg/dL (normal fibrinogen levels are 200 mg/dL and higher).

3. Because cryoprecipitate does not contain factor V, it should not be the sole replacement therapy for disseminated intravascular coagulopathy (DIC).

4. Cryoprecipitate has been withdrawn from many European countries due to safety concerns, primarily the transmission of pathogens (instead, commercial fibrinogen preparations are available for fibrinogen replacement therapy).

G. **Platelet Concentrates**
   1. Platelets that are used clinically are either pooled random-donor platelet concentrates or single-donor apheresis and can be stored for up to 5 days.
   2. In medical patients, a platelet count of $10,000/\mu L$ is a typical threshold for prophylactic platelet transfusion (normal platelet count ranges from 150,000 to 400,000 platelets per μL). The platelet count for therapeutic transfusions to control or prevent bleeding with trauma or surgical procedures requires a higher transfusion trigger of $100,000/\mu L$ for neurosurgical procedures and between $50,000/\mu L$ and $100,000/\mu L$ for other invasive procedures or trauma.
   3. There remains significant risk of bacterial infection with platelet administration because they are stored at $22°C$ rather than at the $4°C$ storage used for red cell storage.
H. **Alloimmunization**. An immunocompetent recipient often develops variable immune responses to the transfused agents that include graft versus host disease. Multiple other antigens that are not routinely crossmatched for platelets may be responsible for alloimmunization.
I. **Leukoreduction**. Leukoreduced platelet and RBC products decrease the risk of alloimmunization. Cytomegalovirus transmission is reduced by reducing leukocyte burden, and as a result, there is also a reduction in febrile transfusion reactions.

III. **Graft versus host disease (GVHD) is a potentially fatal complication that occurs more commonly after a bone marrow or stem cell transplant, or following platelet transfusions where viable white cells from the donor regard the recipient's body as foreign and create acute inflammatory responses and tissue and organ injury by attacking the recipient's body (γ-irradiation is performed for prevention of GVHD).**

IV. **Indications for Platelet Transfusions and Transfusion Triggers**
   A. In medical patients, a platelet transfusion trigger of approximately 10,000 platelets/μL in efforts to prevent bleeding is often described (yet data and prospective studies to evaluate the effects of platelet dose on hemostasis and rates of platelet use overall for perioperative management are often based on consensus guidelines rather than clinical studies).
   B. There are three important areas of controversy regarding the use of platelet transfusions without active bleeding. First, the optimal prophylactic platelet dose to prevent

thrombocytopenic bleeding even in medical patients is not well known. Second, the exact platelet count threshold that requires transfusion of platelets is not known. Finally, whether prophylactic platelet transfusions are superior to therapeutic platelet transfusions in surgical patients is not known.

1. In most surgical patients, there is little data to support prophylactic platelet transfusions; the exceptions are massive transfusion coagulopathy and certain closed procedures where bleeding may be highly problematic such as intracranial hemorrhage.

2. Dilutional thrombocytopenia often occurs as an early manifestation of massive transfusion.

C. **Platelet Counts for Surgery and Invasive Procedures**

1. For surgery or following trauma, expert recommendations suggest that a platelet count of greater than or equal to 50,000/μL be maintained (little data to support these recommendations).

2. In neurosurgical patients or patients with intracerebral bleeding and for neurosurgical procedures, expert recommendations suggest that platelet counts should be maintained at greater than 100,000/μL.

3. With platelet counts between 50,000 and 100,000/μL, clinical decisions to transfuse platelets should be based on the type of surgery, trauma, rates of bleeding, risk of bleeding, use of platelet inhibitors, and other potential coagulation abnormalities.

4. If platelet dysfunction is present in the face of trauma or surgery, platelet transfusions may be necessary, even in the presence of a normal platelet count.

5. **ABO Compatibility**

a. Red cell antigens are expressed on platelets, and ABO-incompatible platelets have reduced posttransfusion platelet count recoveries but normal platelet survival.

b. Patients who receive ABO-incompatible platelets become refractory to additional platelet transfusions at a higher rate than the ABO-compatible recipients because sensitization produces anti–human leukocyte antigen (HLA) and platelet-specific alloantibodies.

V. **Purified Protein Concentrates**

A. **Fibrinogen Concentrates.** Fibrinogen is a critical clotting protein (cryoprecipitate is routinely administered as the source of fibrinogen). Fibrinogen concentrate administration in patients with hypofibrinogenemia and disseminated intravascular coagulation should be avoided.

B. **Prothrombin complex concentrates** are recommended for reversal in patients with life-threatening bleeding and an increased international normalized ratio when urgent reversal is required (warfarin reversal in the United States occurs with FFP).

C. **von Willebrand Factor** is indicated in adult and pediatric patients with von Willebrand's disease for (a) treatment of spontaneous and trauma-induced bleeding episodes and (b) prevention of excessive bleeding during and after surgery.

VI. Hereditary Angioedema and C1 Esterase Inhibitor Concentrates

A. Hereditary angioedema (HAE) is a life-threatening disease resulting from the absence or genetic mutation of a complement component inhibitor called C1 esterase inhibitor (C1 INH).

B. Angioedema produces increased permeability of submucosal or subcutaneous capillaries and postcapillary venules leading to plasma extravasation and subsequent swelling of critical airway structures.

VII. Adverse Effects of Transfusions. The risks of allogeneic transfusion extend beyond viral transmission, and include allergy, alloimmunization, anaphylaxis, bacterial sepsis, graft versus host disease, TRALI, transfusion-related acute circulatory overload, renal failure, volume overload, and immunosuppression (Table 28-4).

A. **Transfusion as an Inflammatory Response**. Transfusion of allogeneic blood has multiple immunomodulatory effects including immunosuppression (in cardiac surgical patients who are already immunosuppressed by surgical trauma, added inhibition of immunomodulation may have harmful effects).

B. **Transfusion-associated circulatory overload** is a volume overload state, where the rate of volume infusion of blood products is in excess of what the patient's cardiovascular status can handle.

C. **Transfusion-Related Acute Lung Injury** (Table 28-5)

1. The most widely accepted current concept is that TRALI results from neutrophil and/or endothelial activation via multiple mechanisms in the lung, resulting in pulmonary vascular injury and pulmonary edema.

Table 28-4

Presentation of Transfusion-Associated Circulatory Overload

Dyspnea
Elevated jugular venous pressure
Hypertension or hypotension
Tachycardia
Rales on lung auscultation
Pulmonary edema
Increased brain natriuretic peptide
Echocardiography: hypervolemia, mitral regurgitation due to volume overload

---

2. Multiple pathogenic transfused factors are associated with TRALI (Fig. 28-1).

D. **Acute Pulmonary Edema and Management**. The multiple signaling mechanisms and inflammatory mediators in TRALI result in increased permeability and the eventual development of noncardiogenic pulmonary edema.

E. **Decreasing the Incidence of TRALI**. Policy changes made to mitigate TRALI have targeted antibody-mediated TRALI.

1. **Plasma from Male Donors**. Because TRALI is usually secondary to donor HLA or human neutrophil antigen antibodies, which are more common in females than

---

Table 28-5

Transfusion-Related Acute Lung Injury

Onset within 6 hours, usually more acute, following transfusion
Bilateral infiltrates seen on frontal chest radiograph
Hypoxemia/ ratio of Pao_2/Fio_2 300 mm Hg regardless of positive end-expiratory pressure level, or oxygen saturation of 90% on room air
Pulmonary artery occlusion $\leq$18 mm Hg when measured, or lack of clinical evidence of left atrial hypertension (volume overload)
Pathophysiologic mechanisms: human neutrophil antigen (HNA) and human leukocyte antigen (HLA) class I and II antibodies, CD40-ligand (CD40L), biologically active lipids

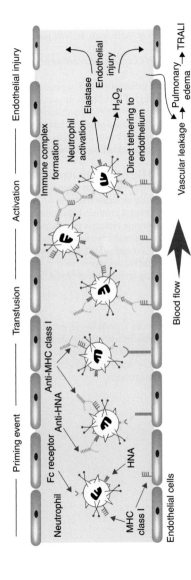

FIGURE 28-1 Transfusion-related acute lung injury (TRALI). Multiple priming events may or may not be required for TRALI but appear to be important factors in the inflammatory process that causes TRALI and may significantly potentiate the acute vasculitis that occurs. Transfusion of blood products from multiparous donors or other donors containing antibodies against white blood cell antigens that include human neutrophil antigen (HNA) and major histocompatibility complex (MHC) class I can result in direct binding and activation of intravascular polymorphonuclear leukocytes. These antibodies may also directly bind and tether neutrophils to the endothelium independent of the adhesion molecules, selectin and integrin. The antigen–antibody binding also produces immune complexes of multiple white blood cell antigens that may also be recognized by the Fc receptors (tail receptors of antibodies) resulting in neutrophil activation. The activated neutrophils bind to the pulmonary vascular endothelium, and aggregated clumps of neutrophils may lodge in the pulmonary microcirculation. Activated neutrophils release multiple proinflammatory substances including proteolytic enzymes, oxygen free radicals, thromboxane, and other inflammatory mediators both locally at the site of vascular injury and systemically. This complex series of events results in damage to endothelial cells, vascular leakage, and pulmonary edema.

521

males, the United Kingdom began using male donor plasma and resuspension of buffy coat–derived platelets in male-donated plasma.

2. These changes resulted in a decrease in number of TRALI reports and deaths.

F. **Transfusion-Related Acute Inflammatory Responses and Immunomodulation**. Although TRALI is an important example of the complex inflammatory responses associated with transfusions, multiple blood products have the potential for proinflammatory responses including acute hypersensitivity responses and anaphylaxis that may not affect the lung.

   1. **Role of Neutrophils and Other Inflammatory Cells**

      a. Polymorphonuclear leukocytes are an important element of the innate immune response (neutrophil-mediated events produce inflammatory responses that often become systemic producing widespread tissue damage and adverse sequelae).

      b. Neutrophil activation is responsible for multiple inflammatory events, including reperfusion injury, a common issue following restoration of blood flow in occluded vessels.

VIII. **Summary**

A. Blood products and transfusions should be considered in the same manner that we consider use of other drug therapies by carefully weighing their risks and benefits.

B. TRALI has emerged as a major cause of morbidity and mortality associated with transfusions.

CHAPTER 29

Procoagulants

I. **Introduction.** Bleeding in a perioperative setting, following trauma or surgery, can arise from numerous causes (activation of the coagulation, fibrinolytic, and inflammatory pathways; dilutional changes; hypothermia; surgical factors). When patients bleed following surgery and trauma, multiple therapeutic approaches are often required in addition to blood transfusion (procoagulants are now increasingly used to treat bleeding in the perioperative setting).

II. Antifibrinolytic Agents: Lysine Analogs
   A. The two synthetic antifibrinolytic agents available are the lysine analogs epsilon aminocaproic acid (EACA) and tranexamic acid (TXA). These agents competitively inhibit activation of plasminogen to plasmin, an enzyme that degrades fibrin clots, fibrinogen, and other plasma proteins.
   B. EACA does not consistently reduce transfusion requirements or surgical reexploration, especially in cardiac surgery.
   C. One of the potential complications of TXA is seizures.
   D. Antifibrinolytic agents also have been studied in other procedures, including orthopedic surgery, and all three agents reduce blood loss.

III. **Antifibrinolytic Agents: Aprotinin.** Aprotinin, a polypeptide serine protease inhibitor, inhibits plasmin and other serine proteases. In Canada, aprotinin is authorized for patients undergoing coronary artery bypass graft surgery.

IV. **Protamine** is a basic protein that inactivates the acidic heparin molecule via a simple acid–base interaction (does not reverse low-molecular-weight heparin).
   A. Excess protamine should be avoided when reversing heparin as it can contribute to coagulopathy (Fig. 29-1).
   B. When protamine is dosed based on the exact amount needed to reverse circulating heparin levels, it produces the lowest activated clotting time values.

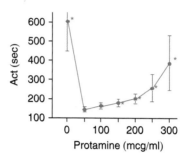

FIGURE 29-1 Excess protamine contributes to elevations in the activated clotting time (ACT), at excesses of the exact dose required to reverse systemic anticoagulation. Thus, overdosage of protamine should be strictly avoided. (Modified from Mochizuki T, Olson PJ, Szlam F, et al. Protamine reversal of heparin affects platelet aggregation and activated clotting time after cardiopulmonary bypass. *Anesth Analg.* 1998;87[4]:781–785.)

C. Protamine can cause adverse reactions including anaphylaxis, acute pulmonary vasoconstriction and right ventricular failure, and hypotension.
   1. Patients at an increased risk for adverse reactions are sensitized, often from exposure to neutral protamine Hagedorn, which contains insulin and protamine.
   2. Other individuals reported at risk for protamine reactions include patients with vasectomy, multiple drug allergies, and prior protamine exposure.

V. **Desmopressin (DDAVP) is the V2 analog of arginine vasopressin that stimulates the release of ultra large von Willebrand factor (vWF) multimers from endothelial cells.**
   A. DDAVP shortens the bleeding time of patients with mild forms of hemophilia A or von Willebrand's disease (the most frequent inherited bleeding disorder).
   B. The specific surgical patients that might benefit from use of DDAVP are not clear.
   C. DDAVP should be administered by slow intravenous infusion to avoid hypotension because it stimulates endothelial cells releasing vasoactive mediators in addition to vWF.

VI. **Fibrinogen is synthesized in the liver and a critical component of effective clot formation. It is the substrate of three** important enzymes involved in clot formation: thrombin, factor (F) XIIIa, and plasmin.

A. Fibrinogen also acts as the binding site (ligand) for glycoprotein IIb/IIIa receptors, found on the platelet surface, which are responsible for platelet aggregation.

B. During major hemorrhage, hemodilution after blood loss and subsequent volume replacement leads to reduced fibrinogen levels impairing fibrin polymerization and reduces clot stability (fibrinogen supplementation to restore plasma fibrinogen is key to normalizing clotting function).

1. Fibrinogen is an underrecognized coagulation factor that is critical for producing effective clot in surgical patients (hypofibrinogenemia is a predictor of perioperative bleeding).

2. Normal fibrinogen levels are 200 to 400 mg/dL (during the third trimester of pregnancy, fibrinogen levels are elevated to >400 mg/dL).

C. A major problem with managing bleeding is that many transfusion algorithms recommend therapy only when fibrinogen levels are less than 100 mg/dL. Cryoprecipitate or fibrinogen concentrates are a better option to restore adequate plasma levels (~200 mg/dL) and need to be considered when treating life-threatening bleeding.

VII. Recombinant coagulation products are used to manage bleeding in hemophilia, von Willebrand's disease, and in patients with acquired antibodies/inhibitors.

A. Recombinant activated factor VIIa (rFVIIa) is most widely known and approved for hemophilia patients with inhibitors to treat bleeding. The incidence of thrombotic complications among patients who received rFVIIa is relatively low. rFVIIa can normalize elevated international normalized ratio (INR)/prothrombin time values without actually correcting the coagulation defect, especially in patients receiving warfarin and other vitamin K antagonists.

B. **Factor XIII (FXIII)** is an important final step in clot formation that stabilizes the initial clot (reductions in FXIII during cardiopulmonary bypass and an inverse relationship between postoperative blood loss and postoperative FXIII levels).

C. **Prothrombin complex concentrates (PCCs)** include factors II, VII, IX, and X in variable concentrations (indicated for prevention/control of bleeding in patients with hemophilia B).

       1. It is considered preferable to give a PCC containing all four vitamin K–dependent coagulation factors and the natural anticoagulants antithrombin and activated protein C (APC) for anticoagulation reversal.

   D. Although warfarin reversal in the United States is typically achieved with fresh frozen plasma (FFP), most other countries use PCCs. Compared with FFP, PCCs provide quicker INR correction, have a lower infusion volume, and are more readily available without crossmatching.

   E. **Topical hemostatic agents** are used intraoperatively to promote hemostasis at the site of vascular injury and include physical and mechanical agents, caustic agents, biologic physical agents, and physiologic agents.

       1. Absorbable agents include gelatin sponges (Gelfoam), derived from purified pork skin gelatin that increase contact activation to help create topical clot. Surgicel or Oxycel are oxidized regenerated cellulose that work like Gelfoam. Avitene is microfibrillar collagen derived from bovine skin.

       2. Collagen sponges are available in different commercial forms and are derived from bovine Achilles tendon or bovine skin. Gelatin foam should not be used near nerves or in confined spaces but can be administered topically with thrombin.

       3. Topically applied thrombin preparations are used extensively.

       4. Fibrin sealants (biologic glue or fibrin tissue adhesives) are component products that combine thrombin (mostly human) and fibrinogen.

VIII. **Summary**

   A. The potential for bleeding in surgical patients represents an ongoing problem for clinicians (increasing use of anticoagulation agents creates a need for multiple pharmacologic approaches).

   B. Therapy should be multimodal when managing perioperative hemostasis (Fig. 29-2).

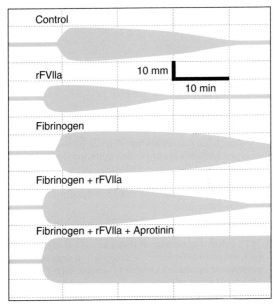

FIGURE 29-2 Thromboelastography recordings obtained with the ROTEM device after the addition of rFVIIa and/or fibrinogen in the presence of tissue-type plasminogen activator in volunteer plasma. Tissue-type plasminogen activator was added to stimulate fibrinolysis. rFVIIa, rFVIIa in a final concentration 1.5 μg/mL; fibrinogen, fibrinogen in a final concentration 100 mg/dL. The maximum clot firmness (the width of clot tracing) was only improved after the addition of fibrinogen. The onset of clotting was shorter after the addition of rFVIIa, but the extent of lysis (i.e., decreased clot firmness) was increased in contrast to the samples with fibrinogen. Fibrinolysis was observed after the addition of rFVIIa and fibrinogen, and the clot structure was improved after the addition of an antifibrinolytic aprotinin. (Modified from Tanaka KA, Taketomi T, Szlam F, et al. Improved clot formation by combined administration of activated factor VII [NovoSeven] and fibrinogen [Haemocomplettan P]. *Anesth Analg.* 2008;106[3]: 732–738, table of contents.)

CHAPTER 30

Anticoagulants

I. Anticoagulants are drugs that delay or prevent the clotting of blood (patients receive anticoagulation for cardiovascular procedures, thromboprophylaxis, or for cardiovascular disease and/or atrial fibrillation). The therapeutic potential of anticoagulation must be considered against risks for increased bleeding.

II. Heparin acts as an anticoagulant by binding to antithrombin (AT), enhancing the rate of thrombin–AT complex formation by 1,000 to 10,000 times (anticoagulation depends on the presence of adequate amounts of circulating AT) (Fig. 30-1). Standardization of heparin potency is based on in vitro comparison with a known standard. Because the potency of different commercial preparations of heparin may vary greatly, the heparin dosing should always be prescribed in units, and most heparin is porcine in origin.

A. **Pharmacokinetics**

1. Heparin is a highly charged acidic molecule administered by intravenous (IV) or subcutaneous injection.
2. The precise pathway of heparin elimination is uncertain, and the influence of renal and hepatic disease on its pharmacokinetics is less than with other anticoagulants.
3. Heparin binds to many different proteins, which can affect its anticoagulant activity and contributes to heparin resistance.

B. **Laboratory Evaluation of Coagulation**. The anticoagulant response to heparin varies widely especially in critically ill patients. Different tests are used to monitor unfractionated heparin (UFH) and other anticoagulants as follows.

1. **Activated Partial Thromboplastin Time**
   a. Heparin treatment is usually monitored to maintain the ratio of the activated partial thromboplastin time (aPTT) within a defined range of approximately

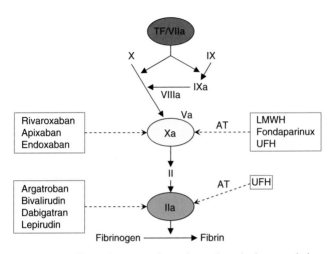

FIGURE 30-1 The major targets for anticoagulants in the coagulation pathway are directed against either factor Xa or thrombin (IIa). Unfractionated heparin (UFH) and low-molecular-weight heparin (LMWH) require circulating antithrombin (AT) as a cofactor, and only UFH will inhibit thrombin. Fondaparinux is a synthetic pentasaccharide and, like LMWH, indirectly inhibits factor Xa, requiring AT as a cofactor. The direct factor Xa inhibitors are AT-independent and include rivaroxaban, apixaban, and endoxaban. Both oral direct thrombin inhibitors (dabigatran) and IV agents directly inhibit thrombin. Vitamin K antagonists, such as warfarin, inhibit the activation of factors II, VII, IX, X, as factors are made but are not activated by the posttranslational carboxylation that is inhibited (mechanism not shown). (Modified from Levy JH, Key NS, Azran MS. Novel oral anticoagulants: implications in the perioperative setting. *Anesthesiology.* 2010;113:726–745.)

    1.5 to 2.5 times normal values (typically 30 to 35 seconds).

b. An excessively prolonged aPTT ($>$120 seconds) is readily shortened by omitting a dose because heparin has a brief elimination half-time.

c. When low-dose heparin is used, laboratory tests may not be required to monitor treatment because the dosage and schedule are well known. However, some hospital laboratories have changed to anti-Xa assays instead of aPTT monitoring because of the variability of responses, with low-dose regimens.

2. **Activated Clotting Time**
   a. At higher heparin concentrations like those typically used during cardiopulmonary bypass, the activated clotting time (ACT) is used to monitor anticoagulation.
   b. Commercially available timing systems are used clinically to measure the ACT and are based on detecting the onset of clot formation (results between different commercial devices to measure the ACT may not be interchangeable).
   c. Heparin effect and its antagonism by protamine are commonly monitored in patients undergoing cardiovascular procedures by measuring the ACT.
   d. In addition to the presence of a heparin effect, the ACT may be influenced by hypothermia, thrombocytopenia, presence of contact activation inhibitors (aprotinin), and preexisting coagulation deficiencies (fibrinogen, factor XII, factor VII).
   e. For cardiac surgery, a baseline value for the ACT is determined (a) before the IV administration of heparin, (b) 3 to 5 minutes after administration, and (c) at 30-minute intervals thereafter. During cardiopulmonary bypass, the target ACT value is still controversial but often considered adequate if the ACT is longer than 350 seconds, although most cardiac surgical centers target an ACT of longer than 400 seconds.
   f. The need to measure ACT repeatedly is emphasized by the fourfold variation in heparin sensitivity between patients and the threefold variation in the rate at which heparin is metabolized.

III. **Clinical Uses.** Heparin is used extensively for multiple purposes and when administered IV has an immediate onset of action, whereas subcutaneous administration results in variable bioavailability with an onset of action in 1 to 2 hours.
   A. **Heparin-Induced Thrombocytopenia**
      1. Thrombocytopenia due to UFH is common and can begin within hours in patients exposed to heparin.
      2. A more severe and even life-threatening syndrome develops in 0.5% to 6.0% of patients, manifesting as severe thrombocytopenia (50% drop in platelet count or <100,000 cells/mm^3), that can be associated with thrombotic events (heparin-induced thrombocytopenia with thrombosis). This severe response typically

develops after 4 to 5 days of heparin therapy and is caused by heparin-dependent antibodies to platelet factor IV that trigger platelet aggregation and result in thrombocytopenia.

B. **Allergic Reactions**. Heparin can cause allergic reactions, but these are rare and present in a manner typical of other hypersensitivity reactions.

C. **Anticoagulation with Protamine**
   1. Positively charged alkaline protamine combines with the negatively charged acidic heparin to form a stable complex that is devoid of anticoagulant activity. These heparin–protamine complexes are removed by the reticuloendothelial system. Clearance of protamine by the reticuloendothelial system (within 20 minutes) is more rapid than heparin clearance and that may explain, in part, the phenomenon of heparin rebound.
   2. The dose of protamine required to antagonize heparin is typically 1 mg for every 100 units of circulating heparin activity.

IV. **Low-Molecular-Weight Heparins. Enoxaparin and dalteparin are two commonly administered low-molecular-weight heparins (LMWHs) derived from standard commercial-grade UFH by chemical depolymerization to yield fragments with a mean molecular weight of 4,000 to 5,000 daltons. The pharmacokinetics of enoxaparin and dalteparin between patients are more consistent than heparin because these drugs bind less avidly to proteins than heparin. This contributes to better bioavailability at low doses. Protamine does not neutralize LMWH.**

   A. **Spinal and Epidural Hematomas**. The risk of spontaneous hematoma formation may be increased in the presence of LMWH (a consideration when selecting regional anesthesia in patients being treated with LMWH preparations).

V. **Prophylaxis against Venous Thromboembolism. The incidence of deep vein thrombosis is 10% to 40% among general surgery patients and higher still in high-risk surgery patient populations (orthopedic, thoracic, cardiac, vascular surgery). Thromboprophylaxis is known to effectively reduce venous thromboembolism in a cost-effective manner (subcutaneous heparin and LMWH are commonly used).**

VI. **Direct Thrombin Inhibitors: Parenteral Agents. An important class of anticoagulants that high-risk surgery patients at** risk for HIT may receive are the direct thrombin inhibitors, including bivalirudin, argatroban, lepirudin, and desirudin (Table 30-1).

VII. **Oral Anticoagulants**
   A. **Vitamin K Antagonists—Warfarin**. Warfarin is the most frequently used oral anticoagulant because of its predictable onset and duration of action and its excellent bioavailability after oral administration. Treatment usually begins with an oral warfarin dose of 5 to 10 mg, and the average maintenance dose is 5 mg; however, the dose varies widely among individuals due to pharmacogenetic differences. Disadvantages of warfarin include delayed onset of action, the need for regular laboratory monitoring, difficulty in reversal should a surgical procedure create concern about bleeding.
   1. **Mechanism of Action**
      a. Warfarin inhibits vitamin K epoxide reductase that converts the vitamin K–dependent coagulation proteins (factors II [prothrombin], VII, IX, and X) to their active form.
      b. The anticoagulant effect of oral or IV warfarin is delayed for 8 to 12 hours, reflecting the onset of inhibition of clotting factor synthesis and the elimination half-time of previously formed clotting factors that are not altered by the oral anticoagulant.
   2. **Pharmacokinetics**
      a. Warfarin is rapidly and completely absorbed, with peak concentrations occurring within 1 hour after ingestion.
      b. Warfarin crosses the placenta and produces exaggerated effects in the fetus, who has limited ability to synthesize clotting factors.
   3. **Laboratory Evaluation**
      a. Treatment with oral anticoagulants is best guided by measurement of the prothrombin time (particularly sensitive to three of the four vitamin K–dependent clotting factors [prothrombin and factors VII and X].
      b. The problem of variability in the responsiveness of prothrombin time reagents has been overcome by the introduction of a standardized system of reporting known as the international normalized ratio (INR).
      c. For most indications, a moderate anticoagulant effect with a targeted INR of 2.0 to 3.0 is appropriate including prosthetic valve prophylaxis.

Table 30-1

Direct Thrombin Inhibitors Currently Available

Drug	Dose	Clinical Status	Indications: Current (Future)	Recommended Monitoring	Time to Stop before Surgery
Bivalirudin	Intravenous	Available in United States, Europe, and Canada	• PCI in patients with HIT • PTCA • Cardiac surgery (Canada) • Acute coronary syndromes (Europe)	ACT	~4–6 h
Argatroban	Intravenous	Available in United States and Europe	• Prophylaxis and treatment of thrombosis in HIT • PCI in patients with HIT	aPTT ACT (PCI)	~4–6 h
Lepirudin	Intravenous	Available in United States and Europe	• HIT and prevention of further VTE	aPTT	~24 h: Lepirudin and desirudin are irreversible thrombin inhibitors

(continued)

Table 30-1

Direct Thrombin Inhibitors Currently Available *(continued)*

Drug	Dose	Clinical Status	Indications: Current (Future)	Recommended Monitoring	Time to Stop before Surgery
Desirudin	Subcutaneous	Available in United States and Europe for hip arthroplasty	• Total hip arthroplasty • (HIT)	aPTT	~24 h
Ximelagatran	Oral	No longer in clinical development		None	
Dabigatran etexilate	Oral	Available in United States for stroke prevention for atrial fibrillation; approved in Europe and Canada for hip and knee arthroplasty	• Total hip or knee arthroplasty • VTE • Atrial fibrillation	Thrombin times, aPTT	~48 h with normal renal function, ~72–96 h or more if abnormal renal function. Drug effects can actually be measured as noted and potentially can be used to guide decision making.

ACT, activated clotting time; aPTT, activated partial thromboplastin time; HIT, heparin-induced thrombocytopenia; PCI, percutaneous coronary intervention; PTCA, percutaneous transluminal coronary angioplasty; VTE, venous thromboembolism.

    d. An excessively prolonged prothrombin time is not readily shortened by omitting a dose because of the long elimination half-time of oral anticoagulants.

    e. Unexpected fluctuations in the dose response to warfarin may reflect changes in diet, undisclosed drug use, poor patient compliance, surreptitious self-medication, or intermittent alcohol consumption.

4. **Clinical Uses**. Vitamin K antagonists (VKAs) are effective in the prevention of venous thromboembolism, the prevention of systemic embolization and resultant stroke in patients with prosthetic heart valves or atrial fibrillation, and for treatment of patients with thrombophilia who are hypercoagulable.

5. **Management before Elective Surgery**

    a. In patients receiving a VKA, the INR should be checked preoperatively. Although minor surgical procedures can be safely performed in patients receiving oral anticoagulants, for major surgery, discontinuation of oral anticoagulants 1 to 3 days preoperatively is recommended to permit the prothrombin time to return to within 20% of its normal range. This approach, followed by reinstitution of the oral anticoagulant regimen 1 to 7 days postoperatively, is not accompanied by an increased incidence of thromboembolic complications in vulnerable patients. Patients at high risk, such as those with prosthetic heart valves, may require bridging with UFH.

    b. Bleeding is the main complication of the VKAs (risk of bleeding is influenced by the intensity of the anticoagulant therapy, the patient's underlying disorder, and the concomitant use of aspirin).

    c. In emergency situations, oral or IV administration of vitamin K is utilized but will not immediately reverse the anticoagulant effect.

B. **New oral agents** (dabigatran, rivaroxaban) have a rapid onset with therapeutic anticoagulation within hours of administration and do not need routine monitoring (Table 30-2).

1. **Perioperative Management of the New Oral Anticoagulants**

    a. The newer therapeutic agents have a rapid onset with therapeutic anticoagulation within hours of administration and do not need routine monitoring.

    b. Newer oral anticoagulants may increase surgical bleeding, they have no validated antagonists, they

Table 30-2

Current and Emerging Factor Xa Inhibitors and Vitamin K Antagonist

Drug	Administration	Clinical Status	Indications: Current (Future)	Monitoring	Time to Stop before Elective Surgery
Apixaban	Oral	Phase III	(Atrial fibrillation) (DVT) (Acute coronary syndrome) (Total knee arthroplasty)	None	Not yet approved, should be similar to rivaroxaban, half-life ~12 h
Danaparoid	Intravenous or subcutaneous	No longer available	Treatment of HIT; thromboprophylaxis in HIT patients	Calibrated plasma anti-Xa activity	No longer available
Low-molecular-weight heparin (LMWH)	Intravenous or subcutaneous	Available in Canada, Europe, and United States	Multiple: thromboprophylaxis, acute coronary syndromes	Plasma anti-Xa activity	At least 12 h before surgery, longer if renal dysfunction as elimination is prolonged, not reversible

Table 30-2

Current and Emerging Factor Xa Inhibitors and Vitamin K Antagonist *(continued)*

Drug	Administration	Clinical Status	Indications: Current (Future)	Monitoring	Time to Stop before Elective Surgery
Fondaparinux	Intravenous or subcutaneous	Available in Canada, Europe, and United States	Thromboprophylaxis and treatment of pulmonary embolism	Calibrated plasma anti-Xa activity	Long half-life of 17–21 h, should be stopped at least 2 d, longer if renal dysfunction
Rivaroxaban	Oral	Available in Canada, Europe, and United States	Total hip or knee arthroplasty (Treatment of DVT and PE) (Atrial fibrillation) (Acute coronary syndromes)	None current	At least 24 h based on prescribing information, but drug half-life may be prolonged with renal dysfunction and recommend holding ~48 h preoperatively with normal renal function and longer if abnormal.

(continued)

Table 30-2

Current and Emerging Factor Xa Inhibitors and Vitamin K Antagonist *(continued)*

Drug	Administration	Clinical Status	Indications: Current (Future)	Monitoring	Time to Stop before Elective Surgery
Unfractionated heparin	Intravenous or subcutaneous			aPTT, heparin levels (plasma anti-Xa)	4–6 h before the procedure if possible but may need to continue for cardiovascular surgery; also reversible with protamine
Warfarin	Oral and intravenous		Anticoagulation for multiple reasons and treatment of thrombophilia	Prothrombin time/INR	~5 d before procedure to allow INR <1.5; patients may require bridging with heparin

aPTT, activated partial thromboplastin time; DVT, deep vein thrombosis; HIT, heparin-induced thrombocytopenia; INR, international normalized ratio; PE, pulmonary embolism.

cannot be monitored by simple standardized laboratory assays, and their pharmacokinetics vary significantly between patients.

c. For procedures with low hemorrhagic risk, a therapeutic window of 48 hours (last administration 24 hours before surgery, restart 24 hours after) is proposed. For procedures with medium or high hemorrhagic risk, stopping therapy 5 days before surgery is recommended.

d. In patients at high thrombotic risk (atrial fibrillation with a history of stroke), bridging with heparin (LMWH) is proposed.

VIII. Platelet Inhibitors

A. **Aspirin**

1. Antiplatelet agents are the mainstay therapy for patients with atherosclerotic vascular disease and coronary artery disease (consistent with the role of platelets in atherosclerosis).

2. Treatment with aspirin reduces the incidence of occlusive arterial vascular events.

3. Aspirin irreversibly acetylates cyclooxygenase and thereby prevents formation of thromboxane A_2. Despite rapid clearance from the body, the effects of aspirin on platelets are irreversible and last for the life of the platelet, 7 to 10 days.

   a. In patients who require temporary interruption of aspirin- or clopidogrel-containing drugs before surgery or a procedure, stopping this treatment 7 to 10 days before the procedure is recommended.

   b. In patients who have had temporary interruption of aspirin therapy because of surgery or a procedure, resuming aspirin approximately 24 hours (or the next morning) after surgery when there is adequate hemostasis is recommended.

B. **Thienopyridines: Clopidogrel, Prasugrel, and Ticagrelor** (Table 30-3)

1. Thienopyridines irreversibly bind to $P2Y_{12}$ receptors thereby blocking adenosine diphosphate (ADP) binding. This $P2Y_{12}$ receptor antagonism inhibits ADP-mediated platelet activation and aggregation.

2. Dual antiplatelet therapy that includes a thienopyridine coadministered with aspirin is commonly used for improving clinical outcomes in patients with ACS and undergoing percutaneous intervention.

Table 30-3

Drugs Used for Platelet Inhibition Therapy

	Clopidogrel	Prasugrel	Ticagrelor	Aspirin
Drug Class Mechanism of Action	Thienopyridine Selective, irreversible binding to and inhibition of $P2Y_{12}$ receptor on platelets	Thienopyridine Selective, irreversible binding to and inhibition of $P2Y_{12}$ receptor on platelets	Thienopyridine Selective, reversible binding to and inhibition of $P2Y_{12}$ receptor on platelets	Acetylsalicylate Cyclooxygenase inhibition
Comments	Prodrug, metabolized to active form by two different metabolic steps, resistance due to metabolism	Prodrug, metabolized to active form by one metabolic step, more potent and resistance rare	Direct-acting agent	Active drug but resistance can occur, likely due to absorption and other factors

3. Current recommendations are to discontinue thienopyridines 7 days before elective surgery and to avoid regional anesthesia until the effects of these drugs have dissipated. Guidelines for management of patients with coronary stents on antiplatelet agents have been proposed (Table 30-4).

C. **Dipyridamole** is most frequently administered in combination with aspirin to prevent stroke in patients who cannot take a thienopyridine. It can increase bleeding and should be stopped preoperatively, but the aspirin component has a longer half-life than dipyridamole.

IX. Platelet Glycoprotein IIb/IIIa Antagonists. An important advance in managing ischemic cardiovascular disease was the development of platelet glycoprotein (GP) IIb/IIIa receptor inhibitors (now often replaced with newer therapies) (Table 30-5).

X. Perioperative Management of Patients on Platelet Inhibitors. The risks and benefits of discontinuing antiplatelet therapy must be carefully considered for each individual patient, especially prior to elective surgery (see Table 30-4).

XI. Thrombolytic Drugs

A. Pharmacologic thrombolysis is produced by drugs that act as plasminogen activators to convert the endogenous proenzyme plasminogen to the fibrinolytic enzyme plasmin that lysis clot and other proteins. The goal of thrombolytic therapy is to restore circulation through a previously occluded artery or vein, most often a coronary artery.

B. Fibrinolytics are injected systemically or directly into the affected arterial lesion.

C. In clinical practice, total plasminogen activator is most commonly used because of its localized catalytic effect on plasminogen activation in the presence of fibrin.

D. Thrombolytic agents have an associated risk of bleeding (particularly intracranial hemorrhage).

E. Angioedema occurs in 1% to 5% of patients receiving IV rt-PA, and the use of angiotensin-converting enzyme inhibitors is strongly associated with this complication.

Table 30-4

Antiplatelet Therapy following Stent Placement (AHA/ACC Recommendations)

1. Before implantation of a stent, the physician should discuss the need for dual-antiplatelet therapy. In patients not expected to comply with 12 months of thienopyridine therapy, whether for economic or other reasons, strong consideration should be given to avoiding a DES.

2. In patients who are undergoing preparation for PCI and who are likely to require invasive or surgical procedures within the next 12 months, consideration should be given to implantation of a bare-metal stent or performance of balloon angioplasty with provisional stent implantation instead of the routine use of a DES.

3. A greater effort by healthcare professionals must be made before patient discharge to ensure that patients are properly and thoroughly educated about the reasons they are prescribed thienopyridines and the significant risks associated with prematurely discontinuing such therapy.

4. Patients should be specifically instructed before hospital discharge to contact their treating cardiologist before stopping any antiplatelet therapy, even if instructed to stop such therapy by another healthcare provider.

5. Healthcare providers who perform invasive or surgical procedures and who are concerned about periprocedural and postprocedural bleeding must be made aware of the potentially catastrophic risks of premature discontinuation of thienopyridine therapy. Such professionals who perform these procedures should contact the patient's cardiologist if issues regarding the patient's antiplatelet therapy are unclear, to discuss optimal patient management strategy.

6. Elective procedures for which there is significant risk of perioperative or postoperative bleeding should be deferred until patients have completed an appropriate course of thienopyridine therapy (12 months after DES implantation if they are not at high risk of bleeding and a minimum of 1 month for bare-metal stent implantation).

   For patients treated with DES who are to undergo subsequent procedures that mandate discontinuation of thienopyridine therapy, aspirin should be continued if at all possible and the thienopyridine restarted as soon as possible after the procedure because of concerns about late stent thrombosis.

ACC, American College of Cardiology; AHA, American Heart Association; DES, drug-eluting stent; PCI, percutaneous coronary intervention.

Table 30-5

Properties of Glycoprotein IIb/IIIa Antagonists

Drug	Structure	Route of Administration	Elimination Half-Time (h)	Excretion	Clinical Uses	Stop before Surgery (h)	Prolong PT/PTT	Antidote
Abciximab	Monoclonal antibodies	Intravenous	12–24	Plasma proteases	ACS PCI	72	No/No	Dialysis
Eptifibatide	Peptide	Intravenous	2–4	Renal	ACS PCI	24	No/No	Dialysis
Tirofiban	Nonpeptide	Intravenous	2–4	Renal (30%–60%) Biliary (40%–70%)	ACS	24	No/No	Dialysis

ACS, acute coronary syndrome; PCI, percutaneous coronary intervention; PT, prothrombin time; PTT, partial thromboplastin time.

CHAPTER 31

Physiology and Management of Massive Transfusion

I. **Introduction.** Hemorrhage due to uncontrolled bleeding (*massive transfusion coagulopathy* or *trauma-induced coagulopathy*) is a clinical problem commonly faced by clinicians managing traumatic injury, surgical patients, and obstetrical patients. The management of hemostasis following traumatic injury and life-threatening hemorrhage has significantly changed over the years from initial resuscitation with crystalloid/colloids and red blood cells to routine administration of plasma/fresh frozen plasma (FFP) and platelets in addition to red cells.

II. Pathophysiology of Hemostatic Abnormalities Associated with Trauma. Hemorrhage is a major cause of mortality following traumatic injury and responsible for approximately 50% of deaths within 24 hours of injury and approximately 80% of intraoperative trauma deaths. Therapy in the past was based on treating coagulopathy after the initial resuscitation and stabilization of the patient. More recent observations in trauma victims found prompt administration of plasma resulted in earlier improvement while the use of large crystalloid volumes was associated with increased bleeding and lower survival.

A. **Trauma and Endothelial Dysfunction**
   1. The term *endotheliopathy of trauma* has been proposed to describe the systemic endothelial injury and dysfunction that contributes to coagulopathy, inflammation, vascular permeability, tissue edema, and multiorgan system dysfunction associated with hemorrhagic shock.
   2. Inflammatory activation following tissue injury contributes to the endothelial dysfunction as does the critical role of fibrinolysis. With tissue injury, the fibrinolytic system is activated converting plasminogen to plasmin, a critical enzyme that cleaves fibrin.
   3. As a result of this pathologic activation, antifibrinolytic therapy is a critical component of a multimodal approach.

III. Massive transfusion is defined as greater than 10 units of
red blood cells within 24 hours after initiating treatment.
Patients who acutely bleed and receive greater than 10 units
of red blood cells within 6 hours of a trauma have a higher
mortality. The massive transfusion itself is likely a marker
for more severe injury rather than a direct effect of the transfusions. The development of massive transfusion strategies
and use of specific protocols improves survival.

A. **Therapeutic Approaches for Massive Transfusion and
Coagulopathy**

1. Transfusion services, blood bankers, clinicians, and
hospitals have developed and implemented protocols
to rapidly provide blood products for patients suffering
acute and massive hemorrhage.

2. Observational studies and retrospective analyses initially
reported improved outcomes with the administration of
whole blood or whole blood equivalents with massive
transfusion that include transfusion ratios of 1:1:1
for red blood cells, plasma, and platelets (there is also
conflicting data suggesting increased morbidity and
mortality associated with plasma product transfusion).

B. **Adverse Effects of Transfusions**

1. Major life-threatening risks of plasma administration
include transfusion-related acute lung injury, transfusion-associated circulatory overload, hemolytic transfusion reactions, and anaphylaxis.

2. Deciphering the causes of adverse outcomes following
transfusions can be difficult because more critically
injured patients who have worse outcomes will also
require more transfusions.

C. **Hemostatic Changes Associated with Massive Transfusion Coagulopathy**

1. Hemostatic abnormalities following massive transfusions and/or trauma can develop as a result of multiple factors not necessarily directly related to blood
administration.

2. Coagulopathy, hypothermia, and acidosis are the triad
that results in higher mortality in the management of
acute trauma.

a. Volume resuscitation with crystalloids, colloids,
and red blood cells (RBC) or the use of cell salvage
systems following blood loss can lead to dilutional
coagulopathy. The hemostatic balance between anticoagulant and procoagulant activity may be lost due
to tissue injury following trauma.

    b. Hypothermia can be a critical factor that precipitates or worsens coagulopathy, as enzymatic cascades are impaired (may appear even as high as 35°C). Platelet function may also be impaired with hypothermia, and platelet dysfunction can also occur due to increased fibrinogen degradation products (FDP) and D-dimer levels.

IV. **Perioperative Hemostatic Changes. Blood loss up to 30% of total blood volume is generally well tolerated with the fluid resuscitation alone. Coagulation factors are progressively diluted to 30% of normal after a loss of one blood volume, and down to 15% after a loss of two blood volumes.**

  A. **Massive Transfusion Coagulopathy**

    1. Because standard laboratory tests often take too long to obtain, laboratory testing plays an uncertain role in decision making in many settings where massive transfusion is necessary.

    2. Transfusion protocols have been developed where fixed doses of FFP and platelets are administered after a specific number of RBC units have been given, often in a 1:1:1 ratio (with life-threatening hemorrhage, transfusion of fixed ratios of RBCs, FFP, and platelets should be administered).

  B. **Role of Red Blood Cells and Anemia**. Anemia may also contribute to bleeding due to multiple mechanisms (nitric oxide scavenging, margination of platelets). The ideal hematocrit to minimize this risk is not clear.

  C. **Causes of Bleeding in the Setting of Massive Transfusion Coagulopathy**

    1. Risk factors for developing massive transfusion coagulopathy are often related to the surgical or traumatic injury that causes the hemorrhage.

    2. Patients should be evaluated for use of additional medications that can affect coagulation.

    3. Many of the standard coagulation tests used for evaluating hemorrhage cannot adequately determine the effects of antiplatelet agents (aspirin, clopidogrel, prasugrel, ticagrelor).

  D. **Hypothermia, Acidosis, and Coagulopathy**

    1. Hypothermia has multiple effects because coagulation is an enzymatic process. As patient temperature decreases, the enzymatic processes that function maximally at normal body temperature are impaired.

2. Hypothermia can produce multiple hemostatic defects that include reversible platelet dysfunction and increased fibrinolysis.
3. Prothrombin time (PT) and activated partial thromboplastin time (aPTT) are prolonged at temperatures of 34°C or less.

E. **Dilutional Coagulopathy**. Before the development of massive transfusion protocols, dilutional coagulopathy was a common cause of bleeding in the actively hemorrhaging patient.

F. **Fibrinolysis** is a critical component of preventing excessive clot formation and balances for hemostasis, but excessive fibrinolysis as occurs commonly in trauma patients can cause bleeding.
1. Fibrinolysis is initiated by mechanisms that include stimulating tissue plasminogen activator (tPA) release in response to vascular endothelial damage, stress responses, and other mechanisms.
2. Plasmin degrades fibrinogen and von Willebrand's factor (vWF) and cleaves receptors from platelets (glycoprotein Ib), thus interfering with platelet function.

G. **Hypofibrinogenemia**
1. Fibrinogen circulates in the highest concentration of all of the coagulation factors (normal values for plasma levels are ~200 to 400 mg/dL).
2. If fibrinogen levels fall to approximately 80 to 100 mg/dL, standard clot-based coagulation tests including PT and partial thromboplastin time (PTT) can be affected. These changes may not be corrected by transfusion of FFP/plasma.

V. **Monitoring Hemostasis during Massive Transfusion.** PTs and aPTTs are often used for monitoring coagulopathy during massive transfusion. PT is considered proportional to coagulation factor loss and/or hemodilution but other factors may also be responsible. These standard coagulation tests have limitations for evaluating bleeding because of the multiple coagulation defects that occur. Whole blood viscoelastic measurements (thromboelastography or thromboelastometry) continue to expand for management of trauma, perioperative bleeding, and massive transfusion coagulopathy.

A. **Treatment of Coagulopathy during Massive Transfusion** (Figs. 31-1 and 31-2).

B. **Plasma/fresh frozen plasma** contains multiple factors for hemostasis and has increasingly been considered a critical component (see Fig. 31-1).

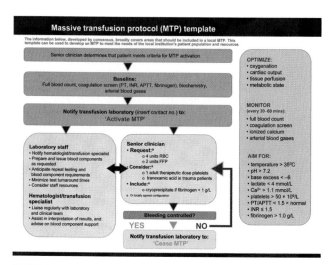

FIGURE 31-1 Massive transfusion protocol (MTP) template. (From http://www.blood.gov.au/pubs/pbm/module1/transfusion.html; accessed 091214, with permission.)

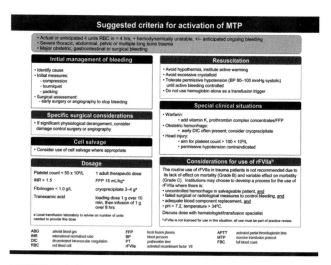

FIGURE 31-2 Suggested criteria for activation of massive transfusion protocol (MTP) template. (From http://www.blood.gov.au/pubs/pbm/module1/transfusion.html; accessed 091214, with permission.)

C. **Platelet Administration**
1. Following traumatic injury or significant postoperative bleeding, the critical platelet count for transfusion is often based on consensus therapy rather than true objective data. Although a count of 50,000 or more is recommended, the threshold for administration of platelets, especially in cases of dilutional coagulopathy, remains unclear as do the ideal ratio of platelets to other blood components.
2. Most protocols attempt to develop a strategy that mimics whole blood replacement with RBC:plasma/FFP:platelets at a 1:1:1 ratio with massive bleeding.
3. Assessing platelet function in the bleeding patient is not possible; therefore, empiric platelet administration is often undertaken.

D. **Antifibrinolytic Agents**
1. Because of the critical role of fibrinolysis with severe bleeding and trauma, the antifibrinolytic agent tranexamic acid is increasingly used as a therapeutic strategy.
2. Inhibiting fibrinolysis during acute bleeding has many beneficial effects including preserving initial clot formation at a bleeding site that may otherwise be broken down.

VI. **Postpartum hemorrhage is an important cause of life-threatening hemorrhage and continues to be a major cause of maternal mortality. As in all life-threatening bleeding, a treatment algorithm that includes a massive transfusion protocol is important.**

VII. **Multimodal Resuscitation: Damage Control Resuscitation**
A. Managing life-threatening and uncontrolled bleeding is a clinical problem that can occur following traumatic injury, during major surgical procedures, and following delivery.
B. A multimodal and multispecialty approach has evolved for the optimal resuscitative approach to hemorrhagic shock (Table 31-1).

VIII. **Summary**
A. Coagulopathy associated with massive transfusion is a complex, multifactorial clinical problem. The role of hypothermia, dilutional coagulopathy, platelet dysfunction, and fibrinolysis should also be considered.
B. Evaluating fibrinogen levels represents a critical aspect of all transfusion algorithms, especially for patients with massive transfusion and life-threatening hemorrhage.

Table 31-1

Multimodal and Multispecialty Approach to Hemorrhagic Shock

Early and increased use of plasma, platelets, and red blood cells while minimizing crystalloid use

Hypotensive resuscitation strategies

Avoiding hypothermia and acidosis

Use of adjuncts (calcium, THAM as an alternate alkalizing agent to sodium bicarbonate), use of tranexamic acid, and off-label uses of procoagulation agents

THAM, tris(hydroxymethyl)aminomethane.

C. Transfusion algorithms provide adequate factor and hemostatic replacement, although the ideal ratio of various blood components and factor concentrates are still being determined.

D. Crystalloids are no longer a primary means of resuscitation; the primary strategy now is replacing acute blood loss with plasma and platelet-containing products instead of early and large amounts of crystalloids and RBCs (see Figs. 31-1 and 31-2).

PART VI

CHAPTER 32

Gastrointestinal Physiology

I. **Liver** (Table 32-1)
   A. **Anatomy**
      1. The liver is divided into four lobes consisting of 50,000 to 100,000 individual hepatic lobules (Fig. 32-1).
      2. Each hepatocyte is also located adjacent to bile canaliculi, which coalesce to form the common hepatic duct. This duct and the cystic duct from the gallbladder join to form the common bile duct, which enters the duodenum at a site surrounded by the sphincter of Oddi (Fig. 32-2).
      3. Hepatic lobules are lined by macrophages, which phagocytize 99% or more of bacteria in the portal venous blood (crucial because the portal venous blood drains the gastrointestinal tract and usually contains colon bacteria).
   B. **Hepatic Blood Flow**
      1. The liver receives a dual afferent blood supply from the hepatic artery and portal veins (Fig. 32-3).
      2. Total hepatic blood flow is approximately 1,450 mL per minute or approximately 29% of the cardiac output (portal vein provides 75% of the total flow but only 50% to 55% of the hepatic oxygen supply, and the hepatic artery provides only 25% of total hepatic blood flow but provides 45% to 50% of the hepatic oxygen requirements).
      3. Hepatic artery blood flow maintains nutrition of connective tissues and walls of bile ducts (loss of hepatic artery blood flow can be fatal because of ensuing necrosis of vital liver structures).
   C. **Control of Hepatic Blood Flow**
      1. Portal vein blood flow, combined with the resistance to portal vein blood flow within the liver, determines portal venous pressure (normally 7 to 10 mm Hg).

Table 32-1

Functions of Hepatocytes

Absorb nutrients from portal venous blood
Store and release carbohydrates, proteins, and lipids
Excrete bile salts
Synthesize plasma proteins, glucose, cholesterol, and fatty
  acids
Metabolize exogenous and endogenous compounds

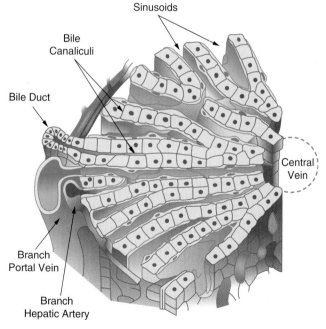

FIGURE 32-1 Schematic depiction of a hepatic lobule with a central vein and plates of hepatic cells extending radially. Blood from peripherally located branches of the hepatic artery and vein perfuses the sinusoids. Bile ducts drain the bile canaliculi that pass between the hepatocytes.

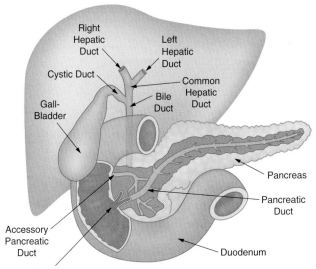

FIGURE 32-2 Connections of the ducts of the gallbladder, liver, and pancreas.

    2. Sympathetic nervous system innervation is from T3 to T11 and is mediated via α-adrenergic receptors (principally responsible for resistance and compliance of hepatic venules).

    3. Fibrotic constriction characteristic of hepatic cirrhosis (most often due to chronic alcohol abuse and hepatitis C) can increase resistance to portal vein blood flow as evidenced by portal venous pressures of 20 to 30 mm Hg (portal hypertension).

       a. The resulting increased resistance to portal vein blood flow may result in development of shunts (varices) to allow blood flow to bypass the hepatocytes.

       b. Ascites results when increased portal venous pressures cause transudation of protein-rich fluid through the outer surface of the liver capsule and gastrointestinal tract into the abdominal cavity.

       c. Hepatic artery blood flow is influenced by arteriolar tone that reflects local and intrinsic mechanisms

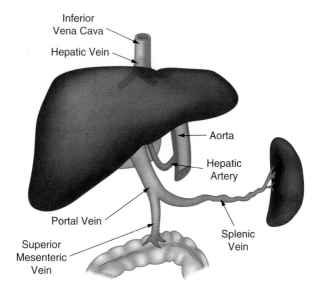

FIGURE 32-3 Schematic depiction of the dual afferent blood supply to the liver provided by the portal vein and hepatic artery.

(autoregulation). A decrease in portal vein blood flow is accompanied by an increase in hepatic artery blood flow by as much as 100%.

d. Surgical stimulation may decrease hepatic blood flow, independent of the anesthetic drug administered. The greatest decreases in hepatic blood flow occur during intraabdominal operations, presumably due to mechanical interference of blood flow produced by retraction in the operative area, as well as the release of vasoconstricting substances such as catecholamines.

D. **Reservoir Function**. The liver normally contains approximately 500 mL of blood or approximately 10% of the total blood volume (may accommodate as much as 1 L of extra blood with increased venous pressure).

1. As such, the liver acts as a storage site when blood volume is excessive, as in congestive heart failure, and is capable of supplying extra blood when hypovolemia occurs.

2. The liver is the single most important source of additional blood during strenuous exercise or acute hemorrhage.

E. **Bile Secretion** (see Fig. 32-2). Hepatocytes continually form bile (500 mL daily) and then secrete it into bile canaliculi, which empty into progressively larger ducts ultimately reaching the common bile duct. The most potent stimulus for emptying the gallbladder is the presence of fat in the duodenum, which evokes the release of the hormone cholecystokinin by the duodenal mucosa (this hormone causes selective contraction of the gallbladder smooth muscle).

1. **Bile salts** combine with lipids in the duodenum to form water-soluble complexes (micelles) that facilitate gastrointestinal absorption of fats (triglycerides) and fat-soluble vitamins (vitamin K is necessary for activation of several clotting factors).

2. **Bilirubin**. After approximately 120 days, the cell membranes of erythrocytes rupture and the released hemoglobin is converted to bilirubin in reticuloendothelial cells (Fig. 32-4).

   a. **Jaundice** is the yellowish tint of body tissues that accompanies accumulation of bilirubin in extracellular fluid. Skin color usually begins to change when the plasma concentration of bilirubin increases to approximately three times normal.

   b. The most common types of jaundice are hemolytic jaundice, due to increased destruction of erythrocytes, and obstructive jaundice, due to obstruction of bile ducts.

F. **Cholesterol** is an important component of cell walls and is transported from the periphery to the liver as high-density lipoproteins (HDL). Once cholesterol has reached the liver, it can be excreted in the bile in association with bile acids (may precipitate as gallstones).

G. **Metabolic Functions**. Metabolism of carbohydrates, lipids, and proteins depends on normal hepatic function. Degradation of certain hormones (catecholamines and corticosteroids), as well as drugs, is an important function of the liver. Hepatocytes are the principal site for synthesis of all the coagulation factors with the exception of von Willebrand factor and factor VIIIC. Because the half-life of clotting factors produced in the liver is short, coagulation is particularly sensitive to acute hepatocellular damage.

1. **Carbohydrates**. Regulation of blood glucose concentration is an important metabolic function of the liver

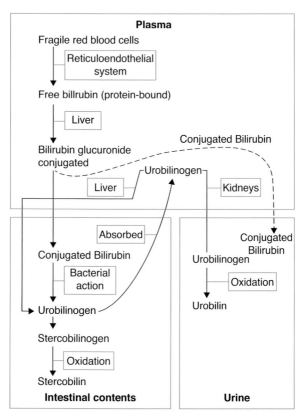

FIGURE 32-4 Schematic depiction of bilirubin formation and excretion. (From Guyton AC, Hall JE. *Textbook of Medical Physiology*. 10th ed. Philadelphia, PA: Saunders; 2000, with permission.)

(when hyperglycemia is present, glycogen is deposited in the liver, and when hypoglycemia occurs, glycogenolysis provides glucose).

2. **Lipids**. The liver is responsible for β-oxidation of fatty acids and formation of acetoacetic acid. Synthesis of fats from carbohydrates and proteins also occurs in the liver.

3. **Proteins**

a. The most important liver functions in protein metabolism are oxidative deamination of amino acids, formation of urea for removal of ammonia, formation of plasma proteins and coagulation factors, and interconversions (transfer of one amino group to another amino acid) among different amino acids.

b. Albumin formed in the liver is critically important for maintaining plasma oncotic pressure as well as providing an essential transport role (half-time for albumin is about 21 days such that plasma albumin concentrations are unlikely to be significantly altered in acute hepatic failure).

II. **Gastrointestinal Tract.** The primary function of the gastrointestinal tract is to provide the body with a continual supply of water, electrolytes, and nutrients. Overall, approximately 9 L of fluid and secretions enters the gastrointestinal tract daily, and all but approximately 100 mL is absorbed by the small intestine and colon (Fig. 32-5). The pH of gastrointestinal secretions varies widely (Table 32-2).

A. **Anatomy.** The smooth muscle of the gastrointestinal tract is a syncytium such that electrical signals originating in one smooth muscle fiber are easily propagated from fiber to fiber.

B. **Blood Flow.** Most of the blood flow to the gastrointestinal tract is to the mucosa to supply energy needed for producing intestinal secretions and absorbing digested materials. Stimulation of the parasympathetic nervous system increases local blood flow, whereas stimulation of the sympathetic nervous system causes vasoconstriction (permits shunting of blood from the gastrointestinal tract for brief periods during exercise or when increased blood flow is needed by skeletal muscles or the heart).

1. **Portal Venous Pressure**

a. The liver offers modest resistance to blood flow from the portal venous system. As a result, the pressure in the portal vein averages 7 to 10 mm Hg, which is considerably higher than the almost zero pressure in the inferior vena cava.

b. Cirrhosis of the liver, most frequently caused by alcoholism, is characterized by increased resistance to portal vein blood flow due to replacement of hepatic cells with fibrous tissue that contracts around the blood vessels.

c. The gradual increase in resistance to portal vein blood flow produced by cirrhosis of the liver causes large collateral vessels to develop between the portal

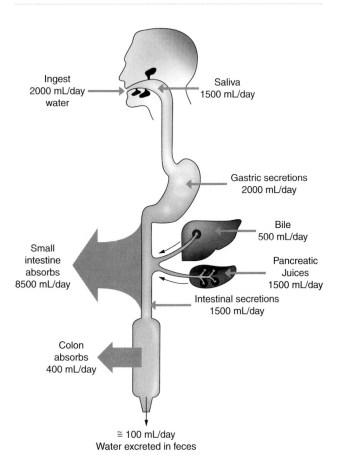

FIGURE 32-5 Overall fluid balance in the human gastrointestinal tract. Approximately 2 L of water are ingested each day and approximately 7 L of various secretions enter the gastrointestinal tract. Of this 9 L, about 8.5 L are absorbed from the small intestine. Approximately 0.5 L passes to the colon, which normally absorbs 80% to 90% of the water presented to it. (From Berne RM, Levy M, Koeppen BM, et al. *Physiology*. 5th ed. St. Louis, MO: Mosby; 2004, with permission.)

Table 32-2

pH and Gastrointestinal Secretions

Secretions	pH
Saliva	6–7
Gastric fluid	1.0–3.5
Bile	7–8
Pancreatic fluid	8.0–8.3
Small intestine	6.5–7.5
Colon	7.5–8.0

veins and the systemic veins. The most important of these collaterals are from the splenic veins to the esophageal veins. These collaterals may become so large that they protrude into the lumen of the esophagus, producing esophageal varicosities. The esophageal mucosa overlying these varicosities may become eroded, leading to life-threatening hemorrhage.

d. In the absence of the development of adequate collaterals, sustained increases in portal vein pressure may cause protein-containing fluid to escape from the surface of the mesentery, gastrointestinal tract, and liver into the peritoneal cavity (ascites).

2. **Splenic Circulation**

a. The splenic capsule in humans, in contrast to that in many lower animals, is nonmuscular, which limits the ability of the spleen to release stored blood in response to sympathetic nervous system stimulation.

b. The spleen functions to remove erythrocytes from the circulation; erythrocytes pass through splenic pores that may be smaller than the erythrocyte (fragile cells do not withstand this trauma, and the released hemoglobin that results from their rupture is ingested by the reticuloendothelial cells of the spleen).

C. **Innervation**. The gastrointestinal tract receives innervation from both divisions of the autonomic nervous system as well as from an intrinsic nervous system (myenteric plexus).

1. The cranial component of parasympathetic nervous system innervation to the gastrointestinal tract (esophagus, stomach, pancreas, small intestine, colon

to the level of the transverse colon) is by way of the vagus nerves.

2. The distal portion of the colon is richly supplied by the sacral parasympathetics via the pelvic nerves from the hypogastric plexus.

D. **Motility**

1. The two types of gastrointestinal motility are mixing contractions and propulsive movements characterized as *peristalsis*.

2. The usual stimulus for peristalsis is distension. Peristalsis is also decreased by increased parasympathetic nervous system activity and anticholinergic drugs.

E. **Ileus**. Adynamic ileus can be relieved by a tube placed into the small intestine and aspiration of fluid and gas until the time when peristalsis returns.

F. **Salivary Glands**. The principal salivary glands (parotid and submaxillary) produce 0.5 to 1.0 mL per minute of saliva (pH 6 to 7), largely in response to parasympathetic nervous system stimulation.

G. **Esophagus**. The upper and lower ends of the esophagus function as sphincters (*upper esophageal [pharyngoesophageal] sphincter* and *lower esophageal [gastroesophageal] sphincter*).

1. **Lower Esophageal Sphincter**. The normal lower esophageal sphincter pressure is 10 to 30 mm Hg at end-exhalation (gastric barrier pressure is calculated as lower esophageal sphincter pressure minus intragastric pressure). This barrier pressure is considered the major mechanism in preventing reflux of gastric contents into the esophagus.

   a. Cricoid pressure decreases lower esophageal sphincter pressure, presumably reflecting stimulation of mechanoreceptors in the pharynx created by the external pressure on the cricoid cartilage (Fig. 32-6).

   b. The administration of anesthetic drugs may decrease upper esophageal sphincter pressure even before the loss of consciousness.

   c. The influence, if any, of changes in lower esophageal sphincter tone and barrier pressure (lower esophageal sphincter tone minus gastric pressure) and subsequent inhalation of gastric fluid during anesthesia remains undocumented.

2. **Gastroesophageal Reflux Disease**. Transient relaxation of the lower esophageal sphincter, rather than decreased lower esophageal sphincter pressure, is the major

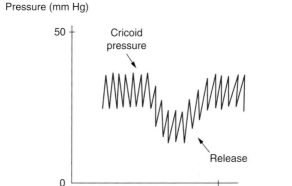

FIGURE 32-6 Application of cricoid pressure causes the lower esophageal sphincter pressure to decrease. (From Chassard D, Tournadre JP, Berrada KR, et al. Cricoid pressure decreases lower esophageal sphincter tone in anaesthetized pigs. *Can J Anaesth.* 1996;43:414–417, with permission.)

mechanism of gastroesophageal reflux disease (GERD). It is estimated that approximately 20% of adults in the United States experience symptoms of GERD.

3. **Hiatal Hernia**. The majority of patients with moderate to severe gastroesophageal reflux have a hiatal hernia (may promote gastroesophageal reflux by trapping gastric acid in the hernia sac).

H. **Stomach** (Fig. 32-7). The ability to secrete hydrogen ions in the form of hydrochloric acid is a hallmark of gastric function.

1. **Gastric Secretions**
   a. Total daily gastric secretion is approximately 2 L with a pH of 1.0 to 3.5 (stomach secretes only a few milliliters of gastric fluid each hour during the periods between digestion).
   b. Strong emotional stimulation, such as occurs preoperatively, can increase interdigestive secretion of highly acidic gastric fluid to >50 mL per hour.

2. **Gastric Fluid Volume and Rate of Gastric Emptying**
   a. Neural and humoral mechanisms greatly influence gastric fluid volume and gastric-emptying time (parasympathetic nervous system stimulation

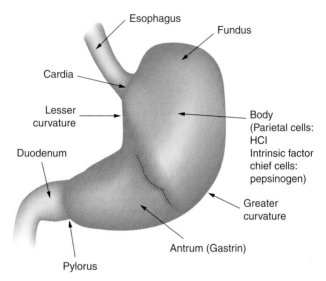

FIGURE 32-7 Anatomy of the stomach indicating the site of production of secretions. Mucus is secreted in all parts of the stomach.

enhances gastric fluid secretion and motility, whereas sympathetic nervous system stimulation has an opposite effect).

b. The elimination of nonnutrient liquids is an exponential process (volume of liquid emptied per unit of time is directly proportional to the volume present in the stomach), whereas the emptying of solids is a linear process (Fig. 32-8). Emptying of liquids from the stomach begins within 1 minute of ingestion, whereas emptying of solids typically begins after a lag time of 15 to 137 minutes (median 49 minutes).

c. Gastric emptying is not delayed after ingestion of 300 mL of water. High lipid and/or caloric content (glucose) slows the emptying of solids from the stomach.

d. Delayed gastric emptying of solids is the most consistent abnormality in diabetic patients with gastroparesis.

e. Certain drugs (opioids, β-adrenergic agonists, and tricyclic antidepressants) may slow gastric emptying.

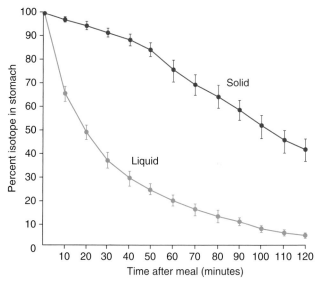

FIGURE 32-8 Gastric emptying of liquids is exponential, whereas emptying of solids is a linear process. (From Minami H, McCallum RW. The physiology of gastric emptying in humans. *Gastroenterology*. 1984;86:1592–1610, with permission.)

Alcohol, at least in concentrations present in wine, does not significantly affect gastric emptying of liquids or solids. Higher concentrations of alcohol, such as present in whiskey, do cause slowing of gastric emptying. Cigarette smoking has been shown to delay emptying of solids, although it may accelerate emptying of liquids.

f. Gastric prokinetic drugs such as metoclopramide may speed the emptying of solids and liquids.

3. **Gastric Emptying Prior to Elective Surgery**

a. Clear liquids can be administered to adult patients scheduled for elective operations until 2 hours before induction of anesthesia without increasing gastric fluid volume.

b. It takes 3 to 4 hours for the stomach to empty following a light breakfast (one slice of white bread with butter and jam, 150 mL of coffee without milk or sugar, 150 mL of pulp-free orange juice). These data are consistent with the recommendation that a 6-hour fast should be enforced after a light breakfast.

4. **Vomiting**
   a. The blood–brain barrier is poorly developed around the chemoreceptor trigger zone and emetic substances present in the circulation are readily accessible to this site.
   b. Serotonin acting at 5-hydroxytryptamine receptors (5-HT$_3$) is an important emetic signal via neural pathways from the gastrointestinal tract ending at the chemoreceptor trigger zone (pharmacologic antagonism of this emetic signal results in antiemetic effects).

I. **Small Intestine**. The small intestine is presented with approximately 9 L of fluid daily (2 L from the diet and the rest representing gastrointestinal secretions), but only 1 to 2 L of chyme enters the colon. The small intestine is the site of most of the digestion and absorption of proteins, fats, and carbohydrates (Table 32-3).

J. **Colon**
   1. The functions of the colon are absorption of water and electrolytes from the chyme and storage of feces (Fig. 32-9).

Table 32-3

Site of Absorption

	Duodenum	Jejunum	Ileum	Colon
Glucose	++	+++	++	0
Amino acids	++	+++	++	0
Fatty acids	+++	++	+	0
Bile salts	0	+	+++	0
Water-soluble vitamins	+++	++	0	0
Vitamin B$_{12}$	0	+	+++	0
Sodium	+++	++	+++	+++
Potassium	0	0	+	++
Hydrogen	0	+	++	++
Chloride	+++	++	+	0
Calcium	+++	++	+	?

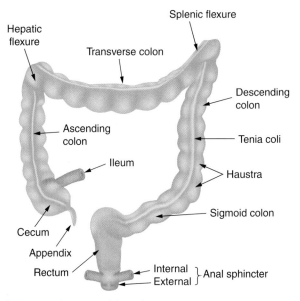

FIGURE 32-9 Anatomy of the colon.

2. Vagal stimulation causes segmental contractions of the proximal part of the colon and stimulation of the pelvic nerves causes explosive movements. Activation of the sympathetic nervous system inhibits colonic activity. Bacteria are predictably present in the colon.

K. **Pancreas** serves as both an endocrine (insulin or glucagon) and exocrine gland (bicarbonate ions to neutralize duodenal contents and digestive enzymes to initiate breakdown of carbohydrates, proteins, and fats).

CHAPTER 33

Metabolism

I. **Metabolism of Nutrients.** One of the gastrointestinal tract's most important functions is for the ingestion of nutrients (carbohydrate, protein, lipid, minerals, vitamins, and water) that the organism uses for production of energy, creation of complex proteins and lipid moieties, and maintenance of electrolytes and total body water stores. The production of energy involves the oxidation of nutrients (carbohydrates, fats, and proteins) that results in creation of high-energy phosphate bonds in which energy is stored for life processes, with carbon dioxide and water produced as side products. The most important high-energy phosphate bond is adenosine triphosphate (ATP) (Table 33-1) (Figs. 33-1 and 33-2).

II. Carbohydrate Metabolism. Carbohydrates comprise a group of organic compounds that include sugars and starches and, in addition to carbon, contain hydrogen and oxygen in the same ratio as water (2:1). Sugars are an important energy source for the body and the sole source of energy for the brain. The liver is the site of carbohydrate metabolism where regulation storage and production of glucose takes place.
   A. **Glycogen**
      1. After entering cells, glucose can be used immediately for release of energy to cells or it can serve as a substrate for glycogen synthase.
      2. The liver and skeletal muscles are particularly capable of storing large amounts of glycogen but all cells can store at least some glucose as glycogen. The liver stores glycogen for release of glucose during fasting, and muscle, which can store as much as 90% of the glucose contained in a meal, catabolizes glycogen during strenuous exercise.
   B. **Gluconeogenesis** is the formation of glucose from amino acids and the glycerol portion of fat. Gluconeogenesis is stimulated by hypoglycemia.

Table 33-1

Estimates of Energy Expenditure in Adults

Activity	Calorie Expenditure (kcal/minute)
Basal	1.1
Sitting	1.8
Walking (2.5 miles/hour)	4.3
Walking (4 miles/hour)	8.2
Climbing stairs	9.0
Swimming	10.9
Bicycling (13 miles/hour)	11.1

C. **Energy Release from Glucose**
   1. Glucose is progressively broken down into two molecules of pyruvate, both of which can enter the citric acid cycle.
   2. The most important means by which energy is released from the glucose molecule is by glycolysis (splitting of the glucose molecule and subsequent oxidative phosphorylation). Oxidative phosphorylation occurs

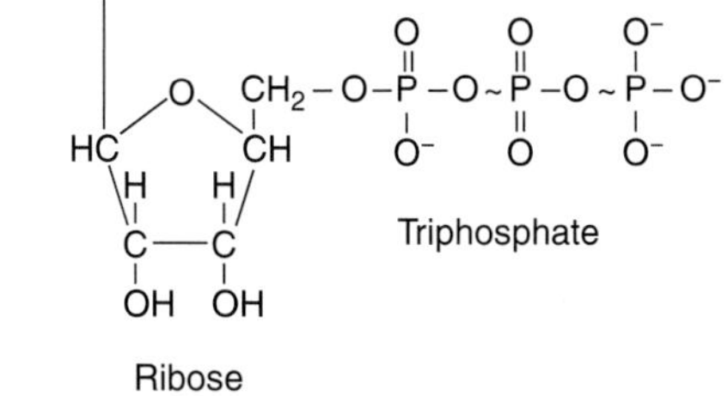

FIGURE 33-1 Metabolism of nutrients in cells is directed toward the ultimate synthesis of adenosine triphosphate (ATP). Energy necessary for physiologic processes and chemical reactions is derived from the high-energy phosphate bonds of ATP.

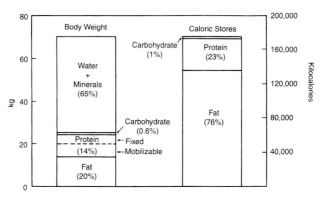

FIGURE 33-2 Comparison of the composition of body weight to caloric stores. (From Berne RM, Levy MN, Koeppen BM, et al. *Physiology*. 5th ed. St. Louis, MO: Mosby; 2004, with permission.)

only in the mitochondria and in the presence of adequate amounts of oxygen.

D. **Anaerobic Glycolysis**
1. In the absence of adequate amounts of oxygen, a small amount of energy can be released by anaerobic glycolysis (glucose is the only nutrient that can serve as a substrate for the formation of ATP without oxygen).
2. Severe liver disease may interfere with the ability of the liver to convert lactic acid to glucose, leading to metabolic acidosis.

III. **Lipid Metabolism**
A. Lipids contain a high amount of potential energy, but are also important as structural components of cell membranes, in signaling pathways, and as precursors to a number of cytokines.
B. A glycerol stem to which three fatty acid molecules are bound is known as a triglyceride. A triglyceride molecule to which one of the terminal fatty acids is replaced with a phosphate ion is known as a phospholipid. Phospholipids are the building blocks of cell membranes and myelin.
1. Triglycerides, after absorption from the gastrointestinal tract, are transported in the lymph and then, by way of the thoracic duct, into the circulation in droplets known as **chylomicrons**.

2. Triglycerides are used in the body mainly to provide energy for metabolic processes similar to those fueled by carbohydrates.

C. Molecules that are part lipid and part protein, lipoproteins, are also synthesized primarily in the liver (Table 33-2).

1. All the cholesterol in plasma is found in lipoprotein complexes, with low-density lipoproteins (LDLs) representing the major cholesterol component in plasma.

2. These LDLs provide cholesterol to tissues, where it is an essential component of cell membranes and is used in the synthesis of corticosteroids and sex hormones.

3. An intrinsic feedback control system increases the endogenous production of cholesterol when exogenous intake is decreased, explaining the relatively modest lowering effect on plasma cholesterol concentrations produced by low-cholesterol diets.

   a. If endogenous increase in cholesterol synthesis is blocked by drugs that inhibit hydroxymethylglutaryl coenzyme A (HMG-CoA) reductase, then there is an appreciable decrease in the plasma cholesterol concentration.

   b. Drugs that selectively inhibit HMG-CoA are known as statins (effectively lower plasma LDL cholesterol concentrations and seem to provide protection against acute cardiac events, perhaps reflecting anti-inflammatory effects).

IV. **Protein Metabolism (Table 33-3). All proteins are composed of the same 20 amino acids, and several of these must be supplied in the diet because they cannot be formed endogenously (essential amino acids) (Table 33-4). Amino acids are relatively strong acids and exist in the blood principally in the ionized form.**

A. **Storage of Amino Acids**

1. Immediately after entry into cells, amino acids are conjugated under the influence of intracellular enzymes into cellular proteins. These proteins can be rapidly decomposed again into amino acids under the influence of intracellular liposomal digestive enzymes. The resulting amino acids can then be transported out of cells into blood to maintain optimal plasma amino acid concentrations.

2. Tissues can synthesize new proteins from amino acids in blood. This response is especially apparent in relation to protein synthesis in cancer cells. Cancer cells are prolific

Table 33-2

Composition of Lipids in the Plasma

	Phospholipid (%)	Triglyceride (%)	Free Cholesterol (%)	Cholesterol Esters	Protein (%)	Density
Chylomicrons	3	90	2	3	2	0.94
LDL	21	6	7	46	20	1.019–1.063
HDL	25	5	4	16	50	1.063–1.21
IDL	20	40	5	25	10	1.006–1.019
VLDL	17	55	4	18	8	0.94–1.006

HDL, high-density lipoprotein; IDL, intermediate-density lipoprotein; LDL, low-density lipoprotein; VLDL, very-low-density lipoprotein.

Table 33-3

Types of Proteins

Globular	Fibrous	Conjugated
Albumin	Collagen	Mucoprotein
Globulin	Elastin fibers	Structural components of cells
Fibrinogen	Keratin	
Hemoglobin	Actin	
Enzymes	Myosin	
Nucleoproteins		

users of amino acids, and, simultaneously, the proteins of other tissues become markedly depleted contributing to cachexia.

B. **Plasma proteins** are represented by (a) albumin, which provides colloid osmotic pressure; (b) globulins necessary for innate and acquired immunity; and (c) fibrinogen, which polymerizes into long fibrin threads during coagulation of blood. Essentially, all plasma albumin and fibrinogen and 60% to 80% of the globulins are formed in the liver. Because of the reversible equilibrium between plasma proteins and other proteins of the body, one of the most effective of all therapies for acute protein deficiency is the intravenous

Table 33-4

Amino Acids

Essential	Nonessential
Arginine	Alanine
Histidine	Asparagine
Isoleucine	Aspartic acid
Leucine	Cysteine
Lysine	Glutamic acid
Methionine	Glutamine
Phenylalanine	Glycine
Threonine	Proline
Tryptophan	Serine
Valine	Tyrosine

administration of plasma proteins. Within hours, amino acids of the administered protein become distributed throughout cells of the body to form proteins where they are needed.

1. **Albumin** is the most abundant plasma protein and is principally responsible for maintaining plasma osmotic pressure. In addition, albumin is important as a transporter of plasma-bound substances often including exogenously administered drugs.
   a. Normal daily synthesis of albumin is about 10 g and the half-time for this protein may be as long as 22 days (serum albumin concentrations may not be noticeably decreased in early states of acute hepatic failure).
   b. Despite the fact that low serum albumin is a poor prognostic factor in critical illness, supplementation has not been shown to improve prognosis.

2. **Coagulation Factors**
   a. Hepatocytes synthesize all coagulation factors with the exception of von Willebrand factor and factor VIIIC.
   b. Coagulation may be rapidly impaired by acute liver failure reflecting the short plasma half-time for many critical component (factor VII, 100 to 300 minutes).

3. **Use of Proteins for Energy**
   a. Once cells contain a maximum amount of amino acids, any additional amino acids are deaminated (oxidative deamination) to keto acids that can enter the citric acid cycle.
   b. Ammonia resulting from deamination is converted to urea in the liver for excretion by the kidneys.
   c. The conversion of amino acids to glucose or glycogen is *gluconeogenesis*, and the conversion of amino acids into fatty acids is *ketogenesis*.

V. **Effects of Stress on Metabolism**
   A. Carbohydrate, lipid, and protein metabolism are significantly altered by stress.
   B. In response to stress, the body increases secretion of cortisol, catecholamines, and glucagon, resulting in increased endogenous glucose production (hepatic gluconeogenesis) and hyperglycemia (to provide glucose to cells for ATP production in those cells involved in the fight or flight response).
   C. Exogenous glucose administered to injured or septic patients has a minimal effect on gluconeogenesis and lipolysis. Conversely, administration of glucose in the presence of starvation decreases gluconeogenesis and lipolysis.

VI. Obesity
   A. The ability to conserve energy in the form of adipose tissue
      would at one time have conferred a survival advantage.
      Today, the combination of easy access to calorically dense
      foods and a sedentary lifestyle has made the metabolic
      consequences of these presumed genes maladaptive. In ad-
      dition, certain medications are commonly associated with
      weight gain (Table 33-5).
   B. Obesity is the most common and costly nutritional problem
      in the United States.
      1. Based on body mass index (BMI) (weight in kilograms
         divided by the square of the height in meters), 67% of
         adult males and 62% of adult females are overweight
         (BMI ≥25).
      2. Individuals with a BMI >35 have class II obesity, and
         class III obesity if the BMI is >40.
      3. A BMI of ≥28 is associated with a three to four times
         increase in the risk of ischemic heart disease, stroke, and
         diabetes mellitus compared with the general population.
         Increased waist circumference (>102 cm in adult males
         and >88 cm in adult females) is associated with an in-
         creased risk for ischemic heart disease, diabetes mellitus,
         and systemic hypertension.
      4. The increased risk for morbidity and mortality extend
         beyond measurements of BMI and fat distribution, as

Table 33-5

Drugs Commonly Associated with Weight Gain

Classification	Drug	Alternative Drug
Antidepressants	Tricyclic antidepressants	Selective serotonin reuptake inhibitors
	Monoamine oxidase inhibitors	
Antidiabetics	Insulin	Metformin
	Sulfonylureas	Acarbose
	Thiazolidinediones	
Antiepileptics	Gabapentin	Lamotrigine
	Valproic acid	Topiramate
Antipsychotics	Clozapine	Haloperidol
Steroids	Glucocorticoids	

Table 33-6

Criteria for Diagnosis of Metabolic Syndrome
(Any Three of the following Characteristics)

Characteristic	Specific Finding
Waist circumference	Males >102 cm (40 inches) Females >88 cm (35 inches)
Blood glucose concentration (fasting)	>110 mg/dL
Increased systemic blood pressure	Systolic >130 mm Hg Diastolic >85 mm Hg
Serum triglyceride concentration	>150 mg/dL
High-density lipoprotein cholesterol concentration	Males <40 mg/dL Females <50 mg/dL

reflected by the diagnosis of **_metabolic syndrome_**, which is present if a patient has three of the following five risk factors: increased waist circumference, low levels of HDL cholesterol, increased triglycerides, hypertension, and glucose intolerance (Table 33-6).

5. The risk of anesthesia may be increased in classes II and III obese patients, reflecting mechanical difficulties (airway, positioning, and ventilation) and increased incidence of comorbid conditions (diabetes mellitus, systemic hypertension).

6. Treatment of obesity by decreasing caloric intake and increasing metabolic rate (exercise) directed toward a long-term decrease in body weight is largely ineffective. Both proteins and carbohydrates can be metabolically converted to fat, and there is no evidence that changing the relative proportions of protein, carbohydrate, and fat in the diet without decreasing caloric intake will promote weight loss.

C. **Pharmacologic Treatment**

1. Orlistat inhibits lipases in the gastrointestinal lumen, thus antagonizing triglyceride hydrolysis and decreasing fat absorption by about 30% (weight loss with orlistat is modest, an average of 2.9 kg at 1 to 4 years).

2. Lorcaserin is a selective 5-HT_{2C} agonist which activates proopiomelanocortin production and promotes weight loss through satiety.

CHAPTER 34

Antiemetics

I. **Introduction.** Along with pain, postoperative nausea and vomiting (PONV) is the most important complaint patients report following surgery under anesthesia and is the leading cause of unanticipated hospital admission following outpatient surgery. Without prophylaxis, nausea occurs in up to 40% of patients who undergo general anesthesia but can be as high as 80% in high-risk patients.

II. **Definition**
   A. Although nausea and emesis are intimately related, one can have one without the other or vice versa. Some drugs are more effective in treating one than the other.
   B. A patient who experiences nausea or has emesis within 24 hours of a surgical procedure that required anesthesia meets the criteria for the diagnosis of PONV. The classification is further divided into early PONV (within 6 hours of emergence from anesthesia) or late PONV (6 to 24 hours after the procedure).

III. **Incidence.** From a patient satisfaction point of view, PONV is a major issue (patients rated emesis as the most important clinical anesthesia outcome to avoid). PONV has been associated with morbidity including dehydration, electrolyte abnormalities, wound dehiscence, bleeding, esophageal rupture, and airway compromise.

IV. **Pathophysiology**
   A. Patients with nausea have a subjective feeling of the need to vomit.
   B. Emesis, which is the expulsion of stomach contents up the esophagus to the mouth, may or may not be preceded by nausea. Emesis is different from regurgitation in which acidic gastric material passively reflexes into the esophagus

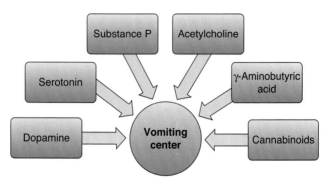

FIGURE 34-1 Pharmacological systems that interact with the vomiting center.

because of an incompetent esophageal sphincter and elevated abdominal pressure.

1. The sequence of events that occur during emesis are controlled by the vomiting center, which lies in the medulla oblongata. A number of neurotransmitters modulate the activity of the vomiting center (Fig. 34-1). Agonists and antagonists of these neurotransmitters are used to prevent nausea and vomiting.

2. Slightly cephalad to the vomiting center is the chemoreceptor trigger zone (CRTZ), which detects noxious chemicals in the bloodstream (ethanol at high concentration).

V. **Prophylaxis.** Antiemetic agents should be used for the prevention and treatment of nausea and vomiting when indicated but not routinely. In order to determine whether prophylaxis is indicated, it is important to assess a patient's propensity to develop PONV according to risk factors that increase or decrease a patient's chances of experiencing PONV.

A. **Patient Factors.** Women, nonsmokers, and those with a history of motion sickness or of previous episodes of PONV are at an increased risk of experiencing PONV.

B. **Surgical Factors**

1. The longer the surgical procedure, the greater is the risk for a patient to develop PONV.

2. Independent of duration, certain surgical procedures have been associated with an increased incidence of PONV (gynecologic surgeries; laparoscopic procedures;

ear, nose, and throat; breast; plastic; and orthopedic surgical procedures).
3. Among adults, risk is reduced with aging.
C. **Anesthetic Factors**. Inhalation anesthetic agents nitrous oxide, neostigmine, and opioids have all been implicated in the genesis of PONV (correlation is limited and most scoring systems used to identify patients at risk of PONV do not use anesthetic factors as risk factors).

VI. **Pharmacologic Interventions. A multimodal approach for prophylaxis in patients at high risk for developing PONV and as rescue therapy in patients who develop PONV in the postanesthetic care unit works well because of the complexity of systems involved in the pathogenesis of PONV (Table 34-1).**
A. **Anticholinergics: Scopolamine**
1. **Prevention of Motion-Induced Nausea and of PONV**. Transdermal absorption of scopolamine provides sustained therapeutic plasma concentrations

Table 34-1

Pharmacologic Therapies for Treatment of Nausea and Vomiting

Anticholinergics	Atropine
	Hyoscine
	Scopolamine
Benzamides	Metoclopramide
Benzodiazepines	Midazolam
Butyrophenones	Droperidol
	Haloperidol
Cannabinoids	Dronabinol
	Nabilone
Glucocorticoids	Dexamethasone
5-HT$_3$ antagonists	Dolasetron
	Granisetron
	Ondansetron
	Palonosetron
	Ramosetron
	Tropisetron
Neurokinin-1 antagonists	Aprepitant
	Fosaprepitant
Phenothiazines	Prochlorperazine
	Promethazine
	Chlorpromazine

that protect against motion-induced nausea usually without introducing prohibitive side effects such as sedation, cycloplegia, or drying of secretions. Transdermal application of a scopolamine patch has been shown to exert significant antiemetic effects in patients treated with patient-controlled analgesia or epidural morphine for the management of postoperative pain.

2. **Central Anticholinergic Syndrome**. Scopolamine and atropine can enter the central nervous system and produce symptoms characterized as the central anticholinergic syndrome. Symptoms range from restlessness and hallucinations to somnolence and unconsciousness.

   a. Physostigmine, a lipid-soluble tertiary amine anticholinesterase drug administered in doses of 15 to 60 μg/kg intravenously (IV), is a specific treatment for the central anticholinergic syndrome.

   b. The central anticholinergic syndrome is often mistaken for delayed recovery from anesthesia or confusion.

3. **Overdose**

   a. Deliberate or accidental overdose with an anticholinergic drug produces a rapid onset of symptoms characteristic of muscarinic cholinergic receptor blockade (dry mouth, swallowing and talking is difficult, vision is blurred, photophobia is present, and tachycardia is prominent). The skin is dry and flushed, and a rash may appear especially over the face, neck, and upper chest (blush area). Body temperature is likely to be increased by anticholinergic drugs, especially when the environmental temperature is also increased. Small children are particularly vulnerable to drug-induced increases in body temperature (atropine fever).

   b. Physostigmine, administered in doses of 15 to 60 μg/kg IV, is the specific treatment for reversal of symptoms (repeated doses of this anticholinesterase drug may be necessary due to its rapid metabolism).

4. **Decreased Barrier Pressure**. Administration of atropine, 0.6 mg IV, or glycopyrrolate, 0.2 to 0.3 mg IV, decreases lower esophageal sphincter pressure and thus decreases barrier pressure and the inherent resistance to reflux of acidic fluid into the esophagus.

B. **Benzamides: Metoclopramide** stimulates the gastrointestinal tract via cholinergic mechanism that results in increased gastric and small intestinal motility.

   1. Because of its antidopaminergic activity, metoclopramide should be used with caution if at all in patients with Parkinson's disease, restless leg syndrome, or who have movement disorders related to dopamine inhibition or depletion.

   2. Akathisia, a feeling of unease and restlessness in the lower extremities, may follow the IV administration of metoclopramide, sometimes so severe that it can result in cancellation of surgery or which may manifest in the postanesthesia care unit.

C. **Benzodiazepines: Midazolam**, if used for its antiemetic effect, should be administered IV toward the end of the surgical procedure or by continuous infusion in intubated and ventilated patients in the intensive care unit.

D. **Butyrophenones: Droperidol and Haloperidol**

   1. The U.S. Food and Drug Administration's (FDA) "black box" restriction on droperidol was for higher doses than are necessary for the treatment of PONV. Because of its efficacy at low dose, the use of droperidol has increased over the last several years for prophylaxis and as rescue therapy as an antiemetic. Prophylactic doses of droperidol of 0.625 to 1.25 mg IV are effective for the prevention and treatment of PONV.

   2. Haloperidol also has antiemetic properties when used in low doses, 0.5 to 2 mg IV.

   3. Extrapyramidal symptoms are a risk of these medications (should be used with caution if at all in patients with Parkinson's disease, restless leg syndrome, and other diseases related to dopaminergic activity).

   4. For patients in whom dopamine antagonism is not a concern, droperidol is as effective as dexamethasone or ondansetron in preventing and treating PONV.

E. **Corticosteroids: Dexamethasone** has efficacy similar to ondansetron and droperidol and with a minimal side effect profile associated with one-time use. Obese and diabetic patients are at increased risk for perioperative hyperglycemia when they receive a single dose of dexamethasone.

F. **5-HT$_3$ receptor antagonists** result in an antiemetic effect.

   1. **Clinical Uses**

      a. The 5-HT$_3$ receptor antagonists represent (ondansetron, tropisetron, granisetron, dolasetron) a significant advance in the prophylaxis and treatment of nausea and vomiting because they are highly specific and evoke minimal side effects.

b. Drugs that act as competitive antagonists at 5-HT$_3$ receptors are useful antiemetics in the prophylaxis and treatment of chemotherapy- and radiation therapy–induced nausea and vomiting.

c. The convenience of use, efficacy, and safety profile are some of the reasons for the popularity of 5-HT$_3$ receptor antagonists for management of PONV.

2. **Comparison with Other Antiemetics**. Ondansetron (4 mg), dexamethasone (4 mg), and droperidol (1.25 mg) administered IV as prophylactic therapy before induction of general anesthesia are equally effective in decreasing the incidence of PONV.

3. **Pharmacokinetics**. The 5-HT$_3$ receptor antagonists are readily absorbed after oral administration and readily cross the blood–brain barrier. Following IV administration, the maximum brain concentration is achieved quickly.

4. **Ondansetron** is structurally related to serotonin and possesses specific 5-HT$_3$ subtype receptor antagonist properties without altering dopamine, histamine, adrenergic, or cholinergic receptor activity. As a result, ondansetron is free of neurologic side effects common to droperidol and metoclopramide.

a. Ondansetron is effective when administered orally or IV. The most significant feature of ondansetron prophylaxis and treatment is the relative freedom from side effects.

b. Ondansetron and other 5-HT$_3$ receptor antagonists can cause slight prolongation of the QTc interval on the electrocardiogram (ECG) of treated patients (has not created concern).

c. Ondansetron, 4 to 8 mg IV (administered over 2 to 5 minutes immediately before the induction of anesthesia), is highly effective in decreasing the incidence of PONV in a susceptible patient population (ambulatory gynecologic surgery, middle ear surgery). Oral (0.15 mg/kg) or IV (0.05 to 0.15 mg/kg) administration of ondansetron is effective in decreasing the incidence of postoperative vomiting in preadolescent children undergoing ambulatory surgery, including tonsillectomy and strabismus surgery.

5. **Tropisetron** shares the beneficial effects and side effects of ondansetron. This drug is also effective in the treatment of symptoms related to carcinoid syndrome and may also possess gastrokinetic properties.
6. **Granisetron** is effective orally and IV (0.02 to 0.04 mg/kg IV is effective in prevention of chemotherapy-induced emesis and PONV).
7. **Dolasetron** is a highly potent and selective 5-HT$_3$ receptor antagonist that is effective in the prevention of chemotherapy-induced nausea and vomiting and PONV following either oral or IV administration (a single IV dose of dolasetron, 1.8 mg, is equivalent to ondansetron, 32 mg IV, and granisetron, 3 mg IV, in preventing chemotherapy-induced nausea and vomiting).

G. **Histamine Receptor Antagonists**
   1. Dimenhydrinate (marketed as Dramamine) is effective in the prevention of PONV as well as motion sickness.
   2. Administration of dimenhydrinate, 20 mg IV, in adults decreases vomiting after outpatient surgery. In children, dimenhydrinate, 0.5 mg/kg IV, significantly decreases the incidence of vomiting after strabismus surgery.

CHAPTER 35

Gastrointestinal Motility Drugs

I. **Introduction.** Aspiration during general anesthesia occurs in approximately 1 in 8,500 adults and 1 in 4,400 children younger than 16 years of age (increased risk for emergency operations, especially bowel obstruction). Factors associated with pulmonary complications of aspiration include the volume and acidity of the aspirated gastric contents. Drugs that increase the pH of gastric contents (antacids) and that decrease the volume of gastric contents (prokinetic drugs) have a role in decreasing the severity of the sequelae of aspirating gastric contents. Enforcement of the American Society of Anesthesiologist Task Force Fasting Recommendations can also reduce the risk of pulmonary aspiration.

II. **Oral Antacids.** Antacids are drugs that neutralize (remove hydrogen ions) acid from gastric contents or decrease the secretion of hydrogen chloride into the stomach. Occasional failure of particulate antacids to increase gastric fluid pH may reflect inadequate mixing with stomach contents or an unusually large volume of gastric fluid. Pneumonitis associated with functional and histologic changes in the lungs may reflect a foreign body reaction to inhaled particulate antacid particles.

   A. Nonparticulate (clear) antacids (sodium citrate) are less likely to cause a foreign body reaction if aspirated, and their mixing with gastric fluid is more complete than is that of particulate antacids.

   B. The onset of effect is more rapid with sodium citrate than with particulate antacids that require a longer time for adequate mixing with gastric fluid.

   C. Sodium citrate, 15 to 30 mL of a 0.3-mol per liter solution administered 15 to 30 minutes before the induction of anesthesia, is effective in reliably increasing gastric fluid pH in pregnant and nonpregnant patients.

III. **Complications of Antacid Therapy** (Table 35-1)

Table 35-1

Complications of Antacid Therapy

Bacterial overgrowth in the small intestine
Urinary tract infections
Urolithiasis (chronic administration)
Altered renal elimination of drugs (reflects increased urinary pH)
Acid rebound (unique to calcium-containing antacids)
Milk-alkali syndrome (hypercalcemia, systemic alkalosis)
Hypophosphatemia (osteomalacia, osteoporosis)
Drug interactions (speed delivery and absorption of drugs such
   as salicylates, indomethacin, naproxen, decreased availability
   of cimetidine)

IV. **Histamine Receptor Antagonists.** Histamine induces contraction of smooth muscles in the airways, increases the secretion of acid in the stomach, and stimulates release of neurotransmitters in the central nervous system (CNS). Histamine receptor antagonists bind to receptors on effector cell membranes, to the exclusion of agonist molecules, without themselves activating the receptor (histamine receptor antagonists do not inhibit release of histamine).

   A. **H_1-Receptor Antagonists.** H_1-receptor antagonists are characterized as first-generation and second-generation receptor antagonists. First-generation drugs tend to produce sedation, whereas second-generation drugs are relatively nonsedating (Table 35-2). The selectivity of the second-generation antagonists for H_1 receptors decreases CNS toxicity.

      1. **Pharmacokinetics.** H_1-receptor antagonists are well absorbed after oral administration, often reaching peak plasma concentrations within 2 hours (Table 35-3).

      2. **Clinical Uses**

         a. H_1-receptor antagonists prevent and relieve the symptoms of allergic rhinoconjunctivitis (sneezing, nasal and ocular itching, rhinorrhea, tearing, and conjunctival erythema) but they are less effective for the nasal congestion characteristic of a delayed allergic reaction. First-generation H_1-receptor antagonists have sedating effects that result in delayed reaction times.

Table 35-2

Pharmacokinetics of H_1-Receptor Antagonists

	Time to Peak Plasma Level (h)	Elimination Half-Time (h)	Clearance Rate (mL/kg/minute)
First-generation receptor antagonists			
Chlorpheniramine	2.8	27.9	1.8
Diphenhydramine	1.7	9.2	23.3
Hydroxyzine	2.1	20.0	98
Second-generation receptor antagonists			
Loratadine	1.0	11.0	202
Acrivastine	0.85–1.4	1.4–2.1	4.56
Azelastine	5.3	22	8.5

Data from Simons FE, Simons KJ. The pharmacology and use of H_1-receptor antagonist drugs. *N Engl J Med.* 1994;330:1663–1670.

    b. Diphenhydramine is prescribed as a sedative, an antipruritic, and as an antiemetic (in combination with systemic or neuraxial opioids to control nausea and pruritus, there is the conceptual risk of depression of ventilation but diphenhydramine counteracts to some extent the opioid-induced decreases in the slope of the ventilatory response to CO_2 and does not exacerbate the opioid-induced depression of the hypoxic ventilatory response during moderate hypercarbia).

    c. Use of antihistamines in the acute treatment of anaphylactic reactions is directed at blocking further histamine-mediated vasodilation and resulting hemodynamic instability, as well as decreasing respiratory and other systemic complications. As such, the administration of H_1-receptor antagonists plus the administration of epinephrine is indicated in the treatment of acute anaphylaxis. These drugs may also be administered prophylactically for anaphylactoid reactions to radiocontrast dyes.

3. **Side Effects**

    a. First-generation H_1 antagonists often have adverse effects on the CNS, including somnolence, diminished alertness, slowed reaction time, and impairment of cognitive function.

Table 35-3

Pharmacokinetics of H$_2$-Receptor Antagonists

	Cimetidine	Ranitidine	Famotidine	Nizatidine
Potency	1	4–10	20–50	4–10
EC$_{50}$ (µg/mL)[a]	250–500	60–165	10–13	154–180
Bioavailability (%)	60	50	43	98
Time to peak plasma concentration (hours)	1–2	1–3	1.0–3.5	1–3
Volume of distribution (L/kg)	0.8–1.2	1.2–1.9	1.1–1.4	1.2–1.6
Plasma protein binding (%)	13–26	15	16	26–35
Cerebrospinal fluid:plasma	0.18	0.06–0.17	0.05–0.09	Unknown
Clearance (mL/minute)	450–650	568–709	417–483	667–850
Hepatic clearance (%)				
Oral	60	73	50–80	22
Intravenous	25–40	30	25–30	25
Renal clearance (%)				
Oral	40	27	25–30	57–65
Intravenous	50–80	50	65–80	75
Elimination half-time (hours)	1.5–2.3	1.6–2.4	2.5–4	1.1–1.6
Decrease dose in presence of renal dysfunction	Yes	Yes	Yes	Yes
Hepatic dysfunction	No	No	No	No
Interfere with drug metabolism by cytochrome P450 enzymes	Yes	Minimal	No	No

[a]EC$_{50}$ denotes the plasma concentration of the drug necessary to inhibit the pentagastrin-stimulated secretion of hydrogen ions by 50%.
Data from Feldman M, Burton ME. Histamine-2-receptor antagonists. *N Engl J Med.* 1990;323:1672–1680.

b. Tachycardia is common, and prolongation of the QTc interval on the electrocardiogram (ECG), heart block, and cardiac arrhythmias have occurred.

c. Second-generation H_1 antagonists are unlikely to produce CNS side effects and enhancement of the effects of diazepam or alcohol is unlikely by second-generation drugs.

d. Antihistamine intoxication is similar to anticholinergic poisoning and may be associated with seizures and cardiac conduction abnormalities resembling tricyclic antidepressant overdose.

B. **H_2-Receptor Antagonists.** Cimetidine, ranitidine, famotidine, and nizatidine are H_2-receptor antagonists that produce selective and reversible inhibition of H_2 receptor–mediated secretion of hydrogen ions by parietal cells.

1. **Mechanism of Action.** The histamine receptors on the basolateral membranes of acid-secreting gastric parietal cells are of the H_2 type and thus are not blocked by conventional H_1 antagonists.

   a. The relative potencies of the four H_2-receptor antagonists for inhibition of secretion of gastric hydrogen ions varies from 20- to 50-fold, with cimetidine as the least potent and famotidine the most potent (see Table 35-3).

   b. The duration of inhibition ranges from approximately 6 hours for cimetidine to 10 hours for ranitidine, famotidine, and nizatidine.

2. **Pharmacokinetics.** The absorption of cimetidine, ranitidine, and famotidine is rapid after oral administration. Because of extensive first-pass hepatic metabolism, however, the bioavailability of these drugs is approximately 50% (see Table 35-3).

   a. Hepatic dysfunction does not seem to significantly alter the pharmacokinetics of H_2-receptor antagonists.

   b. Increasing age must be considered when determining the dose of H_2-receptor antagonists (cimetidine clearance decreases 75% between the ages of 20 years and 70 years.)

3. **Clinical Uses**

   a. In the preoperative period, H_2-receptor antagonists have been administered as chemoprophylaxis to increase the pH of gastric fluid before induction of anesthesia. However, the American Society of Anesthesiologists' practice guidelines for preoperative fasting and the use of pharmacologic agent to reduce the risk of pulmonary aspiration state that the routine preoperative use of medications that block gastric acid secretion to decrease the risks of pulmonary aspiration in patients who have no apparent increased risk for pulmonary aspiration is not recommended.

b. When indicated though, H_2-receptor antagonists have been advocated as useful drugs in the preoperative period to decrease the risk of acid pneumonitis if inhalation of acidic gastric fluid were to occur in the perioperative period (cimetidine, 300 mg orally, 1.5 to 2.0 hours before the induction of anesthesia, with or without a similar dose the preceding evening; famotidine given the evening before and the morning of surgery or on the morning of surgery).

c. H_2-receptor antagonists, in contrast to antacids, have no influence on the pH of the gastric fluid that is already present in the stomach.

d. H_2-receptor antagonists cross the placenta but do not adversely affect the fetus when administered before cesarean section.

e. Preoperative preparation of patients with allergic histories or patients undergoing procedures associated with an increased likelihood of allergic reactions (radiographic contrast dye administration) may include prophylactic oral administration of an H_1-receptor antagonist (diphenhydramine, 0.5 to 1.0 mg/kg) and an H_2-receptor antagonist (cimetidine, 4 mg/kg) every 6 hours in the 12 to 24 hours preceding the possible triggering event. A corticosteroid administered at least 24 hours earlier is commonly added to this regimen.

4. **Side Effects** (Table 35-4)

5. **Drug Interactions** (Table 35-5)

V. **Proton pump inhibitors are the most effective drugs available for controlling gastric acidity and volume (Table 35-6).**

A. **Omeprazole** provides prolonged inhibition of gastric acid secretion, regardless of the stimulus, and it inhibits daytime and nocturnal acid secretion and meal-stimulated acid secretion to a significantly greater degree than do the H_2-receptor antagonists. This drug heals duodenal and, possibly, gastric ulcers more rapidly than do the H_2-receptor antagonists.

Table 35-4

Side Effects of H_2-Receptor Antagonists

Interaction with cerebral H_2 receptors (headache, somnolence, confusion)
Interaction with cardiac H_2 receptors (bradycardia, hypotension, heart block)
Hyperprolactinemia
Acute pancreatitis
Increased hepatic transaminases
Alcohol dehydrogenase dehydration
Thrombocytopenia
Agranulocytosis
Interstitial nephritis
Interfere with drug metabolism by cytochrome P450

B. **Preoperative Medication**
   1. Omeprazole effectively increases gastric fluid pH and decreases gastric fluid volume in children and adults (onset of the gastric antisecretory effect of omeprazole after a single 20 mg oral dose occurs within 2 to 6 hours).
   2. Oral omeprazole should be administered >3 hours before anticipated induction of anesthesia to ensure adequate chemoprophylaxis.
C. **Side Effects**. Omeprazole crosses the blood–brain barrier and may cause headache, agitation, and confusion.

VI. **Gastrointestinal Prokinetics.** Motility-modulating drugs exert their therapeutic effects by increasing lower esophageal sphincter tone, enhancing peristaltic contractions, and accelerating the rate of gastric emptying.
   A. **Dopaminergic Blockers**
      1. **Metoclopramide** acts as a gastrointestinal prokinetic drug that increases lower esophageal sphincter tone and stimulates motility of the upper gastrointestinal tract in normal persons and parturients (only drug approved by the U.S. Food and Drug Administration for the treatment of diabetic gastroparesis).
         a. Gastric hydrogen ion secretion is not altered.
         b. The net effect is accelerated gastric clearance of liquids and solids (decreased gastric emptying time)

Table 35-5

Drug Interactions with Cimetidine

Drug	Effect of Cimetidine on Plasma Concentration	Clearance of Drug (% Decrease)	Mechanism
Ketoconazole	Decreased	No change	Decreased absorption due to increased gastric fluid pH that slows dissolution
Warfarin[a]	Increased	23–36	Decreased hydroxylation of dextrorotatory isomer
Theophylline[a]	Increased	12–34	Decreased methylation
Phenytoin[a]	Increased	21–24	Decreased hydroxylation (?)
Propranolol	Increased	20–27	Decreased hydroxylation
Nifedipine	Increased	38	Unknown
Lidocaine	Increased	14–30	Decreased N-dealkylation
Quinidine	Increased	25–37	Decreased 3-hydroxylation (?)
Imipramine	Increased	40	Decreased N-demethylation
Desipramine	Increased	36	Decreased hydroxylation in rapid metabolizers
Triazolam	Increased	27	Decreased hydroxylation
Meperidine	Increased	22	Decreased oxidation
Procainamide[a]	Increased	28	Competition for renal tubular secretion

[a]Lesser drug interactions also occur with ranitidine.
Data from Feldman M, Burton ME. Histamine-2-receptor antagonists. *N Engl J Med.* 1990;323:1672–1680.

Table 35-6

Pharmacokinetics of Proton Pump Inhibitors

	Bioavailability	Time to Peak Plasma Concentration (h)	Protein Binding	Elimination Half-Time (h)	Hepatic Metabolism	Interfere with Cytochrome P450
Omeprazole	60%	2–4	>90%	0.5–1.0	Yes	Minimal
Esomeprazole	60%	2–4	>90%	0.5–1.0	Yes	Minimal
Lansoprazole	85%	1.5–3.0	97%	1.5	Yes	Minimal
Pantoprazole	77%	2.5	98%	1.9	Yes	No
Rabeprazole	85%	2.9–3.8	96%	1	Yes	No

and a shortened transit time through the small intestine.

2. **Mechanism of Action**

   a. Metoclopramide produces selective cholinergic stimulation of the gastrointestinal tract (gastrokinetic effect).

   b. Metoclopramide does cross the blood–brain barrier and, within the CNS, metoclopramide inhibition of dopamine receptors can produce significant extrapyramidal side effects.

3. **Pharmacokinetics**. Metoclopramide is rapidly absorbed after oral administration, reaching peak plasma concentrations in 40 to 120 minutes. Extensive first-pass hepatic metabolism limits bioavailability to about 75%.

4. **Clinical uses** of metoclopramide include (a) preoperative decrease of gastric fluid volume, (b) production of an antiemetic effect, (c) treatment of gastroparesis, and (d) symptomatic treatment of gastroesophageal reflux.

   a. **Preoperative Decrease in Gastric Fluid Volume**. Metoclopramide, 10 to 20 mg IV over 3 to 5 minutes administered 15 to 30 minutes before induction of anesthesia, results in increased lower esophageal sphincter tone and decreased gastric fluid volume. This gastric emptying effect of metoclopramide may be of potential benefit before the induction of anesthesia in (a) patients who have recently ingested solid food, (b) trauma patients, (c) obese patients, (d) patients with diabetes mellitus and symptoms of gastroparesis, and (e) parturients, especially those with a history of esophagitis ("heartburn"), suggesting lower esophageal sphincter dysfunction and gastric hypomotility. Regardless of the effects of gastric fluid volume, the administration of metoclopramide does not reliably alter gastric fluid pH. It is important to recognize that opioid-induced inhibition of gastric motility may not be reversible with metoclopramide. The beneficial cholinergic stimulant effects of metoclopramide on the gastrointestinal tract may be offset by concomitant administration of atropine in the preoperative medication.

   b. **Production of an Antiemetic Effect**. Metoclopramide decreases chemotherapy-induced nausea and vomiting (probably results from antagonism of dopamine's effects in the chemoreceptor trigger zone). Gastric stasis induced by morphine is reversed by metoclopramide, and opioid-induced nausea and vomiting, which can accompany preoperative medication or postoperative pain management, are blunted.

5. **Side Effects**

a. Metoclopramide should not be administered to patients with known Parkinson's disease, restless leg syndrome, or who have movement disorders related to dopamine inhibition or depletion.

b. Akathisia, a feeling of unease and restlessness in the lower extremities, may follow the IV administration of metoclopramide.

c. IV administration of metoclopramide may also be associated with hypotension, tachycardia, bradycardia, and cardiac arrhythmias.

d. Metoclopramide may increase the sedative actions of CNS depressants.

e. It would seem prudent not to administer metoclopramide to a patient with a suspected or known mechanical obstruction to gastric emptying. Likewise, metoclopramide is not administered after gastrointestinal surgery such as pyloroplasty or intestinal anastomosis because it stimulates gastric motility and may delay healing.

f. Metoclopramide has an inhibitory effect on plasma cholinesterase activity (may explain occasional observations of prolonged responses to succinylcholine). The metabolism of ester local anesthetics could be slowed by metoclopramide-induced decreases in plasma cholinesterase activity.

B. **Macrolides**. The antibiotic erythromycin, as well as other macrolide antibiotics (i.e., azithromycin), increases lower esophageal sphincter tone, enhances intraduodenal coordination, and promotes emptying of gastric liquids and solids in patients with diabetic gastroparesis, in patients awaiting emergency surgery, in normal patients, and in patients in the intensive care unit with food intolerance (Fig. 35-1). Side effects of the macrolide compounds are the same as for any antibiotic (erythromycin should be used if all other prokinetic agents have failed).

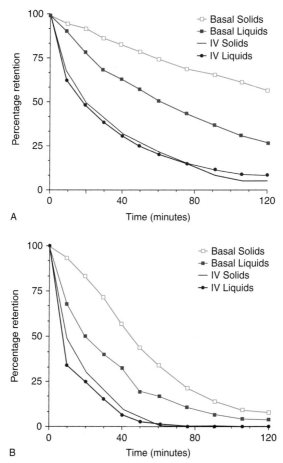

FIGURE 35-1 Erythromycin, 200 mg intravenously over 15 minutes, followed by ingestion of a radioactive-labeled meal (scrambled egg, toast, and water) resulted in more rapid emptying of solids and liquids (IV solids and IV liquids) in patients with diabetic gastroparesis **(A)** and patients without diabetes **(B)** compared with gastric emptying times in the absence of erythromycin (basal solids and basal liquids). (From Urbain JLC, Vantrappen G, Janssens J, et al. Intravenous erythromycin dramatically accelerates gastric emptying in gastroparesis diabeticorum and normal and abolishes the emptying discrimination between solids and liquids. *J Nucl Med.* 1990;31:1490–1493, with permission.)

CHAPTER 36

Nutrition

I. Enteral and Parenteral Nutrition

A. Enteral nutrition is defined as providing nourishment to a patient utilizing a diet that is delivered directly into the gastrointestinal tract (nasogastric tube, nasointestinal tube, gastrostomy tube, jejunostomy tube).

B. Parenteral nutrition is defined as delivery of nutrients directly into the venous circulation (peripheral vein or central vein). The term *total parenteral nutrition* (TPN) is utilized when the only source of nutrient supply is via the parenteral route.

C. Nutritional support is characterized as the use of enteral or parenteral nutrition rather than or in addition to an oral diet.

D. Preexisting TPN should be continued during the perioperative period, whereas enteral nutrition should be discontinued about 6 hours before surgery (reflecting recommendations for food ingestion prior to elective surgery).

II. Nutritional Support

A. Total parenteral nutrition is intended to supply all the essential inorganic and organic nutritional elements necessary to maintain optimal body composition. Alimentation by the gastrointestinal tract (enteral nutrition) is preferred to intravenous (IV) alimentation (parenteral nutrition).

1. Even if the patient's caloric and nitrogen requirements cannot be met with luminal nutrition, the enteral route of feeding should be used unless it is contraindicated (bowel obstruction, inadequate bowel surface area, intractable diarrhea).

2. The enteral and parenteral routes may be used simultaneously to meet nutritional requirements although there is no evidence that the combination of the two to meet caloric needs improves outcome.

Table 36-1

Established Indications for Use of Nutritional Support

Major elective surgery in severely malnourished patients
Major trauma (blunt or penetrating injury, head injury)
Burns
Hepatic dysfunction
Renal dysfunction
Bone marrow transplant recipients undergoing intensive
   chemotherapy
Patients unable to eat or absorb nutrients for an indefinite period
   (neurologic impairment, pharyngeal dysfunction, or short
   bowel syndrome)
Well-nourished, minimally stressed patients unable to eat for
   7 to 10 days

Adapted from Souba WW. Nutritional support. *N Engl J Med*. 1997;336:41–48.

    B. Preoperative nutritional support should be reserved for malnourished patients undergoing major elective surgery.
      1. Most patients do not need nutritional support, and clear-cut benefits of this expensive intervention have been established for only a select group of patients (Table 36-1).
      2. Patients not expected to resume adequate oral feedings within 7 to 10 days of surgery should begin nutritional support within 2 to 4 days postoperatively, within 1 to 2 days if they are in an intensive care unit.

  III. **Enteral nutrition is almost always preferred over parenteral nutrition. Goals include meeting and attenuating the metabolic response to stress, and in addition attenuating cellular injury, and modulating the immune response to injury.**
    A variety of enteral solutions containing various amounts of protein (amino acids), carbohydrates (glucose), fat (medium and long chain triglycerides), micronutrients, macronutrients, and electrolytes are available.
    A. **Enteral tube feeding** may be necessary when patients are unable to consume nutritionally complete, liquefied food orally. Most often, patients receive continuous infusions of enteral nutrition through a nasoenteric tube positioned in the stomach, duodenum, or jejunum. Surgical placement of an esophagostomy or gastrostomy tube may be indicated

for long-term feeding. The rate of infusion is typically 100 to 120 mL per hour (slow rate of infusion prevents the dumping syndrome).

B. **Side Effects**
1. Enteral feeding is frequently stopped because of patient's complaints (bloating or distention, emesis, high gastric residuals [usually 200 to 250 mL]). Osmotic diarrhea in this situation is a diagnosis of exclusion (*Clostridia difficile*). If clinically indicated, serum electrolyte levels should be measured to identify excessive loss or signs of dehydration.
2. Pulmonary aspiration is always a danger when enteral tube feeding is used. Patients should be maintained in a semi-sitting position (head of bed elevated 30 degrees) and in patients at the highest risk of aspiration, the feeding tube should be placed through the pylorus.

IV. **Parenteral nutrition is indicated for patients who are unable to ingest or digest nutrients or to absorb them from the gastrointestinal tract. Parenteral nutrition using isotonic solutions delivered through a peripheral vein is acceptable when the patient requires less than 2,000 calories daily and the anticipated need for nutritional support is brief. When nutritional requirements are greater than 2,000 calories daily or prolonged nutritional support is required, a catheter is placed in the central venous system to permit infusion of a hypertonic (1,900 mOsm/L) nutrition solution.**
A. **Short-term parenteral therapy** (3 to 5 days in patients without nutritional deficits) after uncomplicated surgical procedures is most often provided by hypocaloric, non-nitrogen glucose-electrolyte solutions.
B. **Long-term (total) parenteral nutrition** (IV hyperalimentation) is the technique of providing total nutrition needs by infusion of amino acids combined with glucose and varying amounts of lipids. These hypertonic solutions must be infused into a central vein with a high blood flow to provide rapid dilution. Because the solutions in current use are not nearly as hypertonic and hypercaloric as they once were, there is little concern about the patient becoming hypoglycemic if the infusion is discontinued abruptly but should be considered. Serum electrolytes, blood glucose concentrations, and blood urea nitrogen should be measured periodically during total parenteral nutrition. Tests of hepatic and renal function are also

recommended but can be performed at less frequent intervals.

1. **Side effects** of total parenteral nutrition include infectious (catheter sepsis), mechanical (pneumothorax, catheter thrombosis), and metabolic complications (Table 36-2).

   a. **Sepsis**. Total parenteral nutrition solutions infused through an IV catheter can support the growth of bacteria and fungi (spiking temperature most likely reflects contamination via the delivery system or catheter). In view of the hazard of contamination, the use of a central venous hyperalimentation catheter for administration of medications, as during the perioperative period, or for sampling of blood is not recommended.

   b. **Hyperglycemia**. Blood glucose concentrations should be monitored until glucose tolerance is demonstrated, which usually occurs after 2 to 3 days of therapy as endogenous insulin production increases. Current guidelines suggest a target blood glucose concentration of 140 to 200 mg/dL and avoidance of targets below 140 mg/dL.

   c. **Hypoglycemia**. Accidental, sudden discontinuation of the infusion of total parenteral nutrition solutions containing large amounts of glucose (catheter kink or disconnection) may cause hypoglycemia.

   d. **Metabolic acidosis** may occur because most of the amino acids in TPN are administered as their chloride salts.

   e. **Hypercarbia**. In a patient with inadequate respiratory reserve, respiratory failure can develop with

---

Table 36-2

Metabolic Complications of Parenteral Nutrition

Early Complications	Late Complications
Volume overload	Metabolic bone disease
Hyperglycemia	Hepatic steatosis
Hypophosphatemia (refeeding syndrome)	Hepatic cholestasis
	Trace mineral deficiency
Hypokalemia	Vitamin deficiency
Hypomagnesemia	
Hyperchloremic acidosis	

aggressive nutritional support that increases carbon dioxide production.

2. **Monitoring during Total Parenteral Nutrition**. Access sites are observed for signs of infection. Substitution of sodium or potassium acetate (metabolized to bicarbonate) for sodium or potassium chloride may be helpful should signs of hyperchloremic metabolic acidosis appear. Vitamin K may need to be added to the TPN or administered intravenously based on measurement of prothrombin and plasma thromboplastin times.

V. **Immunonutrition**. Cellular immunity decreases during acute stress as may accompany multiple organ system failure, sepsis, and shock. Immunonutrition is an attempt to enhance immunity and cellular integrity by incorporating specific additives (omega-3 fatty acids, arginine to enhance lymphocyte cytotoxicity, purines as a precursor of RNA and DNA, and antioxidants) into enteral diets.

VI. **Vitamins, Dietary Supplements, and Herbal Remedies**
   A. **Vitamins** are a group of structurally diverse organic substances (water soluble or fat soluble) that must be provided in small amounts in the diet for subsequent synthesis of cofactors that are essential for various metabolic reactions (Table 36-3).
   B. **Water-Soluble Vitamins** (Fig. 36-1)
      1. **Thiamine (vitamin B$_1$)** is converted to a physiologically active coenzyme that is essential for the decarboxylation of α-keto acids such as pyruvate (increased plasma concentrations of pyruvate are a diagnostic sign of thiamine deficiency).
         a. **Causes of Deficiency**. The requirement for thiamine is related to the metabolic rate and is greatest when carbohydrate is the source of energy (important in patients maintained by hyperalimentation in which the majority of calories are provided in the form of glucose).
         b. **Symptoms of deficiency** (beriberi) include loss of appetite, skeletal muscle weakness, a tendency to develop peripheral edema, decreased systemic blood pressure, and low body temperature. Severe thiamine deficiency (Korsakoff syndrome), which may occur in alcoholics, is associated with peripheral polyneuritis. High-output cardiac failure with extensive peripheral edema reflecting hypoproteinemia is often prominent.

Table 36-3

Vitamins

	Function	Deficiency	Toxic Effects	Sources
Thiamine (B₁)	Metabolism of carbohy-drates, alcohol, amino acids	Beriberi Wernicke-Korsakoff syndrome	None	Grains Legumes Poultry Meat
Riboflavin (B₂)	Cellular oxidation-reduction reactions	Stomatitis Dermatitis Anemia	None	Grains Dairy products Meat Eggs Green vegetables
Nicotinic acid (niacin, B₃)	Oxidative metabolism Decreases LDL cholesterol Increases HDL cholesterol	Pellagra	Flushing Headaches Pruritus Hyperglycemia Hyperuricemia	Meat Poultry Fish Grains Peanuts Tryptophan in foods
Pyridoxine (B₆)	Amino acid metabolism Heme synthesis Neuronal excitability Decreases blood homo-cysteine levels	Anemia Cheilosis Dermatitis	Neurotoxicity	Liver Poultry Fish Grains Bananas

(continued)

Table 36-3

Vitamins *(continued)*

	Function	Deficiency	Toxic Effects	Sources
Pantothenic acid	Metabolic processes	Rare	None	Many foods
B_{12} (cobalamin, cyanocobalamin)	DNA synthesis Myelin synthesis Decreases blood homocysteine levels	Megaloblastic anemia Peripheral neuropathies	None	Liver Poultry Fish Dairy products
Folic acid	DNA synthesis Decreases blood homocysteine levels	Megaloblastic anemia Birth defects	None	Legumes Grains Fruit Poultry Meat
Ascorbic acid (vitamin C)	Collagen synthesis Possible protection against certain cancers	Scurvy	Nephrolithiasis Diarrhea	Fruits Green vegetables Potatoes Cereals
Vitamin A (retinol, retinoic acid)	Vision Epithelial integrity	Night blindness Susceptibility to infection	Teratogenicity Hepatotoxicity Cerebral edema	Liver Dairy products Green vegetables

Table 36-3

Vitamins *(continued)*

	Function	Deficiency	Toxic Effects	Sources
Vitamin D (calciferol)	Intestinal calcium absorption	Osteomalacia Rickets	Hypercalcemia	Dairy products Fish Eggs Liver
Vitamin E (tocopherol)	Decreases peroxidation of fatty acids Possible protection against atherosclerosis	Rare	Antagonism of vitamin K Headaches	Vegetable oils Wheat germ Nuts
Vitamin K	Synthesis of clotting factors (VII, IX, X)	Hemorrhagic diathesis	None	Green vegetables Intestinal bacteria

LDL, low-density lipoprotein; HDL, high-density lipoprotein.

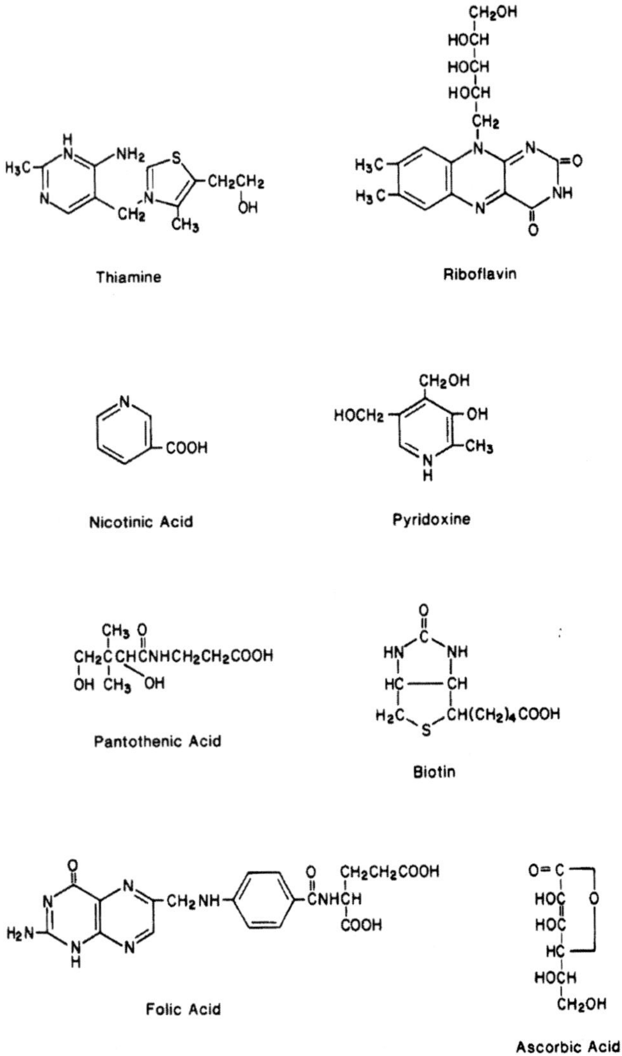

FIGURE 36-1 Chemical structure of water-soluble vitamins.

    c. **Treatment of Deficiency**. Severe thiamine deficiency is treated with IV administration of the vitamin.

2. **Riboflavin (vitamin B$_2$)**. Riboflavin is converted in the body to one of two physiologically active coenzymes that primarily influence hydrogen ion transport in oxidative enzyme systems. Pharyngitis and angular stomatitis are typically the first signs of riboflavin deficiency. Treatment is with oral vitamin supplements that contain riboflavin.

3. **Nicotinic acid (niacin, B$_3$)** is converted to the physiologically active coenzymes that are necessary to catalyze oxidation-reduction reactions essential for tissue respiration.

    a. **Symptoms of Deficiency**. Chronic niacin deficiency is manifested by pellagra (tongue becomes red and swollen). In addition to dementia, motor and sensory disturbances of the peripheral nerves also occur, mimicking changes that accompany a deficiency of thiamine.

    b. The relationship between nicotinic acid requirements and the intake of tryptophan explains the association of pellagra with tryptophan-deficient corn diets. Carcinoid syndrome is associated with diversion of tryptophan from the synthesis of nicotinic acid to the production of serotonin (5-hydroxytryptamine), leading to symptoms of pellagra. Isoniazid inhibits incorporation of nicotinic acid into nicotinamide adenine dinucleotide and may produce pellagra. Pellagra is uncommon in the United States, reflecting the supplementation of flour with nicotinic acid.

4. **Pyridoxine (vitamin B$_6$)** is converted to pyridoxal phosphate that serves an important role in metabolism as a coenzyme for the conversion of tryptophan to serotonin and methionine to cysteine.

    a. **Symptoms of Deficiency**. Pyridoxine deficiency is uncommon, and when present is associated with deficiencies of other vitamins, and if seen is more likely to be seen in the elderly, patients with alcoholism, and in patients who are severely malnourished.

    b. **Drug Interactions**. Isoniazid and hydralazine act as potent inhibitors of pyridoxal kinase, thus preventing synthesis of the active coenzyme form of the vitamin (administration of pyridoxine decreases the incidence of neurologic side effects associated with the administration of these drugs).

5. **Pantothenic acid** is converted to coenzyme A, which serves as a cofactor for enzyme-catalyzed reactions that are important in the oxidative metabolism of carbohydrates, gluconeogenesis, and the synthesis and degradation of fatty acids. Pantothenic acid deficiency in humans is rare, reflecting the ubiquitous presence of this vitamin in ordinary foods as well as its production by intestinal bacteria.

6. **Biotin** functions as a coenzyme for enzyme-catalyzed carboxylation reactions and fatty acid synthesis. Seborrheic dermatitis of infancy is most likely a form of biotin deficiency.

7. **Cyanocobalamin (cobalamin, vitamin B_{12})** is a generic designation to describe several cobalt-containing compounds (cobalamins). Dietary vitamin B_{12} in the presence of hydrogen ions in the stomach is released from proteins.

   a. **Causes of Deficiency**. Gastric achlorhydria and decreased gastric secretion of intrinsic factor are the most likely causes of vitamin B_{12} deficiency in adults. Surgical resection or disease of the ileum predictably interferes with the absorption of vitamin B_{12}. Nitrous oxide irreversibly oxidizes the cobalt atom of vitamin B_{12} such that the activity of two vitamin B_{12}–dependent enzymes, methionine synthetase and thymidylate synthetase, are decreased.

   b. **Diagnosis of Deficiency**. The plasma concentration of vitamin B_{12} (cobalamin) is less than 200 pg/mL when there is a deficiency state. Measurements of gastric acidity may provide indirect evidence of a defect in gastric parietal cell function, whereas the Schilling test (radioactivity in the urine measured after oral administration of labeled vitamin B_{12}) can be used to quantitate ileal absorption of vitamin B_{12}.

   c. **Symptoms of Deficiency**. Deficiency of vitamin B_{12} results in defective synthesis of DNA (symptoms of vitamin B_{12} deficiency manifest most often in the hematopoietic and nervous systems). Clinically, the earliest sign of vitamin B_{12} deficiency is megaloblastic (pernicious) anemia (may be so severe that cardiac failure occurs). Encephalopathy is a well-recognized complication of vitamin B_{12} deficiency manifesting as myelopathy, optic neuropathy, and peripheral neuropathy, either alone or in any combination. Folic acid therapy corrects the hematopoietic, but not nervous system, effects produced by vitamin B_{12} deficiency.

  d. **Treatment of Deficiency**. In the patient with neurologic changes, leukopenia, or thrombocytopenia, treatment must be aggressive with intramuscular administration of vitamin B_{12} and oral administration of folic acid. Neurologic damage after pernicious anemia develops that is not reversed after 12 to 18 months of therapy is likely to be permanent.

8. **Folic acid** is transported and stored as 5-methylhydrofolate after absorption from the small intestine. Conversion to the metabolically active form, tetrahydrofolate, is dependent on the activity of vitamin B_{12}. Virtually all foods contain folic acid, but protracted cooking can destroy up to 90% of the vitamin.

  a. **Causes of Deficiency**. Alcoholism is the most common cause of folic acid deficiency, with decreases in the plasma concentrations of folic acid manifesting within 24 to 48 hours of continuous alcohol ingestion. Drugs that inhibit dihydrofolate reductase (methotrexate, trimethoprim) or interfere with absorption and storage of folic acid in tissues (phenytoin) may cause folic acid deficiency.

  b. **Symptoms of Deficiency**. Megaloblastic anemia is the most common manifestation of folic acid deficiency. This anemia cannot be distinguished from that caused by a deficiency of vitamin B_{12} but is confirmed by the presence of a folic acid concentration in the plasma of less than 4 ng/mL.

  c. **Treatment of Deficiency**. Folic acid is available as an oral preparation alone or in combination with other vitamins and either an oral preparation or as a parenteral injection. In the presence of megaloblastic anemia because of folic acid deficiency, the administration of the vitamin is associated with a decrease in the plasma concentration of iron within 48 hours, reflecting new erythropoiesis.

  d. **Leucovorin** (citrovorum factor) is a metabolically active, reduced form of folic acid. After treatment with folic acid antagonists, such as methotrexate, patients may receive leucovorin (rescue therapy), which serves as a source of tetrahydrofolate that cannot be formed due to drug-induced inhibition of dihydrofolate reductase.

9. **Ascorbic Acid (Vitamin C)**. Ascorbic acid acts as a coenzyme and is important in a number of biochemical reactions, mostly involving oxidation (synthesis of

collagen, carnitine, and corticosteroids). Despite contrary claims, controlled studies do not support the efficacy of even large doses of ascorbic acid in treating viral respiratory tract infections. A risk of large doses of ascorbic acid is the formation of kidney stones resulting from the excessive secretion of oxalate.

a. **Symptoms of Deficiency.** Humans, in contrast to many other mammals, are unable to synthesize ascorbic acid, emphasizing the need for dietary sources of the vitamin to prevent scurvy (gingivitis, rupture of the capillaries with formation of numerous petechiae, failure of wounds to heal). Scurvy is encountered among the elderly, alcoholics, and drug addicts. Patients receiving TPN should receive supplemental ascorbic acid.

C. **Fat-soluble vitamins** (A, D, E, and K) are absorbed from the gastrointestinal tract and any condition that causes malabsorption of fat, such as obstructive jaundice, may result in deficiency of one or all these vitamins (Fig. 36-2).

1. **Vitamin A (retinol, retinoic acid)** is important in the function of the retina, integrity of mucosal and epithelial surfaces, bone development and growth, reproduction, and embryonic development. Sufficient vitamin A is stored in the liver of well-nourished persons to satisfy requirements for several months.

   a. **Symptoms of Deficiency.** The most recognizable manifestation of vitamin A deficiency is night

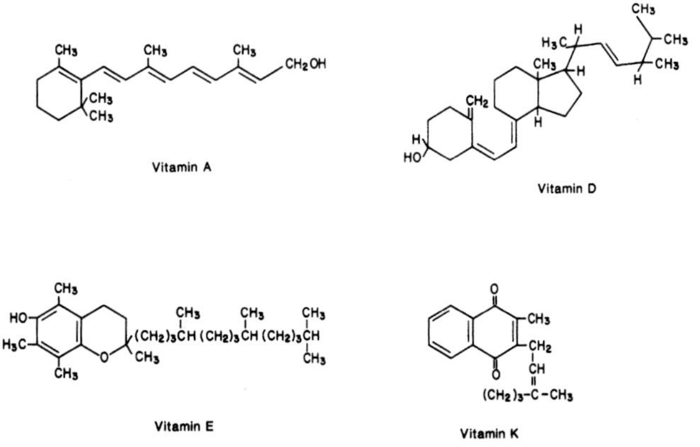

FIGURE 36-2 Chemical structure of fat-soluble vitamins.

blindness (nyctalopia), which occurs only when the depletion is severe. Pulmonary infections are increased as mucous secretion from bronchial epithelium is decreased because the epithelial cells undergo gelatinization.

b. **Hypervitaminosis A** is the toxic syndrome that results from excessive ingestion of vitamin A, particularly in children. Early signs and symptoms of vitamin A intoxication include irritability, vomiting, and dermatitis. Intracranial pressure may be increased, and neurologic symptoms, including papilledema, may mimic those of a brain tumor (pseudotumor cerebri).

2. **Vitamin D's (calciferol)** primary function is to maintain calcium and phosphorous homeostasis.

a. **Symptoms of Deficiency.** A deficiency of vitamin D results in decreased plasma concentrations of calcium and phosphate ions, with the subsequent stimulation of parathyroid hormone secretion.

b. **Hypervitaminosis D** manifests as hypercalcemia, skeletal muscle weakness, fatigue, headache, and vomiting. Early impairment of renal function from hypercalcemia manifests as polyuria, polydipsia, proteinuria, and decreased urine-concentrating ability.

3. **Vitamin E (α-tocopherol)** is not a single molecule but rather a group of fat-soluble substances occurring in plants. There is little persuasive evidence that vitamin E is nutritionally significant in humans. An important chemical feature of the tocopherols is that they are antioxidants (prevents oxidation of essential cellular constituents or prevents the formation of toxic oxidation products).

4. **Vitamin K** is a lipid-soluble dietary compound that is essential for the biosynthesis of several factors required for normal blood clotting.

a. **Mechanism of Action.** Vitamin K functions as an essential cofactor for the hepatic microsomal enzyme that converts glutamic acid residues to γ-carboxyglutamic acid residues in factors II (prothrombin), VII, IX, and X. The γ-carboxyglutamic acid residues make it possible for these coagulation factors to bind calcium ions and attach to phospholipid surfaces, leading to clot formation. Vitamin K activity is assessed by monitoring the prothrombin time.

b. **Clinical Uses**. Vitamin K is administered to treat its deficiency and attendant decrease in plasma concentrations of prothrombin and related clotting factors. Vitamin K replacement therapy is not effective when severe hepatocellular disease is responsible for the decreased production of clotting factors.

c. **Phytonadione** (vitamin K_1) is the preferred drug to treat hypoprothrombinemia. A frequent indication for phytonadione is to reverse the effects of oral anticoagulants.

d. **Menadione** has the same actions and uses as phytonadione and does not require the presence of bile salts for their systemic absorption after oral administration (important when malabsorption of vitamin K is due to biliary obstruction).

VII. **Dietary Supplements. Dietary supplements (vitamins, minerals, herbs, amino acids, enzymes) are products ingested orally and intended to supplement the diet with nutrients thought to improve health. These products are not subject to U.S. Food and Drug Administration (FDA) approval because they are considered nutrients (do not undergo scientific testing to prove efficacy and plants and parts of plants are not patent-eligible) although they cannot be promoted specifically for treatment, prevention, or cure of disease.**

A. **Adverse Effects and Drug Interactions** (Tables 36-4 and 36-5). The most serious side effects associated with these substances include cardiovascular instability, bleeding tendency particularly in conjunction with other anticoagulants such as warfarin, and delayed awakening from anesthesia.

1. Ephedra (ma huang) is a common ingredient in herbal weight-loss products, stimulants, decongestants, and bronchodilators (active moiety in ephedra is ephedrine). The FDA banned sales of dietary supplements containing ephedra in April 2004.

2. Ginseng may cause tachycardia or systemic hypertension particularly in combinations with other cardiac stimulant drugs. In addition, ginseng may decrease the anticoagulant effects of warfarin.

3. St. John's wort that is alleged to be a natural antidepressant has been shown to inhibit serotonin, dopamine, and norepinephrine reuptake and thus present the possibility of interactions with monoamine oxidase inhibitors and other serotoninergic drugs.

Table 36-4

Suggested Uses, Potential Toxicities, and Drug Interactions of Dietary Supplements and Herbal Remedies

	Suggested Uses	Potential Toxicity	Drug Interactions
Black cohosh	Menopausal symptoms	Gastrointestinal discomfort	
Chaste tree berries	Premenstrual symptoms	Pruritus	Dopamine-receptor antagonists
Cranberry	Urinary tract infections	Nephrolithiasis	
Dong quai	Menopausal symptoms	Rash	Warfarin
Echinacea	Upper respiratory infections	Hypersensitivity reactions	
		Hepatic inflammation	
Evening primrose	Eczema	Nausea	Antiepileptic drugs
	Irritable bowel syndrome	Vomiting	
	Premenstrual symptoms	Diarrhea	
	Rheumatoid arthritis	Flatulence	
Feverfew	Prevent migraine	Hypersensitivity reactions	Warfarin
	Arthritis	Inhibits platelet activity	
	Allergies		
Garlic	Hypertension	Gastrointestinal discomfort	Warfarin
	Hypertriglyceridemia	Hemorrhage	
	Hypercholesterolemia		

(continued)

Table 36-4

Suggested Uses, Potential Toxicities, and Drug Interactions of Dietary Supplements and Herbal Remedies *(continued)*

	Suggested Uses	Potential Toxicity	Drug Interactions
Ginger	Motion sickness Vertigo		Warfarin
Ginkgo biloba	Dementia Claudication Tinnitus	Gastrointestinal discomfort Headache Dizziness Bleeding Seizures	Warfarin
Ginseng	Fatigue Diabetes	Tachycardia Hypertension	Warfarin
Goldenseal	Laxative	Hypertension Edema	
Kava-kava	Anxiety	Rash Sedation Liver toxicity	Benzodiazepines Alcohol Anesthetic drugs

Table 36-4

Suggested Uses, Potential Toxicities, and Drug Interactions of Dietary Supplements and Herbal Remedies *(continued)*

	Suggested Uses	Potential Toxicity	Drug Interactions
Kola nut	Fatigue	Irritability Insomnia	Stimulants
Licorice	Gastric ulcers	Hypertension Gastrointestinal discomfort	
Saw palmetto	Prostatic hyperplasia	Headache Insomnia Dizziness	Digoxin Oral contraceptives
St. John's wort	Depression Anxiety	Gastrointestinal discomfort	Serotonin antagonists Anesthetic drugs Benzodiazepines
Valerian	Insomnia	Headaches	Anesthetic drugs Antiepileptic drugs

Table 36-5

Suggested Uses, Potential Toxicities, and Drug Interactions of Nonherbal Dietary Supplements

	Suggested Uses	Potential Toxicity	Drug Interactions
Coenzyme Q10	Congestive heart failure Hypertension	Dyspepsia Nausea Diarrhea	Warfarin
Glucosamine	Osteoarthritis	Gastrointestinal discomfort	Warfarin
Melatonin	Insomnia Jet lag	Fatigue Sedation	
S-adenosylmethionine	Osteoarthritis Depression	Nausea Gastrointestinal discomfort	Tricyclic antidepressants

CHAPTER 37

Normal Endocrine Function

I. **Normal Endocrine Function.** Patients may present with an endocrinopathy requiring surgery or more commonly have an endocrine abnormality, which complicates surgical and anesthetic management. Management of endocrinopathies includes hormone replacement and medical or surgical reduction of hormone levels produced by tumors.

II. **Mechanism of Hormone Action.** Hormones bind to membrane and nuclear receptors to trigger selective and diverse cellular responses.

III. **Hypothalamus and Pituitary Gland.** Hormones designated as hypothalamic-releasing or hypothalamic-inhibitory hormones originate in the hypothalamus and control secretions from the anterior pituitary (Table 37-1). The pituitary gland lies in the sella turcica at the base of the brain and is connected to the hypothalamus by the pituitary stalk. Physiologically, the gland is outside the blood–brain barrier and is divided into the anterior pituitary (adenohypophysis) and posterior pituitary (neurohypophysis). The anterior pituitary synthesizes, stores, and secretes six tropic hormones. The posterior pituitary stores and secretes two hormones—arginine vasopressin, formerly designated antidiuretic hormone (ADH), and oxytocin (Table 37-2).

   A. **Anterior Pituitary** (see Table 37-2)

   1. **Growth hormone (somatotropin; GH)** stimulates growth of all tissues in the body (linear bone growth) and evokes intense metabolic effects (protein synthesis, mobilization of fatty acids, antagonism of insulin action, sodium and water retention; Fig. 37-1).

      a. Releasing (GH-releasing hormone) and inhibitory (somatostatin) hormones, physiologic events (perioperative anxiety), and medications regulate GH secretion (Table 37-3).

613

Table 37-1

Hypothalamic Hormones

Hormone	Target Anterior Pituitary Hormone
Human growth hormone–releasing hormone	HGH
Human growth hormone–inhibiting hormone (somatostatin)	HGH, prolactin, TSH
Prolactin-releasing factor	Prolactin
Prolactin-inhibiting factor	Prolactin
Luteinizing hormone–releasing hormone	LH, FSH
Corticotropin-releasing hormone	ACTH, β-lipotropins, endorphins
Thyrotropin-releasing hormone	TSH

ACTH, adrenocorticotrophic hormone; FSH, follicle-stimulating hormone; HGH, human growth hormone; LH, luteinizing hormone; TSH, thyroid-stimulating hormone.

  b. Large doses of corticosteroids suppress secretion of GH (inhibitory effects on growth observed in children receiving high doses of corticosteroids).

2. **Prolactin** promotes the growth and development of the breast in preparation for breast-feeding (Table 37-4). Preoperative anxiety also increases plasma concentrations of prolactin.

3. **Gonadotropins** (luteinizing hormone and follicle-stimulating hormone) are responsible for pubertal maturation and secretion of steroid sex hormones by the gonads of either sex.

4. **Adrenocorticotrophic hormone (ACTH)** regulates secretions of the adrenal cortex, especially cortisol. Secretion of ACTH responds dramatically to stress under the control of corticotropin-releasing hormone from the hypothalamus, as well as a negative feedback mechanism from the circulating plasma concentration of cortisol (Table 37-5).

  a. In the absence of ACTH, the adrenal cortex undergoes atrophy, but the zona glomerulosa, which secretes aldosterone, is least affected (hypophysectomy has minimal effects on electrolyte balance because of the continued release of aldosterone from the adrenal cortex).

  b. Chronic administration of corticosteroids suppresses corticotropin-releasing hormone and leads to atrophy

Table 37-2		
Pituitary Hormones		
Hormone	**Cell Type**	**Principal Action**
Anterior pituitary		
Human growth hormone (HGH, somatotropin)	Somatotropes	Accelerates body growth; insulin antagonism
Prolactin	Lactotropes	Stimulates secretion of milk and maternal behavior, inhibits ovulation
Luteinizing hormone (LH)	Gonadotropes	Stimulates ovulation in females and testosterone secretion in males
Follicle-stimulating hormone (FSH)	Gonadotropes	Stimulates ovarian follicle growth in females and spermatogenesis in males
Adrenocorticotrophic hormone (ACTH)	Corticotropes	Stimulates adrenal cortex secretion and growth; steroid production
Thyroid-stimulating hormone (TSH)	Thyrotropes	Stimulates thyroid secretion and growth
β-Lipoprotein	Corticotropes	Precursor of endorphins
Posterior pituitary		
Arginine vasopressin	Supraoptic nuclei	Promotes water retention and regulates plasma osmolarity
Oxytocin	Paraventricular nuclei	Causes ejection of milk and uterine contraction

the hypothalamic-pituitary axis. Several months may be required for recovery of this axis after removal of the suppressive influence. In such patients, stressful events during the perioperative period might evoke life-threatening hypotension.

c. It is a common practice to administer supplemental exogenous corticosteroids (based on the magnitude of stress) to patients considered at risk for suppression of the hypothalamic-pituitary axis

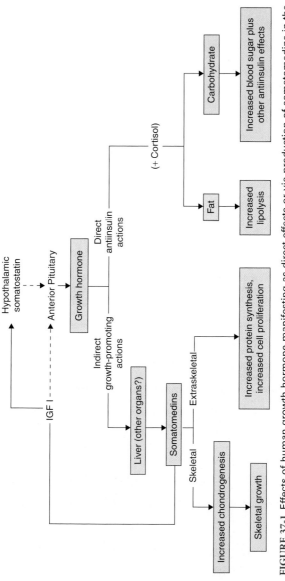

FIGURE 37-1 Effects of human growth hormone manifesting as direct effects or via production of somatomedins in the liver. (From Ganong WF. *Review of Medical Physiology*. 21st ed. New York, NY: Lange Medical Books/McGraw Hill; 2003, with permission.)

Table 37-3

Regulation of Growth Hormone Secretion

Stimulation	Inhibition
GH-releasing hormone	GH-inhibiting hormone (somatostatin)
Stress	Insulin-like growth factor 1 (IGF-1)
Physiologic sleep	Pregnancy
Hypoglycemia	Hyperglycemia
Free fatty acid decrease	Free fatty acid increase
Amino acid increase	Cortisol
Fasting	Obesity
Estrogens	
Dopamine	
α-Adrenergic agonists	

GH, growth hormone.

(little evidence, however, that supplemental corticosteroids in excess of normal daily physiologic secretion are necessary or beneficial intra- or postoperatively).
5. **Thyroid-stimulating hormone (TSH)** accelerates all the steps in the formation of thyroid hormones and causes proteolysis of thyroglobulin in the follicles of thyroid cells to release thyroid hormones into the circulation.
   a. Secretion of TSH from the anterior pituitary is under the control of thyrotropin-releasing hormone from

Table 37-4

Regulation of Prolactin Secretion

Stimulation	Inhibition
Prolactin-releasing factor	Prolactin-inhibiting factor
Pregnancy	Prolactin
Suckling	Dopamine
Stress	L-dopa
Physiologic sleep	
Metoclopramide	
Cimetidine	
Opioids	
α-Methyldopa	

Table 37-5

Regulation of Adrenocorticotrophic Hormone Secretion

Stimulation	Inhibition
Corticotropin-releasing hormone	ACTH
Cortisol decrease	Cortisol increase
Stress	Opioids
Sleep–wake transition	Etomidate
Hypoglycemia	Suppression of the hypothalamic-pituitary axis
Trauma	
α-Adrenergic agonists	
β-Adrenergic antagonists	

ACTH, adrenocorticotropic hormone.

the hypothalamus as well as a negative feedback mechanism, depending on the concentrations of thyroid hormones circulating in plasma.

  b. Hypothyroidism with increased plasma concentrations of TSH indicates a primary defect at the thyroid gland (primary hypothyroidism) and an attempt by the anterior pituitary to stimulate hormonal output by releasing TSH.

  c. A defect at the hypothalamus or anterior pituitary is indicated by low concentrations of both TSH and thyroid hormones circulating in plasma (secondary hypothyroidism).

B. **Posterior Pituitary**. Arginine vasopressin (AVP) and oxytocin are transported in secretory granules along axons from corresponding nuclei in the hypothalamus to the posterior pituitary for subsequent release in response to appropriate stimuli.

  1. **Arginine Vasopressin**. The physiologic functions of AVP include vasoconstriction, water retention, and corticotropin secretion. Decreases in blood volume, increased plasma osmolality, and decreased arterial pressure stimulate AVP release (Table 37-6).

  a. Administration of morphine, or other opioids, in the absence of painful stimulation does not evoke the release of AVP.

  b. Decreases in urine output and fluid retention previously attributed to release of AVP during positive pressure ventilation of the lungs are more

Table 37-6

Regulation of Arginine Vasopressin Secretion

Stimulation	Inhibition
Increased plasma osmolarity	Decreased plasma osmolarity
Hypovolemia	
Pain	Ethanol
Hypotension	α-Adrenergic agonists
Hyperthermia	Cortisol
Stress	Hypothermia
Nausea and vomiting	
Opioids (?)	

      likely the result of changes in cardiac filling pressures that impair the release of atrial natriuretic hormone.

    c. Destruction of neurons in or near the supraoptic and paraventricular nuclei of the hypothalamus from pituitary surgery, trauma, cerebral ischemia, or malignancy may decrease vasopressin release to cause central diabetes insipidus (diabetes insipidus from lack of vasopressin release during pituitary surgery is usually transient).

    d. Unnecessary or excessive secretion of AVP with subsequent retention of water and dilutional hyponatremia may result from head injuries, intracranial tumors, meningitis, or pulmonary infections.

  2. **Oxytocin**. Breast suckling and cervical and vaginal dilation stimulate oxytocin secretion. Large amounts of oxytocin cause sustained uterine contraction as necessary for postpartum hemostasis. Oxytocin has only 0.5% to 1.0% the antidiuretic activity of AVP and can be released abruptly and independently of AVP.

IV. **Thyroid Gland**. The thyroid gland maintains optimal metabolism for normal tissue function. The principal hormonal secretions of the thyroid gland are thyroxine (T_4) and triiodothyronine (T_3) (Fig. 37-2). In addition to thyroid hormones, the thyroid gland secretes calcitonin, which is important for calcium ion use. The thyroid hormones increase oxygen consumption in nearly all tissues, except for the brain (consistent with the minimal changes in anesthetic

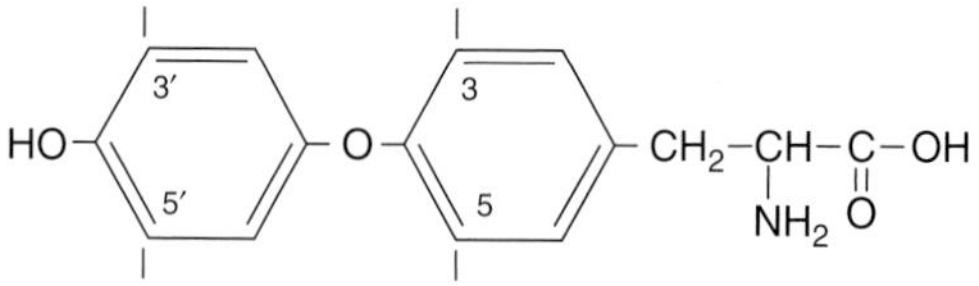

3,5,3′,5′,- Tetraiodothyronine (thyroxine, T_4)

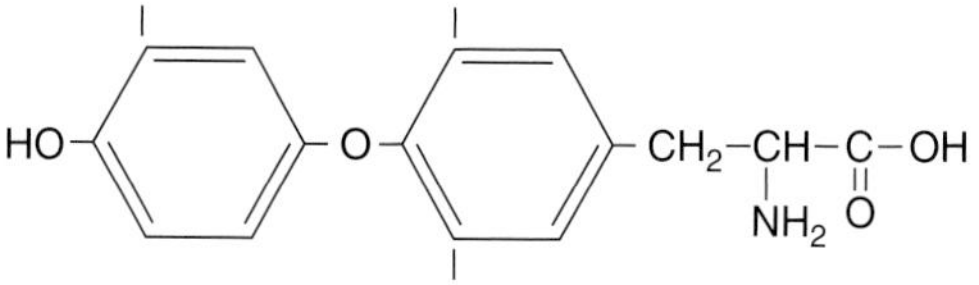

3,5,3′,- Triiodothyronine (T_3)

FIGURE 37-2 Chemical structure of thyroid hormones.

requirements [MAC]) that accompany hyperthyroidism or hypothyroidism. Cardiovascular changes are often the earliest clinical manifestations of abnormal thyroid hormone levels. Thyroid hormones are stored in combination with thyroglobulin. Stimulation of proteases by TSH results in cleavage of hormones from thyroglobulin and their release into the systemic circulation.

A. **Mechanism of Action**
   1. When thyroid hormones enter cells, T_3 binds to nuclear receptors. T_4 also binds to these receptors but not as avidly and rather serves principally as a prohormone for T_3.
   2. Sympathomimetic effects that accompany thyroid hormone stimulation most likely reflect a greater number and sensitivity of β-adrenergic receptors to release of T_4 and T_3. When thyroid hormones accelerate metabolism, tissues vasodilate and blood flow delivers necessary oxygen and carries away metabolites and heat. As a result, cardiac output often increases but systemic blood pressure is unchanged because peripheral vasodilation offsets the impact of more blood flow.
   3. Excess protein catabolism associated with greater secretion of thyroid hormones is the mechanism behind skeletal muscle weakness characteristic of hyperthyroidism.
   4. The fine muscle tremor that accompanies hyperthyroidism stems from the sensitivity of neuronal synapses in the area of the spinal cord that controls skeletal muscle tone.

B. **Calcitonin**
   1. Is a polypeptide hormone secreted by the thyroid gland that decreases the concentration of calcium ions in plasma by weakening the activity of osteoclasts and strengthening the activity of osteoblasts.
   2. A total thyroidectomy and subsequent absence of calcitonin does not measurably influence the plasma concentration of calcium because of the predominance of parathyroid hormone.

V. **Parathyroid Glands**
   A. The four parathyroid glands secrete parathyroid hormone (PTH) that regulates plasma concentration of calcium ions. Secretion of PTH is inversely related to plasma ionized calcium concentration. Small declines in the plasma concentration of calcium ions stimulate the release of PTH.
   B. PTH exerts its effect on target cells in bones, renal tubules, and the gastrointestinal tract by stimulating the formation of cyclic adenosine monophosphate (cAMP). Because a portion of cAMP synthesized in the kidneys escapes into the urine, its assay serves as a measure of parathyroid gland activity.

VI. **Adrenal Cortex. The adrenal cortex secretes three major classes of corticosteroids: mineralocorticoids, glucocorticoids, and androgens. More than 30 different corticosteroids have been isolated from the adrenal cortex, but only two are important: aldosterone, a mineralocorticoid, and cortisol, the principal glucocorticoid (Table 37-7).**
   A. **Mineralocorticoids: Aldosterone** accounts for approximately 95% of the mineralocorticoid activity of the corticosteroids.
      1. **Physiologic Effects.** Aldosterone sustains extracellular fluid volume by conserving sodium and by maintaining a normal plasma concentration of potassium. Sodium ions are absorbed at the same time potassium ions are secreted by the lining of epithelial cells of the distal renal tubules and collecting ducts.
         a. If aldosterone secretion is excessive, extracellular fluid volume, cardiac output, and systemic blood pressure increase.
         b. If plasma concentration of potassium decreases approximately 50% after excess secretion of aldosterone, skeletal muscle weakens or paralysis occurs because nerve and muscle membranes are hyperpolarized and the transmission of action potentials is prevented.

Table 37-7

Physiologic Effects of Endogenous Corticosteroids (mg)

	Daily Secretion	Sodium Retention[a]	Glucocorticoid Effect[a]	Antiinflammatory Effect[a]
Aldosterone	0.125	3,000	0.3	Insignificant
Desoxycorticosterone	—	100	0	0
Cortisol	20	1	1	1
Corticosterone	Minimal	15	0.35	0.3
Cortisone	Minimal	0.8	0.8	0.8

[a]Relative to cortisol.

2. **Mechanism of Action**. Aldosterone diffuses to the interior of renal tubular epithelial cells, where it induces DNA to form messenger RNA (mRNA) necessary for the transport of sodium and potassium ions. It takes as long as 30 minutes before the new mRNA appears and approximately 45 minutes before the rate of sodium ion transport begins to increase.

3. **Regulation of Secretion**. The most important stimulus for aldosterone secretion is an accumulation of potassium in the plasma.

B. **Glucocorticoids: Cortisol**. At least 95% of the glucocorticoid activity results from the secretion of cortisol.

   1. **Physiologic Effects**
      a. Cortisol (a) increases gluconeogenesis, (b) breaks down protein, (c) mobilizes fatty acid, and (d) has antiinflammatory effects.
      b. Cortisol may improve cardiac function by increasing the number or responsiveness of β-adrenergic receptors.
      c. Cortisol promotes the normal responsiveness of arterioles to the constrictive action of catecholamines.

   2. **Developmental Changes**. Plasma concentrations of cortisol increase progressively during the last trimester of pregnancy to reach a peak plasma concentration at term, so that systems critical for survival are mature for the onset of extrauterine life (pulmonary surfactant, maturation of various enzyme systems in the liver, and the expression of the enzyme necessary for the synthesis of epinephrine from norepinephrine).

   3. **Gluconeogenesis**. Cortisol stimulates gluconeogenesis by the liver as much as 10-fold. Amino acids are mobilized from extrahepatic sites and transferred to the liver for conversion to glucose.

   4. **Protein Catabolism**. Cortisol breaks down protein stores in nearly all cells except hepatocytes, to mobilize amino acids for gluconeogenesis. When excesses of cortisol are sustained, skeletal muscle weakness may become pronounced.

   5. **Antiinflammatory Effects**. In large amounts, cortisol stabilizes lysosomal membranes, stops migration of leukocytes into the inflamed area, and lessens capillary permeability to prevent loss of plasma into tissues. This effect of cortisol is useful for disease states with inflammation such as rheumatoid arthritis and acute glomerulonephritis. In the treatment of allergic reactions, cortisol prevents the life-threatening inflammatory responses of allergic reactions such as

laryngeal edema (does not alter the antigen–antibody interaction or histamine release associated with allergic reactions).

6. **Mechanism of Action**. Cortisol stimulates DNA-dependent synthesis of mRNA in the nuclei of responsive cells, leading to the synthesis of necessary enzymes.

7. **Regulation of Secretion**
   a. The most important stimulus for the secretion of cortisol (13 to 20 mg daily) is the release of ACTH from the anterior pituitary (see Table 37-5).
   b. The secretion of ACTH in the anterior pituitary is determined by two hypothalamic neurohormones, diurnal release of corticotropin-releasing hormone and AVP that act synergistically.
   c. Cortisol is secreted and released by the adrenal cortex at a basal rate of approximately 20 to 30 mg daily. In response to maximal stressful stimuli (sepsis, burns), the output of cortisol is increased to approximately 150 mg daily.

8. **Effect of Anesthesia and Surgery**
   a. Perioperative stress stimulates hormonal secretion of ACTH and cortisol. This response may be diminished by surgeries such as laparoscopy and blunted by choice of anesthetic technique.
   b. Plasma cortisol concentrations typically return to normal levels within 24 hours postoperatively but may remain elevated for as long as 72 hours, depending on the severity of the surgical trauma (disturbances in the circadian rhythm may be associated with postoperative fatigue and debility).
   c. In addition to surgical trauma, the choice of anesthetic drugs and techniques may influence the hypothalamic-pituitary-adrenal response. Large doses of opioids may attenuate the cortisol response to surgical stimulation. Volatile anesthetics do not suppress the stress-induced endocrine response as much. Etomidate, unique among drugs administered to induce anesthesia, inhibits cortisol synthesis even in the absence of surgical stimulation.

VII. **Reproductive Glands. In both sexes, the reproductive glands (testes and ovaries) produce germ cells and steroid sex hormones.**
   A. **Testes**
      1. The testes secrete male sex hormones, which are collectively designated *androgens*.

2. Testosterone, the most potent and abundant of the androgens, develops and maintains male sex characteristics.

3. Testosterone production continues throughout life, although the amount produced lessens gradually after 40 years (at age 80 years, it is approximately one-fifth the peak value).

4. The adrenal cortex also secretes androgens, but the effects of these hormones are usually inconsequential unless a hormone-secreting tumor develops.

B. **Ovaries**

1. **Estrogens** give the female sexual characteristics.

2. Progesterone prepares the uterus for pregnancy and the breasts for lactation.

C. **Menstruation**

1. The overall duration of a normal menstrual cycle is 21 to 35 days and consists of three phases designated as follicular, ovulatory, and luteal.

2. The increase in body temperature (approximately 0.5°C) that accompanies ovulation most likely reflects a thermogenic effect of progesterone.

D. **Pregnancy**

1. During pregnancy, the placenta forms large amounts of estrogens, progesterone, chorionic gonadotropin, and chorionic somatomammotropin.

2. The first key hormone of pregnancy, chorionic gonadotropin, which can be detected in the maternal plasma within 9 days after conception, is the basis for pregnancy tests. After approximately 12 weeks, the placenta secretes sufficient amounts of progesterone and estrogens to maintain pregnancy and the corpus luteum involutes.

3. Greater concentrations of progesterone in plasma and associated sedative effects during pregnancy may explain why requirements for volatile anesthetics lessen in gravid animals. In animals, anesthetic requirements return to nonpregnant values within 5 days postpartum, whereas the plasma concentration of progesterone remains increased, suggesting that the decrease in MAC cannot be attributed entirely to progesterone.

4. The parturient with asthma may experience unpredictable changes in airway reactivity.

E. **Menopause**. Between the ages of 45 and 55 years, a woman's ovaries gradually become unresponsive to the stimulatory effects of luteinizing hormone (LH) and follicle-stimulating hormone, and the sexual cycles disappear. Sensations of warmth spreading from the trunk to the face (hot flashes) coincide with surges of LH secretion and are prevented by exogenous administration of estrogens.

VIII. **Pancreas.** The exocrine pancreas secretes digestive substances into the duodenum. The islets of Langerhans are organized endocrine cells that secrete four hormones (insulin, glucagon, somatostatin, and pancreatic polypeptide) into the systemic circulation. The pancreas contains 1 to 2 million islets (each islet receives a generous blood supply, which unlike any other endocrine organ, drains into the portal vein).

  A. **Insulin** is a 51-amino acid peptide hormone synthesized in the β cells of the islets of Langerhans (Fig. 37-3). The amount of insulin secreted daily is equivalent to approximately 40 units. In the systemic circulation, insulin has an elimination half-time of approximately 5 minutes, with greater than 80% degraded in the liver and kidneys.

    1. **Regulation of Secretion**

      a. The principal control of insulin secretion is via a negative feedback effect of the blood glucose concentration in the pancreas (Table 37-8). Virtually no insulin is secreted by the pancreas when the blood glucose

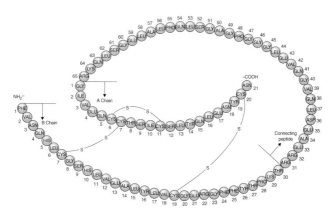

FIGURE 37-3 Proinsulin, which is converted to insulin by proteolytic cleavage of amino acids 31, 32, 64, 65, and the connecting peptide. (From Larner J. Insulin and oral hypoglycemic drugs: glucagon. In: Gilman AG, Goodman LS, Rall TW, et al, eds. *The Pharmacological Basis of Therapeutics.* 7th ed. New York, NY: Macmillan; 1985, with permission.)

Table 37-8	
Regulation of Insulin Secretion	
Stimulation	**Inhibition**
Hyperglycemia	Hypoglycemia
β-Adrenergic agonists	β-Adrenergic antagonists
Acetylcholine	α-Adrenergic agonists
Glucagon	Somatostatin
	Diazoxide
	Thiazide diuretics
	Volatile anesthetics
	Insulin

concentrations are less than 50 mg/dL, and maximum stimulation for release of insulin is at concentrations greater than 300 mg/dL (Fig. 37-4).

b. Oral glucose is more effective than glucose administered intravenously in evoking the release of insulin, suggesting the presence of an anticipatory signal from the gastrointestinal tract to the pancreas.

c. Glycosuria is more likely after intravenous rather than oral glucose administration.

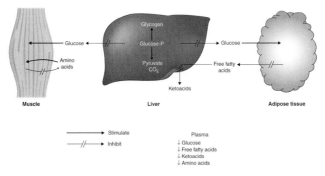

FIGURE 37-4 Insulin stimulates tissue uptake of glucose and amino acids, whereas release of fatty acids is inhibited. As a result, the plasma concentrations of glucose, free fatty acids, amino acids, and ketoacids decrease. (From Berne RM, Levy MN, Koeppen BM, et al. *Physiology.* 5th ed. St. Louis, MO: Mosby; 2004, with permission.)

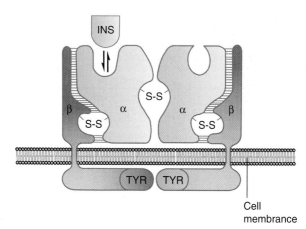

FIGURE 37-5 Schematic depiction of the insulin receptor consisting of two α and two β subunits joined by disulfide bonds (-S-S-). Insulin (INS) attaches to the α subunits, which triggers autophosphorylation of the tyrosine kinase (TYR) portions of the β subunits inside the cell and the resultant effects of insulin. (From Ganong WF. *Review of Medical Physiology.* 21st ed. New York, NY: Lange Medical Books/ McGraw Hill; 2003, with permission.)

2. **Physiologic Effects**
   a. Insulin receptor expression is highest in tissues, which regulate glucose, lipid, and protein metabolism (adipose, skeletal muscle, and liver) via insulin (Fig. 37-5).
   b. Insulin promotes the use of carbohydrates for energy while depressing the use of fats and amino acids.
   c. Insulin facilitates glucose uptake and storage in the liver through effects on specific enzymes (induces the activity of glucokinase).
   d. Resting skeletal muscles are almost impermeable to glucose except in the presence of insulin. Exercise increases the permeability of skeletal muscle membranes to glucose, perhaps because insulin is released from within the skeletal muscle itself or its vasculature.
   e. Brain cells are unique in that the permeability of their membranes to glucose does not depend on the presence of insulin. This characteristic is crucial because brain cells use only glucose for energy, thus the importance of maintaining blood glucose concentrations above a critical level of approximately 50 mg/dL.

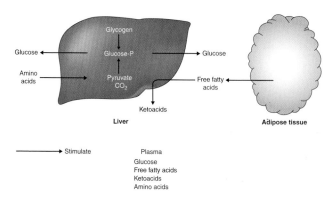

FIGURE 37-6 Glucagon stimulates tissue release of glucose, free fatty acids, and ketoacids and hepatic uptake of amino acids. (From Berne RM, Levy MN, Koeppen BM, et al. *Physiology*. 5th ed. St. Louis, MO: Mosby; 2004, with permission.)

      f. Deficiencies in insulin signaling are associated with insulin resistance.

   B. **Glucagon** is a catabolic hormone acting to mobilize glucose, fatty acids, and amino acids into the systemic circulation (Fig. 37-6). These responses are the reciprocal of the insulin effects, emphasizing that these two hormones are also reciprocally secreted (Table 37-9). The principal stimulus for secretion of glucagon is hypoglycemia. Glucagon abruptly increases the blood glucose concentration by stimulating glycogenolysis in the liver.

Table 37-9

Regulation of Glucagon Secretion

Stimulation	Inhibition
Hypoglycemia	Hyperglycemia
Stress	Somatostatin
Sepsis	Insulin
Trauma	Free fatty acids
β-Adrenergic agonists	α-Adrenergic agonists
Acetylcholine	
Cortisol	

CHAPTER 38

Drugs that Alter Glucose Regulation

I. **Diabetes Mellitus (Table 38-1)**

   A. Diabetes mellitus is classified by the underlying disease etiology (type 1 vs. type 2) rather than by age-of-onset (juvenile-onset vs. adult-onset diabetes) or treatment modality (insulin-dependent vs. non–insulin-dependent diabetes).

      1. The insulin deficiency in type 1 diabetes is the result of autoimmune-mediated destruction of pancreatic beta cells.

      2. Onset of type 1 diabetes is at a younger age than onset of type 2 diabetes, and sensitivity to insulin is normal. In contrast, the peripheral insulin resistance of type 2 diabetes is often coupled with a failure to secrete insulin because of pancreatic β cell dysfunction.

      3. Oral hypoglycemic drugs are alternatives to exogenous administration of insulin to patients with type 2 diabetes.

   B. Low plasma concentrations of insulin, although inadequate to prevent hyperglycemia, may block lipolysis. This differential effect of insulin explains why hyperglycemia can exist without the presence of ketone bodies. Ketosis can be reliably prevented by continuously providing all diabetic patients with glucose and insulin. Prevention is uniquely important in the perioperative period when nutritional intake is altered.

   C. The goals of therapy for patients with diabetes mellitus include preventing the adverse consequences of hypoglycemia and hyperglycemia, avoiding weight gain, and reducing microvascular and macrovascular complications.

      1. Symptoms often resolve when blood glucose levels are less than 200 mg/dL.

      2. Long-term metabolic control of diabetes is best monitored by measurement of glycosylated hemoglobin (HbA_{1c}), which reflects glucose control over the previous 2 to 3 months. In general, HbA_{1c} values less than 6.0% to 7.0% are associated with fewer microvascular complications.

Table 38-1

Etiologic Classification of Diabetes Mellitus

Type 1 diabetes mellitus (absolute insulin deficiency from pancreatic β cell destruction)
Type 2 diabetes mellitus (insulin resistance vs. insulin deficiency)
Gestational diabetes mellitus
Exocrine pancreas disease (pancreatitis, pancreatectomy, cystic fibrosis, hemochromatosis)
Drug-induced (glucocorticoids, thiazides, thyroid hormone, β-adrenergic agonists)
Endocrinopathies (acromegaly, Cushing syndrome, glucagonoma)
Genetic defects in pancreatic β cell function
Genetic defects in insulin action (resistance)
Infections (congenital rubella, cytomegalovirus)
Uncommon immune-mediated diabetes ("stiff man" syndrome, anti-insulin receptor antibodies)

II. **Insulin.** Patients with type 1 diabetes mellitus do not produce insulin and require insulin therapy to survive. Insulin is prescribed for patients with type 2 diabetes mellitus if treatment with oral glucose regulators fails. Insulin therapy mirrors the normal pattern of insulin secretion (pulsatile secretion that occurs under basal conditions and in response to meals) with basal supplementation and by short-acting insulin taken before food absorption. Insulin receptors become fully saturated with low concentrations of insulin (continuous infusion of insulin, 1 to 2 units per hour, has the same or even greater pharmacologic effect than a single larger intravenous [IV] dose that is cleared rapidly from the circulation).

   A. **Pharmacokinetics**

   1. Insulin is metabolized in the kidneys and liver (~50% of the insulin that reaches the liver through its portal vein is metabolized in a single passage). Nevertheless, renal dysfunction alters the disappearance rate of circulating insulin to a greater extent than does hepatic disease (unexpected prolonged effects of insulin are found in patients with renal disease, reflecting impairment of both its metabolism and excretion by the kidneys).

   2. Despite rapid clearance from plasma after IV injection of insulin, the pharmacologic effect lasts for 30 to 60 minutes

because insulin is tightly bound to tissue receptors. Insulin administered subcutaneously releases slowly into the circulation to produce a sustained biologic effect.

3. Insulin is secreted into the portal venous system in the basal state at a rate of approximately 1 unit per hour. After food intake, the rate of insulin secretion increases 5- to 10-fold. The total daily secretion of insulin is approximately 40 units.

4. The sympathetic and parasympathetic nervous systems innervate the insulin-producing islet cells to influence the basal rate of hormone secretion as well as the response to stress (α-adrenergic stimulation decreases and β-adrenergic or parasympathetic nervous system stimulation increases the basal secretion of insulin).

5. The insulin response to glucose is greater after oral ingestion than after IV infusion because glucose-dependent insulinotropic polypeptide is released after oral ingestion of glucose and the pancreatic β cell response is augmented.

6. To gain adequate glycemic control in type 1 diabetes, at least two daily subcutaneous injections of intermediate- or long-acting insulin combined with rapid-acting insulin are nearly always required.

B. **Insulin Preparations and Delivery** (Table 38-2). Human insulin manufactured using recombinant DNA technology has replaced insulin extracted from beef and pork pancreas. Allergy or immunoresistance to animal insulins is no longer a serious problem.

1. The basic principle of replacement is to provide a slow, long-acting, continuous supply of insulin (neutral protamine Hagedorn [NPH] insulin, insulin glargine, insulin detemir, or insulin degludec) that mimics the nocturnal and interprandial basal secretion of normal pancreatic β cells.

2. Commercially prepared insulin is bioassayed, and its physiologic activity (potency), based on the ability to decrease blood glucose concentration, is expressed in units. The potency of insulin is 22 to 26 U/mg.

   a. Insulin U-100 (100 U/mL) is the most commonly used commercial preparation. The total daily exogenous dose of insulin for treatment of type 1 diabetes mellitus is usually in the range of 0.5 to 1 U/kg/day.

   b. This insulin requirement may be increased dramatically by stress associated with sepsis or trauma.

3. Continuous subcutaneous insulin infusion (CSII) through an external pump delivers basal insulin (0.01 to

Table 38-2

Classification of Insulin Preparations

Insulin Preparation	Hours after Subcutaneous Administration		
	Onset	Peak	Duration (h)
Very rapid–acting			
Lispro	5–15 min	45–75 min	2–4
Insulin aspart	5–15 min	45–75 min	2–4
Glulisine	5–15 min	45–75 min	2–4
Rapid-acting			
Regular	30 min	2–4 h	6–8
Intermediate-acting			
NPH	2 h	4–12 h	18–28
Long-acting			
Detemir	2 h	3–9 h	6–24
Glargine	1.5 h	None	20–>24
Ultra long-acting			
Degludec	2 h	None	>40

NPH, neutral protamine Hagedorn.

0.015 U/kg/hour) and bolus doses before meals. With this system, nocturnal versus daytime basal requirements can be accommodated, infusions can be altered during exercise, and doses can be calculated via algorithms of previous glucose values and insulin delivery. Short-acting insulin (regular) and ultra rapid-acting insulins (lispro, aspart, and glulisine) are the only preparations used for CSII delivery pumps.

C. **Lispro** is a short-acting insulin analogue that more closely parallels physiologic insulin secretion and needs (injected subcutaneously begins to act within 15 minutes, the peak effect is reached in 45 to 75 minutes, and the duration of action is only 2 to 4 hours).

1. Lispro injected just before eating provides a postprandial plasma insulin concentration profile similar to that of normal insulin secretion.

2. An important benefit of lispro is a decrease in postprandial hyperglycemia and less risk of hypoglycemia, which may follow injection of regular insulin.

D. **Insulin aspart and glulisine** are synthetic rapid-acting analogues with a profile of action and therapeutic benefits similar to those of lispro.

E. **Regular insulin (crystalline zinc insulin)** is a fast-acting preparation and is the only form of insulin that can be administered IV as well as subcutaneously.

   1. Administration of regular insulin is preferred for treating the abrupt onset of hyperglycemia or the appearance of ketoacidosis.

   2. In the perioperative period, regular insulin is administered as a single IV injection (1 to 5 units) or as a continuous infusion (0.5 to 2.0 units per hour) to treat metabolic derangements associated with diabetes mellitus.

F. **Neutral protamine Hagedorn** is an intermediate-acting preparation whose absorption from its subcutaneous injection site is delayed because the insulin is conjugated with protamine.

G. **Side Effects**

   1. **Hypoglycemia** is the most serious side effect of insulin therapy (patients are vulnerable to hypoglycemia if they receive exogenous insulin in the absence of carbohydrate intake, as during a perioperative period, especially before surgery).

      a. The first symptoms of hypoglycemia are the compensatory effects of increased epinephrine secretion: diaphoresis, tachycardia, and hypertension. Symptoms of hypoglycemia involving the central nervous system (CNS) include mental confusion progressing to seizures and coma.

      b. The diagnosis of hypoglycemia during general anesthesia is difficult because anesthetic drugs mask the classic signs of sympathetic nervous system stimulation (signs of sympathetic nervous system stimulation are likely to be confused with responses evoked by painful surgical stimulation in an anesthetized patient).

      c. Severe hypoglycemia is treated with 50 to 100 mL of 50% glucose solution administered IV (alternatively, glucagon, 0.5 to 1.0 mg IV).

   2. **Allergic Reactions**

      a. Use of human insulin preparations has eliminated the problem of systemic allergic reactions that could result from administration of animal-derived insulins.

      b. Local allergic reactions are characterized by an erythematous indurated area that develops at the site of insulin injection (cause is likely to be noninsulin materials in the insulin preparation).

c. Chronic exposure to low doses of protamine in NPH insulin may stimulate the production of antibodies against protamine. Patients remain asymptomatic until a large dose of protamine is administered IV to antagonize the anticoagulant effects of heparin.

3. **Lipodystrophy** results when fat atrophies at the site of subcutaneous injection of insulin.

4. **Insulin Resistance**
   a. Patients requiring greater than 100 units of exogenous insulin daily are in a state of insulin resistance.
   b. Acute insulin resistance is associated with trauma from infection or surgery.

5. **Drug Interactions**
   a. There are hormones administered as drugs that counter the hypoglycemic effect of insulin (adrenocorticotrophic hormone, estrogens, glucagon).
   b. Epinephrine inhibits the secretion of insulin and stimulates glycogenolysis.
   c. Certain antibiotics (tetracycline or chloramphenicol), salicylates, and phenylbutazone increase the duration of action of insulin and may have a direct hypoglycemic effect.
   d. The hypoglycemic effect of insulin may be potentiated by monoamine oxidase inhibitors.

III. **Oral Glucose Regulators. Oral drugs with different mechanisms of action are available for controlling plasma glucose concentrations in patients with type 2 diabetes mellitus (Table 38-3). None of these drugs will adequately control hyperglycemia indefinitely (use of combinations of oral drugs from the onset of treatment may be indicated). The effect on HbA$_{1c}$ is similar for these drugs.**

A. **Metformin** is an oral biguanide that is often prescribed as the initial agent to prevent hyperglycemia in patients with type 2 diabetes. Metformin decreases blood glucose concentrations in both the fasting and postprandial state and rarely causes hypoglycemia. Metformin should not be prescribed for patients with lactic acidosis, acute kidney injury, gastrointestinal intolerance, or acute hepatic disease.

   1. **Pharmacokinetics**. In contrast to sulfonylureas, metformin is not bound to plasma proteins and does not undergo metabolism. It is eliminated by the kidneys, with 90% of an oral dose excreted in approximately

Table 38-3

Oral Drugs for Treatment of Type 2 Diabetes Mellitus

Sulfonylureas (stimulate insulin secretion; hypoglycemia a risk)
Glyburide
Glipizide
Glimepiride
Gliclazide
Tolbutamide
Tolazamide
Chlorpropamide
Acetohexamide
Meglitinides (stimulate insulin secretion; hypoglycemia a risk)
Repaglinide
Nateglinide
Biguanides (inhibit glucose production by the liver; hypoglycemia not a risk)
Metformin
Thiazolidinediones (increase sensitivity to insulin for glucose uptake by skeletal muscles and adipose tissues; hypoglycemia not a risk)
Rosiglitazone
Pioglitazone
α-Glucosidase inhibitors (slow digestion and absorption of carbohydrates from the diet; hypoglycemia not a risk)
Acarbose
Miglitol

12 hours. In view of its dependence on renal clearance, metformin is prescribed with caution, if at all, to patients with renal dysfunction.

2. **Mechanism of Action**
   a. The blood glucose–lowering effect of metformin is not mediated through stimulation of endogenous insulin secretion.
   b. Metformin activates adenosine monophosphate–activated protein kinase to suppress hepatic glucose production by decreasing gluconeogenesis and glycogenolysis.

3. **Side Effects**
   a. The most common side effects of metformin are anorexia, nausea, and diarrhea, which are dose related. In contrast to sulfonylureas, metformin does not cause hypoglycemia.

b. **Lactic acidosis** is a possible side effect associated with metformin that has been described during the intraoperative period (some have recommended discontinuing metformin 48 hours or longer before elective operations). If metformin cannot be discontinued before surgery, the patient is monitored for the development of lactic acidosis (arterial blood gases and pH, serum lactate concentrations, renal function) in the perioperative period.

B. **Sulfonylureas** are capable of lowering blood glucose concentrations even to hypoglycemic levels. The sulfonylureas have no effect on and no role in the treatment of patients with type 1 diabetes mellitus. Although sulfonylureas are derivatives of sulfonamides, they have no antibacterial actions. These drugs should not be administered to patients with known allergy to sulfa drugs.

1. **Mechanism of Action**. Sulfonylureas inhibit adenosine triphosphate–sensitive potassium ion channels (now known as the *sulfonylurea receptor-1*) on pancreatic β cells. As a result, there is an influx of calcium and stimulation of exocytosis (release) of insulin storage granules.

2. **Pharmacokinetics**. Oral hypoglycemics are readily absorbed from the gastrointestinal tract, with the most important distinguishing features being differences in duration of action and elimination half-time (Table 38-4).

3. **Side Effects**

a. The most common severe complication of these drugs is hypoglycemia (greatest risk of hypoglycemia occurs with drugs with the longest elimination half-times).

b. Although hypoglycemia from sulfonylureas may be infrequent, it is often more prolonged and more dangerous than hypoglycemia from insulin (Table 38-5).

c. Hypoglycemia caused by sulfonylureas is treated with prolonged infusion of glucose-containing solutions.

d. Risk factors for sulfonylurea-induced hypoglycemia include (a) impaired nutrition, as in the perioperative period, (b) age older than 60 years, (c) impaired renal function, and (d) concomitant drug therapy that potentiates sulfonylureas (phenylbutazone, sulfonamide antibiotics, warfarin) or itself produces hypoglycemia (alcohol or salicylates).

Table 38-4

Classification and Pharmacokinetics of Sulfonylurea Oral Hypoglycemics

	Equivalent Daily Dose (mg)	Daily Dose Range (mg)	Doses/Day	Duration of Action (h)	Elimination Half-Time (h)[a]
Glyburide	2.5–5	2.5–20	1–2	18–24	4.6–12
Glipizide	5–10	5–40	1–2	12–24	4–7
Glimepiride	2	2–4	1	24+	5–8
Tolbutamide	1,000	500–1,000	2–3	6–12	4–8
Tolazamide	250	200–1,000	1–2	16–24	7
Acetohexamide	500	250–1,500	2	12–18	1.3–6
Chlorpropamide	100–250	100–750	1	36	30–36

[a]Approximate.

Table 38-5	
Comparison of Sulfonylurea Therapy with Insulin Therapy	
Sulfonylurea	**Insulin**
Failed initial response in 10% to 15% of patients	No maximum dose
Secondary failure rate each year among treated patients is about 10%	
Hypoglycemia may be more severe	Hypoglycemia may be more frequent
Associated cardiac complications	Lipid levels lowered
Patients may prefer oral medication	Patients may resist injections

C. **Glyburide** stimulates insulin secretion over a 24-hour period after a morning oral dose. When administration is discontinued, the drug is cleared from plasma in about 36 hours.

D. **Glipizide** stimulates insulin secretion over a 12-hour period after a morning oral dose. Relatively rapid clearance from the plasma minimizes the potential for long-lasting hypoglycemia.

E. **Tolbutamide** is the shortest acting and least potent sulfonylurea (see Table 38-4). Of all the sulfonylureas, tolbutamide probably causes the fewest side effects, although it can produce hypoglycemia and hyponatremia.

F. **Acetohexamide** differs from other sulfonylureas in that most of its hypoglycemic action comes from its principal metabolite hydroxyhexamide, which is 2.5 times as potent as the parent compound. This drug is not recommended for patients with renal disease because the kidneys excrete the active metabolite. Acetohexamide is the only sulfonylurea with uricosuric properties (uricosuric drugs increase the excretion of uric acid in the urine), making it an appropriate drug for the diabetic patient with gout.

G. **Chlorpropamide** is the longest acting sulfonylurea with a duration of action that may approach 72 hours (see Table 38-4).

  1. The maximal effect of chlorpropamide may not be apparent for 7 to 14 days, and several weeks are needed for complete elimination of the drug.

2. Because 20% of a dose is excreted unchanged, impaired renal function can lead to accumulation and an enhanced hypoglycemic effect.

3. Chlorpropamide is associated with reactions similar to those produced by disulfiram (facial flushing after ingestion of alcohol) and can cause severe hyponatremia.

H. **Meglitinides**

1. Repaglinide and the phenylalanine derivative, nateglinide, differ in structure and timing of action from sulfonylurea drugs. Although these drugs exert effects on β cells similar to those of sulfonylurea drugs, their peak effect is about 1 hour and duration of action is about 4 hours.

2. The short duration of action and activity only in the presence of glucose should decrease the risk of prolonged hypoglycemic episodes.

I. **α-Glucosidase Inhibitors**

1. Acarbose and miglitol are α-glucosidase inhibitors that decrease carbohydrate digestion and absorption of disaccharides by interfering with intestinal glucosidase activity.

2. These drugs are useful only as monotherapy when postprandial hyperglycemia is the main problem.

J. **Thiazolidinediones** act principally at skeletal muscle, liver, and adipose tissue to decrease insulin resistance and hepatic glucose production and to increase use of glucose by the liver.

1. Like metformin, thiazolidinediones act in the presence of insulin and are especially effective in obese patients.

2. The possibility of drug-induced liver dysfunction is the reason that plasma concentrations of hepatic transaminases must be measured periodically.

K. **Glucagon-like peptide-1 (GLP-1) receptor agonists** are injectable agents that bind to receptors in the pancreas, gastrointestinal tract, and brain to increase insulin secretion from β cells (glucose dependent), decrease glucagon production from α cells, and reduce gastric emptying. The risk of hypoglycemia increases when GLP-1 receptor agonists are combined with sulfonylureas.

CHAPTER 39

Drugs for the Treatment of Hypothyroidism and Hyperthyroidism

I. **Hypothyroidism.** In primary hypothyroidism, thyroid-stimulating hormone (TSH) concentrations can be used to monitor this treatment (free T_4 is an insensitive indicator and may be within the normal range when TSH is inhibited). Measurement of free T_4 is warranted in secondary hypothyroidism when TSH release is impaired.

A. **Synthetic Thyroxine (T_4: Levothyroxine).** Synthetic thyroxine (T_4) is the treatment of choice for primary hypothyroidism. In the peripheral tissues, T_4 is deiodinated to form T_3 (the active form of thyroid hormone).

B. **T_3 formulations (liothyronine)** is the levorotatory isomer of T_3 and is 2.5 to 3.0 times as potent as levothyroxine. Its rapid onset and short duration of action preclude the use of liothyronine for long-term thyroid replacement.

II. **Hyperthyroidism.** The treatments for hyperthyroidism are antithyroid drugs, radioiodine, and/or surgery. Measuring free T_3 and T_4 is necessary to assess the efficacy of treatment.

A. **Thionamides (methimazole, propylthiouracil, carbimazole)** are antithyroid drugs that inhibit the formation of thyroid hormone by inhibiting thyroid peroxidase to prevent incorporation of iodine into tyrosine residues of thyroglobulin. Antithyroid drugs are useful in the treatment of hyperthyroidism before elective thyroidectomy.

1. **Side Effects.** Granulocytopenia and agranulocytosis are serious but rare side effects that are most likely to occur in the first 3 months of therapy with an antithyroid drug. Fever or pharyngitis may be the earliest manifestation of the development of agranulocytosis. Recovery is likely if the antithyroid drug is discontinued at the first sign of this side effect.

B. **Iodine (Saturated Potassium Iodide Solutions [SSKI], Potassium Iodide-Iodine [Lugol's Solution])**

1. Iodide is the oldest available therapy for hyperthyroidism, providing a paradoxical treatment that is effective

for reasons that are not fully understood (the most important clinical effect of high doses of iodide is inhibition of the release of thyroid hormone).

2. Iodide is particularly useful in the treatment of hyperthyroidism before elective thyroidectomy. The combination of oral potassium iodide and propranolol is a recommended approach.

3. The vascularity of the thyroid gland is also decreased by iodide therapy.

C. **Radioactive iodine** is administered as the therapy of choice for Graves' hyperthyroidism.

1. Among the radioactive isotopes of iodine, ^{131}I is the most frequently administered. This isotope is rapidly and efficiently trapped by thyroid gland cells, and the subsequent emission of destructive β rays acts almost exclusively on these cells, with little or no damage to surrounding tissue.

2. It is possible to completely destroy the thyroid gland with ^{131}I within 6 to 18 weeks.

3. Most thyroid cancers except for follicular cancer accumulate little radioactive iodine. As a result, the therapeutic effectiveness of ^{131}I for treatment of thyroid cancer is limited.

CHAPTER 40

Other Endocrine Drugs

I. **Introduction.** Preparations that contain synthetic hormones identical to those secreted endogenously by endocrine glands may be administered as drugs. Typically, the clinical application of these drugs is for hormone replacement to provide a physiologic effect. Recombinant DNA technology permits the incorporation of synthetic genes that code for the synthesis of specific human hormones by bacteria, thus permitting production of pure hormones devoid of allergic properties.

II. **Corticosteroids.** The actions of corticosteroids are classified according to the potencies of these compounds to (a) evoke distal renal tubular reabsorption of sodium in exchange for potassium ions (mineralocorticoid effect) or (b) produce an antiinflammatory response (glucocorticoid effect). Naturally occurring corticosteroids are cortisol (hydrocortisone), cortisone, corticosterone, desoxycorticosterone, and aldosterone (Fig. 40-1).

A. **Structure–Activity Relationships**
1. Modifications of structure, such as introduction of a double bond in prednisolone and prednisone, have resulted in synthetic corticosteroids with more potent glucocorticoid effects than the two closely related natural hormones, cortisol and cortisone, respectively (Table 40-1).
2. At the same time, mineralocorticoid effects and the rate of hepatic metabolism of these synthetic drugs are less than those of the natural hormones.

B. **Mechanism of Action**
1. Glucocorticoids attach to cytoplasmic receptors to enhance or suppress changes in the transcription of DNA and thus the synthesis of proteins. Glucocorticoids also inhibit the secretion of cytokines via posttranslational effects.
2. Mineralocorticoid receptors are present in distal renal tubules, colon, salivary glands, and the hippocampus.

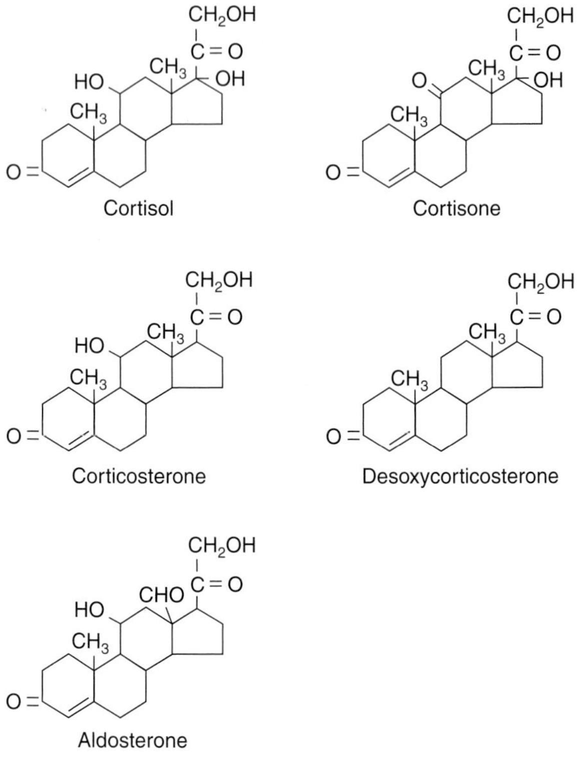

FIGURE 40-1 Endogenous corticosteroids.

Cortisol

Cortisone

Corticosterone

Desoxycorticosterone

Aldosterone

In contrast, glucocorticoids receptors are more widely distributed and do not bind aldosterone making these receptors glucocorticoid-selective.

C. **Maintenance of Homeostasis**. Permissive and protective effects of glucocorticoids are critical for the maintenance of homeostasis during severe stress.

1. **Permissive actions** of glucocorticoids occur at low physiologic steroid concentrations and serve to prepare the individual for responding to stress.

2. **Protective actions** of glucocorticoids occur when high plasma concentrations of steroids exert antiinflammatory and immunosuppressive effects. This protective

Table 40-1

Comparative Pharmacology of Endogenous and Synthetic Corticosteroids

	Antiinflammatory Potency	Sodium Retaining Potency	Equivalent Dose (mg)	Elimination Half-Time (h)	Duration of Action (h)	Route of Administration
Cortisol	1	1	20	1.5–3.0	8–12	Oral, topical, IV, IM, IA
Cortisone	0.8	0.8	25	0.5	8–36	Oral, topical, IV, IM, IA
Prednisolone	4	0.8	5	2–4	12–36	Oral, topical, IV, IM, IA
Prednisone	4	0.8	5	2–4	12–36	Oral
Methylprednisolone	5	0.5	4	2–4	12–36	Oral, topical, IV, IM, IA, epidural
Betamethasone	25	0	0.75	5	36–54	Oral, topical, IV, IM, IA
Dexamethasone	25	0	0.75	3.5–5.0	36–54	Oral, topical, IV, IM, IA
Triamcinolone	5	0	4	3.5	12–36	Oral, topical, IV, IM, epidural
Fludrocortisone	10	250	2	—	24	Oral, topical, IV, IM
Aldosterone	0	3,000				

IV, intravenous; IM, intramuscular; IA, intraarticular.

response prevents the host-defense mechanisms that are activated during stress from overshooting and damaging the organism.

D. **Pharmacokinetics**

1. Synthetic cortisol and its derivatives are effective orally (see Table 40-1).

2. Water-soluble cortisol succinate can be administered intravenously (IV) to achieve prompt increases in plasma concentrations. More prolonged effects are possible with intramuscular (IM) injection.

3. Cortisone acetate may be given orally or IM but cannot be administered IV. The acetate preparation is a slow-release preparation lasting 8 to 12 hours. After release, cortisone is converted to cortisol in the liver.

4. Corticosteroids are also promptly absorbed after topical application or aerosol administration.

III. **Synthetic Corticosteroids (see Table 40-1) (Figs. 40-1 and 40-2).**

A. **Prednisolone** is an analogue of cortisol that is available as an oral or parenteral preparation. The antiinflammatory effect of 5 mg of prednisolone is equivalent to that of 20 mg of cortisol. Cortisol and prednisone are suitable for sole replacement therapy in adrenocortical insufficiency because of the presence of glucocorticoid and mineralocorticoid effects.

B. **Prednisone** is rapidly converted to prednisolone after its absorption from the gastrointestinal tract (antiinflammatory effect and clinical uses are similar to those of prednisolone).

C. **Methylprednisolone** is the methyl derivative of prednisolone. The antiinflammatory effect of 4 mg of methylprednisolone is equivalent to that of 20 mg of cortisol. The acetate preparation administered intraarticularly has a prolonged effect.

D. **Betamethasone** is a fluorinated derivative of prednisolone. The antiinflammatory effect of 0.75 mg is equivalent to that of 20 mg of cortisol. Betamethasone lacks the mineralocorticoid properties of cortisol (not acceptable for sole replacement therapy in adrenocortical insufficiency).

E. **Dexamethasone** is a fluorinated derivative of prednisolone and an isomer of betamethasone. The antiinflammatory effect of 0.75 mg is equivalent to that of 20 mg of cortisol. This corticosteroid is commonly chosen to treat certain types of cerebral edema.

F. **Triamcinolone** is a fluorinated derivative of prednisolone. The antiinflammatory effect of 4 mg is equivalent to

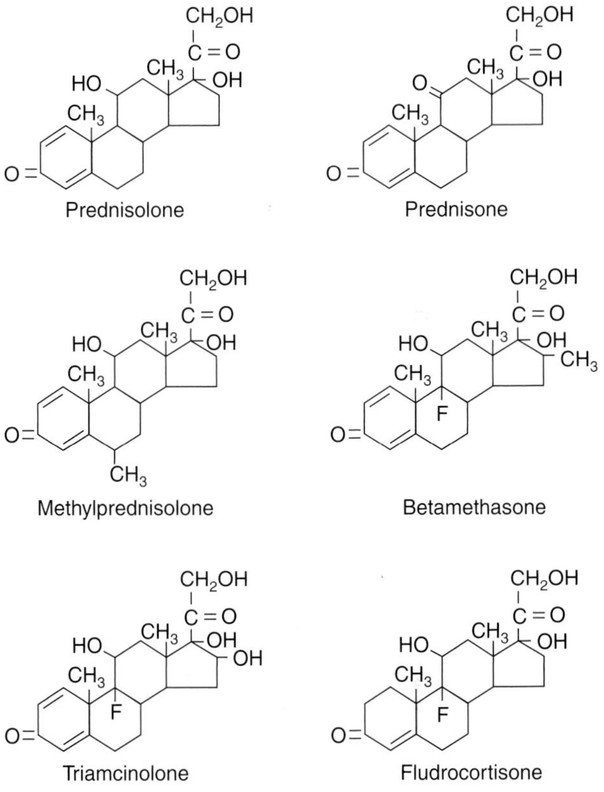

FIGURE 40-2 Synthetic corticosteroids.

that of 20 mg of cortisol. The hexacetonide preparation injected intraarticularly may provide therapeutic effects for 3 months or longer.

1. This drug is often used for epidural injections in the treatment of lumbar disk disease.

2. An unusual adverse side effect of triamcinolone is an increased incidence of skeletal muscle weakness. Anorexia rather than appetite stimulation, and sedation rather than euphoria may accompany administration of triamcinolone.

IV. Clinical Uses. The only universally accepted clinical use of corticosteroids and their synthetic derivatives is as replacement therapy for deficiency states. The safety of corticosteroids is such that it is acceptable to administer a single large dose in a life-threatening situation on the presumption that unrecognized adrenal or pituitary insufficiency may be present. Prednisolone or prednisone are recommended when an antiinflammatory effect is desired (antiinflammatory effect of corticosteroids is palliative because the underlying cause of the response remains yet suppression of the inflammatory response may be lifesaving in some situations). Masking of the symptoms of inflammation may delay diagnosis of life-threatening illness, such as peritonitis due to perforation of a peptic ulcer.

A. **Deficiency States**

1. Acute adrenal insufficiency requires electrolyte and fluid replacement as well as supplemental corticosteroids (cortisol is administered at a rate of 100 mg IV every 8 hours after an initial injection of 100 mg).

2. Management of chronic adrenal insufficiency in adults is with the daily oral administration of cortisone, 25.0 to 37.5 mg. A typical regimen is 25.0 mg in the morning and 12.5 mg in the late afternoon (mimics the normal diurnal cycle of adrenal secretion).

B. **Allergic Therapy**. Topical corticosteroids are capable of potent antiinflammatory effects and are the mainstay of allergic therapy. Unlike antihistamines that provide pharmacologic effects within 1 to 2 hours, topical corticosteroids may require 3 to 5 days of treatment to produce a therapeutic effect.

C. **Asthma** is an inflammatory disease of the lungs and inhaled glucocorticoids are often recommended as first-line therapy for controlling the symptoms.

1. Inhaled glucocorticoids have oropharyngeal side effects that include dysphonia and candidiasis.

2. Parenteral corticosteroids are important in the emergent preoperative preparation of patients with active reactive airway disease and in the treatment of intraoperative bronchospasm. Doses equivalent to 1 to 2 mg/kg of cortisol (or the equivalent dose of prednisolone) are commonly recommended. Preoperative corticosteroid administration 1 to 2 hours before induction of anesthesia is important because the beneficial effects of corticosteroids may not be fully manifest for several hours.

D. **Antiemetic Effect**
1. Dexamethasone prevents postoperative nausea and vomiting only when administered near the beginning of surgery, probably by reducing surgery-induced inflammation due to inhibition of prostaglandin synthesis.
2. Administration of higher doses (8 to 10 mg) of dexamethasone has a similar antiemetic effect to lower doses (4 to 5 mg). Dexamethasone is also effective in suppressing chemotherapy-induced nausea and vomiting.

E. **Postoperative Analgesia**
1. Glucocorticoids peripherally inhibit phospholipase enzyme that is necessary for the inflammatory chain reaction along both the cyclooxygenase and lipoxygenase pathways. As a result, glucocorticoids may be effective in decreasing postoperative pain but with a different side effect profile than nonsteroidal antiinflammatory drugs.
2. Perioperative IV dexamethasone at doses more than 0.1 mg/kg decreases acute postoperative pain and reduces opioid use, especially when administered preoperatively.

F. **Cerebral Edema**
1. Corticosteroids in large doses are of value in the reduction or prevention of vasogenic cerebral edema and the resulting increases in intracranial pressure that may accompany intracranial tumors and metastatic lesions and bacterial meningitis.
2. Dexamethasone, with minimal mineralocorticoid activity, is frequently selected to decrease cerebral edema and associated increases in intracranial pressure.
3. The administration of glucocorticoids to patients with severe head injury, cerebral infarction, and intracranial hemorrhage is not useful.

G. **Aspiration Pneumonitis**. Despite the absence of confirming evidence that corticosteroids are beneficial, it is not uncommon for the treatment of aspiration pneumonitis to include the empiric use of pharmacologic doses of these drugs.

H. **Lumbar Disk Disease**
1. An alternative to surgical treatment of lumbar disk disease is the epidural placement of corticosteroids. Corticosteroids may decrease inflammation and edema of the nerve root that has resulted from compression.
2. A common regimen is epidural injection of 25 to 50 mg of triamcinolone, or 40 to 80 mg of methylprednisolone, in a solution containing lidocaine at or near the interspace corresponding to the distribution of pain.

3. Injection of triamcinolone, 80 mg, into the lumbar epidural space of patients with lumbar disk disease results in acute suppression of plasma concentrations of adrenocorticotropic hormone (ACTH) and cortisol. Exogenous corticosteroid coverage during this potentially vulnerable (<1 month) period should be considered in patients undergoing major stress

I. **Immunosuppression.** In organ transplantation, high doses of corticosteroids are often administered at the time of surgery to produce immunosuppression and decrease the risk of rejection of the newly transplanted organ.

J. **Arthritis**
1. The criterion for initiating corticosteroid therapy in patients with rheumatoid arthritis is rapid control of symptomatic flares and progressive disability despite maximal medical therapy. Corticosteroids are administered in the smallest dose possible that provides significant but not complete symptomatic relief.
2. Painless destruction of the joint is a risk of this treatment.

K. **Collagen Diseases.** Manifestations of collagen diseases (except for scleroderma) are decreased and longevity is improved by corticosteroid therapy.

L. **Ocular Inflammation**
1. Corticosteroids are used to suppress ocular inflammation (uveitis and iritis) and thus preserve sight (instillation of corticosteroids into the conjunctival sac results in therapeutic concentrations in the aqueous humor).
2. Topical and intraocular corticosteroid therapy often increases intraocular pressure and is associated with cataractogenesis.
3. Corticosteroids are not recommended in herpes simplex infections (dendritic keratitis) of the eye.
4. Topical corticosteroids should not be used for treatment of ocular abrasions because delayed healing and infections may occur.

M. **Cutaneous Disorders.** Topical administration of corticosteroids is frequently effective in the treatment of skin diseases. Systemic absorption is also occasionally enhanced to the degree that suppression of the hypothalamic-pituitary-adrenal (HPA) axis occurs or manifestations of Cushing syndrome appear.

N. **Postintubation Laryngeal Edema**
1. Treatment of postintubation laryngeal edema may include administration of corticosteroids, such as dexamethasone,

0.1 to 0.2 mg/kg IV (efficacy of corticosteroids for treatment of this condition has not been confirmed).

2. Dexamethasone, 0.6 mg/kg orally is an effective treatment for children with mild croup.

O. **Myasthenia Gravis**. Corticosteroids are usually reserved for patients with myasthenia gravis who are unresponsive to medical or surgical therapy. These drugs seem to be most effective after thymectomy.

P. **Respiratory Distress Syndrome**
1. Administration of corticosteroids at least 24 hours before delivery decreases the incidence and severity of respiratory distress syndrome in neonates born between 24 and 36 weeks' gestation.
2. Dexamethasone administered for prolonged periods (42 days) improves pulmonary and neurodevelopmental outcome of low-birth-weight infants at risk for bronchopulmonary dysplasia.

Q. **Cardiac Arrest**. Administration of glucocorticoids (along with vasopressin and epinephrine) during a cardiac arrest may improve survival and is associated with better neurologic outcomes.

V. **Side Effects.** The side effects of chronic corticosteroid therapy include (a) suppression of the HPA axis, (b) electrolyte and metabolic changes, (c) osteoporosis, (d) peptic ulcer disease, (e) skeletal muscle myopathy, (f) central nervous system dysfunction, (g) peripheral blood changes, and (h) inhibition of normal growth. Systemic corticosteroids used for short periods of time (<7 days) even at high doses are unlikely to cause adverse side effects. Inhaled corticosteroids are unlikely to evoke adverse systemic effects.

VI. **Corticosteroid Supplementation in the Perioperative Period**
A. Corticosteroid supplementation should be increased whenever the patient being treated for chronic hypoadrenocorticism undergoes a surgical procedure (based on the concern that these patients are susceptible to cardiovascular collapse because they cannot release additional endogenous cortisol in response to the stress of surgery).
B. More controversial is the management of patients who may manifest suppression of the HPA axis because of current or previous administration of corticosteroids for treatment of a disease unrelated to pituitary or adrenal function.
C. There is no advantage in supraphysiologic glucocorticoid prophylaxis during surgical stress, and replacement doses of

cortisol equivalent to the daily unstressed cortisol production rate are sufficient to allow homeostatic mechanisms to function during surgery.

D. Patients taking greater than 20 mg per day of prednisone or its equivalent for more than 3 weeks have a suppressed HPA axis. Patients taking less than 5 mg per day of prednisone or its equivalent can be considered not to have suppression of their HPA axis. Patients taking 5 to 20 mg per day of prednisone or its equivalent for more than 3 weeks may or may not have suppression of the HPA axis.

1. For patients with a suppressed HPA axis (patients taking >20 mg prednisone per day for more than 3 weeks), glucocorticoid supplementation should consider the stress of surgery. For minor surgical stress (inguinal hernia repair), the daily cortisol secretion rate and static plasma cortisol measurements suggest that a glucocorticoid replacement dose of 25 mg of hydrocortisone or 5 mg of methylprednisolone is sufficient.

2. For moderate surgical stress (nonlaparoscopic cholecystectomy, colon resection, total hip replacement), cortisol production rates suggest the glucocorticoid requirement is about 50 to 75 mg daily of hydrocortisone for 1 to 2 days.

3. For major surgical stress (pancreatoduodenectomy, esophagectomy, cardiopulmonary bypass), the glucocorticoid dose should be 100 to 150 mg of hydrocortisone daily for 2 to 3 days.

4. Maintenance doses of a corticosteroid should be administered with the preoperative medication on the day of surgery. There is no objective evidence to support increasing the maintenance dose of corticosteroid preoperatively.

VII **Electrolyte and Metabolic Changes and Weight Gain**

A. Hypokalemic metabolic alkalosis reflects mineralocorticoid effects of corticosteroids on distal renal tubules, leading to enhanced absorption of sodium and loss of potassium. Edema and weight gain accompany this corticosteroid effect.

B. Corticosteroids inhibit the use of glucose in peripheral tissues and promote hepatic gluconeogenesis (hyperglycemia can usually be managed with diet, insulin, or both).

C. **Osteoporosis**

1. Osteoporosis, vertebral compression fractures, and rib fractures are common and serious complications of

corticosteroid therapy (an indication for withdrawal of corticosteroid therapy).

2. The presence of osteoporosis could predispose patients to fractures during positioning in the operating room.

D. **Skeletal muscle myopathy** characterized by weakness of the proximal musculature is occasionally observed in patients taking large doses of corticosteroids.

E. **Central Nervous System Dysfunction**. Corticosteroid therapy is associated with an increased incidence of neuroses and psychoses. Cataracts develop in almost all patients who receive prednisone, 20 mg daily, or its equivalent for 4 years.

F. **Peripheral Blood Changes**. A single dose of cortisol decreases by almost 70%—the number of circulating lymphocytes, and by more than 90%—the number of circulating monocytes in 4 to 6 hours. This acute lymphocytopenia most likely reflects sequestration from the blood rather than destruction of cells.

VIII. **Drugs that Regulate Calcium. Parathyroid hormone (PTH) regulates extracellular calcium concentration through action on the bone, kidney, and intestine. PTH secretion is activated by hypocalcemia and elevated phosphorous levels. The net effect of PTH is to increase extracellular calcium.**

A. **Hypercalcemia** can be categorized as either parathyroid dependent or non–parathyroid dependent. Hypercalcemia from parathyroid disease is associated with bone loss and osteoporosis. Management of hypercalcemia includes IV fluids, bisphosphonates, calcitonin, and glucocorticoids.

B. **Hypocalcemia**

1. The most common setting for symptomatic hypocalcemia is within 12 to 24 hours after surgery, particularly after total or subtotal thyroidectomy or four-gland parathyroid exploration or removal.

2. Hypocalcemia can cause neuromuscular irritability, arrhythmias, congestive heart failure (decreased myocardial contractility), and hypotension.

3. Acute, severe hypocalcemia (total serum calcium levels <7.5 mg/dL, normal albumin) is a medical emergency associated with death from laryngeal spasm or grand mal seizures. IV calcium is indicated for acute symptomatic hypocalcemia (10% calcium gluconate contains less elemental calcium than calcium chloride but is less likely to cause tissue necrosis during an extravasation).

IX. **Drugs for Pituitary Function—Anterior Pituitary Hormones.**
Perioperative replacement of anterior pituitary hormones
may be necessary for patients receiving exogenous hormones
because of a prior hypophysectomy. Cortisol must be provided
continuously, whereas thyroid hormones have such a long
elimination half-time that they can be omitted for several days
without adverse effects.
   A. **Growth Hormone**
      1. Recombinant growth hormone is administered subcuta-
         neously and daily to treat growth hormone deficiency.
      2. **Octreotide**
         a. Octreotide is a somatostatin analogue that inhibits
            the release of growth hormone, making it an effective
            treatment for patients with acromegaly.
         b. Because somatostatin analogues inhibit the secretion
            of insulin, decreased glucose tolerance and even overt
            hyperglycemia might be expected during treatment
            with octreotide.
         c. Octreotide may be a lifesaving treatment in patients
            experiencing an acute carcinoid crisis although bolus
            injection of this somatostatin analog may be accom-
            panied by bradycardia and second- and third-degree
            heart block.
   B. **Gonadotropins** are used most often for the treatment of
      infertility and cryptorchism. Induction of ovulation can be
      stimulated in females who are infertile because of pituitary
      insufficiency.
   C. **Adrenocorticotrophic Hormone**
      1. The physiologic and pharmacologic effects of ACTH re-
         sult from this hormone's stimulation of secretion of corti-
         costeroids from the adrenal cortex, principally cortisol.
      2. An important clinical use of ACTH is as a diagnostic aid
         in patients with suspected adrenal insufficiency.
      3. Treatment of disease states with ACTH is not physiolog-
         ically equivalent to administration of a specific hormone
         because ACTH exposes the tissues to a mixture of gluco-
         corticoids, mineralocorticoids, and androgens.

X. **Melatonin is the principal substance secreted by the pineal
gland. The mammalian pineal gland is a neuroendocrine
transducer. Photic information from the retina is transmitted to the pineal gland through the suprachiasmatic nucleus
of the hypothalamus and the sympathetic nervous system.**
   A. In humans, the circadian rhythm for the release of melato-
      nin from the pineal gland is closely synchronized with the
      habitual hours of sleep.

B. It is unclear whether the beneficial effect of exogenous melatonin on symptoms of jet lag are due to a hypnotic effect or resynchronization of the circadian rhythm.

XI. **Posterior Pituitary Hormones.** Arginine vasopressin (AVP) (also known as *antidiuretic hormone* [ADH]) and oxytocin are the two principal hormones secreted by the posterior pituitary.

A. **Arginine vasopressin** is the exogenous preparation of AVP used to treat a variety of clinical conditions.

1. **Diabetes insipidus** is due to inadequate secretion of vasopressin by the posterior pituitary. Excessive water loss and hypernatremia via polyuria follow.

    a. Neurotrauma and surgery of the pituitary and hypothalamus, cerebral ischemia, or cerebral malignancy can cause diabetes insipidus.

    b. Nephrogenic diabetes insipidus resulting from an inability of the renal tubules to respond to adequate amounts of centrally produced AVP does not respond to exogenous administration of the hormone or its congeners.

2. **Hypotension during Anesthesia**

    a. Perioperative administration of angiotensin-converting enzyme inhibitors (ACE-I) or angiotensin II receptor blockers (ARB) inhibits the renin-angiotensin system and can cause refractory hypotension after administration of anesthesia.

    b. Vasopressin may be effective to treat hypotension from anaphylaxis and from severe catecholamine deficiency after resection of a pheochromocytoma.

3. **Septic Shock**

    a. Excess generation of nitric oxide, activation of the renin-angiotensin system, and low plasma concentrations of vasopressin contribute to progressive loss of vascular tone during sepsis.

    b. Vasopressin infusion (0.01 to 0.04 unit per minute) can reverse systemic hypotension and decrease norepinephrine dosages in catecholamine-resistant septic shock.

4. **Refractory Cardiac Arrest**

    a. Vasopressin is an alternative to epinephrine for vasopressor therapy during cardiopulmonary resuscitation (vasopressin 40 units IV was similar to epinephrine 1 mg IV for management of ventricular fibrillation and pulseless electrical activity).

    b. Vasopressin is more effective than epinephrine for management of asystole and the treatment of refractory cardiac arrest.

    c. The American Heart Association recommends that vasopressin, as a one-time only dose of 40 units IV be considered instead of epinephrine 1 mg IV every 3 to 5 minutes for patients who are being treated for cardiac arrest.

   5. **Esophageal Varices.** Vasopressin may serve as an adjunct in the control of bleeding esophageal varices and during abdominal surgery in patients with cirrhosis and portal hypertension. Infusion of 20 units over 5 minutes results in marked decreases in hepatic blood flow lasting about 30 minutes.

   6. **Side Effects**

    a. Vasoconstriction and increased systemic blood pressure occur only with doses of vasopressin that are much larger than those administered for the treatment of diabetes insipidus.

    b. Vasopressin, even in small doses, may produce selective vasoconstriction of the coronary arteries, with decreases in coronary blood flow manifesting as angina pectoris, electrocardiographic evidence of myocardial ischemia, and, in some instances, myocardial infarction.

B. **Oxytocin** stimulates uterine muscle and is administered to induce labor at term, reduce and prevent uterine atony, and decrease hemorrhage in the postpartum or postabortion period. All preparations of oxytocin used clinically are synthetic, and their potency is described in units. Synthetic preparations are identical to the hormone normally released from the posterior pituitary but devoid of contamination by other polypeptide hormones and proteins found in natural proteins.

   1. **Side Effects.** High and bolus doses of oxytocin are more likely to decrease systolic and diastolic blood pressure via a direct relaxant effect on vascular smooth muscles.

XII. **Drugs for Reproductive Regulation—Ovarian Hormones**

A. Estrogens are effective in treating unpleasant side effects of menopause. There is no evidence that administration of estrogens delays the progression of atherosclerosis in postmenopausal women. There is evidence that administration of estrogen to postmenopausal women prevents bone loss (protects against osteoporosis) and also prevents vertebral and femoral bone fractures. The presence of receptors for estrogen increases the likelihood of a palliative response to estrogen therapy in women with metastatic breast cancer.

An important use of estrogens is in combination with progestins as oral contraceptives.

1. **Route of Administration**. The absorption of most estrogens and their derivatives from the gastrointestinal tract is prompt and nearly complete.

2. **Side Effects**. The most frequent unpleasant symptom associated with the use of estrogens is nausea. There is an increased incidence of vaginal and cervical adenocarcinoma in daughters of mothers treated with diethylstilbestrol or other synthetic estrogens during the first trimester of pregnancy.

B. **Antiestrogens**. Clomiphene and tamoxifen act as antiestrogens by binding to estrogen receptors. Tamoxifen is administered for a period of 5 years to postmenopausal women with breast cancer that was characterized by estrogen-responsive receptors (tamoxifen has estrogenic activity in some tissues, including bone).

C. **Tissue-Specific Estrogens**. Raloxifene is a nonsteroidal benzothiophene that acts as a selective estrogen-receptor modulator (preserves the beneficial effects of estrogens including prevention of bone loss and lowering of plasma cholesterol concentrations without any associated effects on reproductive organs).

D. **Progesterone**. Orally active derivatives of progesterone are designated *progestins* (often combined with estrogens as oral contraceptives). Dysfunctional uterine bleeding can be treated with small doses of a progestin for a few days, with the goal being induction of progesterone-withdrawal bleeding.

E. **Antiprogestins** inhibit the hormonal effects of progesterone and are the most effective and safest means of medical abortion.

1. Mifepristone (RU 486) can be administered in a single oral dose to produce termination of pregnancy.

2. Mifepristone has been used as a postcoital contraceptive within 72 hours of unprotected intercourse.

F. **Oral contraceptives** are most often a combination of an estrogen and a progestin (inhibits ovulation, presumably by preventing release of follicle-stimulating hormone by estrogen and luteinizing hormone by progesterone).

1. **Side Effects**

a. Estrogens in combined preparations are believed to be responsible for most, if not all of the side effects of oral contraceptives (increased incidence of thromboembolism).

b. Nausea, vomiting, weight gain, and breast discomfort resembling early pregnancy are attributed to the estrogen component of oral contraceptives.

c. The incidence of myocardial infarction and stroke is increased in patients who chronically take oral contraceptives.

d. Oral contraceptives containing high doses of estrogen may produce alterations in the glucose tolerance curves of patients with preclinical diabetes mellitus.

e. An increased incidence of breast cancer in patients taking oral contraceptives has not been documented.

f. Depression of mood and fatigue have been attributed to the progestin component of oral contraceptives.

XIII. Androgens are administered to males to stimulate the development and maintenance of secondary sexual characteristics. The most common indication of androgen therapy in females is palliative management of metastatic breast cancer. Androgens enhance erythropoiesis by stimulation of renal production of erythropoietin. The efficacy of anabolic steroids to improve athletic performance is not documented and is condemned on ethical grounds. Certain androgens may be useful in the treatment of hereditary angioedema.

A. **Route of Administration**. About 99% of testosterone circulating in the plasma is bound to sex hormone–binding globulin. Testosterone administered orally is readily absorbed but is metabolized so extensively by the liver that therapeutic effects do not occur. Testosterone can also be delivered via patch and gels.

B. **Side Effects**
   1. Dose-related cholestatic hepatitis and jaundice are particularly likely to accompany androgen therapy for palliation in neoplastic disease.
   2. Androgens increase the potency of coumarin anticoagulants and the likelihood of spontaneous hemorrhage.

C. **Danazol**. The low androgenic activity of danazol makes it the preferred androgen for treatment of hereditary angioedema. As with other androgens, danazol therapy has been associated with abnormal liver function tests and jaundice.

D. **Finasteride** is administered orally (5 mg once daily) for the treatment of benign prostatic hyperplasia. Treatment of male pattern baldness, hirsutism, and acne may represent other potentially useful applications for finasteride.

CHAPTER 41

Antimicrobials, Antiseptics, Disinfectants, and Management of Perioperative Infection

I. **Introduction.** The excessive use of antimicrobials (antibiotics) for the treatment of conditions for which these drugs provide little or no benefit (upper respiratory tract infections, bronchitis) has contributed to the emergence of bacterial resistance. It is estimated that 21% of all prescriptions written for antimicrobials are for ambulatory patients seen in physicians' offices with the diagnosis of upper respiratory tract infections or bronchitis. Misuse of antibiotics in the general population is in contrast to the proven benefit of antibiotic prophylaxis for selected surgical procedures, which has been part of a national initiative to enhance compliance (Table 41-1).

II. **Antimicrobial Prophylaxis for Surgical Procedures**

A. The use of antimicrobial prophylaxis in surgery involves a risk-to-benefit evaluation, which varies depending on the nature of the operative procedure (Table 41-2). It is recommended that prophylactic antimicrobials should be administered intravenously (IV) within 1 hour of surgical incision (tissue concentration of the antibiotic should exceed the minimum inhibitory concentration [MIC] associated with the procedure and or patient characteristics from the time of incision to the completion of surgery). Antibiotic treatment is not recommended for longer than 24 hours.

B. Because of their wide therapeutic index and low incidence of side effects, cephalosporins (most often a cost-effective first-generation cephalosporin such as cefazolin) are the antimicrobials of choice for surgical procedures in which skin flora and normal flora of the gastrointestinal and genitourinary tracts are the most likely pathogens.

1. Cephalosporins can safely be used in patients with an allergic reaction to penicillins that is not

659

Table 41-1

SCIP Measures Related to Prevention of Surgical Site Infection

SCIP-Inf 1: Prophylactic antibiotic received within 1 h prior to surgical incision

SCIP-Inf 2: Prophylactic antibiotic selection for surgical patients

SCIP-Inf 3: Prophylactic antibiotics discontinued within 24 h after surgery end time (48 h for cardiac patients)

SCIP-Inf 4: Cardiac surgery patients with controlled 6 AM postoperative serum glucose ($\leq$200 mg/dL)

SCIP-Inf 5: Postoperative wound infection diagnosed during index hospitalization

SCIP-Inf 6: Surgical patients with appropriate hair removal

SCIP-Inf 7: Colorectal surgical patients with immediate post-operative normothermia

SCIP, Surgical Care Improvement Project.
From Rosenberger LH, Politano AD, Sawyer RG. The surgical care improvement project and prevention of post-operative infection, including surgical site infection. *Surg Infect (Larchmt)*. 2011;12(3):163–168.

an immunoglobulin E (IgE)–mediated reaction (anaphylaxis, urticaria, bronchospasm) or exfoliative dermatitis (Stevens-Johnson syndrome).

2. In patients with documented IgE-mediated anaphylactic reactions, β-lactam antibiotics can usually be substituted with clindamycin or vancomycin.

3. Routine prophylaxis with vancomycin is not recommended for any patient population in the absence of documented or highly suspected colonization or infection with methicillin-resistant *Staphylococcus aureus* (recent hospitalization or nursing home stay and hemodialysis patients) or known IgE-mediated response to β-lactam antibiotics.

C. Pseudomembranous colitis is the most frequent complication of prophylactic antimicrobials, including the IV cephalosporins (Table 41-3).

III. **Antimicrobial Selection.** Prompt identification of the causative organism is essential for the selection of appropriate antimicrobial drugs to treat ongoing infection. Infections

Table 41-2

Recommended Doses and Redosing Intervals for Commonly Used Antimicrobials for Surgical Prophylaxis

Antimicrobial	Recommended Dose Adults[a]	Pediatrics[b]	Half-life in Adults With Normal Renal Function, h[19]	Recommended Redosing Interval (From Initiation of Preoperative Dose), h[c]
Ampicillin–sulbactam	3 g (ampicillin 2 g/sulbactam 1 g)	50 mg/kg of the ampicillin component	0.8–1.3	2
Ampicillin	2 g	50 mg/kg	1–1.9	2
Aztreonam	2 g	30 mg/kg	1.3–2.4	4
Cefazolin	2 g, 3 g for pts weighing ≥120 kg	30 mg/kg	1.2–2.2	4
Cefuroxime	1.5 g	50 mg/kg	1–2	4
Cefotaxime	1 g[d]	50 mg/kg	0.9–1.7	3
Cefoxitin	2 g	40 mg/kg	0.7–1.1	2
Cefotetan	2 g	40 mg/kg	2.8–4.6	6
Ceftriaxone	2 g[e]	50–75 mg/kg	5.4–10.9	NA
Ciprofloxacin[f]	400 mg	10 mg/kg	3–7	NA
Clindamycin	900 mg	10 mg/kg	2–4	6
Ertapenem	1 g	15 mg/kg	3–5	NA

(continued)

Table 41-2

Recommended Doses and Redosing Intervals for Commonly Used Antimicrobials for Surgical Prophylaxis *(continued)*

Antimicrobial	Recommended Dose Adults[a]	Recommended Dose Pediatrics[b]	Half-life in Adults With Normal Renal Function, h[19]	Recommended Redosing Interval (From Initiation of Preoperative Dose), h[c]
Fluconazole	400 mg	6 mg/kg	30	NA
Gentamicin[g]	5 mg/kg based on dosing weight (single dose)	2.5 mg/kg based on dosing weight	2–3	NA
Levofloxacin[f]	500 mg	10 mg/kg	6–8	NA
Metronidazole	500 mg	15 mg/kg Neonates weighing <1,200 g should receive a single 7.5-mg/kg dose	6–8	NA
Moxifloxacin[f]	400 mg	10 mg/kg	8–15	NA
Piperacillin–tazobactam	3.375 g	Infants 2–9 mo: 80 mg/kg of the piperacillin component Children >9 mo and ≤40 kg: 100 mg/kg of the piperacillin component	0.7–1.2	2
Vancomycin	15 mg/kg	15 mg/kg	4–8	NA

Oral antibiotics for colorectal surgery prophylaxis (used in conjunction with a mechanical bowel preparation)

Erythromycin base	1 g	20 mg/kg	NA
Metronidazole	1 g	15 mg/kg	0.8–3
Neomycin	1 g	15 mg/kg	6–10
			2–3 (3% absorbed under normal gastrointestinal conditions)
			NA
			NA

[a] Adult doses are obtained from the studies cited in each section. When doses differed between studies, expert opinion used the most-often recommended dose.

[b] The maximum pediatric dose should not exceed the usual adult dose.

[c] For antimicrobials with a short half-life (e.g., cefazolin, cefoxitin) used before long procedures, redosing in the operating room is recommended at an interval of approximately two times the half-life of the agent in patients with normal renal function. Recommended redosing intervals marked as "not applicable" (NA) are based on typical case length; for unusually long procedures, redosing may be needed.

[d] Although FDA-approved package insert labeling indicates 1 g, 14 experts recommend 2 g for obese patients.

[e] When used as a single dose in combination with metronidazole for colorectal procedures.

[f] While fluoroquinolones have been associated with an increased risk of tendinitis/tendon rupture in all ages, use of these agents for single-dose prophylaxis is generally safe.

[g] In general, gentamicin for surgical antibiotic prophylaxis should be limited to a single dose given preoperatively. Dosing is based on the patient's actual body weight. If the patient's actual weight is more than 20% above ideal body weight (IBW), the dosing weight (DW) can be determined as follows: DW = IBW + 0.4(actual weight − IBW).

From Bratzler DW, Dellinger, EP, Olsen KM, et al; American Society of Health-System Pharmacists; Infectious Diseases Society of America; Surgical Infection Society; Society for Healthcare Epidemiology of America. Clinical practice guidelines for antimicrobial prophylaxis in surgery. *Am J Health Syst Pharm.* 2013;70(3):195–283. http://www.ashp.org/surgical-guidelines. Accessed February 24, 2014.

Table 41-3

Direct Drug Toxicity Associated with Administration of Antimicrobials

Toxicity	Antimicrobial
Allergic reactions	All antimicrobials but most often with β-lactam derivatives
Nephrotoxicity	Aminoglycosides
	Polymyxins
	Amphotericin B
Neutropenia	Penicillins
	Cephalosporins
	Vancomycin
Inhibition of platelet aggregation	Penicillins (high doses)
Prolonged prothrombin time	Cephalosporins
Bone marrow suppression (aplastic anemia, pancytopenia)	Chloramphenicol
	Flucytosine
	Linezolid (reversible)
Hemolytic anemia	Chloramphenicol
	Sulfonamides
	Nitrofurantoin
	Primaquine
Agranulocytosis	Macrolides
	Trimethoprim-sulfamethoxazole
Leukopenia and thrombocytopenia (folate deficiency)	Trimethoprim
Normocytic normochromic anemia	Amphotericin B
Ototoxicity	Aminoglycosides
	Vancomycin (auditory neurotoxicity)
	Minocycline (vestibular toxicity)
Seizures	Penicillins and other β-lactams (high doses, azotemic patients, history of epilepsy)
	Metronidazole
Neuromuscular blockade	Aminoglycosides
Peripheral neuropathy	Nitrofurantoin (renal failure)
	Isoniazid (prevent with pyridoxine)
	Metronidazole

Table 41-3

Direct Drug Toxicity Associated with Administration of Antimicrobials *(continued)*

Toxicity	Antimicrobial
Benign intracranial hypertension	Tetracyclines
Optic neuritis	Ethambutol
Hepatotoxicity	Isoniazid
	Rifampin
	Tetracyclines (high doses)
	β-Lactam antimicrobials (high doses)
	Nitrofurantoin
	Erythromycin
	Sulfonamides
	Quinupristin-dalfopristin
Increased plasma bilirubin concentrations	Erythromycin
Gastrointestinal irritation	Tetracyclines
Prolongation of QTc interval	Erythromycin
	Fluoroquinolones
Exaggerated sympathomimetic effects in patients receiving monoamine oxidase inhibitors	Linezolid
Hyperkalemia	Trimethoprim-sulfamethoxazole
Tendinitis	Fluoroquinolones
Arthralgias and myalgias	Quinupristin-dalfopristin
Photosensitivity	Sulfonamides
	Tetracyclines
	Fluoroquinolones
Teratogenicity	Tetracyclines
	Metronidazole
	Rifampin
	Trimethoprim
	Fluoroquinolones

behind obstructing lesions such as pneumonia behind a blocked bronchus will not respond to antimicrobials until the obstruction is relieved.

A. **Nosocomial Infections**
   1. Nearly 80% of nosocomial infections occur in three sites (urinary tract, respiratory system, and bloodstream). The incidence of nosocomial infections is highly associated

with the use of devices such as ventilators, vascular access catheters, and urinary catheters. Intravascular access catheters are the most common cause of bacteremia or fungemia in hospitalized patients.

2. The organism infecting access catheters most commonly comes from the colonized hub or lumen and reflect skin flora (*S. aureus* and *Staphylococcus epidermidis*). Initial therapy of suspected intravascular catheter infection usually includes vancomycin because of the high incidence of methicillin-resistant *S. aureus* and *S. epidermidis* in the nosocomial environment.

IV. **Special Patient Groups**
   A. **Parturients** (Table 41-4). Most antimicrobials cross the placenta and enter maternal milk. The immature fetal liver may lack enzymes necessary to metabolize certain drugs such that pharmacokinetics and toxicities in the fetus are often different from those in older children and adults. Teratogenicity is a concern when any drug is administered during early pregnancy.
   B. **Elderly Patients**
      1. Physiologic changes that occur with increasing age can alter oral absorption, distribution metabolism, and excretion of antimicrobials.
      2. Penicillins and cephalosporins, because of their large therapeutic index, obviate the need for significant changes in dosage schedules in elderly patients who have normal serum creatinine concentrations.
      3. Administration of aminoglycosides and vancomycin to elderly patients may require adjustments in dosing regimens.
   C. **HIV-Infected Patients**. There has been concern about increased risk of postoperative infection in HIV-infected patients based on their increased risk for opportunistic infection in the setting of reduced T4 cell counts (goal is preoperative control on an antiretroviral regimen with preserved T4 cell counts).

V. **Antibacterial Drugs Commonly Used in the Perioperative Period**
   A. **Penicillins**. The bactericidal action of penicillins reflects the ability of these antimicrobials to interfere with the synthesis of peptidoglycan, which is an essential component of cell walls of susceptible bacteria. Cell membranes of resistant gram-negative bacteria are in general resistant to penicillins

Table 41-4

Antimicrobials in Pregnancy

Drug	Maternal Toxicity	Fetal Toxicity	Excreted in Colostrum
Considered safe			
Penicillins	Allergic reactions	None known	Trace
Cephalosporins	Allergic reactions	None known	Trace
Erythromycin base	Allergic reactions	None known	Yes
	Gastrointestinal irritation		
Use cautiously			
Aminoglycosides	Ototoxicity	Ototoxicity	Yes
	Nephrotoxicity		
Clindamycin	Allergic reactions	None known	Trace
	Colitis		
Ethambutol	Optic neuritis	None known	Unknown
Isoniazid	Allergic reactions	Neuropathy	Yes
	Hepatotoxicity	Seizures	
Rifampin	Allergic reactions	None known	Yes
	Hepatotoxicity		
Sulfonamides	Allergic reactions	Kernicterus (at term)	Yes
		Hemolysis (G6PD deficiency)	

(continued)

Table 41-4

Antimicrobials in Pregnancy *(continued)*

Drug	Maternal Toxicity	Fetal Toxicity	Excreted in Colostrum
Avoid			
Metronidazole	Allergic reactions Alcohol intolerance Peripheral neuropathy	None known (teratogenic in animals)	Yes
Contraindicated			
Chloramphenicol	Bone marrow depression	Gray syndrome	Yes
Erythromycin estolate	Hepatotoxicity	None known	Yes
Nalidixic acid	Gastrointestinal irritation	Increased intracranial pressure	Unknown
Fluoroquinolones	Gastrointestinal irritation Allergic reactions Peripheral neuropathy	Arthropathies (animals)	Unknown
Nitrofurantoin	Gastrointestinal irritation	Hemolysis (G6PD deficiency)	Trace
Tetracyclines	Hepatotoxicity Nephrotoxicity	Tooth discoloration and dysplasia Impaired bone growth	Yes
Trimethoprim	Allergic reactions	Teratogenicity	Yes

because they prevent access to sites where synthesis of peptidoglycan is taking place.

1. **Clinical Indications**
   a. Penicillin is the drug of choice for treatment of pneumococcal, streptococcal, and meningococcal infections. Penicillin is the drug of choice for treating all forms of actinomycosis and clostridial infections causing gas gangrene.
   b. Prophylactic administration of penicillin is highly effective against streptococcal infections, accounting for its value in patients with rheumatic fever.
   c. Transient bacteremia occurs in the majority of patients undergoing dental extractions, emphasizing the importance of prophylactic penicillin in patients with congenital or acquired heart disease or tissue implants undergoing dental procedures.
   d. Intrathecal administration of penicillins is not recommended because these drugs are potent convulsants when administered by this route.

2. **Excretion.** Renal excretion of penicillin is rapid (60% to 90% of an intramuscular [IM] dose is excreted in the first hour), such that the plasma concentration decreases to 50% of its peak value within 1 hour after injection.

3. **Duration of Action**
   a. Methods to prolong the duration of action of penicillin include the simultaneous administration of probenecid, which blocks the renal tubular secretion of penicillin.
   b. Procaine penicillin contains 120 mg of the local anesthetic for every 300,000 units of the antimicrobial (hypersensitivity to procaine must be considered).

B. **Penicillinase-Resistant Penicillins**
   1. The major mechanism of resistance to the penicillins is bacterial production of β-lactamase enzymes that hydrolyze the β-lactam ring, rendering the antimicrobial molecule inactive (methicillin, oxacillin, nafcillin, cloxacillin, and dicloxacillin are not susceptible to hydrolysis by staphylococcal penicillinases).
   2. Penetration of nafcillin into the central nervous system (CNS) is sufficient to treat staphylococcal meningitis.

C. **Penicillinase-Susceptible Broad-Spectrum Penicillins (Second-Generation Penicillins).** Broad-spectrum penicillins have a wider range of activity than other penicillins, being bactericidal against gram-positive and gram-negative bacteria. They are all inactivated by penicillinase produced by certain gram-negative and gram-positive bacteria. Therefore, these drugs are not effective against most staphylococcal infections.

1. **Ampicillin** (α-aminobenzylpenicillin) has a broader range of activity than penicillin G. Its spectrum encompasses not only pneumococci, meningococci, gonococci, and various streptococci but also a number of gram-negative bacilli, such as *Haemophilus influenzae* and *Escherichia coli*.

   a. Approximately 50% of an oral dose of ampicillin is excreted unchanged by the kidneys in the first 6 hours, emphasizing that renal function greatly influences the duration of action of this antimicrobial.

   b. Among the penicillins, ampicillin is associated with the highest incidence of skin rash (9%), which typically appears 7 to 10 days after initiation of therapy (often due to protein impurities in the commercial preparation of the drug and do not represent true allergic reactions).

2. **Amoxicillin**. Its spectrum of activity is identical to that of ampicillin, but it is more efficiently absorbed from the gastrointestinal tract than ampicillin, and effective concentrations are present in the circulation for twice as long.

D. **Extended-Spectrum Carboxypenicillins (Third-Generation Penicillins)**

1. **Carbenicillin**

   a. The principal advantage of carbenicillin is its effectiveness in the treatment of infections caused by *Pseudomonas aeruginosa* and certain *Proteus* strains that are resistant to ampicillin.

   b. This antimicrobial is penicillinase susceptible and therefore ineffective against most strains of *S. aureus*. Carbenicillin is not absorbed from the gastrointestinal tract; therefore, it must be administered parenterally.

   c. Approximately 85% of the unchanged drug is recovered in urine over 9 hours. Probenecid, by delaying renal excretion of the drug, increases the plasma concentration of carbenicillin by approximately 50%.

   d. The sodium load administered with a large dose of carbenicillin (30 to 40 g) is considerable because greater than 10% of carbenicillin is sodium (about 5 mEq/g). Congestive heart failure may develop in susceptible patients in response to this acute drug-produced sodium load.

    e. Hypokalemia and metabolic alkalosis may occur because of obligatory excretion of potassium with the large amount of nonreabsorbable carbenicillin.

    f. Carbenicillin interferes with normal platelet aggregation such that bleeding time is prolonged but platelet count remains normal.

E. **Extended-spectrum acylaminopenicillins (fourth-generation penicillins)** have the broadest spectrum of activity of all the penicillins. Like the carboxypenicillins, the acylaminopenicillins are derivatives of ampicillin. These drugs are ineffective against penicillinase-producing strains of *S. aureus.*

F. **Penicillin β-Lactamase Inhibitor Combinations**. Clavulanic acid, sulbactam, and tazobactam are β-lactam compounds that bind irreversibly to the β-lactamase enzymes that are produced by many bacteria, thus inactivating these enzymes and rendering the organisms sensitive to β-lactamase–susceptible penicillins.

VI. **Cephalosporins, like the penicillins, are bactericidal antimicrobials that inhibit bacterial cell wall synthesis and have a low intrinsic toxicity. Bacteria can produce cephalosporinases (β-lactamases) that disrupt the β-lactam structure of cephalosporins and thus inhibit their antimicrobial activity. Like the newer penicillins, the new cephalosporins have an extraordinarily broad spectrum of antimicrobial action. Nephrotoxicity owing to cephalosporins, with the exception of cephaloridine, is less frequent than after administration of aminoglycosides or polymyxins. The incidence of allergic reactions in patients being treated with cephalosporins ranges from 1% to 10%. The majority of the allergic reactions consist of cutaneous manifestations that occur 24 hours after drug exposure. Life-threatening anaphylaxis is estimated to occur in 0.02% of treated patients. Because the cephalosporins share immunologic cross-reactivity, patients who are allergic to one cephalosporin are likely to be allergic to others. The possibility of cross-reactivity between cephalosporins and penicillins seems to be very infrequent, and cephalosporins are often selected as alternative antimicrobials in patients with a history of penicillin allergy.**

A. **Cephalosporins and Allergy to Penicillins**

    1. Hypersensitivity is the most common adverse reaction to β-lactam antimicrobials. Allergic reactions are noted in 1% to 10% of patients treated with penicillins,

making these antimicrobials the most allergenic of all drugs.

   a. Most often, the allergic response is a delayed reaction characterized by a maculopapular rash and/or fever.

   b. Less often but more serious is immediate hypersensitivity that is mediated by IgE antibodies. Manifestations of immediate hypersensitivity may include laryngeal edema, bronchospasm, and cardiovascular collapse.

   c. Allergic reactions may occur in the absence of previous known exposure to any of the penicillins. This may reflect prior unrecognized exposure to penicillin, presumably in ingested foods.

   d. Allergic reactions can occur with any dose or route of administration, although severe anaphylactic reactions are more often associated with parenteral than with oral administration.

2. Some patients who experience cutaneous reactions may continue to receive the offending penicillin or receive the same penicillin in the future without experiencing a similar response.

B. **Cross-Reactivity**. The presence of a common nucleus (β-lactam ring) in the structure of all penicillins means that allergy to one penicillin increases the likelihood of an allergic reaction to another penicillin (actual cross-reactivity is rare).

C. **Classification**. Cephalosporins are classified as first-, second-, and third-generation because of their antimicrobial spectrum. First-generation cephalosporins are inexpensive, exhibit low toxicity, and are as active as second- and third-generation cephalosporins against staphylococci and nonenterococcal streptococci (first-generation cephalosporins have been commonly selected for antimicrobial prophylaxis in patients undergoing cardiovascular, orthopedic, biliary, pelvic, and intraabdominal surgery). All cephalosporins can penetrate into joints and can readily cross the placenta.

   1. **First-Generation Cephalosporins**

      a. Cephalothin is the prototype of first-generation cephalosporins (excreted largely unaltered by the kidneys, emphasizing the need to decrease the dose in the presence of renal dysfunction). Oral absorption is poor and IM injection is painful, accounting for its common administration by the IV route. Although cephalothin is present in many tissues and fluids, it does not enter the cerebrospinal fluid in significant

amounts and is not recommended for treatment of meningitis.
   b. Cefazolin has essentially the same antimicrobial spectrum as cephalothin but has the advantage of achieving higher blood levels, presumably due to slower renal elimination (viewed as the drug of choice for antimicrobial prophylaxis for many surgeries). This drug is well tolerated after IM or IV injection.

2. **Second-Generation Cephalosporins**
   a. Cefoxitin and cefamandole are examples of second-generation cephalosporins with extended activity against gram-negative bacteria.
   b. Cefoxitin is resistant to cephalosporinases produced by gram-negative bacteria.
   c. Cefamandole is pharmacologically similar to cefoxitin, but its methylthiotetrazole side chain poses a risk of bleeding and disulfiram-like reactions with concurrent use of alcohol.
   d. Both drugs are excreted predominantly unchanged by the kidneys.

3. **Third-Generation Cephalosporins**
   a. Third-generation cephalosporins have an enhanced ability to resist hydrolysis by the β-lactamases of many gram-negative bacilli.
   b. Unlike older cephalosporins, the third-generation cephalosporins achieve therapeutic levels in the cerebrospinal fluid and can be used to treat meningitis.
   c. Cefotaxime was the first third-generation cephalosporin and has been effective in a broad range of infections, including meningitis caused by gram-negative bacilli other than *Pseudomonas*.
   d. Ceftriaxone has the longest elimination half-time of any third-generation cephalosporin and is highly effective against gram-negative bacilli.
   e. The spectrum of activity of cefixime and a single daily dose make it attractive for upper respiratory tract infections, but less expensive alternatives are available.

VII. Other β-Lactam Antimicrobials

A. **Aztreonam**

1. The antimicrobial activity of this drug is limited to gram-negative bacteria. Aztreonam is not absorbed from the gastrointestinal tract, but therapeutic blood levels are achieved after IM or IV administration in most body tissues and fluids, including cerebrospinal fluid.

2. Clearance is principally by glomerular filtration.
3. Because aztreonam combines the activity of the amino-glycosides with the low toxicity of the β-lactam antimi-crobials, it can replace aminoglycosides in the treatment of many gram-negative infections.

VIII. **Aminoglycoside antimicrobials are poorly lipid-soluble antimicrobials (<1% of an orally administered aminogly-coside is absorbed) that are rapidly bactericidal for aero-bic gram-negative bacteria. There is a linear relationship between the plasma creatinine concentration and the elimi-nation half-time of aminoglycosides.**

   A. **Streptomycin** is rarely selected because of the rapid emer-gence of resistant organisms, the frequent occurrence of vestibular damage during prolonged treatment, and the availability of less toxic antimicrobials.

   B. **Gentamicin** is active against *P. aeruginosa* as well as the gram-negative bacilli (penetrates pleural, ascitic, and sy-novial fluids in the presence of inflammation). Monitoring plasma concentrations of gentamicin is the best approach for recognizing potentially toxic levels (>9 μg/mL).

   C. **Amikacin** is a semisynthetic derivative of kanamycin that has the advantage of not being associated with the develop-ment of resistance. The principal use of amikacin is in the treatment of infections caused by gentamicin- or tobramycin-resistant gram-negative bacilli. The incidence of nephrotoxic-ity and ototoxicity is similar to that produced by gentamicin.

   D. **Neomycin** is commonly used for topical application to treat infections of the skin (as after burn injury), cornea, and mu-cous membranes. Allergic reactions occur in 6% to 8% of patients treated with topical neomycin. Oral neomycin does not undergo systemic absorption and is thus administered to decrease bacterial flora in the intestine before gastroin-testinal surgery and as an adjunct to the therapy of hepatic coma (decreases blood ammonia concentrations).

   E. **Side Effects**
      1. **Ototoxicity** reflects drug-induced destruction of vestib-ular or cochlear sensory hairs that is dose-dependent and most likely occurs with chronic therapy, especially in el-derly patients, in whom renal dysfunction is more likely. Furosemide, mannitol, and probably other diuretics seem to accentuate the ototoxic effects of aminoglycosides.
      2. **Nephrotoxicity**
         a. Aminoglycosides can produce acute tubular necrosis that initially manifests as an inability to concentrate

urine and the appearance of proteinuria and red blood cell casts (usually reversible if the drug is discontinued).

b. Neomycin is the most nephrotoxic of the aminoglycosides and therefore is not administered by the parenteral route.

3. **Skeletal muscle weakness** is most likely because of the ability of aminoglycosides to inhibit the prejunctional release of acetylcholine while also decreasing postsynaptic sensitivity to the neurotransmitter (IV administration of calcium overcomes the effect of aminoglycosides at the neuromuscular junction).

a. Patients with myasthenia gravis are uniquely susceptible to skeletal muscle weakness if treated with an aminoglycoside.

b. Administration of a single dose of an aminoglycoside is unlikely to produce skeletal muscle weakness in an otherwise healthy patient.

IX. **Macrolides are stable in the presence of acidic gastric fluid, and as a result, these antimicrobials are well absorbed from the gastrointestinal tract.**

A. **Erythromycin** has a spectrum of activity that includes most gram-positive bacteria. In patients who cannot tolerate penicillins or cephalosporins, erythromycin or clindamycin are an effective alternative for the treatment of streptococcal pharyngitis, bronchitis, and pneumonia. Severe nausea and vomiting may accompany infusion of erythromycin.

1. **Effects on QTc.** Oral erythromycin prolongs cardiac repolarization and is associated with reports of torsades de pointes.

B. **Azithromycin** resembles erythromycin in its antimicrobial spectrum, but an extraordinarily prolonged elimination half-time (68 hours) permits once-a-day dosing for 5 days.

X. **Clindamycin resembles erythromycin in antimicrobial activity, but it is more active against many anaerobes. Because severe pseudomembranous colitis can be a complication of clindamycin therapy, this drug should be used only to treat infections that cannot be adequately treated by less toxic antimicrobials.**

A. **Side Effects**

1. Clindamycin produces prejunctional and postjunctional effects at the neuromuscular junction, and these effects cannot be readily antagonized with calcium or anticholinesterase drugs.

2. Large doses of clindamycin can induce profound and long-lasting neuromuscular blockade in the absence of nondepolarizing muscle relaxants and after full recovery from the effects of succinylcholine has occurred.

XI. Vancomycin is a bactericidal glycopeptide antimicrobial that impairs cell wall synthesis of gram-positive bacteria. The oral route of administration is used only for the treatment of staphylococcal enterocolitis and antimicrobial-associated pseudomembranous enterocolitis (poorly absorbed from the gastrointestinal tract). Vancomycin is administered IV for the treatment of severe staphylococcal infections or streptococcal or enterococcal endocarditis in patients who are allergic to penicillins or cephalosporins. Concomitant administration of an aminoglycoside is often necessary when vancomycin is used in the treatment of enterococcal endocarditis. Vancomycin is the drug of choice in the treatment of infections caused by methicillin-resistant *S. aureus* (prosthetic heart valve endocarditis). When vancomycin is administered IV, the recommendation is to infuse the calculated dose (10 to 15 mg/kg) over 60 minutes to minimize the occurrence of drug-induced histamine release and hypotension (begin 2 hours prior to surgery for prophylaxis) (Fig. 41-1). Infusion over 60 minutes produces sustained plasma concentrations for up to 12 hours. Vancomycin is principally excreted by the kidneys, with 90% of a dose being recovered unchanged in urine.

A. **Side Effects**

1. Rapid infusion (<30 minutes) of vancomycin has been associated with profound hypotension and even cardiac arrest. Hypotension is often accompanied by signs of histamine release characterized by intense facial and truncal erythema ("red man syndrome"). The red man syndrome may occur even with slow infusion of vancomycin and is not always associated with hypotension.

2. Cardiovascular side effects most likely reflect nonimmunologic histamine release induced by vancomycin (direct myocardial depression does not seem to be important in causing hypotension).

3. Vancomycin may also produce allergic reactions characterized as anaphylactoid with associated hypotension, erythema, and occasionally bronchospasm (plasma tryptase concentrations are not increased following vancomycin-induced anaphylactoid reactions thus permitting a method to distinguish anaphylactic from anaphylactoid reactions).

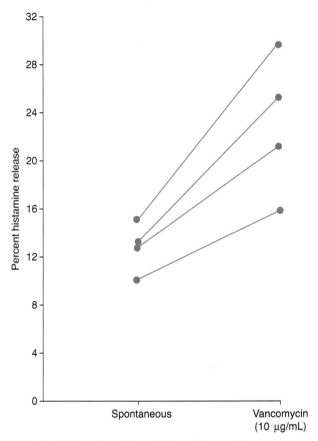

FIGURE 41-1 Histamine release (%) from dispersed human cutaneous mast cells after the administration of vancomycin. (From Levy JH, Kettlekamp N, Goertz P, et al. Histamine release by vancomycin. A mechanism for hypotension in man. *Anesthesiology*. 1987;67: 122–125, with permission.)

4. Arterial hypoxemia manifesting as an unexpected decrease in the Sp_{O_2} may occur in association with vancomycin administration, perhaps reflecting drug-induced vasodilation in the lungs leading to an increase in ventilation to perfusion mismatching.

5. Oral H_1 (diphenhydramine 1 mg/kg) and H_2 (cimetidine 4 mg/kg) receptor antagonists administered 1 hour before induction of anesthesia decrease histamine-related side effects of rapid vancomycin infusion (1 g over 10 minutes). In ambulatory anesthesia settings, as for orthopedic procedures, the time available for vancomycin administration before surgical incision or tourniquet inflation is often limited and may result in inadequate levels of antibiotic in blood and tissues if vancomycin cannot be administered more rapidly than 10 to 15 mg/kg over 60 minutes.

6. Ototoxicity is likely when persistent high plasma concentrations (>30 μg/mL) are present. Particular attention to ototoxicity and nephrotoxicity is required when vancomycin is administered with an aminoglycoside.

7. The administration of vancomycin to a patient recovering from succinylcholine-induced neuromuscular blockade has resulted in a return of neuromuscular blockade.

XII. **Bacitracins** are a group of polypeptide antibiotics effective against a variety of gram-positive bacteria. Use of these antimicrobials is limited to topical application in ophthalmologic and dermatologic ointments.

XIII. **Metronidazole** is bactericidal against most anaerobic gram-negative bacilli and *Clostridium* species. This antimicrobial has been useful in treating a variety of CNS, bone, and joint infections; abdominal and pelvic sepsis; and endocarditis. Metronidazole is a useful part of preoperative prophylactic regimens for elective colorectal surgery. Side effects of metronidazole include dry mouth (metallic taste) and nausea. Concurrent ingestion of alcohol may cause a reaction similar to that produced when alcohol is ingested by patients taking disulfiram.

XIV. **Fluoroquinolones** are broad-spectrum antimicrobials that are bactericidal against most enteric gram-negative bacilli. The dose of the fluoroquinolones should be decreased in the presence of renal dysfunction. Fluoroquinolones have been useful clinically in the treatment of genitourinary and gastrointestinal infections. Fluoroquinolones are associated with an increased risk of tendinitis and tendon rupture.

A. **Ciprofloxacin** is highly effective in the treatment of urinary and genital tract infections, including prostatitis, and gastrointestinal infections.

B. **Moxifloxacin** is long acting for the treatment of acute
bacterial sinusitis, acute bacterial exacerbation of chronic
bronchitis, community-acquired pneumonia, skin infections, and complicated intraabdominal infections. Because
of serious adverse effects including peripheral neuropathy,
syndrome of inappropriate secretion of antidiuretic hormone, tendonitis, acute liver failure, QTc prolongation, toxic
epidermal necrolysis, psychotic reactions, and Stevens-
Johnson syndrome, use is recommended only when less
toxic options are not available.

XV. **Antiseptic and Disinfectant Prophylaxis for Surgical Procedures. Decontamination of the skin with antiseptic preparations reduces the burden of skin flora (Centers for Disease
Control and Prevention guidelines recommend showering
or bathing with an antiseptic solution before surgery). The
main types of disinfectants are alcohols, chlorhexidine, and
iodine-containing preparations which can be used alone or
in combination.**

XVI. Topical Antiseptics
   A. **Alcohols** are applied topically to decrease local cutaneous
bacterial flora (quick drying and antisepsis) before penetration of the skin with needles. On the skin, 70% ethyl alcohol
kills nearly 90% of the cutaneous bacteria within 2 minutes.
Isopropyl alcohol has a slightly greater bactericidal activity
than ethyl alcohol.
      1. **Fire Risks**. Alcohol-based surgical solutions can create
a fire hazard (flash fire) especially if the solution is
allowed to pool (e.g., in the umbilicus) or the patient is
draped before the solution is completely dry resulting in
trapped alcohol vapors being channeled to the surgical
site where a heat source may be used.
   B. **Chlorhexidine** disrupts cell membranes of the bacterial cells and is effective against both gram-positive and
gram-negative bacteria. It persists on the skin to provide
continued antibacterial protection. As a hand wash or
surgical scrub, 2% chlorhexidine causes a greater initial
decrease in the number of normal cutaneous bacteria than
does povidone-iodine or hexachlorophene.
   C. **Iodine** is a rapid-acting antiseptic that, in the absence of
organic material, kills bacteria, viruses, and spores (1% tincture of iodine will kill 90% of the bacteria in 90 seconds,
whereas a 5% solution achieves this response in 60 seconds).
The most important use of iodine is disinfection of the skin

(best used in the form of a tincture of iodine because the alcohol vehicle facilitates spreading and skin penetration).

D. **Iodophors** are a loose complex of elemental iodine with an organic carrier that not only increases the solubility of iodine but also provides a reservoir for sustained release (most widely used iodophor is povidone-iodine).

1. **Clinical Uses**

   a. The iodophors have a broad antimicrobial spectrum and are widely used as hand washes, including surgical scrubs; preparation of the skin before surgery or needle puncture; and treatment of minor cuts, abrasions, and burns.

   b. A standard surgical scrub with 10% povidone-iodine solutions (Betadine) will decrease the usual cutaneous bacterial population by more than 90%, with a return to normal in about 6 to 8 hours. A disinfectant which contains an iodophor in isopropyl alcohol (DuraPrep) is more effective than povidone-iodine in decreasing the number of positive skin cultures.

2. **Corneal Toxicity**

   a. Chemical burns to the cornea may follow exposure (accidental splashes) to a variety of disinfectant solutions (chlorhexidine, hexachlorophene, iodine, alcohol, detergents containing iodine-based solutions).

   b. Povidone-iodine solution without detergent appears to be least toxic to the cornea.

XVII. **Preference for Chlorhexidine or Iodine for Skin Disinfection**

A. Central vascular catheters are a common site of hospital-acquired infection.

B. An iodophor in isopropyl alcohol solution is superior to povidone-iodine for decreasing the number of positive skin cultures immediately after disinfection as well as in bacterial regrowth and colonization of epidural catheters (potential neurotoxicity of chlorhexidine that is inadvertently introduced into the neuraxial space).

XVIII. **Quaternary ammonium compounds are bactericidal in vitro to a wide variety of gram-positive and gram-negative bacteria. Many fungi and viruses are also susceptible.** *Mycobacterium tuberculosis,* **however, is relatively resistant.**

A. Alcohol enhances the germicidal activity of quaternary ammonium compounds so that tinctures are more effective than aqueous solutions.

B. Benzalkonium and cetylpyridinium (mouthwash) are examples of quaternary ammonium compounds.

These compounds may be used preoperatively to decrease the number of microorganisms on intact skin. There is a rapid onset of action, but the availability of more efficacious solutions has decreased their frequency of use.

C. Quaternary ammonium compounds have been widely used for the sterilization of instruments (endoscopes and other instruments made of polyethylene or polypropylene absorb quaternary ammonium compounds, which may decrease the concentration of the active ingredient to below a bactericidal concentration).

XIX. **Hexachlorophene (pHisoHex) is a polychlorinated bisphenol that exhibits bacteriostatic activity against gram-positive but not gram-negative organisms.**

A. Immediately after a hand scrub with hexachlorophene, the cutaneous bacterial population may be decreased by only 30% to 50% compared with greater than 90% following use of an iodophor. After 60 minutes, the bacterial population surviving a hexachlorophene scrub will decrease to about 4%, whereas with the iodophor scrub, the bacterial population will have recovered to about 16% of normal.

B. Because most of the potentially pathogenic bacteria on the skin are gram-positive, 3% hexachlorophene is commonly used to decrease the spread of contaminants from caregivers' hands.

C. Hexachlorophene may be absorbed through intact skin in sufficient amounts to produce neurotoxic effects, including cerebral irritability.

XX. **Methods for Sterilization of Instruments**

A. **Formaldehyde** is a volatile, wide-spectrum disinfectant that kills bacteria, fungi, and viruses by precipitating proteins (used to disinfect surgical instruments). Formaldehyde can be toxic, allergenic, and is a known carcinogen.

B. Glutaraldehyde is superior to formaldehyde as a disinfectant because it is rapidly effective against all microorganisms, including viruses and spores and also possesses tuberculocidal activity.

1. Glutaraldehyde is less volatile than formaldehyde and hence causes minimal odor and irritant fumes.

2. As a sterilizing solution for endoscopes, glutaraldehyde is superior to iodophors and hexachlorophene.

XXI. **Pasteurization (hot water disinfection) is a process that destroys microorganisms in a liquid medium by application** of heat (water temperatures in the range of 55°C to 75°C) will destroy all vegetative bacteria of significance in human disease, as well as many fungi and viruses.

A. Pasteurization kills bacteria by coagulating cell proteins, and water acts as a very effective medium for transferring the heat required to destroy organisms.

B. Equipment (respiratory therapy breathing circuits, anesthesia breathing circuits) should be submerged in water at 68°C for a minimum of 30 minutes.

XXII. Silver nitrate is used as a caustic, antiseptic, and astringent. Solutions of silver nitrate are strongly bactericidal, especially for gonococci, accounting for its frequent use as prophylaxis for ophthalmia neonatorum.

A. Silver sulfadiazine or nitrate is used in the treatment of burns. Hypochloremia may occur reflecting the combination of silver ions with chloride. Hyponatremia also may result because the sodium ions are attracted by chloride ions into the exudate. Absorbed nitrate can cause methemoglobinemia.

XXIII. Ethylene oxide is a readily diffusible gas that is noncorrosive and antimicrobial to all organisms at room temperature. This gaseous alkylating material is widely used as an alternative to heat sterilization. Special sterilizing chambers are required because the gas must remain in contact with the objects for several hours. Adequate airing of sterilized materials, such as tracheal tubes, is essential to ensure removal of residual ethylene oxide and thus minimize tissue irritation.

CHAPTER 42

Chemotherapeutic Drugs

I. Introduction

    A. The effectiveness of chemotherapy requires that there be complete destruction (total cell kill) of all cancer cells because a single surviving cell with the ability to divide can give rise to sufficient progeny to ultimately kill the host.

    B. Use of several chemotherapeutic drugs (also called *antineoplastic drugs*) concurrently or in a planned sequence is commonly done in efforts to eradicate even small residual tumor cell populations that have survived treatment with a single or previous agent.

        1. In practice, combination chemotherapy regimens typically use the largest tolerated doses of each chemotherapeutic drug; drugs that work via different mechanisms and that do not share similar toxic effects are combined.

        2. Using a combination of agents that have different mechanisms also decreases the chances that drug-resistant tumor cell populations will emerge (Fig. 42-1).

    C. It is predictable that clinical manifestations of toxicity caused by chemotherapeutic drugs often include myelosuppression (leukopenia, thrombocytopenia, or anemia), nausea, vomiting, diarrhea, mucosal ulceration, dermatitis, and alopecia as these represent activity at normal rapidly dividing cells. Myelosuppression is the dose-limiting factor for many chemotherapeutic drugs and is the most common toxicity that leads to temporary or permanent withdrawal of therapy (usually reversible with discontinuation of the chemotherapeutic agent).

II. Drug Resistance. Resistance to chemotherapeutic drugs often occurs and has many causes (some chemotherapy agents lead to induction of drug-metabolizing enzymes; many solid tumors grow so rapidly that portions of the tumor are poorly vascularized, preventing therapeutic concentrations from reaching many target cells and mutations in the drug-binding domain of the target enzyme).

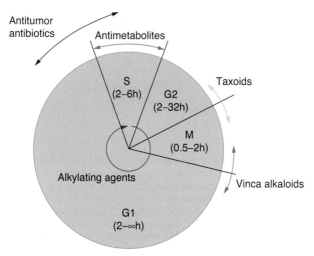

FIGURE 42-1 Cell cycle specificity of chemotherapy agents. The cell cycle is divided into a number of phases, G1 (gap 1, cells increase in size and prepare for DNA synthesis), S (synthesis, DNA replication occurs), G2 (gap 2, cells continue to grow and prepare for mitosis), and M (mitosis, cellular growth stops and preparation for cell division takes place), each of which can vary in length according to the type of cell and the growth rate of the cell. The activity of different classes of certain chemotherapy agents (antibiotics, antimetabolites, taxoids, vinca alkaloids) is optimal in different phases of the cell cycle, whereas alkylating agents are relatively non–phase-specific. (From Caley A, Jones R. The principles of cancer treatment by chemotherapy. *Surgery [Oxford].* 2012;30:186–190, with permission.)

III. Classification (Table 42-1)
   A. Knowledge of drug-induced adverse effects and evaluation of appropriate laboratory tests (hemoglobin, platelet count, white blood cell count, coagulation profile, arterial blood gases, blood glucose, plasma electrolytes, liver and renal function tests, electrocardiogram [ECG], and radiograph of the chest) are useful in the preoperative evaluation of patients being treated with specific chemotherapeutic drugs.
   B. Immunosuppression makes these patients susceptible to iatrogenic infections, thus asepsis and the use of appropriate prophylactic antibiotics is critical.
   C. A history of severe vomiting or diarrhea may be associated with electrolyte disturbances and decreased intravascular fluid volume.

Table 42-1

Chemotherapeutic Drugs, Therapeutic Uses, and Associated Side Effects

Group and Class	Therapeutic Uses	Side Effects (Other than Nausea and Vomiting)
Alkylating Agents		
Nitrogen mustards		
Mechlorethamine	Hodgkin disease Non-Hodgkin lymphoma	Myelosuppression Mucositis Alopecia
Cyclophosphamide	Acute lymphocytic leukemia Chronic lymphocytic leukemia Lymphomas Myeloma Neuroblastoma Breast, ovarian, cervical, and testicular cancer Lung cancer Wilms tumor Sarcoma	Myelosuppression Mucositis Alopecia Hemorrhagic cystitis Skin pigmentation Seizures Renal failure Cardiac failure Inappropriate secretion of vasopressin (ADH)
Melphalan	Myeloma Breast cancer	Myelosuppression
Chlorambucil	Hodgkin disease Non-Hodgkin lymphoma Macroglobulinemia	Myelosuppression Secondary leukemias
Ethyleneimine		
Hexamethylmelamine	Ovarian cancer	Myelosuppression
Thiotepa	Bladder, breast, and ovarian cancer	
Alkyl sulfonates		
Busulfan	Acute myelogenous leukemia Chronic myelogenous leukemia	Myelosuppression Thrombocytopenia

(continued)

Table 42-1

Chemotherapeutic Drugs, Therapeutic Uses, and
Associated Side Effects *(continued)*

Group and Class	Therapeutic Uses	Side Effects (Other than Nausea and Vomiting)
Nitrosoureas		
Carmustine (BCNU)	Hodgkin disease Non-Hodgkin lymphoma Astrocytoma Myeloma Melanoma	Myelosuppression Hepatitis Interstitial pulmonary fibrosis Renal failure Flushing
Lomustine (CCNU)	Hodgkin disease Non-Hodgkin lymphoma Astrocytoma Small lung cell cancer	
Semustine (methyl-CCNU)	Colon cancer	Myelosuppression
Streptozotocin	Insulinoma Carcinoid tumor	Myelosuppression Hepatitis Renal failure
Triazenes		
Dacarbazine (DTIC)	Hodgkin disease Melanoma Sarcomas	Myelosuppression Flulike syndrome
Temozolomide	Astrocytoma Melanoma	Hepatic toxicity Hyperglycemia Anemia Thrombocytopenia Lymphocytopenia
Bioreductive alkylating drugs		
Mitomycin-C	Head and neck, breast, lung, gastric, colon, rectal, and cervical cancer	Myelosuppression Mucositis Cardiac failure Interstitial fibrosis Hemolytic uremic syndrome

Table 42-1

Chemotherapeutic Drugs, Therapeutic Uses, and
Associated Side Effects *(continued)*

Group and Class	Therapeutic Uses	Side Effects (Other than Nausea and Vomiting)
Platinum Compounds		
Cisplatin	Head and neck, thyroid, lung, ovarian, endometrial, cervical, and testicular cancer Neuroblastoma Osteogenic sarcoma	Myelosuppression Peripheral neuropathy Allergic reactions Renal toxicity Electrolyte abnormalities (hypocalcemia, hypomagnesemia, hypophosphatemia)
Carboplatin	As for cisplatin	Myelosuppression
Oxaliplatin	Colon cancer	Myelosuppression Peripheral neuropathy
Antimetabolites		
Folate analogues		
Methotrexate	Head, neck, breast, and lung cancer Acute lymphocytic leukemia Non-Hodgkin lymphoma Osteogenic sarcoma	Myelosuppression Mucositis Pneumonitis Hepatic fibrosis
Pyrimidine analogues		
Fluorouracil (5-FU)	Head and neck, breast, gastric pancreatic, bladder, ovarian, cervical, and prostate cancer Hepatoma	Myelosuppression Mucositis Alopecia Pigmentation Chest pain

(continued)

Table 42-1

Chemotherapeutic Drugs, Therapeutic Uses, and
Associated Side Effects *(continued)*

Group and Class	Therapeutic Uses	Side Effects (Other than Nausea and Vomiting)
Cytarabine	Acute lymphocytic leukemia	Myelosuppression
	Acute myeloid leukemia	Mucositis
	Non-Hodgkin lymphoma	Hepatitis
Gemcitabine	Breast, lung, pancreatic, and bladder cancer	Myelosuppression
		Flulike syndrome
Purine analogues		
Mercaptopurine	Acute lymphocytic leukemia	Myelosuppression
	Acute myeloid leukemia	Anorexia
	Chronic myeloid leukemia	Jaundice
Thioguanine	As for mercapto-purine	Myelosuppression
		Anorexia
Fludarabine	Chronic lympho-cytic leukemia	Myelosuppression
	Non-Hodgkin lymphoma	Optic neuritis
		Peripheral neu-ropathy
		Seizures
		Coma
		Depletion of CD4 cells
Pentostatin	Chronic lympho-cytic leukemia	Myelosuppression
	Cutaneous T-cell lymphoma	Depletion of T cells
	Hairy cell leukemia	Hepatitis

Table 42-1

Chemotherapeutic Drugs, Therapeutic Uses, and
Associated Side Effects *(continued)*

Group and Class	Therapeutic Uses	Side Effects (Other than Nausea and Vomiting)
Cladribine	Chronic lympho-cytic leukemia Cutaneous T-cell lymphoma Hairy cell leukemia Waldenström macroglobu-linemia	Myelosuppression Tumor lysis syndrome Asthenia
Hydroxyurea	Chronic myeloid leukemia Polycythemia vera Thrombocytopenia Melanoma	Myelosuppression Dermatologic changes
Topoisomerase Inhibitors Anthracyclines		
Doxorubicin	Hodgkin disease Non-Hodgkin lymphoma Acute lymphocytic leukemia Neuroblastoma Thyroid, breast, lung, and gas-tric cancer	Myelosuppression Cardiomyopathy Mucositis
Daunomycin	Acute myeloid leukemia Acute lymphocytic leukemia	
Idarubicin	As for daunomycin	

(continued)

Table 42-1

Chemotherapeutic Drugs, Therapeutic Uses, and Associated Side Effects *(continued)*

Group and Class	Therapeutic Uses	Side Effects (Other than Nausea and Vomiting)
Epirubicin	Hodgkin disease Non-Hodgkin lymphoma Acute lymphocytic leukemia Breast, lung, gastric, and bladder cancer	Myelosuppression Cardiomyopathy Alopecia Phlebitis
Anthracenediones Mitoxantrone	Acute myeloid leukemia Breast cancer	Myelosuppression Mucositis
Epipodophyllo-toxins Etoposide	Hodgkin disease Non-Hodgkin lymphoma Acute myeloid leukemia Kaposi sarcoma Breast, lung, and testicular cancer	Myelosuppression Systemic hypotension Hepatitis Mucositis
Teniposide	Acute lympho-cytic leukemia (children) Acute myeloid leukemia (children)	Myelosuppression Systemic hypotension
Dactinomycin	Wilms tumor Rhabdomyosarcoma Choriocarcinoma Kaposi sarcoma Ewing sarcoma Testicular cancer	Myelosuppression Mucositis Cheilitis Glossitis Alopecia Cutaneous erythema

Table 42-1

Chemotherapeutic Drugs, Therapeutic Uses, and Associated Side Effects *(continued)*

Group and Class	Therapeutic Uses	Side Effects (Other than Nausea and Vomiting)
Camptothecins		
Irinotecan	Colon cancer Ovarian cancer	Myelosuppression Alopecia
Topotecan	Lung cancer Ovarian cancer	As for irinotecan
Antitumor Antibiotics		
Antibiotic		
Bleomycin	Hodgkin disease Non-Hodgkin lymphoma Head and neck cancer Testicular cancer	Interstitial pulmonary fibrosis Allergic reactions Skin pigmentation
Tubulin-Binding Drugs		
Vinca alkaloids		
Vinblastine	Hodgkin disease Non-Hodgkin lymphoma Breast cancer Testicular cancer	Myelosuppression Peripheral neuropathy
Vincristine	Hodgkin disease Non-Hodgkin lymphoma Small cell lung cancer Neuroblastoma Wilms tumor Rhabdomyosarcoma Acute lymphocytic leukemia	Myelosuppression Peripheral neuropathy
Vinorelbine	Breast cancer Lung cancer	Myelosuppression Peripheral neuropathy

(continued)

Table 42-1
Chemotherapeutic Drugs, Therapeutic Uses, and Associated Side Effects *(continued)*

Group and Class	Therapeutic Uses	Side Effects (Other than Nausea and Vomiting)
Taxanes		
Paclitaxel	Breast, lung, bladder, and ovarian cancer	Myelosuppression Peripheral neuropathy Allergic reactions Alopecia totalis
Docetaxel	Breast, lung, bladder, and ovarian cancer	Myelosuppression Peripheral neuropathy Allergic reactions Alopecia totalis Cardiac dysrhythmias Capillary leakage
Signal Transduction Modulators		
Antiestrogens		
Tamoxifen	Breast cancer	Venous thrombosis Weight gain Amenorrhea Hypercalcemia Endometrial cancer Hot flashes
Toremifene	Breast cancer	Venous thrombosis Hot flashes
Raloxifene	Breast cancer	Venous thrombosis Hot flashes

Table 42-1

Chemotherapeutic Drugs, Therapeutic Uses, and Associated Side Effects *(continued)*

Group and Class	Therapeutic Uses	Side Effects (Other than Nausea and Vomiting)
Antiandrogens		
Flutamide	Prostate cancer	Gynecomastia Hot flashes
Bicalutamide	Prostate cancer	Gynecomastia Hot flashes
Nilutamide	Prostate cancer	Gynecomastia Hot flashes Delayed visual adaptation to dark
Monoclonal Antibodies		
Rituximab	Chronic lympho-cytic leukemia Non-Hodgkin lymphoma	Infusion-related chills, rash, and fever Non–infusion-related myalgias, angioedema, broncho-spasm, cardiac dysrhythmias Myelosuppression
Trastuzumab	Breast cancer	Fever and chills
Aromatase Inhibitors		
Aminoglute-thimide	Breast cancer	Orthostatic hypotension Glucocorticoid deficiency Cutaneous rash
Anastrazole	Breast cancer	Asthenia Headache Hot flashes
Letrozole	Breast cancer	Headache Heartburn

(continued)

Table 42-1

Chemotherapeutic Drugs, Therapeutic Uses, and
Associated Side Effects *(continued)*

Group and Class	Therapeutic Uses	Side Effects (Other than Nausea and Vomiting)
Gonadotropin-Releasing Drugs		
Leuprolide	Breast cancer	Impotence
	Prostate cancer	Hot flashes
		Pain at sites of bony metastases (tumor flare)
Buserelin	Breast cancer	As for leuprolide
Progestin		
Megestrol acetate	Breast cancer	Weight gain
	Prostate cancer	
	Endometrial cancer	

ADH, antidiuretic hormone; BCNU, bischloroethylnitrosourea; CCNU, 1-(2-chloroethyl)-3-cyclohexyl-1-nitrosourea; DTIC, dimethyl triazeno imidazole carboxamide.

Adapted from Rubin EH, Hait WN. Principles of cancer treatment. *Sci Am Med.* 2003;12(IV):1–17.

D. The existence of mucositis makes placement of pharyngeal airways, laryngeal mask airways, and esophageal catheters questionable.

E. Theoretically, the effects of succinylcholine may be prolonged if plasma cholinesterase activity is decreased by chemotherapeutic drugs.

IV. Toxicities

A. Chemotherapeutic drugs typically target proteins or nucleic acids that are common to malignant and nonmalignant cells and thus possess a narrow therapeutic index (see Table 42-1).

B. Patients who have a history of chemotherapy-induced nausea and vomiting are not necessarily prone to postoperative nausea and vomiting. Development of serotonin antagonists as effective antiemetics in addition to combination antiemetic regimens has facilitated the tolerance of emetogenic chemotherapeutic drugs.

V. **Alkylating Agents (nitrogen mustards, alkyl sulfonates, nitrosoureas, and triazenes) form covalent alkyl bonds with nucleic acid bases, resulting in intrastrand or interstrand DNA cross-links that are toxic to cells undergoing division.**
   A. **Side Effects**
      1. Bone marrow suppression is the most important dose-limiting factor in the clinical use of alkylating drugs, especially busulfan. Lymphocytopenia is usually present within 24 hours. Variable degrees of depression of platelet and erythrocyte counts may occur. Hemolytic anemia is predictably present.
      2. All alkylating drugs are powerful central nervous system (CNS) stimulants, manifesting most often as nausea and vomiting.
      3. Pneumonitis and pulmonary fibrosis are potential adverse effects of alkylating drugs.
      4. Inhibition of plasma cholinesterase activity may be present for as long as 2 to 3 weeks after administration of chemotherapy regimens that include an alkylating agent and can lead to prolonged skeletal muscle paralysis after administration of succinylcholine.
      5. Rapid drug-induced destruction of malignant cells can produce increased purine and pyrimidine breakdown, leading to uric acid–induced nephropathy (recommend adequate fluid intake, alkalinization of the urine, and administration of allopurinol be established before drug treatment).
   B. **Nitrogen Mustards**
      1. **Mechlorethamine** is a rapidly acting nitrogen mustard administered intravenously (IV) to minimize local tissue irritation (intensely powerful vesicants requiring that gloves be worn by personnel handling the drug).
         a. **Clinical Uses**. Mechlorethamine produces beneficial effects in the treatment of Hodgkin disease and, less predictably, in other lymphomas.
         b. **Side Effects**. The major side effects of mechlorethamine include nausea, vomiting, and myelosuppression (leukopenia and thrombocytopenia constitute the principal limitation on the amount of drug that can be given). Latent viral infections may be unmasked by treatment with mechlorethamine. Thrombophlebitis is a potential complication, and extravasation of the drug results in severe local tissue reactions.
      2. **Cyclophosphamide** is absorbed after oral or parenteral administration and is subsequently activated in the liver

Table 42-2

Side Effects of Cyclophosphamide

Hypersensitivity reactions
Fibrosing pneumonitis
Pericarditis and pericardial effusion (possible cardiac tamponade)
Nausea and vomiting
Hemorrhagic cystitis (dysuria and hematuria are indications to
    discontinue the drug)
Inappropriate secretion of arginine vasopressin (possible water
    intoxication)
Extravasation does not produce thrombophlebitis

to aldophosphamide for transport to target tissues. Target cells are able to convert aldophosphamide to highly cytotoxic metabolites than alkylate DNA.

   a. **Clinical Uses**. Cyclophosphamide is used in the treatment of a wide range of cancers (combination with methotrexate and fluorouracil as adjuvant therapy after surgery for breast cancer) and inflammatory diseases.

   b. **Side Effects** (Table 42-2)

3. **Melphalan** is a phenylalanine derivative of nitrogen mustard with a range of activity similar to other alkylating drugs. It is not a vesicant.

   a. **Side effects** of melphalan are primarily hematologic and are similar to those of other alkylating drugs. It is usually necessary to maintain a significant degree of bone marrow depression (leukocyte count 3,000 to 5,000 cells/mm^3) to achieve optimal therapeutic effects. Pulmonary fibrosis is possible. Nausea and vomiting are not common side effects of melphalan. Alopecia does not occur.

4. **Chlorambucil** is the treatment of choice in chronic lymphocytic leukemia and in primary (Waldenström) macroglobulinemia. A marked increase in the incidence of leukemia and other tumors has been noted with the use of this drug for the treatment of polycythemia vera.

   a. **Side Effects**. Cytotoxic effects of chlorambucil on the bone marrow, lymphoid organs, and epithelial tissues are similar to those observed with other alkylating drugs. Its myelosuppressive action is usually moderate, gradual, and rapidly reversible. Pulmonary fibrosis is possible. Nausea and vomiting are frequent.

C. **Alkyl Sulfonates**

1. Busulfan produces remissions in up to 90% of patients with chronic myelogenous leukemia. The drug is of no value in the treatment of acute leukemia.

   a. **Side Effects**. Busulfan can produce progressive pulmonary fibrosis in up to 4% of patients (prognosis after appearance of clinical symptoms is poor, with a median survival of 5 months). Myelosuppression and thrombocytopenia are important side effects. Hyperuricemia resulting from extensive purine catabolism is possible (allopurinol is recommended to minimize renal complications).

D. **Nitrosoureas** (carmustine, lomustine, semustine, streptozocin) possess a wide spectrum of activity for human malignancies including intracranial tumors, melanomas, and gastrointestinal and hematologic malignancies (high lipid solubility results in passage across the blood–brain barrier and efficacy in the treatment of meningeal leukemias and brain tumors). With the exception of streptozocin, the clinical use of nitrosoureas is limited by profound drug-induced myelosuppression.

1. **Carmustine** is capable of crossing the blood–brain barrier and is used to treat meningeal leukemia and primary as well as metastatic brain tumors.

   a. **Side Effects**. Carmustine has been associated with interstitial pneumonitis and fibrosis much like bleomycin. The incidence of pulmonary toxicity is in the range of 20% to 30% (mortality in those affected of 24% to 90%). The cumulative dose is the major risk factor. A unique side effect of carmustine is a delayed onset (after approximately 6 weeks of treatment) of leukopenia and thrombocytopenia.

2. **Lomustine and Semustine**. Lomustine and its methylated analogue semustine possess similar clinical toxicity to carmustine. Lomustine appears to be more effective than carmustine in the treatment of Hodgkin disease.

3. **Streptozocin** has a unique affinity for β cells of the islets of Langerhans and has proved useful in the treatment of human pancreatic islet cell carcinoma and malignant carcinoid.

   a. **Side Effects**. Approximately 70% of patients receiving this drug develop hepatic or renal toxicity. Hyperglycemia can occur as a result of selective destruction of pancreatic β cells. Myelosuppression is not produced by this drug.

4. **Mitomycin** is of value in the palliative treatment of gastric adenocarcinoma in combination with fluorouracil and doxorubicin.

   a. **Side Effects**. Myelosuppression is a prominent side effect of mitomycin and is characterized by severe leukopenia and thrombocytopenia, which may be delayed in appearance. Mitomycin is capable of inducing pulmonary fibrosis, with an incidence ranging between 3% and 12%. Glomerular damage resulting in renal failure is a rare but well-recognized complication.

VI. **Platinating Drugs**

A. **Cisplatin** results in chemotherapeutic effects resembling DNA alkylating drugs by cross-linking adjacent or opposing guanine bases to disrupt DNA. The drug must be administered IV because oral ingestion is ineffective. High concentrations of cisplatin are found in the kidneys, liver, intestines, and testes, but there is poor penetration into the CNS (treatment of many nonhematologic malignancies, including lung, bladder, testicular, and ovarian cancer).

1. **Side Effects**

   a. Renal toxicity is prominent and becomes the dose-limiting toxic effect of cisplatin.

   b. Hypomagnesemia that is associated with cisplatin's renal tubular injury may predispose to cardiac dysrhythmias and decrease the dose requirements for neuromuscular blocking drugs.

   c. Ototoxicity caused by cisplatin is manifested by tinnitus and hearing loss in the high-frequency range.

   d. Cisplatin is considered highly emetogenic, with marked nausea and vomiting occurring in almost all patients who do not receive antiemetics.

   e. Peripheral sensory neuropathies, paresthesias, and loss of vibratory and position sense are common findings. Most neuropathies are reversible, although symptoms may persist for months.

VII. **Antimetabolites (folate analogues, pyrimidine analogues, purine analogues) are particularly effective in destroying cells during the S phase of the cell cycle, which is when DNA** is synthesized. Side effects (myelosuppression and mucositis) reflect effects on proliferating but nonmalignant cells.

A. **Folate Analogues**

1. **Methotrexate** is a poorly lipid-soluble folate analogue that is effective in the treatment of different hematologic and nonhematologic cancers. Significant metabolism of methotrexate does not seem to occur, with more than 50% of the drug appearing unchanged in urine.

   a. **Clinical Uses.** Methotrexate is a useful drug in the treatment of acute lymphoblastic leukemia in children but not adults. Choriocarcinoma is effectively treated with this drug. Improvement in the clinical manifestations of psoriasis in patients reflects the effect of methotrexate on rapidly dividing epidermal cells. This drug may also be useful in the treatment of rheumatoid arthritis. Methotrexate is poorly transported across the blood–brain barrier, and neoplastic cells that have entered the CNS probably are not affected.

   b. **Side Effects.** Leukopenia and thrombocytopenia reflect bone marrow depression. Ulcerative stomatitis and diarrhea are frequent side effects and require interruption of treatment. Hemorrhagic enteritis and death from intestinal perforation may occur. Pulmonary toxicity may take the form of fulminant non-cardiogenic pulmonary edema, or a more progressive inflammation, with interstitial infiltrates and pleural effusions. Short-term or intermittent therapy with methotrexate results in increases in liver transaminase enzymes. Normal cells can be protected from lethal damage by folate antagonists with sequential administration of folinic acid (leucovorin), thymidine, or both (termed the *rescue technique*).

B. **Pyrimidine analogues** (fluorouracil and cytarabine) prevent the biosynthesis of pyrimidine nucleotides and interfere with synthesis and functioning of nucleic acids.

1. **Fluorouracil** lacks significant inhibitory activity on cells and must be converted enzymatically to a 5′-monophosphate nucleotide. Fluorouracil readily enters the cerebrospinal fluid.

   a. **Clinical Uses.** Fluorouracil may be of palliative value in certain types of carcinoma, particularly of the breast and gastrointestinal tract. The drug is often used for the topical treatment of premalignant keratoses of the skin and superficial basal cell carcinomas.

    b. **Side effects** caused by fluorouracil are difficult to anticipate because of their delayed appearance. Fluorouracil-induced myocardial ischemia is a rare cardiac toxicity that may lead to myocardial infarction up to 1 week after treatment. Myelosuppression, most frequently manifesting as leukopenia between 9 and 14 days of therapy, is a serious side effect. Thrombocytopenia and anemia may complicate treatment with fluorouracil. Loss of hair progressing to total alopecia may occur.

2. **Cytarabine**, like other pyrimidine antimetabolites, must be activated by conversion to the $5'$-monophosphate nucleotide before inhibition of DNA synthesis can occur. Resistance to cytarabine reflects activity of cytidine deaminase, an enzyme capable of converting cytarabine to the inactive metabolite arabinosyl uracil.

    a. **Clinical Uses**. Cytarabine is particularly useful in chemotherapy of acute granulocytic leukemia in adults.

    b. **Side Effects**. Cytarabine is a potent myelosuppressive drug capable of producing severe leukopenia, thrombocytopenia, and anemia. Cerebellar toxicity and ataxia can occur at high doses. Thrombophlebitis at the site of infusion is common.

C. **Purine Analogues (Mercaptopurine, Azathioprine, Thioguanine, Pentostatin, Cladribine)**

1. **Mercaptopurine** is incorporated into DNA or RNA strands and either blocks further strand synthesis or causes structural alterations that damage DNA. This drug is useful in the treatment of acute leukemia in children. Allopurinol, as an inhibitor of xanthine oxidase, prevents conversion of mercaptopurine to 6-thiouric acid and thus increases the exposure of cells to mercaptopurine (dose is decreased by about one-third when the drug is combined with allopurinol).

    a. **Side Effects**. The principal side effect of mercaptopurine is a gradual development of bone marrow depression manifesting as thrombocytopenia, granulocytopenia, or anemia several weeks after initiation of therapy. Jaundice occurs in approximately one-third of patients and is associated with bile stasis and occasional hepatic necrosis. Hyperuricemia and hyperuricosuria may occur during treatment with mercaptopurine, presumably reflecting destruction of cells (may require the use of allopurinol).

2. **Thioguanine** is of particular value in the treatment of acute myelogenous leukemia, especially if given with cytarabine. Minimal amounts of 6-thiouric acid are formed (may be administered concurrently with allopurinol without a decrease in dosage).

3. **Pentostatin and cladribine** are purine analogues that have clinical activity against a variety of indolent lymphoid tumors, with the most dramatic effects occurring in patients with hairy cell leukemia. Patients with acute leukemia and cells with high levels of adenosine deaminase activity are most likely to respond to these drugs.

4. **Hydroxyurea** acts on the enzyme ribonucleoside diphosphate reductase to interfere with the synthesis of DNA. The primary use of hydroxyurea is in the treatment of chronic myelogenous leukemia.

   a. **Side Effects.** Myelosuppression manifesting as leukopenia, megaloblastic anemia, and occasionally thrombocytopenia is the major side effect produced by hydroxyurea.

VIII. **Topoisomerase Inhibitors (Doxorubicin, Daunorubicin, Etoposide, Teniposide). Topoisomerases are enzymes that correct alterations in DNA, which occur during replication and transcription. Because cancer cells possess more topoisomerase activity than normal cells, there is more drug-induced DNA damage and resultant cell death. Toxicity reflects effects of inhibition of topoisomerase enzymes on normal proliferating tissues (myelosuppression, mucositis). These drugs exhibit a broad spectrum of chemotherapeutic activity being useful in the treatment of leukemia, lung, colon, and ovarian cancer.**

A. **Doxorubicin and daunorubicin** are anthracycline antibiotics that are natural products of certain soil fungi. Drug-induced free radicals may overwhelm the heart's antioxidant defenses leading to cardiotoxicity. Daunorubicin and doxorubicin are administered IV, with care taken to prevent extravasation because local vesicant action may result. Ultimately, approximately 40% of daunorubicin and doxorubicin are metabolized (may result in hepatic dysfunction).

1. **Clinical Uses.** Daunorubicin is used primarily in the treatment of acute lymphocytic and myelocytic leukemia. Doxorubicin is one of the most active single drugs for treating metastatic adenocarcinoma of the breast, carcinoma of the bladder, bronchogenic carcinoma,

metastatic thyroid carcinoma, oat cell carcinoma, and osteogenic carcinoma.

2. **Side Effects**. Cardiomyopathy and myelosuppression are side effects of the chemotherapeutic antibiotics.

   a. **Cardiomyopathy** is a unique dose-related and often irreversible side effect of the anthracycline antibiotics (congestive heart failure develops in <3% of patients with a cumulative dose of doxorubicin of <400 mg/m², rising to 18% at 700 mg/m²) (Fig. 42-2). Previous treatment with anthracycline antibiotics may enhance myocardial depressant effects of anesthetic drugs even in patients with normal resting cardiac function.

   b. An acute form of cardiomyopathy occurs in approximately 10% of patients and is characterized by relatively benign changes on the ECG (resolve 1 to 2 months after discontinuation of therapy). There is an associated acute reversible decrease in the ejection fraction within 24 hours after a single dose.

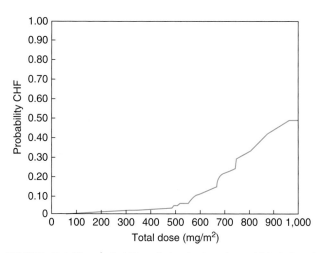

FIGURE 42-2 The probability of developing doxorubicin-induced congestive heart failure (CHF) versus the total cumulative dose of doxorubicin. (From Von Hoff DD, Layard MW, Basa P, et al. Risk factors for doxorubicin-induced congestive heart failure. *Ann Intern Med.* 1979;91:710–707, with permission.)

    c. A second form of cardiomyopathy is characterized by the insidious onset of symptoms such as dry nonproductive cough, suggesting bronchitis, followed by rapidly progressive heart failure that is unresponsive to inotropic drugs and mechanical ventricular assistance (occurs in almost 2% of treated patients and is fatal approximately 3 weeks after the onset of symptoms in nearly 60% of affected patients). Predictive tests to permit early recognition of impending cardiomyopathy are not available, although diminution in QRS voltage on the ECG is consistent with the diffuse character of the myocardial damage. Systolic time intervals and echocardiograms have been used to detect cardiotoxicity before the occurrence of clinically significant damage. Dexrazoxane is a free-radical scavenger that protects the heart from doxorubicin-associated damage.

B. **Dactinomycin** (actinomycin D) is an antibiotic with chemotherapeutic activity resulting from its ability to bind to DNA, especially in rapidly proliferating cells. There is no evidence that the drug undergoes metabolism. Dactinomycin does not cross the blood–brain barrier in amounts sufficient to produce a pharmacologic effect.

    1. **Clinical Uses.** The most important clinical use of dactinomycin is the treatment of Wilms tumor in children and of rhabdomyosarcoma.

    2. **Side Effects.** The toxic effects of dactinomycin include the early onset of nausea and vomiting, often followed by myelosuppression manifesting as pancytopenia 1 to 7 days after completion of therapy.

C. **Bleomycin.** In the presence of oxygen and either iron or copper, bleomycin produces free radicals that create DNA breaks. Bleomycin is eliminated primarily by renal excretion (excessive concentrations of drug occur if usual doses are administered to patients with impaired renal function).

    1. **Clinical Uses.** Bleomycin is effective in the treatment of testicular carcinoma, particularly if administered in combination with vinblastine.

    2. **Side Effects.** The most common side effects of bleomycin are mucocutaneous reactions. In contrast to other chemotherapeutic drugs, bleomycin causes minimal myelosuppression. Unexplained exacerbations of rheumatoid arthritis have occurred. Patients with lymphomas who are receiving bleomycin may develop an acute reaction characterized by hyperthermia, hypotension,

and hypoventilation (likely mechanism is the release of an endogenous pyrogen, presumably from destroyed tumor cells).

a. **Pulmonary Toxicity**. The most serious side effect of bleomycin is dose-related pulmonary toxicity (bleomycin is concentrated preferentially in the lungs and is inactivated by a hydrolase enzyme, which is relatively deficient in lung tissue) (Fig. 42-3). Some form of pulmonary toxicity (most often pulmonary fibrosis) occurs in 4% of patients treated with bleomycin.

b. The first signs of pulmonary toxicity are cough, dyspnea, and basilar rales, which may progress as a mild form of pulmonary toxicity (exertional dyspnea and a normal resting Pao_2) or more severe form of arterial hypoxemia at rest is associated with radiographic findings of interstitial pneumonitis and fibrosis.

c. Acutely increased inhaled concentrations of oxygen facilitate production of superoxide and other free radicals in the presence of bleomycin (it has been recommended that inhaled oxygen concentrations be maintained below 30% in bleomycin-treated patients).

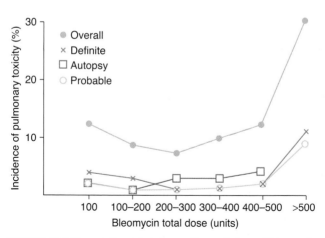

FIGURE 42-3 The relationship between the total dose of bleomycin and the incidence of pulmonary toxicity. (From Ginsberg SJ, Comis RL. The pulmonary toxicity of antineoplastic agents. *Semin Oncol.* 1982;9:34–51, with permission.)

> ### Table 42-3
>
> Risk Factors for Development of Chemotherapy-Induced Pulmonary Toxicity
>
> Total drug dose
> Age
> Concurrent or prior chest radiation
> Oxygen therapy
> Combination chemotherapy
> Preexisting pulmonary disease
> Genetic predisposition
> Cigarette smoking (?)

    d. A more practical question is whether hyperoxia for short periods of time several days after treatment is a risk factor for bleomycin-induced pulmonary damage. Patients with prior exposure to bleomycin but with no risk factors appear to be at a minimum risk from hyperoxia (Table 42-3).

    e. In contrast, those patients with one or more major risk factors (preexisting pulmonary damage from bleomycin, renal dysfunction, prior exposure to bleomycin within a 1- to 2-month period) may be at higher risk for the development of bleomycin-induced hyperoxic pulmonary injury in the operating room. It may be prudent to maintain these patients on the minimum inspired oxygen concentration that can be used safely intraoperatively to provide oxygen saturations of greater than 90%.

    f. The role of excessive crystalloid administration has not received the same scrutiny as increased delivered oxygen concentrations. A consideration in this regard is replacement of fluids with colloids rather than crystalloids to decrease or prevent pulmonary interstitial edema in bleomycin-treated patients undergoing surgery.

    g. In the future, bleomycin may be replaced with phleomycin, an analogue of bleomycin that has lower pulmonary toxicity and a broader effectiveness against multiple types of tumors.

IX. **Tubulin-Binding Drugs. Microtubules are subcellular structures that maintain cell shape; organize the location of** organelles; and mediate intracellular transport and secretion, neurotransmission, and cell motility. Vinca alkaloids bind to depolymerized microtubules and inhibit microtubule formation. Taxanes bind to polymerized microtubules and inhibit their breakdown. The result of these interactions is the failure of the cell to undergo normal mitosis leading to cell death.

A. **Vinca alkaloids** represent the active medicinal ingredients from the pink periwinkle plant (vincristine, vinblastine, vinorelbine, vindesine). Vincristine is highly effective against Hodgkin disease, non-Hodgkin lymphoma, and pediatric solid tumors. Vinorelbine is active against breast and lung cancer. Vinblastine is most often used in the treatment of testicular cancer and non-Hodgkin lymphoma.

1. **Side Effects**
   a. Myelosuppression manifesting as leukopenia, thrombocytopenia, and anemia are the most prominent side effects of vinca alkaloids, appearing 7 to 10 days after initiation of treatment.
   b. Symmetric peripheral sensory–motor neuropathy often occurs during administration of therapeutic doses of vincristine and may become the dose-limiting side effect.
   c. Autonomic neuropathy with orthostatic hypotension, bowel motility dysfunction, and cranial nerve involvement (laryngeal nerve paralysis with hoarseness, weakness of the extraocular muscles) are present in about 10% of treated patients.

B. **Taxanes**. Paclitaxel (active extract from the Pacific yew tree) and docetaxel (more water-soluble semisynthetic derivative) share a broad spectrum of similar chemotherapeutic activity against breast, lung, ovarian, and bladder cancer.

1. **Side Effects**. Taxanes are associated with myelosuppression, peripheral neuropathy, and alopecia. Cardiac effects including dysrhythmias, myocardial ischemia, and transient asymptomatic bradycardia may be more common with paclitaxel than docetaxel. Docetaxel seems to have unique vascular permeability properties that may result in peripheral edema, pleural effusion, and ascites.

X. **Signal transduction modulators (hormones)** that may be useful in the treatment of neoplastic disease include antiestrogens, antiandrogens, aromatase inhibitors, gonadotropin-releasing drugs, and progestin. Mutations in cancer cells result in uncontrolled cell proliferation using activated signaling pathways. Hormonal treatment of cancer disrupts growth factor receptor interactions.

A. **Progestins** act by reducing the production of hormones that stimulate the neoplastic endometrium.

B. **Estrogens and Androgens**
1. Malignant changes in the breast and prostate often depend on hormones for their continued growth. Eventually, prostatic tumors become insensitive to the lack of androgen or the presence of estrogens, presumably because of the survival of progressively undifferentiated cells that favor the emergence of cell types that no longer depend on androgens for their growth.
2. Hypercalcemia may be associated with androgen or estrogen therapy, requiring adequate hydration in an attempt to facilitate renal excretion of calcium (plasma calcium concentrations should be determined in patients receiving treatment with these hormones).

C. **Antiestrogens** such as tamoxifen are useful in the treatment of breast cancer that expresses estrogen or progesterone receptors (binds to estrogen receptors and disrupts receptor interactions with estrogen).

D. **Antiandrogens** (flutamide, bicalutamide, nilutamide) are competitive antagonists of the interactions between androstenedione and androgen receptors.
1. Administered with other drugs that decrease androgen production, flutamide is an effective treatment for hormone-dependent prostate cancer.
2. Skeletal muscle weakness and development of osteoporosis reflect a male menopause-like state.
3. Flutamide can induce methemoglobinemia (pulse oximetry readings in the presence of methemoglobinemia can overestimate the hemoglobin saturation levels).

XI. **Monoclonal antibodies (trastuzumab, alemtuzumab, rituximab, imatinib) target specific antigen sites on cancer cells Vaccines may induce genetic manipulation of cancer cells to make them more antigenic and thus susceptible to immune responses (vaccines against the hepatitis B virus, specific human papillomaviruses).**

XII. **Aromatase inhibitors block the conversion of androgens to estrone in peripheral tissues including breast tissue (results in intense inhibition of estrogen effects on responsive receptors).**

CHAPTER 43

Drugs Used for Psychopharmacologic Therapy

I. **Introduction.** Drugs used for psychopharmacologic therapy include antidepressants, anxiolytics, lithium, antipsychotics, and anticonvulsants. It is well accepted that anesthesia can be safely administered to patients being treated with drugs used to treat mental illness (past recommendations for discontinuation of antidepressant therapy are not justified). It is important to be alert for potential drug interactions.

II. **Antidepressants.** Considering the wide range of disorders for which antidepressant drugs are effective, the term *antidepressant* has become a misnomer (Table 43-1). Antidepressants are logically classified based on their chemical structures and their acute neuropharmacologic effects (Table 43-2). Neurobiologically, reuptake blockade or monoamine oxidase (MAO) inhibition (necessary for breakdown of free norepinephrine and serotonin) occurs promptly after initiation of antidepressant therapy, but clinical improvement typically does not occur for 2 to 4 weeks. Perhaps adaptive changes including downregulation of neurotransmitter receptors are necessary before evidence of clinical improvement appears.

   A. **Selective serotonin reuptake inhibitors (SSRIs)** are the most broadly prescribed class of antidepressants and are the drugs of choice for the treatment of mild to moderate depression. Compared with tricyclic antidepressants, SSRIs lack anticholinergic properties, do not cause postural hypotension or delayed conduction of cardiac impulses, and do not appear to have a major effect on the seizure threshold. Perhaps the most important advantage of SSRIs compared with tricyclic antidepressants is the relative safety of SSRIs when taken in overdose. Abrupt discontinuation of SSRIs with short elimination half-times may be associated with dizziness, paresthesias, myalgias, irritability, insomnia, and visual disturbances. Suicidal tendencies in children and

Table 43-1

Clinical Uses of Antidepressant Drugs

Unipolar and bipolar depression
Panic disorder
Social phobia
Posttraumatic stress syndrome
Neuropathic pain
Migraine prophylaxis
Obsessive-compulsive disorder
Bulimia
Childhood attention deficit hyperactivity disorder

adolescents may be increased in those age groups when they are treated with SSRIs.

1. **Fluoxetine** is commonly administered once daily in the morning to decrease the risk of insomnia. Because fluoxetine has a prolonged elimination half-time (1 to 3 days for acute administration and 4 to 6 days for chronic administration), the drug can be taken every other day.

   a. **Side Effects.** The most common side effects of fluoxetine are nausea, anorexia, insomnia, sexual dysfunction, agitation, and neuromuscular restlessness, which may mimic akathisia. Like tricyclic antidepressants, fluoxetine may be an effective analgesic for treatment of chronic pain as may be associated with rheumatoid arthritis. Fluoxetine does not cause hypotension, and changes in conduction of cardiac impulses seem infrequent. Because of its long elimination half-time, fluoxetine should be discontinued for about 5 weeks before initiating treatment with an MAO inhibitor. The long elimination half-time of fluoxetine appears to prevent withdrawal symptoms induced by abrupt discontinuance of the drug. An overdose with fluoxetine alone is not associated with the risk of cardiovascular and central nervous system (CNS) toxicity.

   b. **Drug Interactions**. Among the SSRIs, fluoxetine is the most potent inhibitor of certain hepatic cytochrome P450 enzymes. As a result, this drug may increase the plasma concentrations of drugs that depend on hepatic metabolism for clearance (addition of fluoxetine to treatment with a tricyclic

Table 43-2

Comparative Pharmacology of Antidepressant Drugs

	Sedative Potency	Anticholinergic Potency	Orthostatic Hypotension
Selective serotonin reuptake inhibitors			
Fluoxetine	+	+	+
Sertraline	+	+	+
Paroxetine	+	+	+
Fluvoxamine	+	+	+
Citalopram	+	+	+
Escitalopram	+	+	+
Bupropion	+		
Venlafaxine	+	+	May cause hypertension in some individuals + +
Trazodone	+ + +	+	Associated with cardiac dysrhythmias + +
Nefazodone	+ + +	+	+ +
Tricyclic and related cyclic compounds[a]			
Amitriptyline	+ + +	+ + + +	+ + +
Amoxapine	+	+ +	+ +

Table 43-2

Comparative Pharmacology of Antidepressant Drugs *(continued)*

	Sedative Potency	Anticholinergic Potency	Orthostatic Hypotension
Clomipramine	+ + +	+ + +	+ + +
Desipramine	+	+	+ + + +
Doxepin	+ + +	+ +	+ + +
Imipramine	+ + αω	+ +	+ + + +
Nortriptyline	+	+	0
Protriptyline	+	+ + +	+ +
Trimipramine	+ + +	+ +	+ +
Mirtazapine			
Monoamine oxidase inhibitors			
Phenelzine	+	+ +	+ + +
Tranylcypromine	+	+	+ + +
Isocarboxazid	+		+ + +

a All tricyclic and related cyclic compounds may produce cardiac dysrhythmias.
0, none; +, mild; + +, moderate; + + +, marked; + + + +, greatest.

antidepressant drug may result in a two- to fivefold increase in the plasma concentration of the tricyclic drug). MAO inhibitors combined with fluoxetine may cause the development of a serotonin syndrome characterized by anxiety, restlessness, chills, ataxia, and insomnia.

2. **Sertraline** has a spectrum of efficacy similar to fluoxetine. This drug has a shorter elimination half-time (25 hours) than fluoxetine and is a less potent inhibitor of hepatic microsomal enzymes. The recommended washout period before starting an MAO inhibitor is 14 days.

3. **Paroxetine** has an efficacy similar to that of fluoxetine. This drug has a relatively short elimination half-time (24 hours), and there are no active metabolites. Side effects resemble those of other SSRIs with the exception of a possibly increased incidence of sedation. Paroxetine produces less inhibition of hepatic cytoplasmic P450 enzymes than is fluoxetine. Enhancement of the anticoagulant effect of warfarin reflects competition for common protein-binding sites. The recommended washout period before starting an MAO inhibitor is 14 days.

4. **Citalopram/Escitalopram (S Isomer of Citalopram).** Citalopram causes dose-dependent QT interval prolongation, which can place patients at risk for torsades de pointes. Escitalopram may also prolong the QT interval but possibly to a lesser degree.

5. **Fluvoxamine** is effective in the management of obsessive-compulsive disorders. Although it produces less inhibition of hepatic cytoplasmic P450 enzymes than the other SSRIs, fluvoxamine may still cause clinically significant drug interactions.

6. **Bupropion** is effective in the treatment of major depression, producing improvement in 2 to 4 weeks. In addition, bupropion is effective for smoking cessation. Unlike the SSRIs, bupropion is not associated with significant drug interactions and is not commonly associated with sexual dysfunction.

7. **Venlafaxine** is perceived to have a profile of efficacy similar to that of the tricyclic antidepressants but does not produce anticholinergic effects or postural hypotension.

8. **Duloxetine.** Indications for its use include major depression, fibromyalgia, and diabetic neuropathy. Duloxetine should be avoided in patients with severe renal

dysfunction and chronic liver disease. The potential for the development of serotonin syndrome is present when this drug is used in conjunction with another serotonergic drug.

9. **Trazodone** is effective in the management of depression but its greatest efficacy may be treatment of insomnia induced by SSRIs or bupropion.

10. **Nefazodone** is chemically related to trazodone but with fewer α_1-adrenergic blocking properties. The risk of sedation and priapism may be less than in patients treated with trazodone. Orthostatic hypotension may occur.

B. **Management of Anesthesia**

1. SSRIs may have antiplatelet activity and increase the risk of bleeding particularly in the setting of antiplatelet medication use.

2. The risks of discontinuing an SSRI may take 2 to 3 weeks for full washout and reinitiation may require 2 to 4 weeks for reestablishment of clinical antidepressant effect. Furthermore, discontinuation of a patient's SSRI may expose them to the risks of a major depressive episode.

C. **Tricyclic and Related Antidepressants**. Before the availability of SSRIs, tricyclic antidepressants and related cyclic antidepressants were the most commonly used drugs to treat depression (see Table 43-2). Although tricyclic antidepressants are highly effective, they have been supplanted as first-line drugs in many clinical situations because of their unfavorable side effect profile (largely resulting from their anticholinergic, antiadrenergic, and antihistaminic properties). Tricyclic antidepressants also have a narrow therapeutic index and are potentially lethal in overdose.

1. **Chronic Pain Syndromes**. The tricyclic antidepressants (especially amitriptyline and imipramine), in doses lower than those used to treat depression, may be useful in the treatment of chronic neuropathic pain and other chronic pain syndromes including fibromyalgia. The efficacy of tricyclic antidepressants on chronic pain syndromes may be limited by a narrow therapeutic index and intolerability of side effects.

2. **Structure–Activity Relationships**. The structure of tricyclic antidepressants resembles that of local anesthetics and phenothiazines.

a. Imipramine, which is the prototype of the tricyclic antidepressants, differs from phenothiazine only in the replacement of the sulfur atom with an ethylene linkage to produce a seven-membered central ring.

b. Desipramine is the principal metabolite of imipramine, and nortriptyline is the demethylated metabolite of amitriptyline.

3. **Mechanism of Action**. Tricyclic antidepressants act at several transporters and receptors, but their antidepressant effect is likely produced by blocking the reuptake (uptake) of serotonin and/or norepinephrine at presynaptic terminals, thereby increasing the availability of these neurotransmitters.

4. **Pharmacokinetics**. Tricyclic antidepressants are efficiently absorbed from the gastrointestinal tract after oral administration, reflecting high lipid solubility. The long elimination half-time (17 to 30 hours) and wide range of therapeutic plasma concentrations make once-daily dosing intervals effective.

5. **Metabolism**. Tricyclic antidepressants are oxidized by microsomal enzymes in the liver with subsequent conjugation with glucuronic acid. Imipramine is metabolized to the active compound desipramine.

6. **Side Effects (see Table 43-2)**

a. **Anticholinergic effects** of tricyclic antidepressants are prominent, especially at high doses. Amitriptyline causes the highest incidence of anticholinergic effects (dry mouth, blurred vision, tachycardia, urinary retention, slowed gastric emptying, ileus), whereas desipramine produces the fewest such effects.

b. **Cardiovascular Effects**. Orthostatic hypotension and modest increases in heart rate are the most common cardiovascular side effects of tricyclic antidepressants (orthostatic hypotension may be particularly hazardous in elderly patients, who are at increased risk of fractures when they fall). The risk of hypotension during general anesthesia in patients treated with tricyclic antidepressants is low. Previous suggestions that tricyclic antidepressants increase the risks of cardiac dysrhythmias and sudden death have not been substantiated in the absence of drug overdose. Atropine is a useful treatment when tricyclic antidepressants dangerously slow atrioventricular or intraventricular conduction of cardiac impulses. Direct cardiac depressant effects may reflect quinidine-like actions of tricyclic antidepressants on the heart.

    c. **Central Nervous System Effects**. Sedation associated with tricyclic antidepressant therapy may be desirable for management of depressed patients with insomnia. Tricyclic antidepressants lower the seizure threshold, raising the question of the advisability of administering these drugs to patients with seizure disorders. Treatment with tricyclic antidepressants may enhance the CNS-stimulating effects of enflurane. Because of their cardiac toxicity, tendency to cause seizures, and depressant properties on the CNS, the tricyclic antidepressants may be fatal if taken in an overdose. The combination of a tricyclic antidepressant and an MAO inhibitor may result in CNS toxicity manifesting as hyperthermia, seizures, and coma.

7. **Drug Interactions**

    a. **Sympathomimetics**. For patients recently started on tricyclic antidepressants, exaggerated pressor responses should be anticipated whether or not direct-acting or indirect-acting sympathomimetics are administered, whereas in individuals chronically treated with tricyclic antidepressants (>6 weeks), administration of either a direct-acting or indirect-acting sympathomimetic is acceptable. Induction of anesthesia may be associated with an increased incidence of cardiac dysrhythmias in patients treated with tricyclic antidepressants. The dose of exogenous epinephrine necessary to produce cardiac dysrhythmias during anesthesia with a volatile anesthetic is decreased by tricyclic antidepressants.

    b. **Anticholinergics**. Because the anticholinergic side effects of drugs may be additive, the use of centrally active anticholinergic drugs for preoperative medication of patients treated with tricyclic antidepressants could increase the likelihood of postoperative delirium and confusion (central anticholinergic syndrome). Glycopyrrolate would theoretically be less likely to evoke this type of drug interaction in patients being treated with tricyclic antidepressants.

    c. **Antihypertensives**. Rebound hypertension after abrupt discontinuation of clonidine may be accentuated and prolonged by concomitant tricyclic antidepressant therapy.

    d. **Opioids**. In animals, tricyclic antidepressants augment the analgesic and ventilatory depressant effects of opioids.

8. **Tolerance** to anticholinergic effects (dry mouth, blurred vision, tachycardia) and orthostatic hypotension develops during chronic therapy with tricyclic antidepressants.

9. **Overdose**
   a. Tricyclic antidepressant overdose is life-threatening, as the progression from an alert state to unresponsiveness may be rapid. Intractable myocardial depression or ventricular cardiac dysrhythmias are the most frequent terminal events.
   b. Presenting features of tricyclic antidepressant overdose include agitation and seizures followed by coma, depression of ventilation, hypotension, hypothermia, and striking evidence of anticholinergic effects including mydriasis, flushed dry skin, urinary retention, and tachycardia. The QRS complex on the electrocardiogram (ECG) may be prolonged to greater than 100 milliseconds.
   c. Treatment of a life-threatening overdose of a tricyclic antidepressant is directed toward management of CNS and cardiac toxicity (Table 43-3).

D. **Monoamine Oxidase Inhibitors**. MAO inhibitors constitute a heterogenous group of drugs that block the enzyme

---

Table 43-3

Pharmacologic Treatment of Tricyclic Antidepressant Overdose

Symptom	Treatment
Seizures	Diazepam
	Sodium bicarbonate
	Phenytoin
Ventricular cardiac dysrhythmias	Sodium bicarbonate
	Lidocaine
	Phenytoin
Heart block	Isoproterenol
Hypotension	Crystalloid or colloid solutions
	Sodium bicarbonate
	Sympathomimetics
	Inotropics

Data from Frommer DA, Kulig KW, Marx JA, et al. Tricyclic antidepressant overdose. *JAMA*. 1987;257:521–526, with permission.

Table 43-4

Dietary Restrictions in Patients Treated with Monoamine Oxidase Inhibitors

Prohibited foods
Cheese
Liver
Fava beans
Avocados
Chianti wine
Prohibited drugs
Cyclic antidepressants
Fluoxetine
Cold or allergy medications
Nasal decongestants
Sympathomimetic drugs
Opioids (especially meperidine)

that metabolizes biogenic amines, increasing the availability of these neurotransmitters in the CNS and peripheral autonomic nervous system. MAO inhibitors are used less commonly because their administration is complicated by side effects (hypotension), lethality in overdose, and lack of simplicity in dosing. Patients treated with MAO inhibitors must follow a specific tyramine-free diet because of the potential for pharmacodynamic interactions with tyramine that can result in systemic hypertension (Table 43-4).

1. **Monoamine oxidase enzyme** system is a flavin-containing enzyme found principally on outer mitochondrial membranes (Fig. 43-1).
2. **Mechanism of Action**
   a. MAO inhibitors act by forming a stable, irreversible complex with MAO enzyme, especially with cerebral neuronal MAO. As a result, the amount of neurotransmitter (norepinephrine) available for release from CNS neurons increases. These effects, however, are not limited to the brain, and the concentration of norepinephrine also increases in the sympathetic nervous system.
   b. Because MAO inhibitors cause irreversible enzyme inhibition, their effects are prolonged as the synthesis of new enzyme is a slow process.

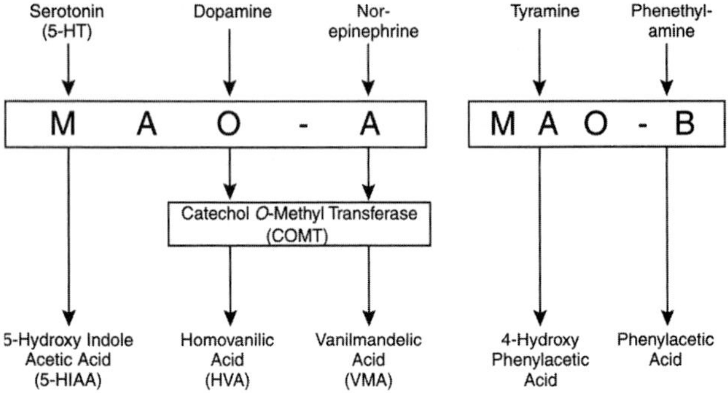

FIGURE 43-1 The two forms of monoamine oxidase enzyme (MAO-A and MAO-B) exhibit substrate selectivity. (From Michaels I, Serrins M, Shier NQ, et al. Anesthesia for cardiac surgery in patients receiving monoamine oxidase inhibitors. *Anesth Analg.* 1984;63:1041–1044, with permission.)

3. **Side Effects**
   a. The most common serious side effect of MAO inhibitors is orthostatic hypotension (may reflect accumulation of the false neurotransmitter octopamine).
   b. Weight gain is a common side effect of treatment with MAO inhibitors.
   c. In contrast with tricyclic antidepressants is the failure of MAO inhibitors to produce cardiac dysrhythmias.

4. **Dietary Restrictions (see Table 43-4)**
   a. MAO enzyme present in the liver, gastrointestinal tract, kidneys, and lungs seems to perform a protective function in deactivating circulating monoamines (initial defense against monoamines absorbed from foods, such as tyramine and β-phenylethanolamine, which would otherwise produce an indirect sympathomimetic response and precipitous hypertension).
   b. MAO-A is found in the gastrointestinal tract and liver, where it acts to metabolize bioactive amines such as tyramine. The MAO inhibitors used in the United States as antidepressants inhibit MAO-A and MAO-B nonselectively.
   c. Because patients treated with MAO inhibitors cannot metabolize dietary tyramine and other monoamines, these compounds can enter the systemic circulation and be taken up by sympathetic

nervous system nerve endings. This uptake can elicit massive release of endogenous catecholamines and result in a hyperadrenergic crisis characterized by hypertension (resembles that which occurs with the release of catecholamines from a pheochromocytoma), hyperpyrexia, and cerebral vascular accident.

d. Treatment of hypertension is with a peripheral vasodilator such as nitroprusside. Cardiac dysrhythmias that persist after control of systemic blood pressure are treated with lidocaine or a β-adrenergic antagonist.

5. **Drug Interactions**. In addition to interacting with foods, MAO inhibitors can interact adversely with opioids, sympathomimetic drugs, tricyclic antidepressants, and SSRIs. These interactions can result in hypertension, CNS excitation, delirium, seizures, and death. In animals, anesthetic requirements for volatile anesthetics are increased, presumably reflecting accumulation of norepinephrine in the CNS.

   a. **Opioids and Monoamine Oxidase Inhibitors**. Administration of meperidine to a patient treated with MAO inhibitors may result in an excitatory (type I) response (agitation, headache, skeletal muscle rigidity, hyperpyrexia) or a depressive (type II) response characterized by hypotension, depression of ventilation, and coma. Derivatives of meperidine (fentanyl, sufentanil, alfentanil) have been associated with adverse reactions in patients treated with MAO inhibitors. Morphine does not inhibit uptake of serotonin, but its opioid effects may be potentiated in the presence of MAO inhibitors.

   b. **Sympathomimetics and Monoamine Oxidase Inhibitors**. There is no experimental evidence to support the recommendation that all sympathomimetic drugs be avoided in patients treated with MAO inhibitors. If needed, the use of a direct-acting sympathomimetic (phenylephrine) is preferable to an indirect-acting drug (decrease the dose to about one-third of normal, with additional titration of doses based on cardiovascular responses).

   c. **Overdose**. Overdose with an MAO inhibitor is reflected by signs of excessive sympathetic nervous system activity (tachycardia, hyperthermia, mydriasis), seizures, and coma. Treatment is supportive in addition to gastric lavage.

6. **Management of Anesthesia**
   a. In the past, it was a common recommendation to discontinue MAO inhibitors 2 to 3 weeks before elective surgery based on the concern that life-threatening cardiovascular and CNS instability could occur during anesthesia and surgery (seems to be based more on anecdotes and isolated responses than on controlled scientific studies). There is growing appreciation that anesthesia can be safely administered in most patients being chronically treated with MAO inhibitors. When anesthesia is administered to patients treated with MAO inhibitors, it remains prudent to consider certain drug interactions and to avoid certain drugs, if possible.
   b. **Selection of Drugs Used during Anesthesia**. The anesthetic technique selected should minimize the possibility of sympathetic nervous system stimulation or drug-induced hypotension. Regional anesthesia as in parturients is acceptable, recognizing the disadvantage of these techniques should hypotension require administration of a sympathomimetic. If regional anesthesia is performed, a cautious approach is not to add epinephrine to the local anesthetic solution. Etomidate and thiopental have been administered to MAO inhibitor–treated patients undergoing electroconvulsive therapy without adverse effects. Responses to nondepolarizing neuromuscular blocking drugs are not altered by MAO inhibitors.

III. **Serotonin syndrome (mild tremor to altered mental status, clonus, and hyperthermia) occurs when there is an excess of serotonin agonism in the central and peripheral nervous systems (Table 43-5).**
   A. Selective serotonin reuptake inhibitors, tricyclic antidepressants, and MAO inhibitors, particularly in combination, have all been associated with serotonin syndrome.
   B. The differential diagnosis includes malignant hyperthermia, neuroleptic malignant syndrome, and anticholinergic poisoning (see Table 43-5).
   C. Management of serotonin syndrome includes hemodynamic and respiratory supportive care, control of agitation with sedatives, and control of hyperthermia

IV. **Anxiolytics**
   A. **Benzodiazepines** are used clinically as anxiolytics, sedatives, anticonvulsants, and muscle relaxants (appear

Table 43-5

Serotonin Syndrome and Commonly Mistaken Diagnoses

Diagnosis	Inciting Agent	Time Course	Fever	Physical Examination
Serotonin syndrome	Serotonergic agonists	<12 h	>41°	Mydriasis, drooling, sweating, hyperactive reflexes, agitation, coma
Anticholinergic syndrome	Muscarinic antagonists	<12 h	<39°	Mydriasis, dry mouth and skin, normal reflexes, delirium
Neuroleptic malignant syndrome	Dopamine antagonists	1–3 d after dosing	>41°	Normal pupils, drooling, pallor, lead-pipe rigidity, hyporeflexia, alert mutism, coma
Malignant hyperthermia	Volatile anesthetic and/or succinylcholine	Onset immediate to 24 h after administration	To 46°	Normal pupils, mottled sweaty skin, total body rigidity, hyporeflexia, agitation

Adapted from Boyer EW, Shannon M. The serotonin syndrome. *N Engl J Med.* 2005;352:11.

to produce all these effects by facilitating the actions of γ-aminobutyric acid [GABA], the major inhibitory neurotransmitter in the nervous system). Benzodiazepines have less of a tendency to produce tolerance, less potential for abuse, and a large margin of safety if taken as an overdose in isolation.

B. **Buspirone** is a nonbenzodiazepine that is effective in the treatment of generalized anxiety disorders but not panic disorder.

1. This drug is a partial agonist at serotonin receptors but has no direct effects on GABA receptors and thus no pharmacologic cross-reactivity with benzodiazepines, barbiturates, or alcohol.

   a. Buspirone lacks sedative, anticonvulsant, and skeletal muscle–relaxing effects characteristic of benzodiazepines.

   b. Buspirone does not produce dependence and does not appear to be highly toxic if taken in overdose.

2. The principal disadvantage seems to be a slow onset of effect (1 to 2 weeks), which may be interpreted as ineffectiveness by patients experiencing acute anxiety.

V. **Lithium, anticonvulsants, and antipsychotics are considered drugs of choice for the treatment of bipolar disorders. Because of the multiple drug interactions with lithium and severe toxicity, alternative drugs are being used frequently in its place in the treatment of bipolar disorder. The goal for treatment of acute mania is to maintain plasma lithium concentrations between 1.0 and 1.2 mEq/L.**

A. **Pharmacokinetics**

1. Lithium is distributed throughout the total body water and is excreted almost entirely by the kidneys (renal excretion is not enhanced by thiazide diuretics, which act selectively on the distal renal tubules).

2. Depletion of sodium as produced by dehydration, decreased sodium intake, and thiazide and loop diuretics may increase reabsorption of lithium by proximal renal tubules, resulting in as much as a 50% increase in the plasma concentration of lithium.

B. **Side Effects**

1. The most common serious side effects of lithium occur at the kidneys, manifesting as polydipsia and polyuria (the potassium-sparing diuretic amiloride is effective in decreasing urine volume without affecting the plasma concentrations of either lithium or potassium).

2. Changes on the ECG characterized by T wave flattening or inversion occur in some patients being treated with lithium, but there seem to be no related clinical effects. Clinically significant lithium-induced cardiac conduction disturbances are rare. Patients with preexisting sinoatrial node dysfunction (sick sinus syndrome) should probably be treated with lithium only if they have an artificial cardiac pacemaker in place.

3. Hypothyroidism develops in about 5% of patients treated with lithium.

4. Clinically important dermatologic toxicities of lithium include acne and exacerbations of psoriasis or a new onset of psoriasis.

5. Patients may complain of memory disturbance and cognitive slowing. Hand tremor occurs in 25% to 50% of treated patients.

6. The association of sedation with lithium therapy suggests that anesthetic requirements for injected and inhaled drugs could be decreased. Responses to depolarizing and nondepolarizing neuromuscular blocking drugs may be prolonged in the presence of lithium.

C. **Drug Interactions (Table 43-6)**

1. **Toxicity (Table 43-7)**

   a. Diuretic therapy, sodium restriction, and sodium wasting increase reabsorption of lithium and thus increase plasma lithium concentrations. Patients being treated with lithium should avoid nonsteroidal antiinflammatory drugs and diuretics.

   b. Mild lithium toxicity is reflected by sedation, nausea, skeletal muscle weakness, and changes on the ECG characterized by widening of the QRS complex. Atrioventricular heart block, hypotension, cardiac dysrhythmias, and seizures may occur when plasma concentrations of lithium are greater than 2 mEq/L.

   c. Significant lithium toxicity is a medical emergency that may require aggressive treatment, including hemodialysis.

D. **Anticonvulsants in Treatment of Bipolar Disorder**

1. The anticonvulsants carbamazepine and valproic acid are used commonly in the treatment of bipolar disorder.

2. Despite a wide array of side effects, valproic acid is often better tolerated than lithium, which has life-threatening side effects.

3. Side effects of carbamazepine, although rare, include leukopenia, aplastic anemia, and hepatitis (recommended

Table 43-6

Drug Interactions with Lithium

Drug	Interaction
Thiazide diuretics	Increased plasma lithium concentration as a result of decreased renal clearance
Furosemide	Usually no change in the plasma lithium concentration
Nonsteroidal antiinflammatory drugs	Increased plasma lithium concentration as a result of decreased renal clearance (exceptions are aspirin and sulindac)
Aminophylline	Decreased plasma lithium concentration as result of increased renal clearance
Angiotensin-converting enzyme inhibitors	May increase plasma lithium concentration
Neuroleptic drugs	Lithium may exacerbate extrapyramidal symptoms or increase the risk of the neuroleptic malignant syndrome
Anticonvulsant drugs (carbamazepine)	Concurrent use with lithium may result in additive neurotoxicity
β-Adrenergic antagonists	Decrease lithium-induced tremor
Neuromuscular blocking drugs	Lithium may prolong the duration of action

Adapted from Price LH, Heninger GR. Lithium in the treatment of mood disorders. *N Engl J Med.* 1994;331:591–598.

that liver function tests and complete blood counts be followed in patients being treated with carbamazepine).

VI. **Antipsychotic (neuroleptic) drugs** are a chemically diverse group of compounds (phenothiazines, thioxanthenes, butyrophenones) that are useful in the treatment of schizophrenia, mania, depression with psychotic features, and certain organic psychoses (Table 43-8). Phenothiazines and thioxanthenes have a high therapeutic index and relatively flat dose-response curve, accounting for the remarkable safety of these drugs over a wide dose range.

A. **Mechanism of action** of antipsychotic drugs is thought to be due to blockade of dopamine receptors. Blockade of

Table 43-7

Signs and Symptoms of Lithium Toxicity

Toxic Effects	Plasma Lithium Concentration (mEq/L)	Signs and Symptoms
Mild	1.0–1.5	Lethargy
		Irritability
		Skeletal muscle weakness
		Tremor
		Slurred speech
		Nausea
Moderate	1.6–2.5	Confusion
		Drowsiness
		Restlessness
		Unsteady gait
		Coarse tremor
		Dysarthria
		Skeletal muscle fasciculations
		Vomiting
Severe	>2.5	Impaired consciousness (coma)
		Delirium
		Ataxia
		Extrapyramidal symptoms
		Seizures
		Impaired renal function

Adapted from Price LH, Heninger GR. Lithium in the treatment of mood disorders. *N Engl J Med.* 1994;331:591–598.

dopamine receptors in the chemoreceptor trigger zone of the medulla is responsible for the antiemetic effect of these drugs.

B. **Pharmacokinetics**. Phenothiazines and thioxanthenes often display erratic and unpredictable patterns of absorption after oral administration (highly lipid soluble and accumulate in well-perfused tissues such as the brain). Passage across the placenta and accumulation of drug in the fetus is possible.

C. **Metabolism** of phenothiazines and thioxanthenes is principally by oxidation in the liver followed by conjugation. Most oxidative metabolites are pharmacologically inactive, with a notable exception being 7-hydroxychlorpromazine.

Table 43-8

Comparative Pharmacology of Antipsychotic (Neuroleptic) Drugs

Category and Drug	Sedative Potency	Anticholinergic Potency	Orthostatic Hypotension Potency	Extrapyramidal Potency
Phenothiazines				
Chlorpromazine	+ + +	+ +	+ + +	+
Triflupromazine	+ + +	+ +	+ + +	+ +
Thioridazine	+ + +	+ + +	+ + +	+
Fluphenazine	+ +	+	+	+ + +
Perphenazine	+	+	+	+ + +
Trifluoperazine	+ +	+	+	+ + +
Thioxanthenes				
Chlorprothixene	+ + +	+ + +	+ + +	+
Thiothixene	+	+	+	+ + +
Dibenzodiazepines				
Clozapine	+ + +	+ + +	+ + +	0
Loxapine	+ +	+ +	+ +	+ +
Butyrophenones				
Haloperidol	+	+	+	+ + +
Droperidol	+	+	+	+ + +
Diphenylbutylpiperidines				
Pimozide	+	+	+	+ + +
Benzisoxazole				
Risperidone	+	+	+ +	+

0, none; +, mild; + +, moderate; + + +, marked.

D. **Side Effects**. Despite the common occurrence of side effects, these drugs have a large margin of safety and overdoses are rarely fatal.

1. **Extrapyramidal Effects**

   a. Tardive dyskinesia may occur in 20% of patients who receive antipsychotic drugs for longer than 1 year. Manifestations of tardive dyskinesia include abnormal involuntary movements (tongue, facial and neck muscles, upper and lower extremities, truncal musculature, and, occasionally, skeletal muscle groups involved in breathing and swallowing). Tardive dyskinesia only rarely remits, and there is no treatment.

   b. Acute dystonic reactions occur in approximately 2% of treated patients and are most likely to occur within the first 72 hours of therapy. Acute skeletal muscle rigidity and cramping may develop, usually in the musculature of the neck, tongue, face, and back. Opisthotonos and oculogyric crises may occur.

   c. The sudden onset of respiratory distress in a patient on neuroleptics may reflect laryngeal dyskinesia (laryngospasm).

   d. Acute dystonia responds dramatically to diphenhydramine, 25 to 50 mg IV.

2. **Cardiovascular Effects**

   a. IV administration of chlorpromazine causes a decrease in systemic blood pressure resulting from (a) depression of vasomotor reflexes, (b) peripheral α-adrenergic blockade, (c) direct relaxant effects on vascular smooth muscle, and (d) direct cardiac depression.

   b. α-Adrenergic blockade produced by chlorpromazine is sufficient to blunt or prevent the pressor effects of epinephrine.

   c. Miosis that occurs predictably may also be due to α-adrenergic blockade.

   d. A cardiac antidysrhythmic effect of chlorpromazine may reflect the potent local anesthetic activity of this drug.

3. **Neuroleptic malignant syndrome** is characterized by (a) hyperthermia; (b) generalized hypertonicity of skeletal muscles; (c) instability of the autonomic nervous system manifesting as alterations in systemic blood pressure, tachycardia, and cardiac dysrhythmias; and (d) fluctuating levels of consciousness. Skeletal muscle rigidity may be severe enough to cause myonecrosis

leading to increased creatine phosphokinase levels, myoglobinuria, and renal failure.

   a. Mortality is 20% to 30%, with common causes of death being ventilatory failure, cardiac failure and/or dysrhythmias, renal failure, and thromboembolism.

   b. The cause of neuroleptic malignant syndrome is not known and, as a result, treatment is empirical and includes supportive measures and the administration of dantrolene and the dopamine agonists bromocriptine or amantadine.

   c. Malignant hyperthermia associated with anesthesia as well as the central anticholinergic syndrome may mimic the neuroleptic malignant syndrome. A distinguishing feature is the ability of nondepolarizing muscle relaxants to produce flaccid paralysis in patients experiencing the neuroleptic malignant syndrome but not in those experiencing malignant hyperthermia.

4. **Sedation** appears to be due to antagonism of α_1-adrenergic, muscarinic, and histamine (H_1) receptors. With chronic therapy, tolerance develops to the sedative effects produced by these drugs.

5. **Antiemetic Effects**. The antiemetic effects of antipsychotic drugs reflect their interaction with dopaminergic receptors in the chemoreceptor trigger zone of the medulla (seem most effective in preventing opioid-induced nausea and vomiting).

6. **Obstructive jaundice** that is considered to be an allergic reaction occurs rarely 2 to 4 weeks after administration of phenothiazines or thioxanthenes.

7. **Skeletal Muscle Relaxation**. Chlorpromazine causes skeletal muscle relaxation in some types of spastic conditions, presumably by actions on the CNS because the drug is devoid of actions at the neuromuscular junction.

E. **Drug Interactions**

1. The ventilatory depressant effects of opioids are likely to be exaggerated by antipsychotic drugs.

2. The miotic and sedative effects of opioids are increased, and the analgesic actions are likely to be potentiated.

F. **Clozapine** is the only antipsychotic that does not seem to cause tardive dyskinesia or extrapyramidal side effects. Among the most common side effects are sedation, nausea and vomiting, and orthostatic hypotension. A presumed manifestation of a parasympatholytic effect is sustained mild sinus tachycardia. Caution is advised in the use of such an anticholinergic drug in patients at risk for glaucoma, ileus, or urinary retention. Agranulocytosis is a particularly serious side effect of clozapine, occurring in less than 1% of patients. The incidence of seizures is 2% to 4% in those treated with high doses of clozapine.

G. **Butyrophenones**. Droperidol is the butyrophenone most often administered in the preoperative period. Haloperidol has a longer duration of action than droperidol and lacks significant α-adrenergic antagonist effects such that decreases in systemic blood pressure are unlikely (principal use is for treatment of agitation and delirium in the intensive care unit).

1. **Pharmacokinetics**. Droperidol is metabolized in the liver, with maximal excretion of metabolites occurring during the first 24 hours.

2. **Side effects** of butyrophenones resemble those described for phenothiazines and thioxanthenes.

   a. **Central Nervous System**. The outwardly calming effect of droperidol may mask an overwhelming fear of surgery. This dysphoric response detracts from the use of droperidol in the preoperative period, especially as preoperative medication. Akathisia (most often a feeling of restlessness in the legs) may accompany administration of droperidol as preoperative medication. As a dopamine antagonist, droperidol evokes extrapyramidal reactions in about 1% of patients and should not be administered to patients who are concurrently being treated for Parkinson disease. Acute laryngeal dystonia (laryngospasm) is a rare extrapyramidal reaction to the butyrophenones. Diphenhydramine administered IV is an effective treatment for droperidol-induced extrapyramidal reactions. Droperidol does not produce amnesia nor does it have an anticonvulsant action.

   b. **Cardiovascular Effects**. Droperidol can decrease systemic blood pressure as a result of actions in the CNS and by peripheral α-adrenergic blockade. Myocardial contractility is not altered by droperidol. Droperidol is a cardiac antidysrhythmic and protects against epinephrine-induced dysrhythmias.

   c. **Prolonged QTc interval** is a malfunction of cardiac ion channels resulting in impaired ventricular repolarization that can lead to a characteristic polymorphic ventricular tachycardia known as torsades de pointes. The single most common cause of the withdrawal or restriction of the use of drugs that are already in clinical use is the prolongation of the QTc interval on the ECG associated with torsades de pointes (polymorphic ventricular tachycardia). Droperidol is capable of prolonging the QTc interval on the ECG (Fig. 43-2). Since droperidol was approved in 1970, there has not been a single case report where droperidol in doses used for the management of postoperative nausea and vomiting has been associated with cardiac dysrhythmias or cardiac arrest. A "black box warning" includes the requirement that all patients should undergo a 12-lead ECG prior to the administration of droperidol to determine if a prolonged QTc interval is present (>440 milliseconds for males and >450 milliseconds for females).

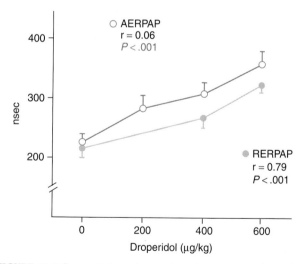

FIGURE 43-2 Droperidol produces dose-dependent prolongation of the antegrade and retrograde effective refractory period of accessory pathways. AERPAP, antegrade effective refractory period of accessory pathways; RERPAP, retrograde effective refractory period of accessory pathways. (From Gomez-Arnau J, Marquez-Montes J, Avello F. Fentanyl and droperidol effects on the refractoriness of the accessory pathway in the Wolff-Parkinson-White syndrome. *Anesthesiology.* 1983;58:307–313, with permission.)

   d. **Ventilation**. Resting ventilation and the ventilatory response to carbon dioxide are not altered by droperidol.
3. **Neuroleptanalgesia** is produced with a 50:1 combination of droperidol with fentanyl. This fixed combination of drugs is not associated with enhanced depression of ventilation as compared with either drug alone.
   a. Neuroleptanalgesia is characterized by trance-like (cataleptic) immobility in an outwardly tranquil patient who is dissociated and indifferent to the external surroundings. Analgesia is intense, allowing performance of a variety of diagnostic and minor surgical procedures such as bronchoscopy and cystoscopy.
   b. The disadvantages of neuroleptanalgesia are prolonged CNS depression and failure to depress sympathetic nervous system responses predictably to painful stimulation.
4. **Antiemetic**. Droperidol is a powerful antiemetic agent as a result of inhibition of dopamine$_2$ receptors in the chemoreceptor trigger zone of the medulla. Despite the black box warning, there is a question whether small antiemetic doses ($\leq$1.25 mg) introduce the risk of prolonged QTc interval on the ECG.

VII. **Cannabis** has been used for thousands of years and is presently the most commonly used illicit drug in the world. The most abundant cannabinoids are δ-9-tetrahydrocannabinol (D9THC), cannabidiol, and cannabinol. Two principal endogenous cannabis receptors (CB1 and CB2) have been identified. CB1 receptors are present in the CNS (especially spinal cord) and CB2 receptors are located peripherally and linked with cells in the immune system.
   A. **Pharmacokinetics**
   1. Cannabinoids undergo substantial hepatic first-pass metabolism following oral administration such that only 10% to 20% of the ingested dose reaches the systemic circulation (produces large amounts of active metabolite, 11-hydroxy-δ-9-tetrahydrocannabinol).
   2. The peak clinical effect after oral administration occurs after 1 to 2 hours and duration of action is 4 to 6 hours. In contrast, inhalation administration results in onset of action within seconds.
   B. **Toxicity**
   1. Euphoria and feeling of relaxation occurs at plasma cannabinoid concentrations of about 3 ng/mL and this can be produced by 2 to 3 mg of D9THC.

2. Acute intoxication may cause perceptual alterations, distortion of time, intensification of normal sensory experiences, decreased reaction times, poor motor skills, increased appetite, impairment of skilled activities, tachycardia, and hypotension.

3. The greatest concern is the creation of long-term toxicity, development of physical dependence associated with withdrawal symptom during a period of abstinence after frequent use.

4. Cannabis is often mixed with tobacco to make it burn more efficiently. Materials that are present in cannabis smoke are carcinogenic.

5. Chronic inhalation of cannabis smoke is associated with an increased incidence of chronic obstructive lung disease and carcinoma of the lung and larynx.

C. **Clinical Uses**

1. D9THC is increasingly used for the long-term treatment of nausea, vomiting, cachexia, and management of chronic pain including migraine.

2. Although use of cannabis for analgesia introduces the potential for psychic and physical dependence, there is considerably less risk of life-threatening side effects compared to those associated with opioids.

3. Pure D9THC may be effective in the treatment of chemotherapy-induced nausea and vomiting and is a recognized appetite stimulant in patients with terminal disease.

VIII. **Psychostimulants**

A. Methylphenidate is a psychostimulant used for the treatment of attention deficit hyperactivity disorder and narcolepsy. Similar to amphetamines, it blocks the reuptake of norepinephrine and dopamine.

B. The risk of intraoperative hemodynamic instability and arrhythmias may be increased.

CHAPTER 44

Physiology of the Newborn

I. **Introduction.** Neonatal physiology is characterized by decreased functional reserve. Increased physiologic demands may place a significant burden on organ systems that have not yet developed normal adult functional reserve.

II. **Neonatal Physiology.** Neonatal oxygen consumption is approximately 6 mL/kg/minute compared to 3 mL/kg/minute in the adult. Even under normal physiologic circumstances, the immature cardiac and respiratory systems operate near the edge of their functional reserve to support this metabolic demand. Immaturity of multiple neonatal organ systems creates important developmental differences in drug handling and response when compared to the older child and adults.

   A. **Neonatal Cardiovascular Physiology**
      1. The newborn infant is in a state of transition from the fetal, intrauterine to the newborn, extrauterine circulatory pattern.
         a. The fetal circulation is characterized by high pulmonary vascular resistance, low systemic vascular resistance (including the placenta), and right-to-left cardiac shunting via the foramen ovale and ductus arteriosus. Expansion of the lungs at birth increases Po_2 and causes a rapid decline in pulmonary vascular resistance and an increase in pulmonary blood flow.
         b. Increasing blood return to the heart via the pulmonary veins raises the pressure of the left atrium above that of the right, causing a functional closure of the foramen ovale. Anatomic closure of the foramen ovale usually occurs between 3 months and 1 year of age, but the foramen remains anatomically patent in 10% to 30% of people throughout life (described as having a "probe patent" foramen ovale).

Individuals with a probe patent foramen ovale are also at risk for systemic air embolism and resultant stroke when air emboli pass from the pulmonary to the systemic circulation.

c. Because the foramen ovale and ductus arteriosus are only functionally closed in the neonatal period, the neonatal circulation is able to readily revert to the fetal pattern, particularly in response to physiologic stresses (hypoxemia, hypercarbia, acidosis).

d. Right-to-left shunting, by causing arterial hypoxemia, causes a further increase in pulmonary vascular resistance, thus creating a vicious cycle (persistent pulmonary hypertension may be seen in premature neonates).

2. The neonatal myocardium contains immature contractile elements and is less compliant than the adult myocardium (Fig. 44-1). Because stroke volume cannot be significantly augmented by volume loading, and because contractile reserve is limited, neonatal cardiac output is exquisitely dependent on heart rate.

a. To meet the elevated metabolic demand, neonatal cardiac output, relative to body weight, is twice that

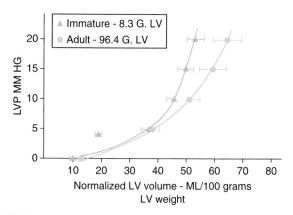

FIGURE 44-1 Pressure volume curve for neonatal and adult heart. Pressure volume curves for adult and neonatal canine heart. The immature heart is less compliant than the adult heart. As a result, the pressure volume curves diverge above a left ventricular pressure (LVP) of about 5 mm Hg.

of the adult. This is achieved with a relatively rapid heart rate (140 beats per minute) because stroke volume cannot be significantly increased.

b. The neonatal circulation is characterized by centralization (increased peripheral vascular resistance and distribution of cardiac output primarily to vital organs), a situation comparable to an adult in compensated shock.

c. The structural and functional immaturity of the neonatal cardiovascular system severely limits the reserve that is available in the face of common perinatal and perioperative events such as hypovolemia, anesthetic-induced depression of contractility, relative bradycardia, and positive pressure ventilation–induced decreases venous return.

d. The marginal cardiovascular reserve of the neonate and leftward shift of the fetal hemoglobin dissociation curve are the rationale underlying the recommendation that the hematocrit be maintained at 30% or higher to prevent tissue ischemia in the newborn.

B. **Respiratory Physiology of the Newborn**

1. The respiratory system of a term neonate at birth is immature and postnatal development continues through early childhood (number of alveoli is reduced at birth and the ratio of alveolar surface area to body surface area is one-third that of the adult).

2. To satisfy increased oxygen demand, neonatal alveolar minute ventilation is twice that of the adult (increasing respiratory rate rather than tidal volume is the most efficient means to increase alveolar ventilation in the newborn).

3. The neonatal chest wall is more compliant and has less outward recoil than that of the adult (neonatal lung has a greater tendency to collapse and the infant is obliged to utilize active mechanisms to maintain normal lung volumes) (Table 44-1).

4. Although airway resistance is relatively low in infants, in absolute terms, the airways are very narrow (minor quantities of secretions or trivial inflammatory disease can produce serious respiratory embarrassment in small infants).

C. **Neonatal Thermoregulation**

1. The neonate tends to become hypothermic during general anesthesia much more rapidly than the adult (neonate primarily relies on nonshivering or chemical

---

Table 44-1

Active Mechanisms Used by Neonates to Maintain Lung Volume[a]

Rapid respiratory rate—early termination of expiration
Intercostal muscle activity in expiration—stabilizes compliant chest wall
Expiration against partially closed glottis—retards expiratory flow

[a]Significantly attenuated by general anesthesia.

---

       thermogenesis in brown adipose tissue for heat production).

2. During anesthesia and surgery, heat loss in the pediatric patient is further enhanced by decrease in the thermoregulatory threshold due to anesthesia, low ambient temperatures of the operating suite (20°C to 22°C), preparation of skin with cold solutions, infusion of cold solutions, anesthesia-induced vasodilatation, and use of dry anesthetic gases in high flow, nonrebreathing systems.

   a. Intraoperative hypothermia will markedly delay emergence.

   b. With the return of the thermostatic reflexes, oxygen consumption increases by three- to fourfold as the metabolic rate is increased in an attempt to generate heat. This additional demand on an immature cardiorespiratory system that is already compromised due to the residual effects of anesthesia and surgery may precipitate cardiorespiratory failure.

   c. Loss of heat during anesthesia and surgery can be prevented by a number of simple measures, such as raising operating room temperature to 28°C to 30°C, radiant heat lamps, wrapping the extremities with insulating material, using nonvolatile warmed solutions for skin preparation, and administration of warmed intravenous fluids and blood products. Inhaled gases should be heated and humidified.

D. **Neonatal Fluid, Electrolyte, and Renal Physiology**

1. The neonate is characterized by an increased total body water, increased extracellular fluid volume, increased water turnover rate, and reduced glomerular filtration rate.

2. Neonates are obligate sodium wasters and require sodium supplementation.

3. Neonates have decreased glycogen stores and are prone to hypoglycemia after relatively brief periods of starvation (glucose is an essential element of the intraoperative fluid plan to maintain serum glucose between 35 and 125 mg/dL).

E. **Neonatal Neurophysiology**

1. Somatosensory evoked potentials can be recorded from the fetal cerebral cortex at 29 weeks' gestation. As such, the functional circuitry required for sensation of pain is likely to be present between 20 and 30 weeks' gestation.

2. The failure to provide analgesia for neonates leads to changes in nociceptive pathways in the dorsal horn of the spinal cord and in the brain.

3. The adequate treatment of pain in the neonatal period is challenging because of the fear of respiratory depression associated with opioid administration (analgesia may be induced by the administration of sucrose and by suckling).

4. Preterm infants are also at risk for retinopathy of prematurity (ROP) in which abnormal growth of retinal vessels can lead to scarring and blindness (gestational age is the primary etiologic factor in the development of ROP, and hyperoxia has been implicated as contributing factor).

CHAPTER 45

Maternal and Fetal Physiology and Pharmacology

I. **Introduction**

   A. As many as 1 out of every 50 pregnant women will undergo some type of surgery during their pregnancy. The pharmacokinetics and pharmacodynamics of many drugs are altered during pregnancy.

   B. When possible, surgery is performed during the second trimester of pregnancy to avoid affecting major organogenesis during the first trimester and to reduce the risk of preterm delivery which is increased in the third trimester.

   C. The effects of anesthesia are normally well tolerated by the fetus.

   1. The fetus does not depend on alveolar ventilation for oxygenation or carbon dioxide removal and has the maternal organs to help manage drug metabolism and excretion (fetal cardiac output is sensitive to depression by anesthetic drugs).

   2. Drugs used in anesthesia cross the placenta to a variable extent. As a general rule, drugs that do not cross the blood–brain barrier do not cross the placenta to any appreciable degree.

II. **Maternal Physiology**

   A. **Physiologic Changes During and Delivery**

   1. **Cardiovascular Changes**. Pregnancy-induced changes in the maternal cardiovascular system include increased blood volume and cardiac output, decreased vascular resistance, and supine hypotension.

   2. **Intravascular Volumes and Hematology**

   a. Maternal intravascular fluid volume begins to increase in the first trimester of pregnancy as the result of increased production of renin, angiotensin, and aldosterone, which together promote sodium absorption and water retention. By term gestation, the plasma volume increases approximately 50%, and the red cell volume increases about 25%. The greater

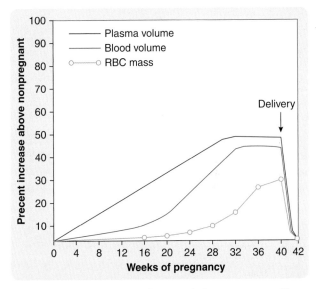

FIGURE 45-1 Blood volume changes during pregnancy. Plasma volume increases during pregnancy more rapidly than red cell mass leading to a physiologic anemia of pregnancy. (Modified from Scott D. Anemia during pregnancy. *Obstet Gynecol Ann.* 1972;1:219.)

increase in plasma volume is the cause of the "physiologic anemia of pregnancy" (Fig. 45-1).

b. The physiologic anemia of pregnancy does not cause a reduction in oxygen delivery because of a coincident increase in cardiac output.

c. The additional intravascular fluid volume (1,000 to 1,500 mL at term) compensates for an average 300 to 500 mL blood loss with vaginal delivery and 800 to 1,000 mL estimated blood loss with cesarean section.

d. Following delivery, uterine contraction creates an autotransfusion of blood often in excess of 500 mL that also compensates for the acute blood loss from delivery.

e. In spite of mild thrombocytopenia, pregnancy is a hypercoagulable state with increases in fibrinogen and factor VII.

B. **Cardiac Output**
   1. By the end of the first trimester, maternal cardiac output increases, on average, by 35% above prepregnancy values and continues to increase to 50% above nonpregnant values by the end of the second trimester (Fig. 45-2).
   2. Labor is associated with further increases in cardiac output, which increases with each uterine contraction.
      a. The largest increase in cardiac output occurs immediately after delivery, when cardiac output can be increased by 80% to 100% above prelabor values.
      b. This massive increase in cardiac output represents a moment of unique risk for patients with

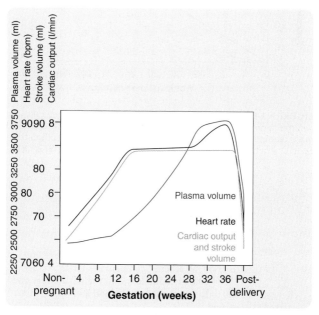

FIGURE 45-2 Maternal hemodynamic changes of pregnancy. Maternal heart rate and cardiac output increase early in the first trimester and plateau in the second trimester. There is an additional increase in heart rate during the third trimester. Plasma volume increases throughout the first and second trimester and reaches a plateau during the third trimester. All values drop rapidly in the days after delivery. (Modified from Thorn SA. Pregnancy in heart disease. *Heart.* 2004;90:450–456.)

cardiopulmonary disease, particularly those with valvular stenosis and pulmonary hypertension.

C. **Systemic Vascular Resistance**. In spite of increases in cardiac output and plasma volume, systemic blood pressure normally decreases secondary to a 20% reduction in systemic vascular resistance by term.

D. **Aortocaval Compression**

1. In the supine position, blood pressure commonly decreases as the result of aortocaval compression by the gravid uterus. Supine hypotension is manifest by symptoms of diaphoresis, nausea, vomiting, and dizziness. At term, there is almost complete occlusion of the inferior vena cava in the supine position, with return of blood from the lower extremities through the epidural, azygos, and vertebral veins.

2. Reduced sympathetic tone resulting from neuraxial or general anesthesia will impair the compensatory sympathetic nervous system response and worsen the hypotensive response to supine positioning.

3. A lateral tilt is used to avoid the hypotension that can be associated with supine positioning with neuraxial techniques for labor analgesia and operative deliveries.

E. **Pulmonary Changes**

1. **Airway**

   a. During pregnancy, there is vascular engorgement with friability and edema of the mucosal lining of the oro- and nasopharynx (danger of bleeding with instrumentation of the airway and increased risk of difficult ventilation and intubation).

   b. Attempts at laryngoscopy should be minimized and a smaller size cuffed endotracheal tube (6.0 to 6.5 mm internal diameter) should be considered to avoid airway edema and bleeding.

2. **Minute Ventilation and Oxygenation**

   a. In order to accommodate the increased oxygen demand and carbon dioxide production of the growing placenta and fetus, minute ventilation is increased 45% to 50% above nonpregnant values during the first trimester and remains at this increased level for the remainder of the pregnancy.

   b. This greater minute ventilation is attained primarily as a result of a greater tidal volume with a small increase in the respiratory rate (Fig. 45-3).

   c. Maternal $Paco_2$ is commonly reduced from 40 mm Hg to approximately 30 mm Hg during the first trimester.

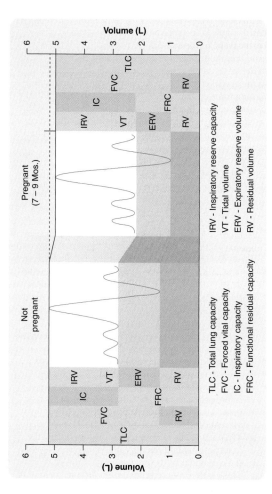

FIGURE 45-3 Changes in maternal pulmonary function. Functional residual capacity (FRC) is reduced by virtue of reductions in expiratory reserve volume (ERV) and residual volume (RV) during pregnancy. Inspiratory capacity (IC) is increased resulting from an increase in tidal volume (VT). (Modified from Hegewald MJ, Crapo RO. Respiratory physiology in pregnancy. *Clin Chest Med.* 2011;32[1]:1–13.)

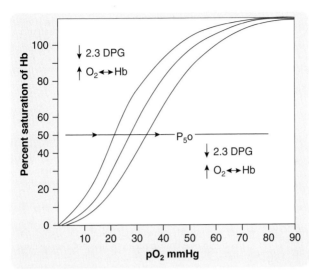

FIGURE 45-4 Right shift of maternal hemoglobin oxygen dissociation curve. Increased interaction with 2,3-DPG results in hemoglobin with lower oxygen affinity and a right shift in the hemoglobin oxygen saturation curve. As a result, oxygen is more easily off-loaded to fetal hemoglobin, which has a left-shifted hemoglobin oxygen dissociation curve. (Modified from Jepson JH. Factors influencing oxygenation in mother and fetus. *Obstet Gynecol.* 1974;44[6]:906–914.)

Arterial oxygenation can be significantly improved by changing position from supine to lateral.

d. Maternal hemoglobin is right-shifted with the P_{50} increasing from 27 to approximately 30 mm Hg (Fig. 45-4). The higher P_{50} in the mother and lower P_{50} in the fetus favors off-loading of oxygen across the placenta.

3. **Lung Volumes**

a. During pregnancy, the growing uterus elevates the diaphragm and causes a reduction in functional residual capacity by 20% at term (see Fig. 45-3).

b. The combination of increased minute ventilation and decreased functional residual capacity results in a greater rate at which changes in the alveolar concentration of inhaled anesthetics can be achieved with spontaneous ventilation in the case of mask induction.

    c. During induction of general anesthesia in a pregnant patient, desaturation occurs more rapidly than in a nonpregnant patient because of decreased functional residual capacity and increased metabolic rate. Administration of 100% oxygen prior to the induction of general anesthesia is critical to allow as much time as possible for safe airway management.

F. **Gastrointestinal Changes**
1. After midgestation, pregnant women are thought to be at increased risk of aspiration pneumonia with administration of general anesthesia.
    a. Increased progesterone and estrogen concentrations during labor, pain, anxiety, and the administration of opioids (including those administered neuraxially) decrease gastric emptying.
    b. All women in labor are considered to have full stomachs and to be at increased risk for pulmonary aspiration with induction of anesthesia.
2. Although blood flow to the liver does not change during pregnancy, markers of liver function all increase to the upper limits of normal.
3. Plasma cholinesterase (pseudocholinesterase) activity is decreased about 30% from the 10th week of gestation up to 6 weeks postpartum, but this decreased cholinesterase activity is not associated with clinically relevant prolongation of neuromuscular blockade.

G. **Renal Changes**. Renal blood flow and the glomerular filtration rate are increased 50% by the second trimester and remain elevated until 3 months postpartum.

H. **Neurobiologic Changes**
1. Pregnant patients are more sensitive to both inhaled and local anesthetic agents (minimum alveolar concentration is reduced by 30% by the first trimester of pregnancy). Unanticipated awareness is more common during cesarean section.
2. Pregnant women are more sensitive to the local anesthetics and a lower dose is able to obtain the same level of either spinal or epidural neuraxial blockade compared to nonpregnant women. At term, distention of epidural veins decreases the size of the epidural space and volume of cerebrospinal fluid (CSF) in the subarachnoid space.

III. **Uteroplacental Physiology. The placenta is composed of both maternal and fetal tissues and is the interface of maternal and fetal circulation systems (Fig. 45-5). It provides a**

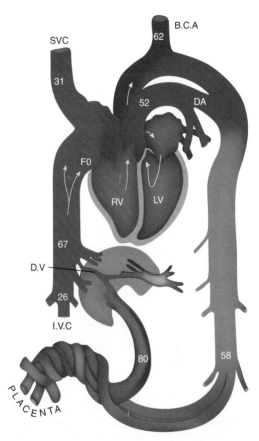

FIGURE 45-5 Diagram of the fetal circulation. Oxygenated blood flows in through the umbilical vein. It passes through the ductus venosus (DV) where it is diluted by deoxygenated blood returning from the inferior vena cava (IVC). Oxygenated blood passes to the right atrium, where little passes through the fetal lungs because of high pulmonary vascular resistance. Part of the circulation passes through the foramen ovale (FO) directly to the left atrium to enter the fetal systemic circulation. Another portion bypasses the lungs by passing from the pulmonary artery through the ductus arteriosus (DA) where it proceeds directly to the aorta. The numbers represent oxygen saturation at various points in the fetal circulation. BCA, brachial cephalic artery; SVC, superior vena cava. (Modified from Meschia G. Fetal oxygenation and maternal ventilation. *Clin Chest Med.* 2011;32[1]:15–19.)

substrate for physiologic exchange between mother and fetus without immunologic rejection.

A. **Uterine blood flow** increases progressively during pregnancy from about 100 mL per minute in the nonpregnant state to 700 mL per minute (about 10% of cardiac output) at term gestation (minimal autoregulation and the vasculature remains essentially fully dilated during normal pregnancy).

1. Uterine and placental blood flows are dependent on maternal cardiac output and are directly related to uterine perfusion pressure. Decreased perfusion pressure can result from maternal hypotension secondary to hypovolemia, aortocaval compression, or decreased systemic resistance from either general or neuraxial anesthesia.

2. Increased uterine venous pressure can also decrease uterine perfusion (supine positioning with vena caval compression).

3. Phenylephrine is not only effective in preventing hypotension but is associated with less fetal acidosis and base deficit than use of ephedrine.

B. **Oxygen Transfer**

1. The fetal oxyhemoglobin dissociation curve is left-shifted (P_{50} = 19 mm Hg, greater oxygen affinity), whereas the maternal oxyhemoglobin dissociation curve is right-shifted (P_{50} = 27 mm Hg, less oxygen affinity).

2. This occurs because fetal hemoglobin does not interact with 2,3-disphosphoglycerate (2,3-DPG), facilitating oxygen transfer to the fetus (see Fig. 45-4).

IV. **Fetal Heart Rate Monitoring. After 25 weeks, variability in fetal heart rate is a reliable sign of well-being. Under general anesthesia and with the use of opioids and maternal cooling, the loss of fetal heart rate variability may not be indicative of fetal academia but may be a result of anesthetic alteration of autonomic tone. Fetal bradycardia is more concerning.**

V. Pain Management

A. Systemic opioids including those used in patient-controlled intravenous analgesia cross the placenta and may reduce fetal heart rate variability (no evidence that this is detrimental to the fetus).

B. If the fetus is born prematurely shortly after exposure to maternal systemic opioids, reversal with naloxone and/or respiratory support may be necessary.

C. Maternal pain control after nonobstetric surgery is of paramount importance to maternal and fetal well-being.

1. Nonsteroidal antiinflammatory drugs should be used with caution in pregnancy (associated with premature

closure of the ductus arteriosus when used after 30 weeks' gestation).

2. Acetaminophen is generally accepted as safe in pregnancy.

D. Following surgery, both the fetal heart rate and uterine activity should be evaluated. Preterm labor can be managed with appropriate tocolytic drugs (postoperative pain medications may make it difficult for the patient to note early contractions).

E. Venous thrombosis prophylaxis should be instituted unless surgically contraindicated.

VI. **Fetal Physiology**

A. **Characteristics of the Fetal Circulation** (see Fig. 45-5). The fetal circulation is characterized by high pulmonary vascular resistance, low systemic vascular resistance (including the placenta), and right-to-left cardiac shunting via the foramen ovale and ductus arteriosus.

B. **Drug Transfer**

1. The maternal blood concentration of a drug is normally the primary determinant of how much drug will ultimately reach the fetus.

2. The high molecular weight and poor lipid solubility of nondepolarizing neuromuscular blocking drugs result in minimal transfer of these drugs across the placenta. Succinylcholine has a low molecular weight but is highly ionized and therefore does not readily cross the placenta unless given in very large doses. Thus, during administration of a general anesthetic for cesarean delivery, the fetus/neonate is not paralyzed.

3. Both heparin and glycopyrrolate have minimal placental transfer because they are highly charged.

4. Placental transfer of volatile agents, benzodiazepines, local anesthetics, and opioids is facilitated by the relatively low molecular weights, neutral charge, and relative lipophilicity of these drugs.

5. Fetal blood is more acidic than maternal and the lower pH creates an environment where weakly basic drugs such as local anesthetics can cross the placenta as a nonionized molecule and become ionized in the fetal circulation (ion trapping). During fetal distress (lower pH in the fetal circulation), higher concentrations of weakly basic drugs such as local anesthetics can be trapped. High concentrations of local anesthetics in the fetal circulation decrease neonatal neuromuscular tone.

C. **Fetal Liver Function and Drug Metabolism**

1. Although fetal liver function is not yet mature, coagulation factors are synthesized independent of the maternal

circulation. These factors do not cross the placenta and their serum concentrations increase with gestational age.

2. The anatomy of the fetal circulation helps to decrease fetal exposure to potentially high concentrations of drugs in umbilical venous blood. Approximately 75% of umbilical venous blood initially passes through the fetal liver, which may result in significant drug metabolism by the fetal liver before the drug reaches the fetal heart and brain (first-pass metabolism).

3. Drugs entering the fetal inferior vena cava via the ductus venosus are initially diluted by drug-free blood returning from the fetal lower extremities and pelvic viscera of the fetus (these anatomic characteristics of the fetal circulation markedly decrease fetal plasma drug concentrations compared to maternal concentrations).

VII. **Anesthetic Toxicity in the Fetus**

A. Although there is no clear evidence for toxicity of specific anesthetic drugs in humans, there is concerning animal data in rodents and primates that suggest that prolonged exposure to general anesthetic drugs (inhaled anesthetics, propofol, ketamine) may induce inappropriate neuronal apoptosis that is associated with long-lasting behavioral abnormalities. Changes in practice have not been recommended in the absence of any anesthetic regimen that has been proven to provide more safety than others.

B. In general, the second trimester is preferred for surgical intervention as this is a period after much organogenesis has taken place and yet minimizes the risk of preterm labor associated with the third trimester.

1. Monitoring for contractions is recommended and, in some situations, suppression with magnesium is recommended after surgery.

2. As the long-term impact of general anesthesia on the fetus is unknown, regional anesthesia is favored when possible for the surgical procedure.

VIII. **Fetal Neurophysiology**

A. **Fetal Pain**

1. The gestational age at which the fetus can feel pain is highly controversial. Afferent sensory fibers required for nociception are in place and a functional spinal reflex is present by 20 weeks' gestation (Fig. 45-6).

2. The functional circuitry required for apprehension of pain is likely to be present between 20 and 30 weeks' gestation (consider for informed decisions about anesthesia for fetal surgery).

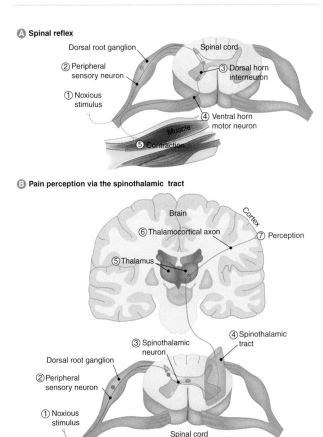

A Spinal reflex

Dorsal root ganglion

Spinal cord

② Peripheral sensory neuron

③ Dorsal horn interneuron

① Noxious stimulus

④ Ventral horn motor neuron

Muscle

⑤ Contraction

B Pain perception via the spinothalamic tract

Brain

Cortex

⑥ Thalamocortical axon

⑦ Perception

⑤ Thalamus

③ Spinothalamic neuron

④ Spinothalamic tract

Dorsal root ganglion

② Peripheral sensory neuron

① Noxious stimulus

Spinal cord

FIGURE 45-6 Spinal reflex and pain perception pathways. **A.** Spinal reflex responses to noxious stimuli occur early in fetal development before cortical connections are functional. **B.** Later in fetal development, a noxious stimulus will activate a peripheral sensory neuron that project to neurons that form the spinothalamic tract. These neurons in turn project to neurons in the thalamus. Thalamic neurons project to neurons in the subplate zone and the somatosensory cortex. This sequence is the anatomic basis for nociception, the sequence of neuronal events that lead to the conscious perception of pain. The functional circuitry required for apprehension of pain is likely to be present between 20 and 30 weeks' gestation. (Modified from Lowery CL, Hardman MP, Manning N, et al. Neurodevelopmental changes in fetal pain. *Semin Perinatol.* 2007;31:275–282.)

CHAPTER 46

Physiology and Pharmacology of the Elderly

I. **Introduction.** Patients older than the age of 65 years comprise 13% of the U.S. population or 40,300,000 people. It is not surprising that variability in physiology increases throughout life resulting in increased pharmacokinetic and pharmacodynamic variability in elderly subjects (clinical result is an increased incidence of adverse drug reactions in elderly patients). The elderly have in common with the newborn limited physiologic reserve.

II. **Aging and the Cardiovascular System.** Heart failure is the most frequent cause of hospitalization in patients older than 65 years of age. It is important to separate the cardiovascular effects of aging from those of common diseases with increased prevalence in the elderly (atherosclerosis, hypertension, diabetes mellitus) (Fig. 46-1). The decline in cardiac function that occurs with aging in the healthy individual appears to be related, in part, to decreasing functional demand.

   A. **Heart**
   1. The heart increases in size during aging as a result of concentric ventricular hypertrophy that occurs in response to the increase in left ventricular afterload.
   2. The heart rate response to severe exercise is diminished (increases in cardiac output in response to severe exertion are attenuated by approximately 20% to 30%).
   3. Cardiac dysfunction in aging is largely related to impaired diastolic left ventricle function with increased prevalence of diastolic heart failure exacerbated by several coexisting diseases (Table 46-1).
   4. Tachycardia and shortened diastolic intervals are associated with marked decreases in ventricular preload in the elderly. Atrial fibrillation is a common rhythm in the elderly. Loss of the atrial "kick" is particularly poorly tolerated by elderly patients.
   5. Perioperative events that reduce venous return, such as hypovolemia, positive pressure ventilation, and

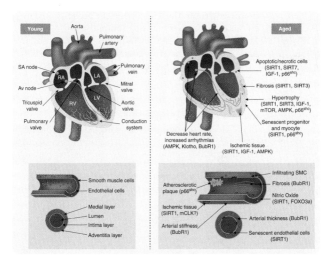

FIGURE 46-1 Age-dependent changes to cardiovascular tissues. Both the heart and vasculature undergo numerous alterations during aging as a result of deregulation of molecular longevity pathways, leading to compromised function. Important functional changes include arterial hypertrophy resulting in increased afterload, ventricular hypertrophy resulting in elevated systolic blood pressure, loss of cells in the electrical conduction system predisposing to arrhythmia, and loss of sensitivity to catecholamines resulting in reduced maximal heart rate and heart rate variability. (Adapted from North BJ, Sinclair DA. The intersection between aging and cardiovascular disease. *Circ Res.* 2012;110[8]):1097–1108. Illustration credit: Cosmocyte/Ben Smith.)

Table 46-1

Diseases Commonly Encountered in the Elderly that Are Associated with Diastolic Dysfunction

Systemic hypertension
Coronary artery disease
Cardiomyopathy
Aortic stenosis
Atrial fibrillation
Diabetes
Chronic renal disease

increased venous capacitance, may be accompanied by significant decreases in cardiac output.

6. Dyspnea in the elderly may indicate congestive cardiac failure and/or pulmonary disease.

B. **Large Vessels**

1. Structural changes in the large vessels (elongated, tortuous, dilated, intima thickened) are an important element of the aging process and contribute significantly to the age-related changes in the heart.

2. In the elderly, the pulse wave is reflected back from the peripheral circulation and augments systolic pressure. Diastolic pressure tends to be lower in the elderly than in younger individuals (pulse pressure are increased and left ventricular afterload is elevated).

C. **Endothelial Function**. Age-related endothelial dysfunction can be characterized as a decrease in the ability of the endothelium to dilate or contract blood vessels in response to physiologic and pharmacologic stimuli.

D. **Conduction System**. There are several important age-related structural and functional changes in the cardiac conduction system (sinoatrial node, atrioventricular node, and conduction bundles also become infiltrated with fibrous and fatty tissue). These changes are responsible for the increased incidence of first- and second-degree heart block, sick sinus syndrome, and atrial fibrillation in the elderly.

E. **Autonomic and Integrated Cardiovascular Responses**

1. Aging is associated with increased norepinephrine entry into the circulation and deficient catecholamine reuptake at nerve endings (elevated circulating concentrations of norepinephrine are usual, generating chronically increased adrenergic receptor occupancy).

2. The cardiovascular response to increased adrenergic stimulation is attenuated by downregulation of postreceptor signaling and reduced contractile response of the myocardium. The number of the β-adrenergic receptors is reduced in the elderly myocardium.

3. Receptor downregulation is responsible for the age-related decline in maximum heart rate during exercise.

4. Orthostatic hypotension is common in the elderly and is associated with syncope, falls, and cognitive decline. Impaired baroreceptor reflexes and attenuated peripheral vasoconstriction are partially responsible.

F. **Anesthetic and Ischemic Preconditioning in the Aging Heart**. Under certain circumstances, exposure to volatile anesthetics (anesthetic preconditioning) or several brief periods of ischemia (ischemic preconditioning) may enhance tolerance to subsequent ischemia, enhance cardiac function, and reduce infarction size. Anesthetic and ischemic preconditioning may be markedly attenuated in the elderly, potentially explaining the difficulty of translating promising preclinical results to treatment.

III. **Aging and the Respiratory System (Tables 46-2 and 46-3). Decreased respiratory reserve may be unmasked by illness, surgery, anesthesia, and other perioperative events. Common respiratory diseases and the effects of smoking and environmental pollution frequently exacerbate the decline in respiratory function with aging (anticipation and amelioration of their effects is critically important to anesthetic management in the elderly as postoperative respiratory complications result in 40% of perioperative deaths in patient older than 65 years).**
   A. **Respiratory System Mechanics and Architecture**
      1. The chest wall becomes less compliant with aging, presumably related to changes in the thoracic skeleton and a decline in costovertebral joint mobility (produce a restrictive functional impairment).
      2. The diaphragm and abdominal muscles assume a greater role in tidal breathing (diaphragmatic function declines with age, predisposing the elderly to respiratory fatigue when required to significantly increase minute ventilation).

Table 46-2

Intrinsic and Extrinsic Events that Influence the Respiratory System during Aging

Intrinsic to the Aging Process	Environmental, Behavioral, and Disease Related
Decreased bronchiolar caliber	Industrial and environmental pollution
Decreased alveolar surface area	Smoking
Increased lung collagen content	General deconditioning
Decreased lung elastin content	Coexisting disease
Kyphoscoliosis	
Increased thoracic cage rigidity	
Decreased diaphragmatic strength	

Table 46-3

Functional Consequences of the Intrinsic and Extrinsic Events that Influence the Respiratory System during Aging

Decrease in lung elastic recoil
Increase in lung compliance
Decrease in oxygen diffusing capacity
Premature airway closure causing V/Q mismatch and increased alveolar-to-arterial oxygen gradient
Small airway closure and gas trapping
Decreased expiratory flow rates

V/Q, ventilation to perfusion.

B. **Lung Volumes and Capacities**
   1. **Vital capacity (VC)** is the volume generated when a maximal inspiration is followed by a maximal expiration. There is a progressive loss of VC with aging.
   2. **Residual Volume.** The residual volume is the volume remaining in the lungs after a maximal expiration. Aging is associated with a progressive increase in residual volume of up to 10% per decade (Fig. 46-2).
   3. **Total lung capacity** is the sum of the residual volume and the VC (remains relatively constant with aging).
   4. **Functional Residual Capacity.** The functional residual capacity (FRC) is the volume remaining in the lungs at the end of a normal expiration. Aging is associated with a progressive increase in FRC that occurs as a result of the decreased elastic recoil force of the lungs.
   5. **Closing Capacity**
      a. Airway closure may occur in small airways (<1 mm) whose caliber is determined by their transmural pressure.
      b. In the elderly, airway closure occurs at approximately 40% of the VC reflecting lung volumes that exceed FRC. Gas exchange impairment due to shunting in regions of airway closure is typical in the elderly during normal tidal breathing. The supine position makes airway closure during normal tidal breathing more likely.
   6. **Expiratory Flow.** There is a progressive decline in forced exhaled volume in 1 second (FEV_1) and forced vital capacity (FVC) with age that is independent of smoking or environmental exposure.

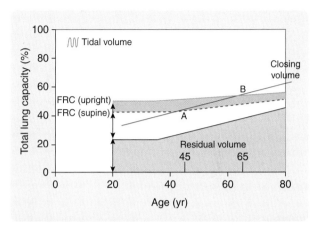

FIGURE 46-2 Effect of aging on lung volumes. Functional residual capacity (FRC) increases with age as a result of increasing residual volume. Closing volume also increases with age and exceeds FRC in the upright position around age 65 years and in the supine position at age 45 years. These changes lead to ventilation perfusion mismatch and shunt, resulting in reduced resting PO_2 with age. (Modified from Sprung J, Gajic O, Warner DO. Review article: age related alterations in respiratory function—anesthetic considerations. *Can J Anaesth.* 2006;53[12]:1244–1257).

7. **Diffusing Capacity and Alveolar-to-Arterial Oxygen Gradient**. Gas exchange efficiency declines with aging as a result of increasing intrapulmonary shunting and decreasing lung diffusing capacity (result is a linear decline in resting supine Pao_2 between early adulthood and 65 years of age) (Fig. 46-3).

8. **Upper Airway Protective Reflexes**. Cough effectiveness is reduced in the elderly because of diminished reflex sensitivity and impaired muscle function. Cough reflex attenuation is associated with an increased incidence of aspiration pneumonia.

9. **Control of Breathing, Chemoreceptors, and Integrated Responses**
   a. The increases in heart rate and minute ventilation in response to elevations in $Paco_2$ or decreases in Pao_2 are markedly attenuated in the elderly.
   b. These important protective reflexes are further attenuated by the administration of opioids and

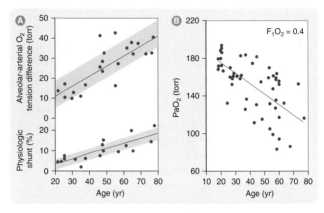

FIGURE 46-3 Effect of aging on gas exchange. **A.** The change in alveolar/arterial oxygen tension with age (shunt fraction or percent shunt). **B.** Relationship of PO_2 with age during spontaneous breathing of 40% oxygen and 60% nitrous oxide under general anesthesia with enflurane. (Modified from Wahba WM. Influence of aging on lung function—clinical significance of changes from age twenty. *Anesth Analg.* 1983;62:764–776).

sedative/hypnotic drugs. The elderly are at particular risk from life-threatening respiratory depression in the perioperative period.

10. **Sleep Disordered Breathing**. The incidence of sleep disordered breathing increases with age, especially in men (estimated that ~20% of elderly people have clinically significant obstructive sleep apnea). Obstructive sleep apnea doubles the risk for postoperative delirium in the elderly.

IV. **Thermoregulation in the Elderly.** Hyperthermia and hypothermia in the elderly are poorly tolerated and extreme cold and heat stress are associated with increased mortality compared to younger individuals (not clear whether the greater susceptibility to thermal stress is related to aging per se or to underlying socioeconomic conditions, general fitness, activity levels, and the effects of coexisting disease in the elderly).

A. **Resting Core Temperature** (Table 46-4)

B. **Response to Cold Stress**

1. Aging is associated with attenuated vasoconstrictor responses to cold. The inability to efficiently conserve heat

Table 46-4

Factors Associated with Reduced Resting Core Temperatures in the Elderly

Neurologic disease
Diabetes
Low body weight
Lack of self-sufficiency
Consumption of less than two meals per day
Smoking
Alcohol consumption

in the elderly is exacerbated by the age-related decrease in skeletal muscle mass.

2. The attenuated cold stress responses of the elderly are further diminished by general and regional anesthesia. Perioperative hypothermia is very likely in the elderly patient unless active measures are taken to maintain normothermia.

V. Gastrointestinal Function in the Elderly

A. **Liver.** Aging is associated with a decrease in liver mass and hepatic blood flow but hepatocellular metabolic function appears to be relatively well preserved throughout life. Because first-pass metabolism is reduced, the oral bioavailability of propranolol and labetalol are increased in the elderly. Conversely, prodrugs, such as the angiotensin-converting enzyme (ACE) inhibitor enalapril, require activation by the liver before they exert their pharmacologic effect, and the bioavailability of these drugs may be decreased in the elderly.

B. **Gastroesophageal Physiology**

1. Gastric emptying of solid material appears to be relatively normal in the healthy elderly population but gastric emptying of liquids may be delayed compared with younger individuals.

2. Emptying of both liquids and solids is commonly delayed in the presence of certain coexisting diseases that are common with aging such as gastroesophageal reflux disease (GERD) (Table 46-5).

3. The typical symptoms of GERD seen in the younger population (heartburn and regurgitation) are less frequent in the elderly, making diagnosis more difficult.

Table 46-5

Factors that Predispose to the Increased Incidence of Gastroesophageal Reflux Disease in the Elderly

Increased prevalence of sliding hiatal hernia
Shortened intraabdominal segment of the lower esophageal sphincter
Impaired clearance of refluxed acid
Use of medications that reduce lower esophageal sphincter pressure
Decreased esophageal peristalsis pressure

Several medications that are commonly prescribed in the elderly population predispose to GERD by decreasing lower esophageal sphincter tone (Table 46-6).

VI. **Renal Function in the Elderly**
   A. Aging is accompanied by a decrease in the cortical nephron population and a reduction in renal mass. Renal blood flow and glomerular filtration rate (GFR) both decline with age.
   B. Despite the significant decline in GFR with aging, the serum creatinine concentration increases minimally because there is also an age-related decrease in skeletal muscle mass.
   C. The renal response to common perioperative stresses may be insufficient to maintain homeostasis.
   D. The elderly are at risk for both dehydration and free water overload because of impaired renal responses.

Table 46-6

Medications that Are Commonly Administered in the Elderly that Reduce Lower Esophageal Sphincter Tone and Predispose to Gastroesophageal Reflux

Anticholinergics
Antidepressants
Nitrates
Calcium channel blockers
Theophylline

Table 46-7

Factors that Are Thought to Be Responsible for the Significant Decrease in Lean Muscle Mass that Occurs with Aging

Decreased motor neuron innervation
Decreased physical activity
Endocrine shift toward catabolism (reduced insulin-like growth factor 1 secretion)
Decreased androgen (testosterone and estrogen) secretion
Decreased total caloric intake
Decreased protein consumption and protein synthesis
Inflammatory mediators and cytokines (interleukins 1 and 6, tumor necrosis factor)

VII. **Skeletal Muscle Mass and Aging**
   A. Aging is associated with a significant decline in neuromuscular performance (causes functional disability and loss of independence). Neuromuscular decline results predominantly from loss of skeletal muscle mass, which declines by approximately 40% between the ages of 20 and 60 years (sarcopenia) (Table 46-7).
   B. Diminished skeletal muscle mass has significant implications for the elderly patient in the perioperative period (Table 46-8).

VIII. **Neurophysiology of Aging**
   A. The elderly demonstrate increased sensitivity to benzodiazepines, opioids, and volatile anesthetic drugs. The

Table 46-8

Perioperative Functional Consequences of the Loss of Skeletal Muscle Mass that Typically Accompanies Aging

Impaired postoperative mobilization and ambulation
Reduced cough effectiveness
Reduced shivering thermogenesis
Altered drug disposition
Reduced neuromuscular functional reserve
Prolonged recovery and hospitalization

minimum alveolar concentration (MAC) of potent volatile anesthetic drugs is decreased by approximately 25% at 80 years of age when compared to MAC values obtained at 40 years of age.

B. Perhaps as a function of limited neurologic reserve, the elderly are at risk for postoperative delirium and postoperative cognitive dysfunction that are strong risk factors for mortality.

1. Postoperative delirium is equally common after both regional and general anesthesia, whereas postoperative cognitive dysfunction may be more common after general anesthesia.

2. Although postoperative cognitive dysfunction is a risk factor for early mortality, it was not found to be a risk factor for dementia.

IX. **Pain and Aging**

A. Pain is a part of daily life for many elderly patients, with about 50% of patients older than the age of 70 years reporting chronic pain.

B. As a general rule, elderly patients are more sensitive to opioids. Morphine and meperidine have active metabolites that accumulate in the elderly. Morphine is metabolized by glucuronidation into two metabolites: Morphine-3-glucuronide and morphine-6-glucuronide will accumulate more in elderly patients, necessitating a reduction in dose of chronically administered morphine.

CHAPTER 47

Physiology and Pharmacology of Resuscitation

I. Introduction

A. The term *resuscitation* for many people means resuscitation from cardiac arrest, so much so that the term *cardiopulmonary resuscitation* and its acronym "CPR" is widely used not only by healthcare professionals but by laypeople as well. In order to improve outcome from cardiac arrest, the American College of Cardiology, American Heart Association, and many other organizations have joined together to educate healthcare professionals and laypeople on how to resuscitate patients who have had a cardiac arrest.

B. Common to all resuscitation scenarios and the actual mechanism by which patients die is inadequate oxygen delivery to tissues (cardiac and brain ischemia if the patient is not resuscitated in a timely and effective fashion).

1. During ventricular tachycardia, ventricular fibrillation, or during asystole, cardiac output decreases to zero as will oxygen delivery to the tissues.

2. During hemorrhagic shock, as hemoglobin levels decrease, the arterial oxygen content decreases and cardiac output falls because of decreased intravascular volume resulting in decreased left ventricular end diastolic volume.

3. During apnea from whatever cause, as whatever oxygen is contained in the functional residual capacity of the lung decreases, the amount of oxygen available to bind with hemoglobin decreases, which also results in a steadily decreasing oxygen delivery and eventually, cell death.

II. Pathophysiology

A. Based strictly on the byproducts of the chemical reactions involved, anaerobic metabolism of pyruvate leads to the production of 4 molecules of ATP, whereas the metabolism of pyruvate in the presence of O_2 can potentially produce 38 molecules of ATP.

1. Anaerobic metabolism is insufficient in the long term to produce enough ATP molecules to maintain cell

integrity. In the absence of oxygen, cells die at a variable rate depending on their metabolic rate (Fig. 47-1).

 a. Typically, neurons are the most sensitive to lack of O_2 and will develop irreversible damage within 3 to 5 minutes; myocytes and hepatocytes on the other hand can survive 1 to 2 hours in the absence of O_2; muscle cells may survive for several hours.

 b. By decreasing metabolic rate, hypothermia can prolong the "safe" ischemic time. Neurons for example decrease their metabolic rate by approximately 7% for every 1°C decrease in temperature.

B. Although temperature has an impact on survivability of ischemic cells, time is the factor that most directly and importantly impacts the reversibility of ischemia—the safe ischemic time.

 1. Independent of all other factors, the number of minutes that cardiac function is arrested, the amount of time that

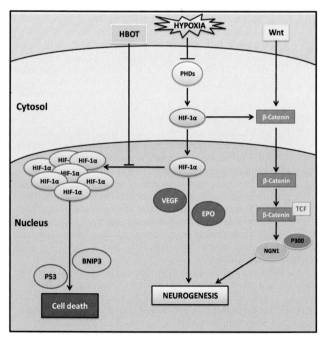

FIGURE 47-1 Events triggered by hypoxia leading to cell death.

the hemoglobin concentration is below 6 g/dL to 7 g/dL, or the duration of apnea or asphyxia all directly correlate with morbidity and mortality.

2. The effect of duration of the arrest on survivability suggests that mortality increases by 8% to 10% for each minute for which there is no cardiac output.

C. From a physiologic perspective, the most vital factor in determining outcome is the timely restoration of normal cardiac, pulmonary, and hemostatic function. Drugs play a limited, but very important, role in the return of the above functions in certain circumstances.

III. Cardiac Arrest

A. Ventricular tachyarrhythmias account for many cardiac arrests (6% to 14% of the time no known structural lesions of the heart can be identified).

1. If no structural cause can be identified, individuals who have a prolonged QT interval are at increased risk of developing polymorphic ventricular tachycardia (*torsades de pointes*) especially if they receive certain drugs that are also known to prolong the QT.

a. Mutations in genes that code for ion channels that generate the cardiac action potential have been identified in patients with the long QT syndrome.

b. The ability of a drug to precipitate a malignant tachyarrhythmia is related not just to the drug itself but also to the dose, to drug interactions, to genetic factors, to the gender of the patient, and to the type and severity of preexisting cardiac disease.

B. Ventricular fibrillation is the cause for most of the other instances of sudden cardiac arrest (true incidence of the precipitating arrhythmia is not known because most sudden cardiac arrests occur out of hospital and typically several minutes pass before the rhythm can be assessed).

C. Independent of the etiology of the cardiac collapse, for resuscitation to be successful, CPR must be initiated as soon as possible.

1. The best outcomes are achieved if the heart is defibrillated within the first 4 minutes after the cardiac arrest, during the electrical phase.

2. In those patients with return of spontaneous circulation (ROSC), the enthusiasm for the ability of hypothermia to attenuate the neurologic injury has been tempered by a more recent well-performed study that did not

demonstrate an improvement in neurologic outcome with hypothermia (33°C vs. 36°C).

3. Once patients enter the metabolic phase after 10 minutes of untreated cardiac arrest, the chances of meaningful recovery are slim.

D. **Hemorrhagic Shock**

1. In patients who sustain traumatic injury, hemorrhage accounts for 30% to 40% of the deaths. Of these, a majority occur before the patients arrive at a hospital. Among traumatized patients who arrive at the hospital, mortality in the first several hours correlates with inadequate resuscitation and the presence of coagulopathy.

2. Improvements in early hemorrhage control and resuscitation and the prevention and aggressive treatment of coagulopathy appear to have the greatest potential to improve outcomes in severely injured trauma patients.

E. **Respiratory Arrest**

1. Respiratory and cardiac arrest are distinct, but if untreated, one inevitably leads to the other. There are a multitude of etiologies of respiratory arrest, and respiratory arrest per se implies any process that inhibits the delivery of sufficient oxygen to the mitochondria to maintain aerobic metabolism.

a. The respiratory centers in the brainstem can be injured by penetrating injury, by increased intracranial pressure due to infection, or intraventricular hemorrhage. Even blunt trauma to the head of sufficient force can produce a similar result.

b. There are a number of drugs that can depress the respiratory centers, most notably opioids, sedatives, and hypnotics. These drugs can suppress ventilation or induce complete apnea even at low doses in patients with central sleep apnea, in patients with chronic obstructive pulmonary disease (COPD) and hypercarbia, and in geriatric patients with comorbid conditions.

c. Although it is true that opioids suppress ventilation, some have used this relationship to justify withholding opioids from patients with severe COPD at the end of their lives.

2. Whatever the cause of respiratory arrest, death does not occur immediately.

a. The hemoglobin in the circulating blood carries enough O_2 for maintenance of aerobic metabolism for 1 to 3 minutes.

    b. In addition, there is O_2 that has already entered the lungs (functional residual capacity), which is enough to meet metabolic demands for a time.

    c. At 3 to 4 minutes of complete apnea, evidence of tissue ischemia would become apparent and at longer than 5 minutes, irreversible damage would occur, especially in the brain. Cardiac arrest would soon follow unless oxygenation and ventilation were immediately rapidly restored.

IV. **Pharmacology**

    A. **Cardiopulmonary Resuscitation**. The primary goal when resuscitating a patient from cardiac arrest is the ROSC that is best achieved with effective chest compressions delivered immediately by a bystander, and if the patient has ventricular fibrillation, the delivery of electroshock therapy to defibrillate the heart. If these maneuvers are unsuccessful in restoring cardiac function and an advanced practitioner is present, drug therapy has been shown to increase the rate of ROSC. Although the drugs currently recommended for advanced cardiac life support improve the likelihood of ROSC, none has improved long-term outcome.

    B. **Epinephrine**

      1. When administered intravenously during a cardiac arrest, epinephrine is thought to increase the ROSC primarily by binding to and activating α-adrenergic receptors. Activation of these receptors on the venules in the periphery increases venous return to the heart, allowing chest compressions to better increase cardiac output.

      2. On the arterial side, the vasoconstriction caused by α receptor activation constricts the peripheral arterial system further centralizing the circulation to perfuse vital organs with the highest oxygen requirement. The increase in cardiac output with an increased systemic vascular resistance is hypothesized to improve coronary artery and carotid artery blood flow.

      3. By activating β receptors within the heart, epinephrine augments cardiac output even further.

      4. Epinephrine has been repeatedly demonstrated to improve ROSC when administered to patients in cardiac arrest but without an improvement in overall outcome.

      5. If the effects of epinephrine are attributed to its effect on α-adrenergic receptors, then drugs with even more α receptor specificity might be indicated, yet studies of epinephrine compared to either norepinephrine or

phenylephrine during cardiac arrest with CPR showed no benefit to the more α receptor–specific drugs.

6. The most recent guidelines of the American Heart Association recommend 1 mg of epinephrine administered intravenously or by the intraosseous injection every 3 to 5 minutes with recognition of the fact that although there may be ROSC, there are no prospective randomized controlled trials that demonstrate an improvement in outcome.

C. **Vasopressin** (antidiuretic hormone) when administered intravenously distributes from the plasma into the extracellular fluid rapidly, exerting its effects within just a few minutes. The current guidelines of the American Heart Association for advanced cardiac life support state that vasopressin (40 units) can be administered intravenously or by the intraosseous route instead of either the first or second dose of epinephrine.

D. **Amiodarone**

1. Amiodarone is the second pharmacologic treatment (after either epinephrine or vasopressin) in patients who have ventricular fibrillation refractory to electric defibrillation (300 mg or 5 mg/kg).

2. The American Heart Association has recommended amiodarone to treat refractory ventricular fibrillation or pulseless ventricular tachycardia.

3. Adverse effects on thyroid gland function are only seen in patients taking the drug in high dose for extended periods of time, not in patients who are administered one or two doses of the drug during sudden cardiac arrest.

V. Hemorrhage

A. The most critical intervention in hemorrhage is to stop the bleeding either by applying a tourniquet in the field to an extremity or if there is massive internal bleeding by transporting the patient as quickly as possible to a level I trauma hospital and from the emergency department directly to the operating room.

B. **Tranexamic acid** is an antifibrinolytic that may be administered to trauma patients (also commonly used in massive hemorrhage during cancer surgery, removal of invasive placenta, and major orthopedic surgery).

VI. Oxygenation/Ventilation. In patients with pulmonary failure or respiratory arrest, immediate assisted ventilation and oxygenation is the intervention most likely to increase the chances of survival. Respiratory arrest secondary to an opioid is reversed with naloxone. Flumazenil antagonizes respiratory arrest secondary to or contributed to by benzodiazepine overdose.

VII. **Summary.** In patients with cardiac arrest, defibrillation in the first 3 minutes and CPR/defibrillation during the next 5 to 7 minutes achieves the best results. In patients with profound hemorrhage, immediate control of bleeding and infusion of red blood cells has the biggest impact on outcome. In patients with pulmonary or respiratory arrest, immediate assisted ventilation and oxygenation is the most likely intervention to increase the chances of survival.

DRUG INDEX

Note: Page numbers followed by *f* indicate figures; page numbers followed by *t* indicate tables.

SUBJECT INDEX

Note: Page numbers followed by *f* indicate figures; page numbers followed by *t* indicate tables.